Bell's Orofacial Pains

Bell's Orofacial Pains
Fifth Edition

Jeffrey P. Okeson, DMD
Professor and Director
Orofacial Pain Center
University of Kentucky
College of Dentistry
Lexington, Kentucky

quintessence
books

Quintessence Publishing Co, Inc
Chicago, Berlin, London, Tokyo, São Paulo, Moscow, Prague, and Warsaw

Library of Congress Cataloging-in-Publication Data

Okeson, Jeffrey P.
    Bell's Orofacial Pains/Jeffrey P. Okeson.
      p. cm.
    Includes bibliographical references and index.
    ISBN 0-86715-293-1
    1. Orofacial pain. I. Bell, Welden E. II. Title. III. Title: Orofacial Pains.
    [DNLM: 1. Temporomandibular Joint Diseases–diagnosis. 2. Facial Pain–
diagnosis. WU 140.5 041b 1995]
    RK322.B44 1994
    617.5'2–dc20
    DNLM/DLC
    for Library of Congress   95-1313
                                         CIP

quintessence
books

Published by Quintessence Publishing Co, Inc
551 North Kimberly Drive
Carol Stream, IL 60188

Editor: Lori A. Bateman
Design / Production: Timothy M. Robbins
Cover design: Jennifer A. Sabella

Printing and binding: BookCrafters, Chelsea, MI
Printed in the USA

This book is dedicated to the memory of

Dr Welden E. Bell (1910–1990)

My teacher,
my mentor,
and
my friend

Contents

Section I The Nature of Pain

Section II Clinical Considerations of Orofacial Pains

Section III Clinical Pain Syndromes

List of Cases

Foreword

The fifth edition of *Bell's Orofacial Pains* continues to meet the high standards achieved in the previous editions and will undoubtedly enjoy the success and reputation that earmark the previous editions. The text deals with a topic that may present distinctive features and difficulties for the patient with orofacial pain and for the clinician trying to treat it. Pain and dysfunction in the orofacial area can be of particular significance, since the orofacial area has special anatomic and physiologic features, and is a region of the body holding unique psychologic and social importance to the individual. Moreover, orofacial pain is a very common experience, and most individuals will have experienced at least one of the two most common pains in the body that occur in the orofacial region, namely toothache and headache.

As Dr Okeson quite rightly points out in the very first page of this book, the dental profession has become extremely effective in managing most forms of acute orofacial pain, but orofacial pain of a chronic or pathologic nature is more problematic. To deal effectively with such pain disorders, the clinician must have a good understanding of the processes underlying the disorders. A lack of knowledge of these processes in the

past, combined with a modus operandi reflecting the traditional training of most dental clinicians that they should be capable of "treating what they see," has often resulted in clinicians "seeing what they treat" and using clinical approaches with which they are comfortable but which may have little if any grounding in scientific fact. While the processes underlying orofacial pain disorders may still be difficult to comprehend because the knowledge base is limited, there have been some remarkable insights into these processes in the last few years as a consequence of an enhanced focus of basic science research, largely using experimental animal models, into pain mechanisms and an increased research interest in behavioral and psychosocial factors influencing pain. This has resulted in a firmer scientific foundation upon which to base diagnosis and management of many of the disorders.

It then follows that extensively reviewed and well-reasoned texts that correlate and reconcile the latest research advances in this field with prudent clinical practice are essential. Such is the approach offered in this book and the reason a fifth edition is warranted. The objective of the book is indeed twofold, since Dr Okeson has aimed to introduce into this edition the most significant recent findings related to the management of orofacial pains, and also to place topics on the neural processes involved in pain early in the text so that a more complete understanding of pain could be appreciated by the reader. Dr Okeson has accomplished the daunting and difficult tasks of reviewing the many research advances of the last few years related to pain and correlating this new knowledge with current diagnostic and therapeutic approaches to orofacial pain disorders. He has produced a text that is not only comprehensive and well-referenced but also well-integrated. The text has been divided into three major sections. The first section, in presenting the normal structure and function of the trigeminal system, provides the clinician with a clear understanding of normal function and a basis upon which to understand and manage dysfunction. The second section provides a classification of orofacial pain disorders and outlines the diagnostic approaches that can be used to differentiate each disorder. The third section deals with management issues for each orofacial pain disorder.

Like its predecessors, this fifth edition of *Bell's Orofacial Pains* is essential reading for those interested in mechanisms of orofacial pain and clinical approaches to diagnose and manage orofacial pain disorders. This book should prove invaluable to dental clinicians and other clinical practitioners dealing with pain problems, as well as to basic and clinical scientists in pain research who are interested in the clinical correlates of what they study.

Barry J. Sessle, BDS, MDS, BSc, PhD
Professor and Dean
Faculty of Dentistry
University of Toronto

Preface

In the early spring of 1982, I first had the opportunity to listen to Dr Welden E. Bell lecture on the subject of orofacial pain. By his written word I had already known him as an international authority on the subject of orofacial pain. I will never forget the first words from his mouth: "Pain is not a sensation," he proclaimed. I squinted slightly, thinking that I had misheard his statement, but then he repeated the seemingly ridiculous remark. I thought, why of course pain is a sensation. How could such an authority make such a misleading statement? He then went on to say that "pain is far more than a simple sensation; pain is an experience." I must admit that at that time in my professional development I really did not appreciate what he was saying. Following that course and after much more reading of his texts and others, I began to better appreciate his words. There is an old saying that "when the student is ready, the teacher will appear." At that moment, Dr Bell became my teacher and later my mentor.

As my career progressed, I learned more and more from Dr Bell. He continued to write even after his retirement from practice, completing seven editions of his two classic texts on orofacial pains and temporomandibular disorders. As I grew to know him more personally, my admiration grew even stronger.

In 1985, I published a textbook on occlusion and temporomandibular disorders. The first letter I received commenting on this new text came from Dr Bell. His praise and complaints meant more to me than he would ever know. Later he honored me by writing the foreword to the third edition of the text.

In October of 1989, I received a letter from Dr Bell informing me that he had just finished the fourth edition of *Orofacial Pains*. He was than 79 years old and asked me if I would consider coauthoring the fifth edition of this text when it came due. His letter presented me with two very different emotions. I immediately felt that I had just received the greatest professional compliment of my career; yet at the same time, I was confronted with the most difficult task I had ever been asked to accomplish. I dared to say yes, but I certainly could not say no. I immediately called Dr Bell to discuss his proposal. I told him of my feelings and he comforted me by explaining that although he would like for me to take the major responsibilities, he would be there for direction and continuity. With a certain amount of pride and a great deal of insecurity, I accepted his invitation.

In the spring of 1990, I had the privilege to meet with Dr Bell on three occasions; two were during meetings that were dedicated to him for his outstanding contributions to the profession. I had the privilege to speak at both these meetings and I felt so proud to have him in the audience. During those three meetings, we were able to take some quiet time to discuss new research findings that altered the current views of muscle pain. He contributed greatly to the muscle pain model you see in this text.

In May of 1990, shortly after the publication of the third edition of his text on temporomandibular disorders, Dr Bell fell suddenly ill and died. His death was a tragic loss to his family and especially his wonderful wife of 58 years, Lucy. His passing was also a tremendous loss to the profession. I personally felt as though I had lost my professional father, and in fact, I had. During the next year I considered and reconsidered how I could accomplish the monumental task of rewriting and updating this text. At times I even considered not attempting it at all, but my admiration for Dr Bell would not let me linger long on such thoughts. In March of 1993, I began the massive task of accumulating the current literature regarding pain. By September of 1994, the task was completed; the product is what you now see.

My goals for this text were twofold. First, I wanted to introduce the latest research findings in the complex study of pain. So much has happened, however, that this has been very difficult. I hope that I have been able to introduce the most significant recent findings related to the management of orofacial pains. The second goal was to introduce the reader to the neuroanatomy and neurophysiology of pain early in the text so that a more thorough understanding of pain may be appreciated. I have added numerous drawings in an attempt to enhance the understanding of this most complex experience we call pain.

This text is divided into three major sections. The first section presents the normal neuroanatomy and function of the trigeminal system. With a clear understanding of normal function, the clinician can begin to understand and manage dysfunction. The second major section presents a classification of the various orofacial pain disorders and describes the history and examination procedures that can be used to differentiate each disorder. This process, called diagnosis, is the most important aspect of orofacial pain management. The third major section presents management considerations for each orofacial pain disorder. It is hoped that this sequence of information will allow the reader to increase his or her skills in this complicated field of study.

The work involved in this revision portrays a labor of love dedicated to Dr Welden Bell. It would not have been possible, however, without the love and support of my wonderful wife Barbara and my sons, Brian and Tyler. It is their love and sacrifice that permitted the accomplishment of this task. I have been greatly blessed with a wonderful family that represents the rock on which I stand.

Terminology

Terms that constitute the language of pain should be defined precisely enough to prevent ambiguity and misunderstandings. Many of the definitions listed below are based on terminology proposed by the Subcommittee on Taxonomy of the International Association for the Study of Pain.[1,2] Some are from a standard medical dictionary.[3] A few are specially defined to express a precise meaning by the author. The reader is urged to become familiar with these definitions.

Algogenic Causing pain.

Allodynia Pain that occurs without noxious stimulation at the site of pain. *(Note: This term applies broadly to all painful sensations, regardless of location, that occur in the absence of noxious stimulation at the site of pain. This would apply, therefore, to spontaneous pain regardless of cause and to pain evoked by nonnoxious stimulation.)*

Analgesia Absence of sensibility to pain. *(Note: Other sensibilities may remain present.)*

Anesthesia Absence of all sensation.

Anesthesia dolorosa Pain in an area that is anesthetic as a result of deafferentation.

Antidromic Conducting impulses in a direction opposite to the normal.

Arthralgia Pain that is felt in joint structures. *(Note: If the site of pain represents the source, the arthralgia would be arthrogenous; otherwise, it would be heterotopic.)*

Arthrogenous pain Pain originating from joint structures.

Causalgia A syndrome of unremitting, burning pain as the result of deafferentation. (Sometimes referred to as reflex sympathetic dystrophy.)

Central pain Pain associated with a lesion of the central nervous system (CNS).

Deafferentation The partial or total loss of afferent neural activity to a particular body region through removal of part of the neural pathway.

Denervation Resection or removal of the nerves to an organ or part.

Dysesthesia An unpleasant abnormal sensation. *(Note: Paresthesia is an abnormal sensation whether unpleasant or not. Paresthesia includes dysesthesia, but not vice versa.)*

Heterotopic pain A general term to designate pain that is felt in an area other than its true site of origin. *(Note: Peripheral heterotopic pain may be felt as projected pain, referred pain, or secondary hyperalgesia.)*

Hypalgesia Diminished sensitivity to stimulation-evoked pain.

Hyperalgesia Increased sensitivity to stimulation-evoked pain. *(Note: Primary hyperalgesia is stimulation-evoked primary pain due to a lowered local pain threshold. Secondary hyperalgesia is stimulation-evoked heterotopic pain that occurs without appreciable change in the local pain threshold.)*

Hyperesthesia Increased sensitivity to stimulation. *(Note: When the sensation is painful, the terms allodynia and hyperalgesia are appropriate.)*

Hypoesthesia Diminished sensitivity to stimulation. *(Note: When the sensation is painful, the terms hypalgesia and analgesia are appropriate.)*

Inflammatory pain Pain that emanates from tissue that is inflamed.

Musculoskeletal pain Deep somatic pain that originates in skeletal muscles, fascial sheaths, and tendons (myogenous pain); in bones and periosteum (osseous pain); in joints, joint capsules, and ligaments (arthralgic pain); and in soft connective tissues (soft connective tissue pain).

Myalgia Pain that is felt in muscle tissue. *(Note: If the site of pain represents the source, the myalgia would be myogenous; otherwise, it would be heterotopic.)*

Myofascial trigger point A hyperirritable spot, usually within a taut band of skeletal muscle or in the muscle fascia, that is painful on compression and that can give rise to characteristic referred pain, tenderness (secondary hyperalgesia), and autonomic phenomena.[4]

Myogenous pain Deep somatic musculoskeletal pain that originates in skeletal muscles, fascial sheaths, or tendons. *(Note: Several types of myogenous pain are identifiable clinically: protective co-contraction, local muscle soreness, myofascial trigger point pain, muscle spasm pain, and muscle inflammation pain.)*

Neuralgia Neuropathic pain felt along the peripheral distribution of a nerve trunk. *(Note: Paroxysmal neuralgia consists of sudden bursts of burning pain. Neuritic neuralgia is persistent, unremitting burning pain.)*

Neuropathic pain Pain that is generated within the nervous system due to some abnormality of neural structures. (Also referred to as neurogenous pain.)

Neuropathy A general term used to designate an abnormality or pathologic change in a peripheral nerve.

Neuroplasticity The dynamic ability of the central nervous system to alter the processing of impulses in response to continued input and/or other factors.

Nociception The mechanism that provides for the reception and conversion of noxious or potentially noxious stimuli into neural impulses and the transmission of such impulses by A-delta and C fibers to the CNS where they are modulated and acted on.

Nociceptive pathway An afferent neural pathway that mediates pain impulses.

Nociceptor A sensory receptor preferentially sensitive to noxious or potentially noxious stimuli.

Noxious stimulus A tissue-damaging stimulus.

Odontalgia Pain that is felt in a tooth. *(Note: If the tooth is the source of the pain, the odontalgia would be odontogenous; if not, it would be heterotopic.)*

Odontogenous pain Deep somatic pain that originates in dental pulps, periodontal ligaments, or both.

Orthodromic Conducting impulses in the normal direction.

Pain The subject's conscious perception of modulated nociceptive impulses that generate an unpleasant sensory and emotional experience associated with actual or potential tissue damage, or described in terms of such damage.

Pain behavior The subject's audible and visible actions that communicate his or her suffering to others.

Pain threshold The lowest stimulus intensity at which a subject perceives pain.

Pain tolerance level The greatest stimulus intensity that a subject is prepared to tolerate.

Paresthesia An abnormal sensation, whether spontaneous or evoked. *(Note: If an abnormal sensation is unpleasant, the term dysesthesia is appropriate.)*

Periodontal pain Odontogenous pain that emanates from the periodontal ligaments.

Primary pain Pain that identifies the true source of nociceptive input.

Projected pain Heterotopic pain that is felt in the anatomic peripheral distribution of the same nerve that mediates the primary pain.

Pulpal pain Odontogenous pain that emanates from the dental pulps.

Referred pain Heterotopic pain that is felt in an area that is innervated by a nerve different from the one that mediates the primary pain. *(Note: Referred pain implies that it occurs without provocation at the site of pain.)*

Reflex sympathetic dystrophy A syndrome of unremitting, burning pain as the result of deafferentation. (Sometimes referred to as causalgia.)

Secondary hyperalgesia Heterotopic pain that is evoked by stimulation at the site of pain.

Secondary pain Heterotopic pain that is induced by deep somatic pain as a central excitatory effect.

Site of pain The anatomic site where pain is felt.

Somatic pain Pain originating in any body structure other than neurogenous structures.

Suffering The emotional response to pain and other factors that reflects the subject's anticipated impending and future threat to his/her well-being. It is influenced by factors that may or may not relate to the initiating pain experience.

Sympathetically maintained pain Pain sustained through activity of the sympathetic nervous system.

Symptoms The objective and subjective evidence of change in structure or function that is indicative of abnormality, dysfunction, or disease.

Vascular pain A type of deep somatic pain of visceral origin that emanates from the afferent nerves that innervate blood vessels. *(Note: Inflammatory vascular pain should be designated as vasculitis [arteritis, phlebitis].)*

Visceral pain Deep somatic pain that originates in visceral structures such as mucosal linings, walls of hollow viscera, parenchyma of organs, glands, dental pulps, and vascular structures.

References

1. Merskey H. Pain terms: A list with definitions and notes on usage. Pain 1979; 6:249.
2. Merskey H. Pain terms: A supplementary note. Pain 1982; 14:205.
3. Dorland's Illustrated Medical Dictionary, ed 26. Philadelphia: WB Saunders Co; 1981.
4. Travell JG, Simons DG. Myofascial Pain and Dysfunction. Baltimore, Md: Williams & Wilkins; 1983.

Section I

The Nature of Pain

1 | Defining the Problem

Pain is an unpleasant experience that perhaps motivates the individual far greater than any other life experience. Pain seriously impairs the lives of millions of people around the world. In 1984, Bonica[1] reported that nearly one-third of the population in industrialized nations suffer to some extent from chronic pain. At that time he estimated that chronic pain costs the American people more than $65 billion annually for health care services, loss of work, decreased productivity, and disability compensation. It is likely that this represents only a fraction of the cost today.

The clinical management of orofacial pain is a primary concern of health professionals all over the world. It is interesting to note that the profession has become extremely effective in the management of acute pain secondary to surgical procedures. The same, however, cannot be said regarding clinical or pathologic pain.

There are reasons for this. The cause of surgical pain is obvious, and its management consists of either suppressing the passage of nociceptive impulses or making the patient insensible to them. Therefore, an effective solution lies within the grasp of the clinician. Clinical pain, however, presents

with different circumstances. For example, the cause of clinical pain may not be easily identified. In fact in some cases the initiating cause may no longer even be present. The mechanisms that are involved with clinical pain appear to be different than surgical pain and are certainly not as well understood. As a rule, orofacial pain from an obvious cause such as a toothache is managed with no difficulty at all. But when a pain occurs spontaneously or without evidence of structural cause, the clinician may become confused and frustrated. For the clinician to effectively manage clinical pain, he or she must have a basic understanding of the mechanisms that create this unpleasant experience. These mechanisms are certainly not easy to understand because our knowledge base falls short of being complete. This text presents the latest information regarding our understanding of clinical pain; however, the reader needs to be constantly accessing current research findings that may shed new light on this most complex problem.

Pain as a Clinical Complaint

Pain, especially chronic pain, is a major health problem. According to the Nuprin Report (Bristol-Myers Co, 1985),[2] of the 1,254 persons questioned, 27% reported having experienced dental pain, and 73% reported headaches during the previous 12 months. Twelve percent of the patients who reported headache seek care from a dentist for the pain. The sample was constructed statistically in such a manner as to allow these figures to reflect the entire adult population of the United States. This report indicates that the task of managing head and neck pain is a very real one indeed. The problem crosses the lines that demarcate the professions; it should be the concern of all health care professionals.

As a clinical symptom, pain is an experience that cannot be shared. It is wholly personal, belonging to the sufferer alone. Different individuals sensing identical noxious stimulation feel pain in different ways and react with different levels of suffering. It is impossible for one person to sense exactly what another feels. Therefore, the examiner is faced with the task of securing enough information from the patient to interpret how the pain feels to and what meaning it has for that patient. The ability to diagnose the disease and treat a person afflicted with pain rests largely on a knowledge of the mechanisms and behavioral characteristics of pain in its various manifestations.

The Dentist's Responsibility

The dentist assumes a great responsibility for the proper management of pains in and around the mouth, face, and neck. He or she must differentiate between pains that stem from dental, oral, and masticatory sources and those that emanate elsewhere. He or she must become an expert in the diagnosis of pain to choose the complaints that are manageable on a dental level with dental methods and techniques. He or she must be able to positively identify complaints that, although related to oral and masticatory functioning, in fact stem from causes that cannot reasonably be resolved with ordinary dental procedures.

The dentist's responsibility in managing pain problems of the mouth and face is twofold. His or her initial responsibility is diagnostic. The dentist should identify those complaints that are correctable with dental therapy. To do this, he or she must have accurate knowledge of pain problems arising from other than oral and masticatory sources. If he or she cannot make a proper diagnosis, it becomes his or her responsibility to refer the patient to a competent specialist.

The second responsibility of the dentist relates to therapy. Once the pain complaint is correctly identified as a condition amenable to dental therapy, treatment by the dentist is in order. Whether or not a consultation with another practitioner is necessary should be considered in the treatment planning. If therapy at any point does not prove effective as planned, it becomes the dentist's responsibility to seek the cause of failure by using, if needed, the aid of colleagues. If the condition presented is clearly one that would not be amenable to dental therapy, the patient should be referred to the appropriate health care practitioner.

Many pain problems require interdisciplinary management and a good working relationship among the therapists. It is important that the dentist understand what his or her responsibilities in treatment are so that he or she can conduct that portion of the therapy effectively. The dentist should not attempt or relinquish more than what his or her fraction of responsibility calls for. A positive, confident competence tempered by a reasonable and cooperative attitude should enable the dentist to work effectively in any multidisciplinary environment.

In recent years, there has been a rapid increase in the dental profession's interest in orofacial pain disorders. This interest has motivated some universities to initiate specialized programs in the field of orofacial pain. It appears as though a new type of clinician is developing with unique experience in managing orofacial pain disorders. This clinician must have a sound understanding of the principles of medicine and dentistry. The role of this professional in the management of pain is being established at this time. Today is certainly an exciting time to be in this field of study.

Historical Note

Merskey[3] reviewed some of the historical background of modern pain concepts. In ancient times, Homer thought that pain was due to arrows shot by the gods. The feeling that pain is inflicted from an outside source seems to be a primitive instinct that has persisted to some degree down through the ages. Aristotle, who probably was the first to distinguish the five physical senses, considered pain to be a "passion of the soul" that somehow resulted from the intensification of other sensory experience. Plato contended that pain and pleasure arose from within the body, an idea that perhaps gave birth to the concept that pain is an emotional experience more than a localized body disturbance.

The Bible makes reference to pain not only in relationship to injury and illness but also as anguish of the soul. Hebrew words used to express grief, sorrow, and pain are used rather interchangeably in the old scriptures.[4] This implies that the early Hebrews considered pain to be a manifestation of concerns that lead also to grief and sorrow. As knowledge of anatomy and physiology increased, however, it became possible to distinguish between pains due to physical and emotional causes.

During the 19th century, the developing field of neurology fostered the concept that pain was mediated by specific pain pathways and not simply due to excessive stimulation of the special senses. Later it was recognized that strict specificity of neural structures for the exclusive mediation of pain did not exist. In recent years, however, some specialization of nociceptive pathways has been identified.[5] Freud developed the idea that physical symptoms could result from thought processes. He considered that symptoms such as pain could develop as a solution to emotional conflicts.

It can be seen therefore that, until very recent years, concepts concerning pain have changed little since ancient times.

Changing Concepts of Pain

The definition of pain found in the medical dictionary summarizes very well the traditional understanding of what pain is like: "A more or less localized sensation of discomfort, distress, or agony, resulting from the stimulation of specialized nerve endings. It serves as a protective mechanism insofar as it induces the sufferer to remove or withdraw from the source."[6] This definition identifies pain as a localized sensation that occurs as the result of noxious stimulation. It suggests that pain is mediated by way of specialized neural structures that are made for that purpose. It indicates that pain is a protective mechanism against injury. Being external to the body, the presumed noxious agent could be avoided by proper evasive action. Such a definition actually describes only one type of pain: superficial somatic pain, which is pain that occurs as the result of noxious stimulation of cutaneous structures by an environmental agent that affects the exteroceptive nociceptors.

During recent years, quite a different concept of pain has evolved. Although the usefulness of pain as a protective mechanism is recognized with regard to purely exteroceptive noxious stimulation, most pain occurs too late to have much protective value. It has to do with events that have already taken place.

Although pain is now recognized as being more an experience than a sensation, it does have a sensory dimension that registers the nature of the initiating stimulus, including its quality, intensity, location, and duration. But it has other dimensions also: *(1)* cognitive, which represents the subject's ability to comprehend and evaluate the significance of the experience; *(2)* emotional, which represents the feelings that are generated; and *(3)* motivational, which has to do with the drive to terminate it. In humans, pain actively involves neocortical processes that have to do with the recognition and interpretation of the consequences of the experience, thus exerting a good measure of influence on the pain and the suffering that

is generated by it.[7] Pain is thought to be more akin to need states such as hunger and thirst; it initiates a drive for action. Pain cannot be sensed in a detached manner; it comes in combination with dislike, anxiety, fear, and urgency.[8] Although pain does result from noxious stimulation, it occurs also from nonnoxious stimuli as well as spontaneously when there is no stimulus at all. The source of stimulation need not be external to the body.

The newer concept of what constitutes pain is expressed in the definition proposed by the Subcommittee on Taxonomy of the International Association for the Study of Pain: "An unpleasant sensory and emotional experience associated with actual or potential tissue damage, or described in terms of such damage."[9] By this definition, pain is understood to represent a subjective psychological state rather than an activity that is induced solely by noxious stimulation. It should be noted that, if the subject regards his or her experience as pain, it should be accepted as pain.

More precisely, pain as presently conceived has a sensory-discriminative dimension to identify the form of energy (thermal, mechanical, chemical) and the spatial, temporal, and intensive aspects of the stimulus. It also has a motivational-affective property by which the consequences of the experience manifest as escape and avoidance behavior, which includes reflex somatic and autonomic motor responses.[10]

When an identifiable cause can be established for pain, management usually entails measures to eliminate this cause if possible. Some pains, however, are behavioral and therefore are learned. Such pains may confuse the clinician who is stimulus-response oriented and thinks only in terms of cause.

Many times, however, the consequences of the experience become the paramount issue in managing the pain problem. In these cases, the proper manipulation of various environmental factors may help the patient unlearn his pain behavior.[11]

It is interesting to note that the more severe the pain and the more distressed the patient, the more emotional are his responses and the greater the impact on his ability to function.[12] The pressure to seek aid for a pain problem increases when the patient is under greater-than-usual stress. It seems that those who find their life situation satisfactory tend to ignore symptoms.[13]

It has also been observed that the intensity of pain from physical injury relates to the *attention* given at the time. Pain and injury may be coincident only when attention is directed to the injury. If one's attention is fully absorbed at the time of injury, no pain at all may be felt. The subject may remain relatively free of pain if he or she is distracted by events having to do with self-preservation, fighting back, escaping, or obtaining aid. Pain may not become an issue until the *consequences* of the injury induce feelings of concern and anxiety that relate more to therapy and recovery processes than to the injury itself.[14,15]

With the changing concepts of pain represented in body, mind, and person, the diagnosis and management of such problems require a broad understanding of people on the part of the attending doctor. Good therapy begins with an attitude of caring and concern for the person more than for his or her body. Human beings are more than patients that have to be treated.[16]

Emergency Nature of Pain

Pain creates for the patient an emergency and therefore becomes a prime motivating cause for seeking aid. When the suffering occurs in and around the mouth, the dentist is usually the first to be called. When it occurs about the ears, face, head, or neck, a physician may be consulted. The actual location of the symptom may well determine who sees the patient initially. Yet the location of the pain can mislead both patient and doctor as to its true source and significance. In the case of obscure pain, the patient may visit several doctors and receive conflicting opinions and treatments. The alarm with which a patient naturally regards his or her own discomfort is increased when a clinician fails to give prompt and lasting relief, so ineffective therapy may intensify the pain and magnify the task of the next therapist to be consulted. It therefore behooves every clinician to become familiar with the mechanisms of pain and the technique of examining patients with pain complaints.

The emergency nature of pain relates to the significance the patient attaches to it. If the cause is obvious, such as a cut finger, little or no alarm ensues because the subject is able to recognize the cause of his suffering and evaluate it realistically. If, however, the pain is located in an area of greater significance, as, for example, the eye, the alarm mounts because it represents a greater threat. Similarly, if the discomfort arises from deeper structures where its cause is less obvious and its seriousness less certain, the patient becomes more concerned. The emergency nature of pain relates more to the fear that it generates than to the actual intensity of the discomfort.

The importance of prompt and effective therapy should not be underestimated, for in this area the therapist proves himself or utterly fails. Whereas competent therapy has as its prime attribute the means of furnishing consolation to a suffering patient, it can be said conversely that incompetence can intensify the patient's alarm. Perhaps there is no area of practice where this is more likely to occur than in the diagnosis and treatment of obscure pain. Nor is any complaint more adversely affected by professional failure. Minor discomfort assumes major significance if the patient believes the problem is so dreadful that it escapes even the "magic abilities of the doctor."

Levels of Pain Processing

It is important early in a discussion of pain to distinguish the differences between four terms: nociception, pain, suffering, and pain behavior. *Nociception* refers to the noxious stimulus originating from the sensory receptor. This information is carried into the central nervous system by the primary afferent neuron.

Pain is an unpleasant sensation perceived in the cortex usually as a result of incoming nociceptive input. The presence or absence of nociceptive input however, does not always relate closely to pain. As will be discussed in detail later (Chapter 4), the central nervous system (CNS) has the ability to alter or modulate nociceptive input before it reaches the cortex for recognition. Therefore, nociceptive input entering the CNS can be modified in a such a manner that the cortex never perceives it as pain. One can quickly appreciate that this ability of the CNS to modulate noxious stimulation is an extremely important function. As will be discussed, modulation of nociceptive input can increase or decrease the perception of pain.

The term *suffering* refers to even another phenomenon. Suffering refers to how the human reacts to the perception of pain. When pain is perceived by the cortex, a very complex interaction of many factors begins. Factors such as past experiences, expectations, perceived threat of the injury, and attention drawn to the injury determine to what degree the subject will suffer. Suffering therefore, may not be proportionally related to nociception or pain. Patients experiencing little pain may suffer greatly while others with significant pain may suffer less.

Pain behavior is still another term with a different meaning. Pain behavior refers to the individual's audible and visible actions that communicate his or her suffering to others. Pain behavior is the only communication the clinician receives regarding the pain experience. This behavior is as individual as people themselves.

It is important for the clinician to recognize that the information related to the therapist by the patient is not nociception nor pain nor even suffering. The patient only relates his or her pain behavior. Yet it is through this communication that the clinician must gain insight into the patient's problem. One can easily see how difficult the clinician's task is when attempting to manage pain disorders.

Phylogenic Considerations

It is interesting that the human being has a brain system that can be functionally

8

divided into three components. The first component is made up of the spinal cord and medulla. This might be thought of as the basic reptilian brain since it functions on a very primitive level and likely represents the only functional brain of the reptile. This portion of the brain provides protective reflex activity against challenges from the environment. For example, if you were to accidently touch a hot stove, your hand would quickly pull away. This reflex activity occurs without thought or cerebral function; there is no evidence in primates that pain is felt. The same activity occurs if you strike a snake with a stick. The snake will coil up or quickly slither away. This primate brain serves a valuable protective function for the individual.

The second functional brain in humans is the mammalian brain. The mammalian brain is made up of the limbic structures wrapped around the upper portion of the medulla and spinal cord. The limbic structures provide the individual with instinctive drives and emotions. This portion of the brain is made up of various centers that instinctively drive the individual toward certain behaviors. These drives do not function on a totally conscious level but rather represent basic needs of the individual: hunger, thirst, sleep, sexual activity. There appears to be a pain/pleasure center in the limbic structures that strongly motivates the individual. When pain is felt, the individual will instinctively direct behavior toward activities that will reduce the pain and when possible stimulate the pleasure side of this center. Stimulating the pleasure side of the pain/pleasure center is a basic drive and can powerfully direct behavior. Addictions to drugs, alcohol, food, and sexual activities are common behaviors that represent instinctive drives to stimulate the pleasure center of the limbic system.

The third functional component of the human brain represents the most complex structure: the cortex. The human not only has the medulla and spinal cord (the primate brain) with the limbic structures (the mammalian brain) but attached to these structures is the cortex. The cortex provides the human with the ability to reason and think. It is at this level that the human who experiences pain begins to apply meaning and consequence to the sensation. For example, the human experiencing pain will evaluate the meaning of this condition as to how it will affect other relationships such as with a spouse or other family members or how it might influence the ability to work or to socialize. It is this phenomenon that makes suffering as we know it so different from that experienced by lower animal life. It is through this mechanism that factors such as attention, anxiety, and fear influence the level of suffering. The effect of one's mental awareness or state of arousal, one's concern for the outcome, and the emotional and/or physical stability of the individual become the dominant modulating influence in every painful experience. We may consider therefore that clinical pain as we know it is a unique experience peculiar to humans.

Anatomic Considerations of the Human

The human being is a phenomenal organism with complexity far beyond the imagination of the best scientific mind. Perhaps it is best to begin a discussion of anatomy from a very broad prospective. The human being is a musculoskeletal system that is encompassed by an envelope that separates it from the environment. The basic structures or cells of the musculoskeletal system as well as the envelope need to receive food or nutrients and so a supply system is present to carry out this task. The functions of all these systems are very complex; therefore, a communication system is needed to coordinate activities of the entire organism.

We have just described the basic systems of the human being. The musculoskeletal system is made up of muscle, bones, and associated structures such as ligaments and tendons. These structures provide the individual with mobility so that food can be procured. The envelope consists of the cutaneous (skin) and mucogingival structures that surround the musculoskeletal system. These structures provide input to the individual from the environment so that appropriate actions can be carried out to preserve the organism.

The supply system is able to take food and air and convert it into energy that can be utilized by the cells. The supply system then transports these essential elements to each individual cell throughout the organism. The supply system comprises the digestive, pulmonary, and circulatory systems.

Because of the complexity of these systems, a master control system is in place to coordinate all these activities. This system is known as the nervous system and is divided into several functional parts. The peripheral nervous system carries information from the musculoskeletal and cutaneous (envelope) structures. There is also a separate nervous system that coordinates activities of the supply system. This is called the autonomic nervous system, which is predominantly responsible for the regulation of blood flow,

breathing, and digestion. Coordination of the peripheral and autonomic nervous systems is carried out by the central nervous system, which is made up of the brain stem and the cortex. The cortex can be thought of as the master computer that stores the data necessary to carry out functions of the individual.

One of the basic concepts in understanding pain is to appreciate that the manner in which the master computer communicates with each of these structures is perceived by the individual differently. As soon as the clinician appreciates this concept, the patient's description of the pain complaint becomes meaningful. As will be discussed, pain originating in each structure has certain clinical characteristics that help differentiate it from others.

In general, the medical and dental professions do not refer to the various systems by using terms such as supply system or envelope. The terms that will be used in this text will be as follows: Somatic structures include all the structures that make up the body (soma) other than the neurologic structures. Somatic structures are divided into two types: the superficial somatic structures, which represent the envelope (skin and mucogingival tissues) and the deep somatic structures, which make up the remainder of the body tissues. The deep somatic structures are then divided into the musculoskeletal structures and the visceral (supply) structures. The nervous system is divided into the three components that have already been presented (peripheral, central, and autonomic).

Neural Pathways of Pain

Fields[17] has described that the subjective experience of pain arises by four distinct processes: transduction, transmission, modulation, and perception.

Transduction is the process by which noxious stimuli lead to electrical activity in the appropriate sensory nerve endings. The body has several types of sensory organs that initiate the process of nociception. These receptors will be discussed in detail in Chapter 2.

The second process is called *transmission* and refers to the neural events that carry the nociceptive input into the central nervous system for proper processing. There are three basic components to the transmission system. The first is the peripheral sensory nerve called the *primary afferent neuron*. This neuron carries the nociceptive input from the sensory organ in to the spinal cord. The second component of the transmission process is the *second order neuron,* which carries the input to the higher centers. Actually this portion of the transmission process can involve a number of neurons that interact as the input is sent to the thalamus. The third component of the transmission system represents interactions of neurons between the thalamus, cortex, and the limbic system as the nociceptive input reaches these higher centers. This process of transmission will be discussed in detail in Chapters 2 and 3.

The third process involved in the subjective experience of pain is called *modulation.* Modulation refers to the ability of the central nervous system to control the pain-transmitting neurons. Several areas of the cortex and brain stem have been identified that can either enhance or reduce nociceptive input arriving by way of the transmitting neurons. The phenomena of modulation will be discussed in Chapter 4.

The final process involved in the subjective experience of pain is *perception.* If nociceptive input reaches the cortex, perception occurs, which immediately initiates a complex interaction of neurons between the higher centers of the brain. It is at this point that suffering and pain behavior begins. This is the least understood aspect of pain and the most variable between individuals. This will discussed in Chapters 5 and 6.

The remaining chapters of this text will review the etiologic, diagnostic, and treatment considerations of orofacial pain disorders.

References

1. Bonica JJ. Pain research and therapy: Recent advances and future needs. In Kruger L, Liebeskind JC (eds): Advances in Pain Research and Therapy, vol 6. New York: Raven Press; 1984: 1–22.

2. Sternbach RA. Survey of pain in the United States: The Nuprin Pain Report. Clin J Pain 1986; 2:49–53.

3. Merskey H. Some features of the history of the idea of pain. Pain 1980; 9:3–8.

4. Strong J. Strong's Exhaustive Concordance of the Bible. Grand Rapids, Mich: Associated Publishers and Authors, Inc.

5. Dubner R. Specialization of nociceptive pathways: Sensory discrimination, sensory modulation, and neural connectivity. In Fields HL, Dubner R, Cervero F (eds): Advances in Pain Research and Therapy, vol 9. New York: Raven Press; 1985: 111–137.

6. Dorland's Illustrated Medical Dictionary, ed 27. Philadelphia: WB Saunders Co; 1988.

7. Melzack R. Psychological concepts and methods for the control of pain. In Bonica JJ (ed): Advances in Neurology, vol 4. New York: Raven Press; 1974: 275–280.

8. Wall PD. Why do we not understand pain? In Duncan R, Weston-Smith M (eds): The Encyclopaedia of Ignorance. Oxford: Pergamon Press; 1977: 361–368.

9. Merskey H. Pain terms: A list with definitions and notes on usage. Pain 1979; 6:249–252.

10. Price DD, Dubner R. Neurons that subserve the sensory-discriminative aspects of pain. Pain 1977; 3:307–338.

11. Fordyce WE. Pain viewed as learned behavior. In Bonica JJ (ed): Advances in Neurology, vol 4. New York: Raven Press; 1974: 415–422.

12. Lipton JA, Marbach JJ. Components of the response to pain and variables influencing the response in three groups of facial pain patients. Pain 1983; 16:343–359.

13. Marbach JJ, Lipton JA. Aspects of illness behavior in patients with facial pain. J Am Dent Assoc 1976; 96:630–638.

14. Wall PD. On the relation of injury to pain. Pain 1979; 6:253–264.

15. Bonica JJ: Letters to the editor. Pain 1975; 7:203–207.

16. Degenaar JJ. Some philosophical considerations on pain. Pain 1979; 7:281–304.

17. Fields HL. Pain. New York; McGraw-Hill; 1987: 5–7.

2 | The Neural Anatomy of Orofacial Pain

The most essential element of managing a patient's pain problem is understanding normal function of the system. This is true of managing any condition. A clinician cannot treat a disorder until he or she has a sound understanding of order. This thought becomes obvious when one considers treatment. When a patient reports to an office with some type of dysfunction, the clinician's therapy should be directed toward reestablishing normal function. How can the clinician expect to be successful without a sound understanding of normal function? The management of pain disorders is too complex to expect "cookbook" therapy to be effective. The clinician must understand the unique characteristics of the system so that therapy can be appropriately designed for each patient.

As mentioned in Chapter 1, the functional process of pain can be grossly separated into four categories: transduction, transmission, modulation, and perception. This chapter will present transduction and transmission. *Transduction* is the process by which noxious stimuli lead to electrical activity in the appropriate sensory nerve endings. The body has several types of sensory organs that initiate the process of nociception.

The second process is called *transmission* and refers to the neural events that carry the nociceptive input into the central nervous system for proper processing. The neuroanatomy of transduction and transmission will be discussed in this chapter. Modulation and perception will be discussed in Chapters 3 and 4.

Neural Structures

A nerve is a cordlike structure that has the ability to convey electrical and chemical impulses. It consists of a connective tissue sheath called *epineurium* that encloses bundles (fasciculi) of nerve fibers, each bundle being surrounded by its own connective tissue sheath called *perineurium*. Within each bundle, the nerve fibers are separated by interstitial connective tissue called *endoneurium*.

An individual nerve fiber consists of a central bundle of neurofibrils in a matrix of nerve protoplasm called *axoplasm* and enclosed in a thin nerve tissue plasma membrane called *axolemma*. Each peripheral nerve fiber is covered by a cellular nerve tissue sheath called *neurolemma* (primary sheath or sheath of Schwann). Some of

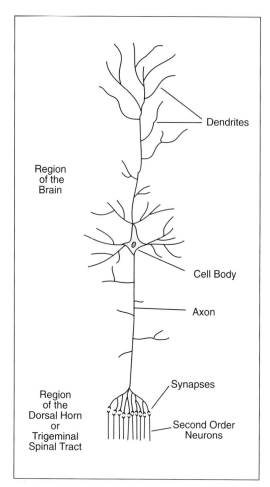

Fig 2-1 The structure of a large neuron of the brain. (Adapted from Guyton: Textbook of Medical Physiology, ed 8. Philadelphia: WB Saunders Co; 1991: 479.)

only neurolemma covers the nerve fiber. Nerve fibers in the central nervous system (CNS) have no neurolemma. Those situated in the white substance are myelinated, whereas those in the gray substance are nonmyelinated.

Myelination of a nerve fiber affects the resting and action potential of the neuron. The myelin acts as insulation so that the action potential of a transferring impulse is only expressed at the node of Ranvier. Therefore the impulse travels from node to node, requiring less time to move down the nerve fiber.[1] Thus myelination increases the conduction velocity of the fiber. The ultrastructure of the primary trigeminal neuron has been well described[2] with electron microscopic techniques.

The structural unit of the nervous system is the nerve cell or *neuron*. It is composed of a mass of protoplasm termed the *nerve cell body* (perikaryon), which contains a spherical nucleus (karyon) and gives off one or more processes. The nerve cell bodies located in the spinal cord are found in the gray substance of the CNS. Cell bodies found outside the CNS are grouped together in *ganglia*. The term *nucleus*, as applied to the gross structure of the CNS, is used to designate a group of nerve cells that bear a direct relationship to the fibers of a particular nerve. Protoplasmic processes from the nerve cell body are called *dendrites* and *axons* (Fig 2-1). A dendrite (from the Greek word dendron, meaning tree) is a branched arborizing process that conducts impulses toward the cell body. An axon (from the Greek word axon, meaning axle or axis) or axis-cylinder is the central core that forms the essential conducting part of a nerve fiber and is an extension of cytoplasm from a nerve cell.

these fibers also have a layer of fatty nerve tissue called the *myelin sheath* (medullary sheath or white substance of Schwann). Fibers with myelin sheaths form the white nerves, those without myelin sheaths the gray nerves. Constrictions called *nodes of Ranvier* occur in myelinated nerves at intervals of about 1 mm. These nodes are caused by the absence of myelin material so that

Depending on the number of axons present, a nerve cell is unipolar, bipolar, or multipolar. Peripheral sensory neurons are unipolar. The single axon leaves the nerve cell body located in the dorsal root ganglion and branches into two parts: a peripheral branch that extends to terminate in a sensory receptor and a central branch that passes through the root of the nerve to terminate in the gray substance of the CNS.

Depending on their location and function, neurons are designated by different terms. An *afferent* neuron conducts the nervous impulse toward the CNS, whereas an *efferent* neuron conducts it peripherally. *Internuncial neurons,* or *interneurons,* lie wholly within the CNS. Sensory or receptor neurons, afferent in type, receive and convey impulses from receptor organs. The first sensory neuron is called the *primary* or *first-order neuron. Second-* and *third-order* sensory neurons are internuncial. *Motor* or *efferent* neurons convey nervous impulses to produce muscular or secretory effects. A *preganglionic neuron* is an *autonomic efferent neuron* whose nerve cell body is located in the CNS and terminates in an autonomic ganglion. A postganglionic neuron has its nerve cell body in the autonomic ganglion and terminates peripherally.

Nervous impulses are transmitted from one neuron to another only at a synaptic junction, or *synapse,* where the processes of two neurons are in proximity. All afferent synapses are located within the gray substance of the CNS. It should be noted that the only synapses that normally occur outside the CNS are those of the efferent preganglionic and postganglionic autonomic fibers, and these are located in the autonomic ganglia. This indicates that there are no anatomic peripheral connections between sensory fibers. All connections are within the CNS, and the peripheral transmission of a sensory impulse from one fiber to another is abnormal. Any artificial or false peripheral synapse, called an *ephapse,* signifies an abnormal or pathologic change.[3]

Functional Neuroanatomy

Information from the tissues outside the central nervous system needs to be transferred into the CNS and on to the higher centers in the brain stem and cortex for interpretation and evaluation. Once this information is evaluated, appropriate action must be taken. The higher centers then send impulses down the spinal cord and back out to the periphery to an efferent organ for the desired action. The primary afferent neuron (first-order neuron) receives stimulus from the sensory receptor. This impulse is carried by the primary afferent neuron into the CNS by way of the dorsal root to synapse in the dorsal horn of the spinal cord with a secondary (second-order) neuron. The cell bodies of all the primary afferent neurons are located in the dorsal root ganglia. The impulse is then carried by the second-order neuron across the spinal cord to the anteriolateral spinothalamic pathway, which ascends to the higher centers. There may be multiple *interneurons* (third-order, fourth-order, etc) that are involved with the transfer of this impulse to the thalamus and cortex. There are also interneurons located in the dorsal horn that may become involved with the impulse as it synapses with the second-order neuron. Some of these neurons may directly synapse with an efferent neuron that is directed out of the CNS by way

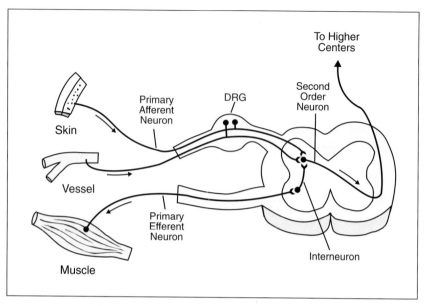

Fig 2-2 A graphic depiction of the peripheral nerve input into the spinal cord. Note the first-order neurons (*primary afferents*) carry input into the dorsal horn to synapses with the second-order neurons. The second-order neuron then crosses over and ascends on to the higher centers. Small interneurons connect the primary afferent neuron with the primary motor (*efferent*) neuron allowing reflex arc activity. The dorsal root ganglion (*DRG*) contains the cell bodies of the primary afferent neurons.

of the ventral root to stimulate an efferent organ such as a muscle (Fig 2-2).

Some neural circuits are simple. For example, an impulse from a sensory receptor is carried into the CNS by the primary afferent neuron and synapses with an interneuron. This interneuron in turn synapses with an efferent motor neuron exiting the CNS to an efferent organ, such as a muscle. A circuit formed by a chain of neurons in such a way that stimulation is followed by an immediate and automatic response is called a *reflex arc*. As will be discussed, most reflex arcs or neural circuits are much more complex, involving several and sometimes vast numbers of interneurons, with many possible responses.

Sensory Receptors

At the distal terminals of afferent (sensory) nerves are specialized *sensory receptors* that respond to physical or chemical stimuli. Once these receptors have been adequately stimulated, an impulse is generated in the primary afferent neuron that is carried centrally into the CNS. Sensory receptors are specific for certain types of stimuli. They can be classified into three main groups: exteroceptors, proprioceptors, and interoceptors.[4]

Exteroceptors. Exteroceptors are sensory receptors that are stimulated by the immediate external environment and are appropriately fashioned and located so as to be exposed to the organism's environment. These receptors provide information from the skin and mucosa (the envelope). Most impulses arising from these receptors are sensed at conscious levels. Some examples of this type of receptor are:

1. Merkel's corpuscles: tactile receptors in the submucosa of the tongue and oral mucosa
2. Meissner's corpuscles: tactile receptors in skin
3. Ruffini's corpuscles: pressure and warmth receptors
4. Krause's corpuscles or end-bulbs: cold receptors
5. Free nerve endings: perceive superficial pain and touch

Proprioceptors. Proprioceptors are sensory receptors that provide information from the musculoskeletal structures concerning the presence, position, and movement of the body. They are involved chiefly with automatic functioning. For the most part, sensations conducted from proprioceptors are below conscious levels even though many such sensations can be brought into consciousness voluntarily. Some examples of this type of receptor are:

1. Muscle spindles: mechanoreceptors found between the skeletal muscle fibers that respond to passive stretch of the muscle, thus signaling muscle length; they are responsible for the myotatic reflex.
2. Golgi tendon organs: mechanoreceptors in the tendons of muscles that signal muscle tension both in contraction and stretching; they are probably responsible for nociceptive and inverse stretch reflexes.

3. Pacinian corpuscles: receptors concerned with the perception of pressure.
4. Periodontal mechanoreceptors: respond to biomechanical stimuli.
5. Free nerve endings: perceive deep somatic pain and other sensations.

Interoceptors. Interoceptors are sensory receptors that are located in and transmit impulses from the viscera (supply system) of the body. Sensation from these receptors for the most part is involved in the involuntary functioning of the body and as such is below conscious levels. Some examples of this type of receptor include the following:

1. Pacinian corpuscles: concerned with perception of pressure
2. Free nerve endings: perceive visceral pain and other sensations

Specialized Receptors and Reflexes

The more highly specialized receptor organs are complex and admirably designed to receive a particular type of stimulus. The neuromuscular endings, or muscle spindles, have their own sensory and motor innervation comprising a monosynaptic reflex system known as the *myotatic* or *stretch reflex.* When muscle spindles are elongated due to passive stretching of the muscle, reflex contraction occurs. This appears to function not only to oppose the forces of gravity but function also during reflex and voluntary contraction of muscles, both flexor and extensor.

Neurotendinous receptors called Golgi tendon organs respond to tendon stretch and muscle contraction. When these receptors are stimulated, an inhibitory reflex occurs that limits contraction and thus protects the muscle from disruption or detachment. The reflex mechanism involved in this activity is called the *nociceptive reflex* and is a polysynaptic relay that involves concurrently the contraction of flexor and inhibition of extensor muscles, resulting in withdrawal of the part stimulated.[5,6]

When a muscle is maximally stretched, stimulation of Golgi tendon organs induces a reflex that causes contraction to cease and the muscle to relax. This reflex is called the *inverse stretch reflex.* Occasional stretching of a muscle that induces this reflex activity is necessary for the muscle to maintain its normal resting length. If conditions prevent normal operation of this reflex, muscular contracture may occur, which causes the muscle to become shortened.[7] Therefore, contracture of elevator masticatory muscles may occur when conditions prevent the full opening of the mouth for extended periods. This phenomenon is also seen to involve the lateral pterygoid muscles in edentulous patients and cause a progressive shift of the mandibular position anteriorly. It results from a lack of the inverse stretch reflex in the lateral pterygoid muscles, which fail to maintain their full resting length. The full intercuspation of natural teeth satisfactorily stimulates the Golgi tendon organs, but artificial dentures may not, because of the resiliency of the interposed underlying soft tissues.

The simplest type of receptor is the nonencapsulated branching of the axon called the *free nerve ending.* These terminations are usually described as naked, and they form a network that is especially dense in the cutaneous layers, mucous membranes, and periodontium. In deeper tissues, the ramification is neither as widely spread nor as dense. The simple free nerve endings

are no doubt the receptors for nociception and pain, but they are not specific for pain only.

Stimulation of the free nerve ending pain receptors can occur as a result of mechanical stimulation, such as pressure; thermal stimulation, such as heat; or by chemical stimulation, such as that produced by substances released following tissue damage.[8] It should be noted that free nerve endings are not required for the reception of noxious stimulation since the nerve fiber itself has the same propensity and the evoked response is similar to that initiated by receptors.

Associated with all vascular tissue, including the endocardium, is a remarkable network of sensory receptors derived from myelinated nerve fibers called the *end-net.*[9] These receptors provide sensory information from the vessels.

The First-Order Neuron

Each sensory receptor is attached to a first-order or primary afferent neuron that carries the impulses to the CNS. The axons of these first-order neurons are found to have varying thickness. It has long been known that a relationship exists between the diameter of nerve fibers and their conduction velocities.[10-12] The larger fibers conduct impulses more rapidly than the smaller ones. A general classification of neurons divides the larger fibers from the smaller ones, calling the larger fibers A fibers and the smaller fibers C fibers. The A fibers are further divided by diameter size into alpha, beta, gamma, and delta. This relationship can be summarized as follows:[13]

Type A fibers

1. Alpha fibers: size, 13 to 20 μm in diameter; velocity, 70 to 120 m/s
2. Beta fibers: size, 6 to13 μm in diameter; velocity, 40 to 70 m/s
3. Gamma fibers: size, 3 to 8 μm in diameter; velocity, 15 to 40 m/s
4. Delta fibers: size, 1 to 5 μm in diameter; velocity, 5 to 15 m/s

Type C fibers

Size, 0.5 to 1 μm; velocity, 0.5 to 2 m/s

There also appears to be a relationship between fiber size and the type of impulse transmitted, although strict specificity has not been proven. It appears that the fast conducting A-alpha, A-beta, and A-gamma fibers carry impulses that induce tactile and proprioceptive responses but not pain. It seems that pain is conducted by A-delta and C fibers, but these are not specific for pain only.

It is recognized that there are two types of cutaneous pain sensation: pricking pain, which is rapidly felt; and burning pain, which is slightly delayed. It is thought by some investigators that these sensations are mediated by different fibers: the pricking sensation by A-delta, the burning sensation by C fibers.[14] It is known, however, that A-delta fibers also conduct touch, warmth, and cold, whereas C fibers also conduct itch, warmth, and cold.[15–17]

There is no general agreement among investigators as to the specificity of function as related to fiber size. It has been demonstrated[18] that the fine peripheral nerve fibers that innervate the cornea are able to convey touch, pain, warmth, and cold. It seems fairly certain that the larger peripheral nerve fibers have specificity of function that excludes pain and that, although small fibers are activated by nonpainful stimuli, the activation of small fibers is necessary for the organism to appreciate pain.[19,20]

Three classes of nociceptive afferent neurons provide the input whereby the brain perceives pain. *(1)* Mechanothermal afferents are primarily A-delta fibers that conduct at a velocity of 12 to 18 m/s and respond to intense thermal and mechanical stimuli. They provide a high degree of discriminative information and are peculiar to primates. *(2)* Polymodal afferents are C fibers that conduct much more slowly, at a velocity of .5 m/s, and respond to mechanical, thermal, and chemical stimuli in all mammals. At this rate, it takes an impulse 2 seconds to go from the big toe to the spinal cord. *(3)* High-threshold mechanoreceptive afferents are chiefly A-delta fibers and normally respond to intense mechanical stimuli in all mammals. They can, however, be sensitized by algogenic substances or repeated noxious stimulation to respond to noxious heat also (see Chapter 4). Only the first two classes of nociceptive afferents normally respond to noxious heat.[21,22]

Second-Order Neuron

The primary afferent neuron carries impulses into the CNS and synapses with the second-order neuron. This second-order neuron is sometimes called a transmission neuron since it transfers the impulse on to the higher centers. The synapse of the primary afferent and the second-order neuron occurs in the dorsal horn of the spinal cord (see Fig 2-2). The specific anatomy of the

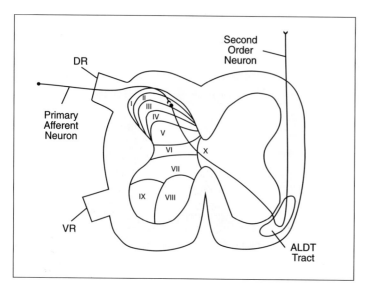

Fig 2-3 Cross-section of the spinal cord, showing the anatomic laminae I through X of the spinal cord gray matter and the ascending sensory anterolateral spinothalamic tract in the white columns (ALDT Tract). (DR) = dorsal root; (VR) = ventral root.

trigeminal system will be reviewed later in this chapter.

There appears to be three specific types of second-order neurons that transfer impulses to the higher centers.[23,24] These neurons are named according to the type of impulses they predominantly carry. The *low-threshold mechanosensitive neurons* (LTM) transfer information of light touch, pressure and proprioception. The *nociceptive specific neurons* (NS) exclusively carry impulses related to noxious stimulation. The third type of second-order neuron is called a *wide dynamic range neuron* (WDR). This neuron is able to respond to a wide range of stimulus intensities from non-noxious to noxious.

Under normal conditions, it is not thought that the low-threshold mechanosensitive neurons are involved in the transfer of nociception. Nociception is primarily carried by the nociceptive-specific and wide dynamic range neurons.

The dorsal horn of the spinal cord is subsided into different layers or *laminae*.[25-27]

These laminae are numbered according to their depth in the dorsal horn from I to VI with the most superficial being I and the deepest lamina VI[24] (Fig 2-3). Studies suggest that nociceptive input enters the dorsal horn by way of the NS and WDR neurons in the area of laminae I, II, and V.[28,29] The LTM neurons that do not carry nociception seemed to be more concentrated in laminae III and IV.

Within the dorsal horn, there are interneurons that transfer impulses to other interneurons or to the ascending neurons. These neurons can be either inhibitory or excitatory. In other words, when some of the neurons are stimulated, they tend to reduce the activity of the neuron to which they synapse. These are called *inhibitory neurons*. Other interneurons, when excited, increase the activity of the neurons on which they synapse. These are called *excitatory neurons*. There are a significant population of these interneurons in laminae II and III and this region is collectively called the *substantia gelatinosa*.

Once the impulses have been transferred from the primary afferents, most of the second-order neurons cross to the opposite side of the spinal cord and enter the *anterolateral spinothalamic tract*, which ascends to the higher centers. Some of the second-order neurons remain on the same side of the dorsal column and ascend by way of the *lemniscal system*. These neurons cross over to the opposite side at the level of the medulla. The dorsal column lemniscal system is composed of large, myelinated nerve fibers that transmit signals to the brain at velocities 30 to 110 m/s. The anterolateral system is composed of much smaller myelinated and unmyelinated fibers that transmit signals at velocities ranging from a few meters per second up to 40 m/s.

These differences immediately characterize the types of sensory information that can be transmitted by these two systems. The dorsal column lemniscal system transmits rapidly information regarding touch, pressure, vibration, and proprioception needed for immediate response of the musculoskeletal system to environmental changes. The anterolateral system transmits impulses at a slower rate but carries a much broader spectrum of sensory information such as pain, warmth, cold, and crude tactile sensations.[30]

Nociceptive input is predominantly carried by the anterolateral system, which is divided into two tracts: the *neospinothalamic tract* and the *paleospinothalamic tract*. The neospinothalamic tract carries the A-delta nociceptive inputs directly to the higher centers. The paleospinothalamic tract predominantly carries the slower C fiber nociception and travels through many other centers before reaching the brain. The significance of these two pathways with regard to fast and slow pain will be discussed in Chapter 3.

Brain Stem and Brain

Once the impulses have been passed to the second-order neurons, these neurons carry them to the higher centers for interpretation and evaluation. There are numerous centers in the brain stem and brain that help give meaning to the impulses. It should also be remembered that numerous interneurons may be involved in transmitting the impulses on to higher centers. In fact, attempting to follow an impulse through the brain stem on to the cortex is no simple task. To intelligently discuss pain in this text, certain functional regions of the brain stem and brain need to be described. The reader should be reminded that the following descriptions will merely be overviews of the what are thought to be the most important functions of each area. The complexity of the organ we call the brain is beyond the scope of this text. In fact, it may be beyond the scope of the human mind itself. A thought-provoking comment by Thibodeau[31] states "Perhaps the capacity of the human brain falls short of the ability to understand its own complexity."

The higher centers of the central nervous system can be subdivided into the following four regions from the most inferior to the most superior:

1. The brain stem made up of the medulla oblongata, the pons, and the midbrain (or mesencephalon).
2. The cerebellum.
3. The diencephalon is made up of the thalamus and hypothalamus.

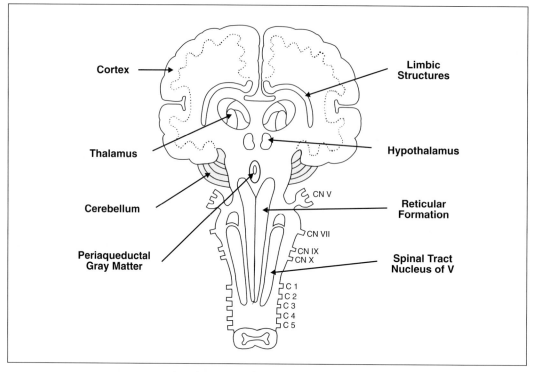

Fig 2-4 A graphic depiction of the brain and brain stem. This figure will be used throughout the text to demonstrate the neuroanatomy and neurophysiology of orofacial pain. *(CN)* = cranial nerve.

4. The cerebrum made up of the cerebral cortex, the basal ganglia, and the limbic structures.

The figures used throughout this text are graphic representations of the brain and brain stem. They are not meant to accurately depict the anatomy of each area but instead to give the reader a functional relationship so that pain processing can be better understood (Fig 2-4).

The Brain Stem. The brain stem is the most superior portion of the spinal cord that attaches to the brain structures. It is divided into three regions: the *medulla*

oblongata, which forms the lowest part of the brain stem; the *midbrain,* which forms the uppermost part; and the *pons,* which lies between them.

The Medulla Oblongata. The medulla oblongata, often referred to as the medulla, is a larger extension of the spinal cord located just above the foramen magnum. It is composed of white matter, which makes up several projection tracts that route impulses directly to the higher centers (ie, spinothalamic tract to the thalamus). The medulla also has a region made up of both white and gray matter called the *reticular formation.* Within the reticular formation are concentrations of cells or *nuclei* that represent centers for various functions. Some of the more important centers are the cardiac, respiratory, and vasomotor centers, which are often referred to as the vital centers. Some of the medullary nuclei bear individual names such as the nucleus gracilis, nucleus cuneatus, and olivary nuclei. Within each nuclei are high concentrations of specific neurotransmitters, which will be discussed in Chapter 3.

The reticular formation plays an extremely important role in monitoring impulses that enter the brain stem. The reticular formation controls the overall activity of the brain by either enhancing or inhibiting the impulses to the brain. As will be discussed in Chapter 3, this portion of the brain stem has an extremely important impact on pain and other sensory input.

Pons. The pons is located just above the medulla and like the medulla is composed of both white matter and reticular formation. Fibers seem to run transversely across the pons into the cerebellum and likely act to communicate with these and other structures. The pons also has centers for reflexes mediated by the fifth, sixth, seventh, and eighth cranial nerves.

Midbrain. The midbrain is appropriately named since it forms the midsection of the brain, lying above the pons and below the cerebrum. It is also referred to as the mesencephalon. The midbrain contains several tracts that relay impulses to the cerebrum. Two other important midbrain structures are the *red nucleus* and the *substantia nigra.* Each of these consists of clusters of cell bodies of neurons involved in muscular control.

Cerebellum. The cerebellum, the second largest part of the brain, is located just below the posterior portion of the cerebrum and is partially covered by it. The outer portion of the cerebellum is made up of gray matter while the inner portion is predominantly white matter. The cerebellum functions to control skeletal muscles in three ways. It acts with the cerebral cortex to produce skilled movements by coordinating the activities of groups of muscles. It also controls skeletal muscles to maintain equilibrium and posture. It also functions below the level of consciousness to make movements smooth instead of jerky; steady instead of trembling; and coordinated instead of inefficient, awkward, and uncoordinated.

Diencephalon. The diencephalon has sometimes been referred to as the "between brain" since it links the brain stem with the cerebrum. The most important structures of the diencephalon are the *thalamus* and *hypothalamus.* Both of these are composed of multiple nuclei that perform many different important functions. In addition to these areas of the diencephalon are two smaller nuclear areas located posterior and inferior to the thalamus, the epithalamus and subthalamus.

Thalamus. The thalamus is located in the very center of the brain with the cerebrum surrounding it from the top and sides and the midbrain below (see Fig 2-4). It is made up of numerous nuclei that function together to interrupt impulses. Almost all impulses from the midbrain and other lower regions of the brain, as well as from the spinal cord, are relayed through synapses in the thalamus before proceeding to the cerebral cortex. The thalamus acts as a relay station for most of the communication between the brain stem, cerebellum, and cerebrum. As impulses arrive at the thalamus, the thalamus makes assessments and directs the impulses to appropriate regions in the higher centers for interpretation and response.

If one were to compare the human brain with a computer, the thalamus would represent the keyboard that controls the functions and directs the signals. The thalamus drives the cortex to activity and enables the cortex to communicate with other regions of the CNS. Without the thalamus, the cortex is useless.

Hypothalamus. The hypothalamus is a small structure in the middle of the base of the brain. Although it is small, its function is great. The hypothalamus is the major center of the brain for controlling internal body functions (the supply system). There are numerous nuclei that make up the hypothalamus, each predominantly controlling a separate function. A few of the important ones are the *preoptic nucleus,* located anteriorly, and primarily concerned with body temperature control. The *supraoptic nucleus* is located anteriorly and inferiorly, and controls the secretion of antidiuretic hormone. This in turn controls the concentration of electrolytes in the body fluids. The *medial nuclei* of the hypothalamus gives a person a sense of satisfaction especially associated with food. Stimulation of the *lateral regions* of the hypothalamus causes a person to become very hungry, while the *anterior lateral regions* causes a person to become very thirsty. Stimulation of the *posterior hypothalamus* excites the sympathetic nervous system throughout the body,

increasing the overall level of activity of many internal parts of the body, especially increasing heart rate and causing blood vessel constriction.

The hypothalamus has neurons that when stimulated can cause secretion of releasing hormones, which are carried by the venous blood directly to the anterior pituitary gland which causes a release of some of the pituitary hormones. These pituitary hormones can cause changes in the body metabolism of carbohydrates, proteins, and fats, as well as alter other body functions.

One can clearly see that this small area of the brain has some powerful effects on functions of the individual. As will be discussed, increased levels of emotional stress can stimulate the hypothalamus to upregulate the sympathetic nervous system and greatly influence nociceptive impulses entering the brain. This simple statement should have extreme meaning to the clinician managing pain.

Cerebrum. The cerebrum is the largest and uppermost division of the brain. It consists of two halves, the right and left cerebral hemispheres. Three major functional units make up the cerebrum: the *cerebral cortex,* the *basal ganglia,* and the *limbic structures.*

Cerebral Cortex. The cerebral cortex represents the outer region of the cerebrum and is made up predominantly of gray matter. The cerebral cortex is the portion of the brain most frequently associated with the thinking process, even though it cannot provide thinking without simultaneous action of deeper structures of the brain. The cerebral cortex is the portion of the brain in which essentially all of our memories are stored, and it is also the area most responsible for our ability to acquire our many muscle skills. We still do not know the basic physiologic mechanisms by which the cerebral cortex stores either memories or knowledge of muscle skills.

In most areas, the cerebral cortex is about 6-mm thick and all together it contains an estimated 50 to 80 billion nerve cell bodies. Perhaps a billion nerve fibers lead away from the cortex as well as comparable numbers leading into it, passing to other areas of the cortex, to and from deeper structures of the brain, and some all the way to the spinal cord.

The surface of the cerebral cortex looks like a group of small sausages, which are each called a *convolution* or *gyrus*. In between each gyrus lies a shallow groove called a *sulcus* or a deeper groove called a *fissure*. Fissures divide each cerebral hemisphere into five lobes. Four of them are named for the bones that lie over them: *frontal lobe, parietal lobe, temporal lobe,* and *occipital lobe*. A fifth lobe, the *insula* (island of Reil), lies hidden from view in the lateral fissure.

Different regions of the cerebral cortex have been identified to have different functions. There is a motor area, which is primarily involved with coordinating motor function. There is a sensory area that receives somatosensory input for evaluation. There are also visual and auditory areas.

Wernicke's area is a region of the cortex that is important for sensory integration. It is in this region that meaning of the sensory input is interpreted. The Wernicke's area interprets the ultimate meanings of almost all the different types of sensory information such as the meanings of sentences and thoughts, whether they are heard, read, felt,

or even generated within the brain itself. This area is well developed in only one of the cerebral hemispheres, usually in the left hemisphere. This unilateral development prevents confusion of thought processes between the two halves of the brain.

Deep to the gray matter of the cerebral cortex lie tracts made up of white matter. There are three types of tracts: *projections tracts, association tracts,* and *commissural tracts.* The projection tracts are extensions of the ascending or sensory spinothalamic tracts and descending or motor corticospinal tracts. The association tracts are the most numerous of the cerebral tracts and extend from one convolution to another in the same hemisphere. Commissural tracts extend from one convolution to a corresponding convolution in the other hemisphere. Commissural tracts comprise the *corpus callosum* by which all direct communication passes between hemispheres.

If one were to again compare the human brain with a computer, the cerebral cortex would represent the hard disc drive that stores all information of memory and motor function. Once again, one should remember that the thalamus (the keyboard) is the necessary unit that calls the cortex to function.

Basal Ganglia. Central to the cerebral cortex is a portion of gray matter called the basal ganglia. The basal ganglia are composed of several nuclei that appear to be intimately involved with coordinating cerebral activities with other brain stem functions. Some of the important nuclei are the *caudate nucleus,* the *putamen,* and the *globus pallidus.* The basal ganglia are important in controlling background gross body movements whereas the cerebral cortex is necessary for performance of the more precise movements of the arms, hands, fingers, and feet. When the hand is performing some precise activity that requires a background stance of the body, the basal ganglia provide the body movements while the cerebral cortex provides the precise movements. The high degree of coordination required among the muscles of the body during most motor functions requires a very complex circuitry of nerve fibers not only between the cerebral cortex and the basal ganglia but also between these structures and the thalamus, cerebellum, the red nucleus, and the substania nigra.

Limbic Structures. The word limbic means border. The limbic system comprises the border structures of the cerebrum and the diencephalon. The limbic structures function to control our emotional and behavioral activities. Within the limbic structures are centers or nuclei that are responsible for specific behaviors. There appears to a pain/pleasure center that on an instinctive level drives the individual toward behaviors that stimulate the pleasure side of the center. These drives are not generally perceived at a conscious level but more as a basic instinct. The instinct, however, will bring certain behaviors to a conscious level. For example, when an individual experiences chronic pain, behavior will be orientated toward withdrawal from any stimulus that may increase the pain. Often the sufferer will withdraw from life itself and mood alterations such as depression will appear. The very important significance of the limbic system and pain will be discussed in later chapters.

The limbic system is divided into the following functional structures that will be discussed in this section: the amygdala, the hippocampus, the mammillary bodies, the septum pellucidum, the cingulate gyrus, the cingulum, the insula, and the parahippocampal gyrus. Many of the limbic structures function in close coordination with the hypothalamus. In some writings, the hypothalamus is considered a limbic structure.

The *amygdala* is a small nuclear structure located deep inside each anterior temporal lobe of the cerebrum. It is believed that this structure functions with the hypothalamus to control the appropriate behavior of the person for each type of social situation.

The *hippocampus* is a primitive portion of the cerebral cortex that lies along the medial-most border of the temporal lobe. It is believed to interpret for the brain the importance of most of our sensory experiences. If the hippocampus determines an experience to be important enough, then the experience will be stored as a memory in the cerebral cortex. Without the hippocampus, a person's ability to store memories becomes very deficient.

The *mammillary bodies* lie immediately behind the hypothalamus and function in close association with the thalamus, hypothalamus, and brain stem to help control many behavioral functions such as the person's degree of wakefulness and perhaps also his feeling of well-being.

The *septum pellucidum* is located anterior to the thalamus, superior to the hypothalamus, and between the basal ganglia. Stimulation of this region can cause many different behavioral effects such as anger and rage.

The *cingulate gyrus*, the *cingulum*, the *insula,* and the *parahippocampal gyrus* form a ring in each hemisphere of the cere-

Fig 2-5 The pathway of cerebrospinal fluid flow from the choroid plexuses in the lateral ventricles to the arachnoidal villi protruding into the dural sinuses. Note the lateral, third, and fourth ventricles. (From Guyton: Textbook of Medical Physiology, ed 8. Philadelphia: WB Saunders Co; 1991: 681. Used with permission.)

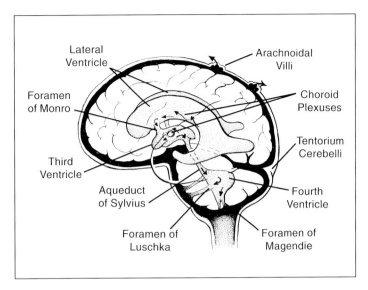

brum around the deeper structures of the limbic system. It is believed that these structures interact and develop associations between the limbic functions and the cerebral functions. This interaction coordinates the conscious cerebral behavioral functions with the subconscious behavioral functions of the deeper limbic system.

Impulses from the limbic system leading into the hypothalamus can modify any one or all of the many internal bodily functions controlled by the hypothalamus. Impulses from the limbic system feeding into the midbrain and medulla can control behavior such as wakefulness, sleep, excitement, attentiveness, and even rage or docility. With this basic understanding of limbic function, one can understand the impact it can have on the overall function of the individual. The limbic system certainly plays a major role in chronic pain problems as will be discussed in later chapters.

Other Important Brain Stem Structures.
This brief summary of brain and brain stem

structures is by no means complete. It is presented so that future discussions regarding pain can have meaning. There are several other structures within the brain stem that should be mentioned before this section is completed. These structures are the ventricles, the periaqueductal gray area, and the raphe magnus nucleus.

Ventricles. The brain, brain stem, and spinal cord are surrounded by cerebrospinal fluid which is encapsulated by the meninges. This fluid acts as a cushion during trauma and also serves as a transport medium for neurotransmitters and other chemicals such as carbon dioxide. Carbon dioxide levels in the cerebrospinal fluid affect neurons of the respiratory center in the medulla and thereby help control respiration.

The cerebrospinal fluid is confined to certain spaces within the brain and brain stem. These spaces are called the *ventricles* and there are four (Fig 2-5). Two of the ventricles are called the lateral ventricles and are located one in each of the cerebral hemispheres. The third ventricle is little more than a lengthwise slit between the right and left thalamus. The fourth ventricle is a diamond-shaped space between the cerebellum posteriorly and the medulla and pons anteriorly.

Formation of the cerebrospinal fluid occurs mainly by filtration from blood in the choroid plexuses. The choroid plexuses are networks of capillaries that project from the inner lining of the meninges (the pia mater) into the lateral ventricles and into the roofs of the third and fourth ventricles. The cerebrospinal fluid then passes from the third ventricle to the fourth by way of a narrow channel called the aqueduct of Sylvius.

Periaqueductal Gray. The *periaqueductal gray area* is a region of the mesencephalon and upper pons surrounding the aqueduct of Sylvius. This region of the brain stem has a high concentration of neurons that are capable of producing power neurotransmitters that can greatly modulate nociceptive impulses. The significance of this region will be discussed in Chapter 4.

Raphe Magnus Nucleus. The *raphe magus nucleus* is a midline nucleus located in the lower pons and upper medulla. Like the periaqueductal gray, it functions to modulate nociceptive input ascending to the thalamus. The importance of this nucleus will be discussed in Chapter 4.

The Trigeminal System

The neural pathways that have been described so far are the common pathways that transmit somatic impulses into the spinal cord and on to the brain. Somatic

input from the face and oral structures does not enter the spinal cord by way of spinal nerves (Fig 2-6). Instead, sensory input from the face and mouth is carried by way of the fifth cranial nerve, the trigeminal nerve. The cell bodies of the trigeminal afferent neurons are located in the large gasserian ganglion. The sensory distribution of this nerve will be discussed later in this chapter. Impulses carried by the trigeminal nerve enter directly into the brain stem in the region of the pons to synapse in the trigeminal spinal nucleus (Fig 2-7). This region of the brain stem is structurally very similar to the dorsal horn of the spinal cord. In fact, it may be considered an extension of the dorsal horn and is sometimes referred to as the medullary dorsal horn.

The brain stem trigeminal nucleus complex consists of the main sensory trigeminal nucleus, which is rostrally located and receives periodontal and some pulpal afferents; and the spinal tract of the trigeminal nucleus, which is more caudally located. The spinal tract is divided into the subnucleus oralis; the subnucleus interpolaris; and the subnucleus caudalis, which corresponds to the medullary dorsal horn. Tooth pulp afferents go to all three subnuclei.[32] The subnucleus caudalis has especially been implicated in trigeminal nociceptive mechanisms on the basis of electrophysiologic observations of nociceptive neurons.[21,28,33] The subnucleus oralis appears to be a significant area of this trigeminal brain stem complex for oral pain mechanisms.[21,34,35]

There is sufficient evidence that facial nociceptive afferents project to the subnucleus caudalis of the massive trigeminal spinal tract nucleus.[36] Evidence at this time supports the concept that the subnucleus caudalis is homologous to the substantia

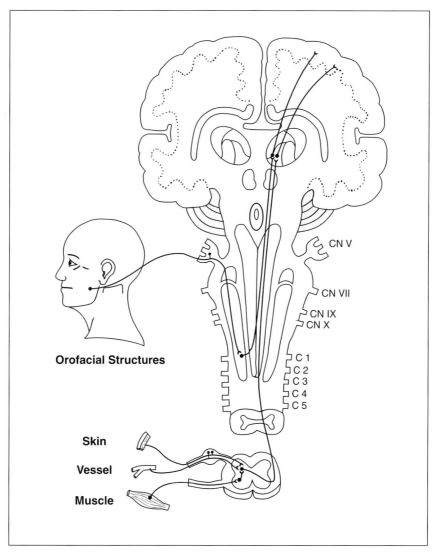

Fig 2-6 The relationship of the trigeminal nerve input and the spinal nerve input as impulses ascend to the higher centers.

gelatinosa of the spinal dorsal horn.[37] Therefore, information concerning the dorsal horn structure can be safely extrapolated and applied to the subnucleus caudalis. The marginal rim of the nucleus corresponds to lamina I of the dorsal horn. The structure of laminae II and III, comprising the substantia gelatinosa of the dorsal horn, should represent the cellular arrangement present in the subnucleus caudalis. Although it is usually presumed that the subnucleus caudalis predominates in trigeminal nociception, no doubt the more rostrally located nuclei are important for nociception also.

Another component of the trigeminal brain stem complex is the motor nucleus of

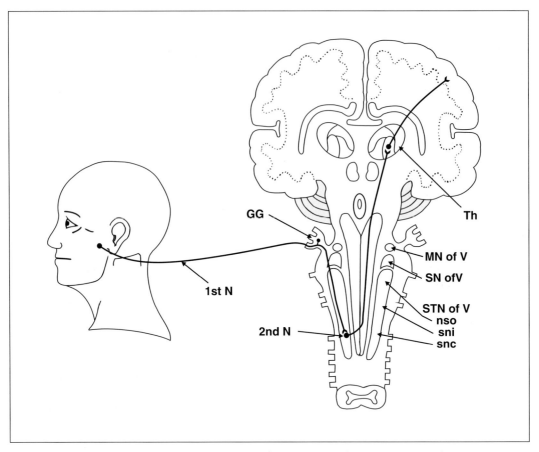

Fig 2-7 A graphic depiction of the trigeminal nerve entering the brain stem at the level of the pons. The primary afferent neuron *(1st N)* enters the brain stem to synapse with a second-order neuron *(2nd N)* in the trigeminal spinal tract nucleus *(STN of V)*. The spinal tract nucleus is divided into three regions; the subnucleus oralis *(nso)*, the subnucleus interpolaris *(sni)*, and the subnucleus caudalis *(snc)*. The trigeminal brain stem complex is also composed of the motor nucleus of V *(MN of V)* and the main sensory nucleus of V *(SN of V)*. The cell bodies of the trigeminal nerve are located in the gasserian ganglion *(GG)*. Once the second-order neuron receives the input it is carried on to the thalamus *(Th)* for interpretation.

the fifth. This area of the complex is involved with interpretation of impulses that demand motor responses. Motor reflex activities of the face are initiated from this area in a similar manner to the spinal reflex activities in the rest of the body.[38]

Second-order trigeminal neurons project to the thalamus from synaptic junctions with primary afferents in the subnucleus caudalis. As in the dorsal horn, these interneurons represent three types of transmission cells: *(1)* wide dynamic range (WDR) neurons that respond to input from tactile and nociceptive fibers are activated by weak and strong stimuli from both nociceptive and myelinated, low threshold mechanoreceptive (LTM) afferents; *(2)* nociceptive-specific (NS) neurons that respond exclusively to input from thin nociceptive fibers are activated by intense noxious mechanical and thermal stimuli. The WDR and NS neurons predominate in laminae I, II, V, and VI and comprise the trigeminal nociceptive pathways. They all receive input from cutaneous structures, and at least half of them receive input from deep structures of the mouth and face also. *(3)* LTM neurons are normally nonnociceptive and respond to light tactile stimuli. They predominate in laminae III and IV but have been found in all the subdivisions of the trigeminal brain stem complex and have especially been implicated in the relay of touch from the face and mouth. The LTM neurons appear to be excited by strong electrical stimulation of tooth pulps and may be involved in some painful pathologic situations.[21] Dubner[22] showed that pain is signaled by specialized central pathways that are exquisitely sensitive to stimulus features. He concluded that the idea that nociceptive pathways merely provide information about the threat of tissue damage should be discarded.

The trigeminal spinal tract nucleus also receives input from nerves other than the trigeminal. Cranial nerves IX and X as well as the upper cervical nerves supply input to the tract (see Fig 2-6). The importance of these multiple innervations will be discussed in Chapter 4.

Autonomic Nervous System

The visceral nervous system is composed of two divisions, the craniosacral portion, known as the parasympathetics, and the thoracolumbar portion, known as the sympathetics. The afferent elements of these nerves receive interoceptive stimuli that normally do not reach the level of consciousness. Under unusual or abnormal conditions, however, such stimuli may be perceived as pain. The efferent elements of these nerves constitute the *autonomic nervous system,* the activities of which are relatively independent of volition. The craniosacral visceral efferents constitute the *parasympathetic autonomics;* the thoracolumbar visceral efferents constitute the *sympathetic autonomics.*

The autonomic nervous system controls various internal functions that are vital to the individual. The autonomic nervous system helps control arterial blood pressure, gastrointestinal motility and secretion, urinary bladder emptying, sweating, body temperature, and many other activities that are controlled in conjunction with other systems. Most of the functions occur continuously and below conscious level. When stimulated, the autonomic nervous system can respond quickly to change body functions. For example, the heart rate can be doubled in 3 to 5 seconds and the arterial pressure can be doubled in 10 to 15 seconds. On the other extreme, the blood pressure can be lowered enough to cause fainting in 4 to 5 seconds. Sweating can begin within seconds and the bladder may empty involuntarily also within seconds. It is these characteristics that allow the body to respond appropriately to environmental challenges.

Since this text is directed toward orofacial pains, only a brief description of the autonomic nervous system will be presented. It is important, however, that the clinician have a basic understanding of this system since some pain conditions are influenced and may even be maintained by activity of the autonomic nervous system (Chapter 17). Other texts should be consulted for a more thorough review of the autonomic nervous system.

The autonomic nervous system (ANS) is activated mainly by centers located in the spinal cord, brain stem, and hypothalamus. Portions of the cortex and limbic system can also influence ANS activity. The efferent impulses are transmitted to various organs by two major subdivisions called the *sympathetic nervous system* and the *parasympathetic nervous system*.

Sympathetic Nervous System

The sympathetic nerves originate in the spinal cord between segments T-1 and L-2 and pass from here first into the sympathetic chain and from there to the tissues and organs that are stimulated by the sympathetic nerves (Fig 2-8). The sympathetic chain is a chain of ganglia that lies to each side of the spinal column. Each sympathetic

pathway, therefore, is composed of two neurons, a preganglionic neuron and a postganglionic neuron. The cell body of each preganglionic neuron lies in the intermediolateral horn of the spinal cord and its fiber passes through an anterior root of the cord into the corresponding spinal nerve. Immediately after the spinal nerve leaves the spinal column, the preganglionic sympathetic fiber leaves the nerve and passes through the white ramus into one of the ganglia of the sympathetic chain. Once it reaches the ganglia, it may immediately synapse with a postganglionic neuron or it may travel up or down the sympathetic chain to synapse with another postganglionic neuron. The postganglionic neuron then transmits the impulse to the target organ.

Some of the postganglionic neurons pass back from the sympathetic chain into the spinal nerves through gray rami at all levels of the spinal cord. These pathways are made up of type C fibers that extend to all parts of the body in the skeletal nerves. They control the blood vessels, sweat glands, and piloerector muscles of the hairs. Approximately 8% of the fibers in the average skeletal nerve are sympathetic fibers. This is a significant finding when considering muscle pain (see Chapter 12).

Some preganglionic sympathetic neurons pass without synapsing all the way from the intermediolateral horn cells of the spinal cord, through the sympathetic chain, through the splanchnic nerve, and finally into the adrenal medullae. There they end directly on modified neuronal cells that secrete epinephrine and norepinephrine into the blood stream. The importance of these neurochemicals will be discussed in Chapter 3.

Fig 2-8 The sympathetic nervous system. Dashed lines represent postganglionic fibers in the gray rami leading into the spinal nerves for distribution to blood vessels, sweat glands, and piloerector muscles. (From Guyton: Textbook of Medical Physiology, ed 8. Philadelphia: WB Saunders Co; 1991: 668. Used with permission.)

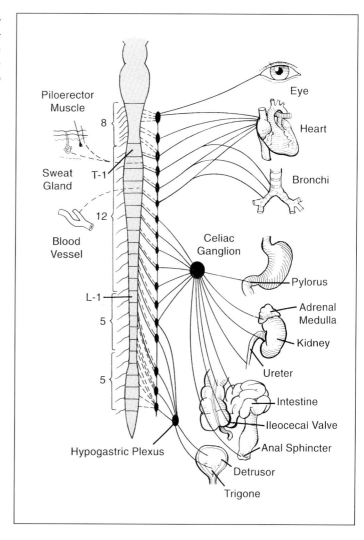

Parasympathetic Nervous System

The parasympathetic nervous system consists of fibers that leave the CNS through cranial nerves III, VII, IX, and X as well as through the second and third sacral spinal nerves and occasionally the first and fourth sacral nerves (Fig 2-9). About 75% of all parasympathetic nerve fibers are in the vagus nerves, passing to the entire thoracic and abdominal regions of the body. In the orofacial region, the parasympathetic nerve fibers travel with the third cranial nerve to the pupillary sphincters and ciliary muscles of the eye. Fibers from the seventh cranial nerve pass to lacrimal, nasal, and submandibular glands, and fibers from the ninth cranial nerve pass to the parotid gland.

Like the sympathetic nervous system, the parasympathetic system also has preganglionic and postganglionic neurons. The dif-

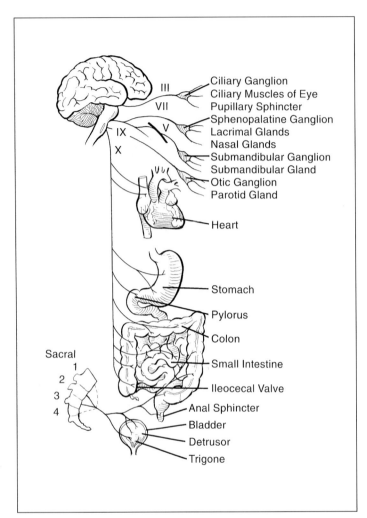

Fig 2-9 The parasympathetic nervous system. (From Guyton: Textbook of Medical Physiology, ed 8. Philadelphia: WB Saunders Co; 1991: 669. Used with permission.)

ference however lies in the location of the synapse. In the parasympathetic nervous system, the preganglionic fiber passes uninterrupted all the way to the organ that is to be controlled. Then in the wall of the organ are located the postganglionic neurons. The preganglionic fibers synapse with these and short postganglionic fibers, 1 mm to several centimeters in length, leave and spread through the substance of the organ.

Functions of the Autonomic Nervous System

As previously mentioned, the function of the autonomic nervous system is to maintain visceral activities of the body. These activities are constantly monitored and when indicated altered to maintain proper function of the body. To maintain this constant influence, both the sympathetic and parasympathetic system remain active at a low level at all times. This base level of activity is called *sympathetic tone or parasympathetic tone.* The value of tone is that it allows a single nervous system to increase or to decrease the activity of a stimulated organ. For example, sympathetic tone normally keeps almost all of the systemic arterioles constricted to approximately half their maximum diameter. By increasing the degree of sympathetic stimulation, these vessels can be constricted even more. On the other hand, by inhibiting the normal tone these same vessels can be dilated. If it were not for this continual sympathetic tone, the sympathetic system could cause only vasoconstriction, never vasodilatation.

The sympathetic nervous system plays a very important role in immediately preparing the individual for environmental challenges. This is commonly called the *fight or flight reaction.* When the individual is physically or emotionally threatened, a mass discharge of the sympathetic nervous system can occur. The results of this discharge permits the person to perform far more strenuous physical activity than would otherwise be possible. This sympathetic mass discharge is characterized by the following changes[39]:

1. Increased arterial pressure
2. Increased blood flow to muscles and away from other organs
3. Increased rates of cellular metabolism throughout the body
4. Increased blood glucose concentration
5. Increased glycolysis in the liver and in muscles
6. Increased muscle strength
7. Increased mental activity
8. Increased rate of blood coagulation

Fig 2-10 Diagrammatic representation of the superficial sensory distribution of the trigeminal nerve: the ophthalmic division (V_1), the maxillary division (V_2), and the mandibular division (V_3).

The importance of this response, especially in its relationship to pain, will be discussed in later chapters.

Peripheral Nociception Pathways

It is important for the clinician to have a sound understanding of the pathways by which nociception can arise. It is the basis for understanding somatic pain. Each of the nerves that innervate the face and oral structures will be reviewed in this section. First afferent or sensory pathways will be discussed (Fig 2-10). Next the efferent or motor pathways will be reviewed (Fig 2-11). Lastly the visceral pathways will be described (Fig 2-12).

Fig 2-11 Diagrammatic representation of the cranial nerves and the structures each subserves. (From Netter FH: The CIBA Collection of Medical Illustrations. Indianapolis: Curtis Publishing Co; 1953. Used with permission.)

Fig 2-12 Diagrammatic representation of the autonomic nerves of the head. (From Netter FH: The CIBA Collection of Medical Illustrations. Indianapolis: Curtis Publishing Co; 1953. Used with permission.)

Afferent (Sensory) Somatic Nerves

Trigeminal Nerve. The chief mediator of somatic sensation from the mouth and face is the fifth cranial nerve, which innervates the face superficially in the region forward of a line drawn vertically from the ears across the top of the head and superior to the level of the lower border of the mandible (Fig 2-10). The ophthalmic division supplies the parietal and frontal areas as well as the upper eyelid and nasal bridge down to the tip of the nose. The maxillary division supplies the anterior portion of the temple, malar, and maxillary areas including the lower eyelid, ala of the nose, and upper lip. The mandibular division supplies the posterior temple, tragus, preauricular area, masseter area, and mandibular region down to the lower border of the mandible, excluding the mandibular angle area. This includes the lower lip and a portion of the auricle and external auditory canal.

The deeper structures of the orofacial region are innervated by branches of the same cranial nerve. The ophthalmic division supplies the orbit and upper part of the nasal cavity. The maxillary division supplies a major portion of the nasal cavity; the palate; the maxillary antrum; the maxillary alveolar process along with the teeth, periodontium, and overlying gingiva; and a small portion of the buccal mucosa in the posterior oral vestibule. The mandibular division supplies sensory innervation to the anterior two-thirds of the tongue; the mandible along with the teeth, periodontium, and overlying gingiva; the mucosa of the floor of the mouth; and most of the oral vestibule. This division also contains proprioceptive sensory fibers that serve the deep sensibility of the mandibular muscles (masseter, temporal, medial pterygoid, lateral pterygoid, mylohyoid, anterior digastric) as well as the tensor muscles of the soft palate and the tympanic membrane. A branch of the mandibular division of the fifth cranial nerve, the auriculotemporal nerve, innervates the temporomandibular joint

Each of the three divisions gives off sensory branches that pass intracranially to supply structures above the tentorium cerebelli.

Facial Nerve. The nervus intermedius contains proprioceptive sensory fibers that serve the deep sensibility of the face except the muscles innervated by the fifth cranial nerve and the 12th cranial nerve. These fibers also serve the deep sensibility of the platysma, stylohyoid, and posterior digastric muscles, which are innervated by the seventh nerve. According to Wolff[40] and Finneson,[41] this nerve contains sensory fibers that supply superficial sensation to the tympanic membrane and part of the external auditory canal.

The facial nerve contains taste fibers to the anterior two thirds of the tongue. These fibers form part of the chorda tympani nerve that is carried in the terminal areas within the sheath of the lingual branch of the trigeminal nerve.

Glossopharyngeal Nerve. Sensory fibers of the ninth cranial nerve innervate the base of the tongue, pharynx, and most of the ear and tympanic membrane. There is considerable overlapping of trigeminal and glossopharyngeal terminal afferent fibers in the throat area so that pain arising from the deeper recesses of the oral cavity may be mediated by either or both nerve trunks. This nerve also contains the taste fibers to the posterior one-third of the tongue. Some intracranial fibers of this nerve mediate sensation below the level of the tentorium cerebelli.

The glossopharyngeal nerve contains proprioceptive sensory fibers that serve the deep sensibility of the pharyngeal area.

Vagus Nerve. Sensory fibers of the tenth cranial nerve innervate the lower part of the pharynx, larynx, posterior part of the external auditory canal, and skin immediately behind the auricle. It also contains taste fibers to the region of the epiglottis.

Cervical Spinal Nerves. The upper three cervical spinal nerves mediate sensory impulses from the superficial structures of the head and face posterior to the trigeminal area and below the lower border of the mandible, including the mandibular angle. This includes most of the auricle as well as the postauricular region except for the skin immediately posterior to the auricle, which is supplied by the vagus nerve. In about 8% of cases, the sensory root of the first cervical nerve is missing.

The upper cervical spinal nerves contain proprioceptive sensory fibers that serve the deep sensibility of the cervical areas except those muscles innervated by other nerves (mylohyoid and anterior digastric by the fifth cranial nerve; platysma, stylohyoid, and posterior digastric by the seventh cranial nerve; tongue muscles by the 12th cranial nerve). Although parts of the sternocleidomastoid and trapezius muscles are innervated by the 11th cranial nerve, actually these fibers arise from the upper cervical segments. These muscles may be considered to be innervated by cervical spinal nerves.

Efferent (Motor) Somatic Nerves

Oculomotor, Trochlear, and Abducent Nerves. The third, fourth, and sixth cranial nerves contain somatic motor fibers to the ocular muscles and to the levator muscle of the upper eyelid.

Trigeminal Nerve. The fifth cranial nerve contains somatic motor fibers that innervate the masseter, temporal, medial pterygoid, lateral pterygoid, mylohyoid, anterior digastric, and the tensor muscles of the soft palate and tympanic membrane. All these motor fibers are part of the mandibular division of this nerve.

Facial Nerve. The seventh cranial nerve contains somatic motor fibers that innervate the muscles of facial expression including the occipitofrontal scalp muscles, the muscles of the auricle, and the platysma. They also supply the stapedius, stylohyoid, and posterior digastric muscles.

Glossopharyngeal Nerve. The ninth cranial nerve contains somatic motor fibers that innervate the stylopharyngeal muscle and along with the vagus supply the constrictor muscles of the pharynx and palatopharyngeal muscle.

Vagus Nerve. The tenth cranial nerve contains somatic motor fibers that innervate musculature of the pharynx and larynx.

Accessory Nerve. The 11th cranial nerve contains somatic motor fibers of both cranial and cervical origin. Those of cranial origin innervate muscles of the larynx and pharynx as branches of the vagus nerve. Those of cervical origin arise from several of

39

the upper cervical segments and innervate parts of the sternocleidomastoid and trapezius muscles.

Hypoglossal Nerve. The 12th cranial nerve contains somatic motor fibers that innervate the intrinsic and extrinsic muscles of the tongue. This nerve also contains motor fibers of cervical origin that innervate some of the hyoid muscles, including the geniohyoid muscle.

Cervical Spinal Nerves. The upper cervical spinal nerves contain somatic motor fibers that supply the cervical and hyoid muscles directly as well as indirectly via the 11th and 12th cranial nerves, as noted earlier. It should be remembered that the mylohyoid and anterior digastric muscles are innervated by the fifth cranial nerve and the platysma, posterior digastric, and stylohyoid muscles by the seventh cranial nerve.

Visceral (Autonomic) Nerves

Sympathetic Nerves

Sympathetic Afferents. The oral and facial structures are supplied with sympathetic visceral afferents[42-44] that are carried within the sheaths of the fifth, seventh, and ninth cranial nerves. All the sympathetic fibers leave these vehicular nerve trunks and pass to the cervical sympathetic chain where they enter the CNS through the sensory roots of the upper thoracic spinal nerves.

Sympathetic Efferents. The dilator of the pupil, the tarsal and orbital muscles, and the salivary glands as well as the blood vessels and skin receive sympathetic autonomic efferents. All sympathetic efferents to the head are postganglionic. The preganglionic fibers are contained within the upper thoracic spinal nerves from which they take leave to join the sympathetic chain at about the level of the stellate ganglion and synapse with the cranial postganglionic fibers in the superior cervical ganglion. These fibers follow the external and internal carotid arteries. Those that follow the internal carotid artery form the internal carotid nerve, which becomes a loose plexus from which fibers join several cranial nerves for terminal distribution to the pupil and orbital muscles as well as to the glands of the nasal cavity, palate, and pharynx. The fibers that follow the external carotid artery supply the smooth muscle of blood vessels and skin as well as the cutaneous glands and large salivary glands.

Parasympathetic Nerves

Parasympathetic Afferents. The oral and facial structures are supplied with parasympathetic visceral afferents that are carried within the trigeminal sheath but exit by way of the sensory roots of the seventh and ninth cranial nerves rather than the fifth. The fibers from the lacrimal, submandibular, and sublingual glands leave the fifth nerve and join with the seventh, whereas those from the parotid gland leave the fifth and join with the ninth.

Parasympathetic Efferents. The sphincter of the pupil, the ciliary muscle of accommodation, the lacrimal gland, and all the salivary glands receive parasympathetic autonomic efferent fibers that are incorporated in the oculomotor, facial, and glossopharyngeal nerves. The preganglionic fibers in the oculomotor nerve leave it to synapse with post-ganglionic fibers in the ciliary ganglion and henceforth are contained within the trigeminal sheath to supply the sphincter of the pupil and the ciliary muscle. The preganglionic fibers in the facial nerve leave it to synapse with postganglionic fibers in the pterygopalatine and submandibular ganglia and henceforth are contained within the trigeminal sheath. Those from the pterygopalatine ganglion supply the lacrimal gland, and those from the submandibular ganglion supply the submandibular and sublingual glands. The preganglionic fibers in the glossopharyngeal nerve leave it to synapse with postganglionic fibers in the otic ganglion and henceforth are contained within the trigeminal sheath to supply the parotid gland. None of the parasympathetic efferents of the vagus nerve supply structures in the masticatory area.

General Considerations of Peripheral Nociceptive Pathways

An understanding of the neural system involved in the sensory and motor innervation of structures of the mouth and face is essential to the effective management of nociceptive activity in that region. A somewhat wider area than just the face, however, is implicated in masticatory function.

Pains arising from peripheral sources are mediated by anatomic structures of the nervous system, namely, sensory receptors and primary sensory neurons. These structures constitute the peripheral pain pathways. In the light of currently held concepts regarding the mechanisms of pain, the clinician should be well informed concerning all the sensory pathways that exist. The brain is constantly receiving an enormous amount of sensory input initiated by stimulation of sensory receptors of all types: exteroceptive, proprioceptive, and interoceptive. Of this volume, only a fraction is ordinarily perceived at conscious levels. Most of this ongoing sensory input is for regulatory purposes to control automatic body functioning. Formerly, the significance of such sensation in pain processes appears not to have been fully appreciated. It is important to be aware of the various routes by which such sensation is conducted. This includes both somatic and visceral pathways that have just been reviewed.

Dentists traditionally have received excellent instruction concerning the trigeminal pathways, which are of great significance in oral and facial pain complaints. Unfortunately the impression is sometimes gained that the trigeminal pathways are exclusively responsible for the mediation of painful sensation from this region. This impression is a fundamental error and may account for some of the confusion that exists in the clinical management of pain complaints. For example, it is a common notion that surgical interruption of the posterior root of the trigeminal nerve will assuredly arrest oral and facial pain, and great consternation may follow the failure of such an operation to be effective.

It should be noted that the oral and masticatory region is innervated by at least six major sensory somatic nerve trunks other than the trigeminal, namely, the seventh, ninth, and tenth cranial nerves and the first, second, and third cervical spinal nerves. It should also be well understood that the visceral nerves actively participate in the mediation of painful sensations. It has been established that all sympathetic afferents and at least the sacral parasympathetic afferents mediate pain at conscious levels.[45] Hannington-Kiff[46] strongly believed that cranial parasympathetic afferent fibers mediate pain, especially that of neurovascular disorders. An understanding of the anatomy of these pathways is important in the management of oral and facial pains. Vast numbers of impulses are conducted to the CNS by afferent visceral nerves. Such ongoing sensory input is normally below conscious levels.

It should be noted that all cranial parasympathetics, although carried in the sheaths of trigeminal branches for peripheral distribution, leave the trigeminal before entering the CNS, and none of them passes through the posterior root of the fifth cranial nerve. The parasympathetic afferents in the trigeminal region enter the CNS by way of the seventh and ninth cranial nerves. It should also be noted that all sympathetic afferents of the head regions, although carried in the sheaths of various cranial nerves including the trigeminal for peripheral distribution, leave these cranial nerves and join the cervical portion of the sympathetic chain and finally enter the spinal cord by way of the posterior roots of the upper thoracic spinal nerves.

It has long been known that the afferent as well as the efferent limb of the myotatic reflex is mediated by motor nerves.[47] Since there is ample evidence of the presence of many afferent fibers in the trigeminal motor root, the motor nerves should be included among nociceptive pathways. It is quite certain that motor nerves mediate normal sensory impulses from the skeletal musculature. This phenomenon may explain why noxious stimulation of motor trunks elicits deep somatic pain felt diffusely in the muscles innervated by those nerves.[48]

It should be evident that painful sensations from the mouth and face can be mediated by many pathways other than the familiar trigeminal route. For this reason, pain from the facial region may not necessarily be arrested by division of the trigeminal sensory root. Such an operation would not affect the mediation of nociceptive sensation conducted by afferents of the seventh, ninth, and tenth cranial nerves or the first, second, and third cervical nerves; afferent neurons carried by motor elements of the trigeminal as well as other cranial and upper cervical nerves; and afferent visceral nerves of the sympathetic and parasympathetic systems.

With this review it becomes obvious that the peripheral nociceptive input from the orofacial structures follows no simple pathway. This complexity certainly adds to the challenge for the clinician.

References

1. Kramer HS, Schmidt WH. Regional anesthesia of the maxillofacial region, in Alling CC, Mahan PE (eds): Facial Pain, ed 2. Philadelphia: Lea & Febiger; 1977: 237–256.

2. Kerr FWL. Fine structure and functional characteristics of the primary trigeminal neuron. In Hassler R, Walker AE (eds): Trigeminal Neuralgia. Stuttgart: Georg Thieme Verlag; 1970: 11–21.

3. Gardner WJ. Trigeminal neuralgia. In Hassler R, Walker AE (eds): Trigeminal Neuralgia. Stuttgart: Georg Thieme Verlag; 1970: 153–174.

4. Guyton, AC. Textbook of Medical Physiology, ed 8. Philadelphia: WB Saunders; 1991: 507.

5. Okeson JP. Managment of Temporomandibular Disorders and Occlusion, ed 3. St Louis: Mosby-YearBook; 1993: 37–38.

6. Widmer CG. Jaw opening reflex activity in the inferior head of the lateral pterygoid muscle in man. Arch Oral Biol 1987; 32:135.

7. Bechtol CO. Muscle physiology. In The American Academy of Orthopedic Surgical Instructional Course Lectures, vol 5. St Louis: CV Mosby; 1948.

8. Feilds HL. Pain. New York: McGraw-Hill; 1987: 26–28.

9. Miller MR. Pain. Morphologic aspects. In Way EL (ed): New Concepts in Pain. Philadelphia: FA Davis; 1967: 7–12.

10. Clark D, Hughes J, Gasser HS. Afferent function in the group of nerves of slowest conduction velocity. Am J Physiol 1935; 114:69–76.

11. Gasser HS, Erlanger J. The role played by sizes of constituent fibers of a nerve trunk in determining the form of its action potential wave. Am J Physiol 1927; 80:522–547.

12. Gasser HS. Conduction in nerves and relation to fiber types. Assoc Res Nerv Dis Proc 1934; 15:35.

13. Guyton, AC. Textbook of Medical Physiology, ed 8. Philadelphia: WB Saunders; 1991: 499.

14. Hallin RG, Wiesenfeld Z, Persson A. Do large diameter cutaneous afferents have a role in the transmission of nociceptive information? Pain 1981; 11(suppl 1):90.

15. Bishop GH. Neural mechanism of cutaneous nerves. Physiol Rev 1946; 26:77–102.

16. Bishop GH. The relationship between nerve fiber size and sensory modality: Phylogenetic implications of the afferent innervation of cortex. J Nerv Ment Dis 1959; 128:89–114.

17. Bishop GH. Fiber size and myelinization in afferent systems. In Knighton RS, Dumke PR (eds): Pain. Boston: Little, Brown; 1966: 83–89.

18. Lele PP, Weddell G. The relationship between neurohistology and coronal sensibility. Brain 1956; 79:119–154.

19. Collins WF, Nulsen FE, Shealy CN. Electrophysiological studies of peripheral and central pathways conducting pain. In Knighton RS, Dumke PR (eds): Pain. Boston: Little, Brown; 1966: 33–45.

20. Ochoa JL, Torebjork HE. Pain from skin and muscle. Pain 1981; 11(suppl 1):87.

21. Sessle BJ. The neurobiology of facial and dental pain: Present knowledge, future directions. J Dent Res 1987; 66:962–981.

22. Dubner R. Specialization of nociceptive pathways: Sensory discrimination, sensory modulation, and neural connectivity. In Fields HL, Dubner R, Cervero F (eds): Advances in Pain Research and Therapy, vol 9. New York: Raven Press; 1985: 111–137.

23. Sessle BJ, Hu JW. Mechanisms of pain arising from articular tissues. Can J Physiol Pharmacol 1991; 69:617–626.

24. Fields HL. Pain. Hightstown, NJ: McGraw-Hill; 1987: 41–78.

25. Rexed B. Cytoarchitectonic atlas of the spinal cord in the cat. J Comp Neurol 1954; 297–379.

26. Gobel S. Neural circuitry in the substantia gelatinosa of Rolands: Anatomical insights. In Bonica JJ, Liebeskind JC, Albe–Fessard DG (eds): Advances in Pain Research and Therapy, vol 3. New York: Raven Press; 1979: 175–195.

27. Kerr FWL. Neuroanatomical substrates of nociception in the spinal cord. Pain 1975; 1:325–326.

28. Dubner R, Bennett GJ. Spinal and trigeminal mechanisms of nociception. Annu Rev Neurosci 1983; 6:381–418.

29. Wall PD. The dorsal horn. In Wall PD, Melzack R (eds): Textbook of Pain. London: Churchill–Livingstone; 1984: 80–87.

30. Guyton, AC. Textbook of Medical Physiology, cd 8. Philadelphia: WB Saunders; 1991: 509.

31. Thibodeau GA. Anatomy and Physiology. St Louis: Times Mirror/Mosby College Publications; 1987: 327.

32. deLaat A. Reflexes excitable in the jaw muscles and their role during jaw function and dysfunction: A review of the literature. Part II. Central connections of orofacial afferent fibers. J Craniomand Pract 1987; 5:247–253.

33. Dubner R, Sessle BJ, Storey AT. The Neural Basis of Oral and Facial Function. New York: Plenum Press; 1978.

34. Gobel S, Hockfield S, Ruda MA. Anatomical similarities between medullary and spinal dorsal horns. In Kawamura Y, Dubner R (eds): Oral-facial sensory and motor functions. Tokyo: Quintessence; 1981: 211–223.

35. Hu JW, Dostrovsky JO, Sessle BJ. Functional properties of neurons in subnucleus caudalis of the cat. I. Responses to oral–facial noxious stimuli and projections to thalamus and subnucleus oralis. J Neurophysiol 1981, 45:173–192.

36. Henry JL, Sessle BJ, Lucier GE, et al. Effects of substance P on nociceptive and nonnociceptive trigeminal brain stem neurons. Pain 1980; 8:33–45.

37. Shigenaga Y, Nakatani J. Distribution of trigeminothalamic projection cells in the caudal medulla of the cat. In Matthew B, Hill RG (eds): Anatomical, Physiological and Pharmacological Aspects of Trigeminal Pain. Amsterdam: Elsevier Biomedical; 1982: 163–174.

38. Lund JP, Donga R, Widmer CG, Stohler CS. The pain-adaptation model: a discussion of the relationship between chronic musculoskeletal pain and motor activity. Can J Physiol 1991; 69:683–694.

39. Guyton AC. Basic Neuroscience: Anatomy and Physiology, ed 2. Philadelphia: WB Saunders; 1992: 282.

40. Wolff HG. Headache and Other Head Pain, ed 2. New York: Oxford University Press; 1963:555–556.

41. Finneson BE. Diagnosis and Management of Pain Syndromes, ed 2. Philadelphia: WB Saunders; 1969.

42. Procacci P, Maresca M. Reflex sympathetic dystrophies and algodystrophies: Historical and pathogenic considerations. Pain 1987; 31:137–140.

43. Paintal AS. The visceral sensations: Some basic mechanisms. In Cervero F, Morrison JFB (eds): Progress in Brain Research, vol 67. Amsterdam: Elsevier Biomedical; 1986: 3–19.

44. Wildicombe JG. Sensory innervation of the lungs and airways. In Cervero F, Morrison JFB (eds): Progress in Brain Research, vol 67. Amsterdam: Elsevier Biomedical; 1986: 49–64.

45. Wolff HG, Wolf S. Pain, ed 2. Springfield, Ill: Charles C Thomas; 1958.

46. Hannington–Kiff JG. Pain Relief. Philadelphia: JB Lippincott; 1974:58–79.

47. McIntyre AK. Afferent limb of the myotatic reflex arc. Nature 1951; 168:168–169.

48. Cailliet R. Neck and Arm Pain. Philadelphia: FA Davis; 1964:1–39.

3 | The Neurophysiology of Orofacial Pain

Now that the anatomy of the central nervous system has been reviewed, the manner by which neural impulses are transferred from one neuron to another will be discussed. This chapter will outline the actual mechanisms that allow for the transfer of impulses from the peripheral sensory receptor into the central nervous system and back out again to receptor organs for appropriate action.

Nerve Action Potential

As discussed in Chapter 2, the neuron is made up of the cell body, the dendrites, and the axon. The *cell body* provides nutrients to the cell. The *dendrites* are multiple branching outgrowths from the cell body that are the main receptors for the neuron. The dendrites provide for communication between adjacent neurons. The *axon* is a single fiber that leaves the cell body to communicate with another neuron at a distant site. The axon is also called the *nerve fiber* and may extend from a few millimeters to as long as a meter. Impulses are carried from the dendrites down the axon by way of an

action potential. The surface of the cell membrane is slightly negatively charged. An action potential begins with a sudden change from the normal resting negative potential to a positive membrane potential and then ends with an almost equally rapid change back to the negative potential. The action potential moves down the cell membrane until it reaches the end of the axon.

The resting state of the cell membrane is said to be *polarized* with a slight negative charge. When the membrane becomes depolarized, there is a sudden permeability to sodium ions, allowing tremendous numbers of sodium ions to flow into the interior of the axon. Within a few 10,000ths of a second after the membrane becomes highly permeable to sodium ions, the sodium channels begin to close, and the potassium channels open more than normally. Then, rapid diffusion of potassium ions to the exterior reestablishes the normal negative resting membrane potential. This is called *repolarization* of the membrane. The depolarization and repolarization of the membrane is dependent on these voltage-gated sodium and potassium channels.

Synapse

Nerve signals are transmitted from one neuron to the next through interneuronal junctions called *synapses*. Synapses occur between different neurons predominantly through contact with the dendrites. There are as many as 100,000 small knobs called *presynaptic terminals* that lie on the surfaces of the dendrites and some on the soma of the neuron. It is thought that in some parts of the brain a single neuron may have synaptic terminals numbering as many as 400,000.[1]

Impulses that cross these synapses create an action potential that is carried down to the terminal end of the axon to synapse with another neuron. Each presynaptic terminal is separated from its adjacent neuron by a small distance called the *synaptic cleft*. The synaptic clefts range from 200 to 300 Å.

Humans have two types of synapses; the chemical synapse and the electrical synapse. Electrical synapses are found in some smooth and cardiac muscles and will not be discussed here. Almost all of the synapses in the central nervous system are chemical.

Within the presynaptic terminals are two important structures; the *synaptic vesicles* and the *mitochondria* (Fig 3-1). The synaptic vesicles contain transmitter substances that when released into the synaptic cleft either excite or inhibit the postsynaptic neuron. In a similar sense the postsynaptic neural membrane has both excitatory and inhibitory receptors. Therefore, if an excitatory transmitter is released in the presence of an excitatory receptor the neuron is excited. If an inhibitory transmitter is released in the presence of inhibitory receptors, the neural activity is inhibited.

The second important structure in the terminal of the neuron is the mitochondrion. The mitochondria provide the adenosine triphosphate (ATP) required to synthesize new transmitter substances.

The synaptic membrane of the presynaptic terminals contain large numbers of *voltage-gated calcium channels*. This is quite different from the other areas of the nerve fiber, which only contain a few of these channels. When the action potential depolarizes the terminal, large numbers of calcium ions, along with the sodium ions that cause most of the action potential, flow into the terminal. The quantity of transmitter substance that is released into the synaptic cleft is directly related to the number of calcium ions that enter the terminal.

At the synapse, the membrane of the postsynaptic neuron contains large numbers of receptor proteins (see Fig 3-1). These *receptor proteins* project out into the synaptic cleft as well as extend into the interior of the postsynaptic neuron. The portion that protrudes into the cleft acts as a binding area for the released neurotransmitters. The portion that extends into the neuron is called the ionophore component and carries neurotransmitters into the neuron that can influence cell activity. The ionophore receptor is one of two types; a chemically activated ion channel or an enzyme that activates an internal metabolic change inside the cell.

The *ion channel* receptors are of three types according to the ions that are involved: sodium, potassium, and chloride. Neurotransmitters that open the sodium channels are generally excitatory transmitters. On the other hand, opening the potassium and chloride channels inhibits the neuron; they are therefore inhibitory transmitters.

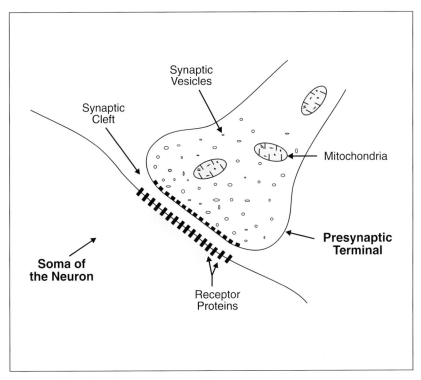

Fig 3-1   The physiologic anatomy of the synapse.

The *enzyme receptors*, when activated, cause changes to occur in the metabolism of the postsynaptic neuron. Stimulation of the enzyme receptors can activate cellular genes which in turn manufacture additional receptors for the postsynaptic membrane. The enzyme receptors can also activate protein kinases, which decrease the number of receptors. Changes such as these can alter the reactivity of the synapse for minutes, days, months, or even years. Transmitters that cause these types of changes in neuron response are called *modulators*. The importance of this feature will be discussed in future chapters.

Neurotransmitters

The neurochemicals that transmit impulses across the synaptic cleft are called *neurotransmitters*. Neurotransmitters are either small rapid-acting molecules or larger slower-acting molecules. The smaller rapidly acting transmitters are the ones that cause most of the acute responses of the nervous system, such as transmission of sensory signals to and inside the brain and motor signals back to the muscles. These larger molecules are the neuropeptides and represent a different group of chemicals. These are not manufactured in the presynaptic terminal but instead in the ribosomes of the neuronal body. The neuropeptides are then transported to the synapse for release

47

in the cleft. These neurotransmitters are much slower acting then the smaller molecules but, when released, have a much longer effect on the postsynaptic neuron.

Rapid-Acting (Small Molecule) Neurotransmitters

Some of the more common small molecule neurotransmitters are listed here with their common locations and effects on the postsynaptic neurons.

Acetylcholine. Acetylcholine is one of the most common neurotransmitters found in the human. It is secreted by neurons in many areas of the brain but specifically by the motor cortex, the basal ganglia, and by the motor neurons that innervate the skeletal muscles. It is also secreted by the preganglionic neurons of the autonomic nervous system, the postganglionic neurons of the parasympathetic nervous system, and by some of the postganglionic neurons of the sympathetic nervous system. In almost all instances, acetylcholine has an excitatory effect on the postsynaptic neuron.

Norepinephrine. Norepinephrine is secreted by many neurons whose cell bodies are in the brain stem and hypothalamus. The highest concentration of norepinephrine-secreting neurons is found in the locus ceruleus of the pons. From this region, these norepinephrine-producing neurons extend to many other regions of the brain and brain stem to influence the overall activity and mood of the mind. Norepinephrine is almost always an excitatory neurotransmitter.

Glutamate. Glutamate is an amino acid that is secreted by the presynaptic terminals in many of the sensory pathways as well as in many areas of the cortex. It has been found in the spinal cord dorsal horn associated with noxious input.[2,3] It is thought to always cause excitation.

Aspartate. Like glutamate, aspartate is an amino acid that is secreted by the presynaptic terminals of many of the sensory pathways in the dorsal horn. It is thought to always cause excitation.

Serotonin. Serotonin is secreted by nuclei that originate in the median raphe of the brain stem and project to many areas of the brain and down into the spinal dorsal horn. Serotonin is a monoamine released by blood platelets. It is synthesized in the central nervous system (CNS) from L-tryptophan, a dietary essential amino acid.[4] It is released when the nucleus raphe magnus in the brain stem is stimulated by sensory input.[5] Peripherally, serotonin is an algogenic agent[6] and is thought to relate especially to vascular pain syndromes (see Chapter 16). In the CNS, serotonin is an important chemical in the endogenous antinociceptive mechanism.[7] Central serotonin is thought to potentiate endorphin analgesia.[4] It reduces stimulation-evoked excitation of nociceptive dorsal horn interneurons.[8] The activation of serotoninergic pathways in the brain stem by tricyclic antidepressants yields paralleling analgesic effects along with its action on depressive states.[9] Descending serotoninergic and norepinephrinergic neurons in the dorsal horn suggest that they provide global suppression or enhancement that enables nociceptive pathways to respond more effectively to incoming sensory information.[10]

Gamma-aminobutyric Acid. Gamma-aminobutyric acid (GABA) is secreted by neurons in the spinal cord, cerebellum, basal ganglia, and parts of the cortex. It is believed to always have an inhibitory effect on the postsynaptic neuron.

Glycine. Glycine is secreted in many areas of the spinal cord and likely to also be secreted in the trigeminal spinal nucleus. It is probably always an inhibitory transmitter.

Dopamine. Dopamine is secreted by neurons that originate in the substantia nigra and extend into the basal ganglia. The normal effect of dopamine is inhibitory.

Histamine. Histamine is a vasoactive amine that derives from the amino acid histadine. Although histamine serves as a neurotransmitter in the CNS, it is probably best know as a vasodilator and its action to increase small-vessel permeability. It also causes contraction of smooth muscle in the lung.

Slow-Acting (Large Molecule) Neurotransmitters

The large molecule neurotransmitters are the neuropeptides. The following is a short description of a few of the important neuropeptides that serve as neurotransmitters.

Substance P. Substance P is a polypeptide composed of 11 amino acids. It is released at the central terminals of primary nociceptive neurons and acts as a transport substance, being found at the distal terminals as well.[11] Centrally, it acts as an excitatory neurotransmitter for nociceptive impulses.[12,13] It is released from spinal cord cells by the stimulation of A-delta and C fiber afferents and excites neurons in the dorsal horn that are activated by noxious stimuli.[14] Its modulating action on pain is both rapid and short-lived.[15] Substance P released from unmyelinated afferents is involved in neurogenic inflammatory phenomena such as cutaneous wheal formation and the hyperemia of reflex axon flare. It is known that the substance P content is highest in the most severely inflamed joints. When injected into a joint, substance P increases both the inflammation and the destructive change that occurs.[16]

Endorphins. The endorphins are polypeptides (chains of amino acids). They are identical to portions of the pituitary hormone beta-lipotropin, which consists of 91 amino acids.[17–19] They behave like morphine and bind to morphine receptors to obtund pain. Like morphine, they are displaced from these receptors by the morphine antagonist naloxone. Repeated injections of enkephalin and beta-endorphin will cause tolerance and physical dependence.[20]

The short-chain enkephalins appear to act chiefly in the cerebrospinal fluid. They have a short, rapid action and serve especially to limit the experience of excessive, sudden pain more than as an analgesic. The longer-chain beta-endorphin appears to be closely related to pituitary function and may act somewhat like a hormone. It is longer lasting, requires the passage of a latent period before it becomes active, and has high antinociceptive potency.[20–22] Evidence exists that the endogenous opiates may act more as neuromodulators of postsynaptic activity than as classic neurotransmitters.[19,23] It has been shown that endorphins are important contributors to pain threshold and pain tolerance.[24] There is considerable interneurotransmitter action associated with the antinociceptive system (see Chapter 4). For example, endorphin is potentiated by serotonin that is released from serotoninergic neurons only in the presence of dopamine, while norepinephrine exerts a deterrent effect.[25,26] It should be noted that Kosterlitz[27] remarked, "While it has been shown in many laboratories that the enkephalins and endorphins have antinociceptive effects, the underlying mechanisms have not been fully analyzed, and, in particular, the conditions controlling the release of opioid peptides are still not understood."

It should be noted that beta-endorphin is appreciably released in long-distance runners.[28] It is also significant that placebo analgesia is endorphin-mediated and naloxone-reversible.[29,30] Analgesia produced by hypnosis, however, is not reversed by naloxone.[31,32] Hypnoanalgesia no doubt is based on other mechanisms.

Bradykinin. Bradykinin is an endogenous polypeptide consisting of a chain of nine amino acids. Released as part of an inflammatory reaction, it is a powerful vasodilator and causes increased capillary permeability. With few exceptions, bradykinin acts as an algogenic agent that excites all types of receptors. It sensitizes some high threshold receptors so that they respond to otherwise innocuous stimuli such as those that occur during normal activities.[33] Bradykinin requires the presence of prostaglandins to act.[34] It is also released during ischemic episodes.[35]

Elimination of the Transmitter from the Synapse

Once the transmitter has been released into the synapse, a mechanism must be present to remove the transmitter. If this does not occur, the transmitter's effect on the postsynaptic neuron is prolonged. In most instances the transmitter is immediately removed, which enables the postsynaptic neuron to return to its normal membrane resting potential. The elimination of the neurotransmitter can occur by one of three methods: diffusion, enzymatic destruction, or re-uptake.

In some instances a released neurotransmitter will merely diffuse out of the synaptic cleft. As the transmitter leaves the synapse, its effect on the postsynaptic neuron is eliminated. This processes is called *diffusion*.

Some neurotransmitters are immediately destroyed by enzymes that are either released or are already present in the synaptic cleft. This process of eliminating the transmitter is called *enzymatic destruction*. For example, when acetylcholine is released, the enzyme cholinesterase is present in the cleft, bound in the proteoglycan matrix that fills the space. This enzyme can very rapidly split the acetylcholine, rendering it immediately inactive.

A third method of eliminating the neurotransmitter from the synapse is by *neurotransmitter re-uptake*. Some neurotransmitters are actively transported back into the presynaptic terminal itself for reuse. This occurs in the presynaptic terminals of the sympathetic nervous system with the re-uptake of norepinephrine.

Neurochemistry of Nociception

The peripheral nociceptor can be activated by thermal, mechanical, and chemical stimulation. When thermal and mechanical stimulation produce nociceptive input, the reason for the pain is usually apparent. Chemical stimulation of the nociceptor, on the other hand, may be less apparent to the sufferer. In fact, once the mechanical or thermal stimulation has terminated, the reason for continued nociceptive input is likely to be neurochemical. There are a variety of compounds that can accumulate near the nociceptor following tissue injury that can be responsible for maintaining nociceptive input. There are at least three sources of these compounds: the damaged cells themselves, secondary to plasma extravasation and lymphocyte migration, or the nociceptor itself.

Damage to tissue cells produces leakage of intracellular contents. Among the substances released by tissue damage are potassium and histamine, both of which either activate or sensitize the nociceptor.[36] These substances have been documented to excite polymodal nociceptors and produce pain when injected into skin.[37,38] Other compounds such as acetylcholine, serotonin, and ATP may be released by tissue damage and are known to either activate or sensitize nociceptors. In fact, there is evidence that several of these compounds can act in combination to sensitize nociceptors.[39]

One of the most potent pain-producing substances that appears in injured tissue is bradykinin. Polymodal nociceptors can be activated by bradykinin[40] and they then can become sensitized to thermal stimuli.

Another group of compounds that are synthesized in the regions of tissue damage are the metabolic products of arachidonic acid. These compounds are considered inflammatory mediators and include both prostaglandins and leukotrienes. These compounds appear whenever animal cells are damaged and are present in increased concentration in inflammatory exudates. The prostaglandins are a group of chemically related long-chain hydroxy fatty acids. There are six types, each designated by a suffix letter. Subscript numerals indicate the degree of saturation of the side chain. Prostaglandin E_2 is metabolized from arachidonic acid through the action of cyclo-oxygenase. This occurs in conjunction with an inflammatory process.

Prostaglandins do not seem to be algogenic substances per se. They sensitize nociceptive nerve endings to different types of stimuli, thus lowering their pain thresholds to all kinds of stimulation.[41] Prostaglandins are required for bradykinin to act[34]; bradykinin in turn stimulates the release of prostaglandins.[42] The two therefore are mutually potentiating. Prostaglandin E also increases the response of slowly adapting A-delta mechanoreceptors to nonnoxious stimuli.[43] There is evidence that a prostaglandin-like substance is released in the CNS during an inflammatory reaction that induces prostaglandin hyperalgesia.[44]

Another important metabolic pathway of arachidonic acid is the lipoxygenase pathway, which produces the leukotrienes. Leukotrienes produce hyperalgesia in animal models and in humans.[45] The hyperalgesia produced by leukotriene B_4 is not blocked by cyclo-oxygenase inhibitors but is blocked by depletion of polymorphonuclear leukocytes.[46] This may suggest that leukocytes contribute to nociceptor activation but this is yet to be documented.

In addition to the chemical mediators that are released from damaged cells or synthesized in the region of damage, the nociceptors themselves can release substances that enhance nociception. One such substance is substance P. Unmyelinated primary afferent neurons seem to produce substance P and, when stimulated, can release this potent excitatory neurotransmitter into the extracellular space.[47] Substance P is a very strong vasodilator and produces edema. Substance P also causes release of histamine from mast cells, which is an excitatory neurotransmitter and also causes vasodilation and edema.[48]

Neuronal Sensitization

When excitatory neurotransmitters are released in the synaptic cleft, the postsynaptic neuron is excited and an impulse is started and carried down the axon. If excitatory neurochemicals remain in the region of the synapse, the neuron can be depolarized quicker with the next release of a neurotransmitter. This process is called *sensitization*. Sensitization is the result of a lowering of the threshold that causes the depolarization of the primary afferent neuron. It is one explanation for the hyperalgesic state that is commonly associated with inflammatory tissues. For example, several hours after a small cut, the individual will develop a region around the injured tissue that is quite sensitive to even light touch. This increased sensitivity of local tissues is due to the neurochemicals that sensitize nearby primary afferent neurons so that even light mechanical stimulation creates depolarization and nociceptive input. This type of sensitization is called peripheral sensitization. As will be discussed, sensitization of neurons can also occur within the central nervous system.

Axon Transport System

The nerve cell body (soma) of the primary trigeminal neuron located in the gasserian ganglion produces peptides and proteins that are moved to the central terminal by an *axon transport system* thought to be via microtubules or microfilaments in the axon. The velocity of this transport system does not seem to vary appreciably between myelinated and nonmyelinated fibers. Some transport substances likely serve as primary afferent neurotransmitters and therefore are essential to the transmission of pain information. The axon transport system is probably involved in this complex neurochemical process. Substance P is thought to be one neurotransmitter released at the central terminal of nociceptive primary neurons. This substance is found also at the distal terminals, having reached there no doubt by way of the axon transport system.[11] Thus, sensory information may be signaled very rapidly to the CNS by transmission of nerve impulses or more slowly by way of neurochemical substances conducted through the axon transport system.[49]

There is evidence that the axon transport system can move neurotransmitters in the primary afferent neurons both centrally (*orthodromically,* in the normal direction of impulses) as well as peripherally (*antidromically,* in the opposite direction of normal impulses). Antidromic activity of the primary afferent neuron results in the release of neurotransmitters into the peripheral terminals, leading to sensitization of other neurons in the adjacent area. This process is called *neurogenic inflammation.* Neurogenic inflammation not only results in peripheral sensitization (hyperalgesia) but can also cause local vasodilation and edema. Local vasodilation caused by neurogenic inflammation is called *flare,* while local edema is called *wheal.*

The sympathetic efferents may also produce neurogenic inflammation as indicated by the fact that sympathetic blockade reduces the inflammation of reflex sympathetic dystrophy as well as that of inflammatory arthritis.[16]

Transmission of Afferent Impulses to the Cortex

When a peripheral nociceptor is stimulated, a series of events occur that carry that impulse into the CNS and to the higher centers for interpretation and evaluation. If the impulse has significance, the higher centers may pass it to the cortex where it is then perceived as pain. This series of events is by no means simple. In fact most of the impulses that enter the CNS never reach the cortex. To better understand orofacial pains we will now follow the pathway of a nociceptive impulse from the peripheral receptor to the cortex.

It would be easy to believe that orofacial nociception begins with a trigeminal nerve pathway. Although this is commonly true, it is only one of many pathways that carry orofacial nociception to the brain. Nociceptive impulses from the face and mouth may be mediated centrally by way of afferent primary neurons that pass through the fifth, seventh, ninth, and tenth cranial nerves as well as the first, second, and third

cervical spinal nerves and by way of visceral afferents that descend through the cervical sympathetic chain to pass through the posterior roots of the upper thoracic spinal nerves. The nerve cell bodies of the primary sensory neurons are located in the posterior root ganglion of the nerve through which they pass, except for the proprioceptive fibers of the fifth cranial nerve, which are located in the mesencephalic nucleus in the midbrain.[50]

To simplify our discussion, we will only discuss the pathway of a single trigeminal primary afferent neuron; for example, coming from the pulp of a mandibular molar. Once the nociceptor located in the pulp is activated, the impulse is carried into the central nervous system by a primary afferent neuron in the mandibular branch of the fifth cranial nerve (Fig 3-2). The cell body of this neuron is located in the gasserian or trigeminal ganglion. This primary afferent neuron enters the brain stem and synapses with a second-order neuron in the subnucleus caudalis of the trigeminal spinal tract nucleus. Although the subnucleus caudalis has been well implemented as the primary location of nociceptive input for the face, recent information suggests that the subnucleus oralis may play an important role in nociception of the intraoral structures.[51] For this discussion, I will continue to use the subnucleus caudalis. The primary neuron will synapse in this subnucleus with one of the three types of second-order neurons. Since this discussion concerns nociception, let us assume the second-order neuron is a nociceptive-specific (NS) neuron. This NS neuron will then be activated and the impulse will be carried to the higher centers by this second-order neuron. In some instances, the neuron may carry the impulse

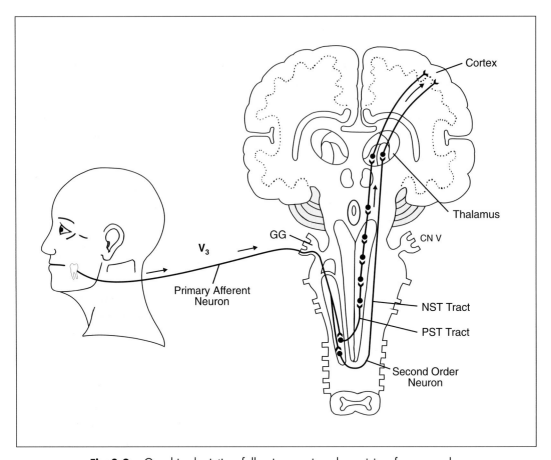

Fig 3-2 Graphic depiction following an impulse arising from a molar to interpretation in the higher centers. The impulse is carried by the primary afferent neuron of the mandibular division of the trigeminal nerve (V₃) through the gasserian ganglion (GG) into the subnucleus caudalis region of the trigeminal spinal tract. At that point, it synapses with a second-order neuron to be transferred to the higher centers for evaluation. If the input is carried by an A-delta fiber it may synapse with a wide dynamic range neuron and be carried to the higher centers by way of the neospinothalamic tract (NST Tract). This input is carried quickly to the higher centers and is therefore referred to as fast pain. If the primary afferent input is carried by a C fiber, it may synapse with a nociceptive specific neuron and be carried up the paleospinothalamic tract (PST Tract). This tract passes through the reticular formation and may therefore be influenced by many modulating interneurons. Nociception carried on this tract is called slow pain.

directly higher on the same side of the brain (see Chapter 2). This is not usually the case with nociception. In most instances, the NS neuron will cross the brain stem and ascend in the anterolateral tract on the opposite side. At this point nociceptive input can be carried by one of two tracts. Nociceptive impulses that have been carried by the faster A-delta primary fibers synapse mainly in lamina I of the subnucleus caudalis. These NS neurons carry these impulses by way of the *neospinothalamic tract* directly to the thalamus. These fibers are mainly carrying mechanical and thermal pain. Since this pathway ascends directly to the thalamus, it is said to carry *fast pain.*

Nociceptive impulses carried by primary afferent C fibers synapse in laminae II, III (substantia gelatinosa), and V. The NS neurons that synapse with these fibers carry impulses by way of the *paleospinothalamic tract.* This tract does not ascend directly to the thalamus but instead projects numerous interneurons into the reticular formation of the brain stem. The impulses are then carried by way of many interneurons through the reticular formation to the thalamus. The nociceptive impulse therefore can be changed or *modulated* by the reticular formation before it ascends to the thalamus. Since the impulse takes longer to reach the thalamus, this type of pain is called *slow pain.*

There are significant functional differences between fast pain and slow pain. The fast pain can be easily localized as to the exact location of its origin. It is likely to be perceived by the individual as sharp pain. It is important that the individual quickly perceive this pain and react in an appropriate manner. Slow pain, in contrast, is much more difficult to locate and is felt as a deep,

dull, aching sensation. This type of pain is likely to be responsible for suffering. Since this type of nociception is thought to be primarily carried by C fibers, substance P is likely to be a major neurotransmitter. Substance P is slow to build up at the synapse and also slow to be destroyed. Therefore, its concentration at the synapse is believed to increase for at least several seconds, and perhaps much longer, after nociceptive stimulation begins. After the impulse is over, the substance P probably persists for many more seconds or perhaps even minutes. The importance of this is that it might explain the progressive increase in intensity of slow-chronic pain with time. It might also explain, at least partially, the persistence of this type of pain even after the painful stimulus has been removed.

If the nociceptive impulse we are following entered the fast pain tract, the thalamus would immediately receive the information and send it to the cortex for evaluation and response. The motor cortex would quickly coordinate a response with the basal ganglia and cerebellum, producing a descending impulse to a motor neuron creating a muscle action. This response may even be a reflex.

If, however, the nociceptive impulse that we are following entered the slow pain tract, a different series of events would occur. As discussed in Chapter 2, the reticular formation is a portion of the brain stem that contains a number of nuclei that can either excite or inhibit the incoming impulses. The reticular formation therefore controls the overall activity of the brain. The area of the reticular formation that seems to increase or excite incoming impulses is called the *bulboreticular facilitory* area. This region contains a group of neurons that secrete acetylcholine, an excitatory transmitter. Fibers passing through this region of the reticular formation travel to the intralaminar nuclei of the thalamus. The level of activity of the brain stem bulboreticular facilitory area (and therefore the level of activity of the entire brain) is determined to a great extent by the sensory signals that enter this area from the periphery. Pain signals, in particular, increase the activity in this area and strongly excite the brain to attention.[52]

Not only does an excited bulboreticular facilitory area quickly send impulses to the thalamus and cortex but return impulses are also influenced. In other words, impulses leaving the cortex travel down to the thalamus and through this facilitory area. When this area is activated, these descending impulses are enhanced. Therefore, any time the cerebral cortex becomes activated by either thinking or motor processes, reverse signals are sent to the brain stem excitatory area, increasing the impulses. This generally provides a positive feedback system that allows any beginning activity in the cerebrum to support still more activity, thus leading to an awake mind. Perhaps it is this mechanism that is responsible for sleep disruption in individuals suffering with chronic pain.

Another important area in the reticular formation that controls brain activity is the *reticular inhibitory area*. This area is located medially and ventrally in the medulla and can reduce the tonic nerve signals transmitted through the spinal cord and trigeminal brain stem complex. This region of the reticular formation has a high concentration of neurons that secrete serotonin, an inhibitory transmitter. This area will be discussed in Chapter 4.

Now to follow our nociceptive impulse and assume that the excitatory area of the reticular formation enhanced it and sent it to the thalamus. (In many instances the impulse may have been terminated in the reticular formation.) Once the impulse reaches the thalamus, it is sent not only to the sensory cortex but signals are simultaneously sent to the limbic structures and hypothalamus. The sensory cortex now recognizes the nociceptive impulse as pain. Along with this recognition comes evaluation of the meaning of this sensation. The cortex may reach back into memory for assistance in evaluating this unpleasant sensation. It is at this point that prior experiences of pain and suffering begin to give meaning to the sensation. If the individual has experienced this sensation and learned it was of little consequence, the pain may be totally ignored. On the other hand, if this same pain sensation has caused considerable alteration in the quality of life, much attention will be drawn to the sensation.

In addition to these responses are still other responses influenced by the limbic system and hypothalamus. As discussed in Chapter 2, the limbic system is responsible for basic instincts and behavior. Within the limbic system are certain centers that determine behavior. These centers influence the *affective* nature of sensory sensation, that is whether the sensory sensations are pleasant or unpleasant. The centers have been described in terms of pain/pleasure, reward/punishment, and satisfaction/aversion centers. Electrical stimulation of certain regions pleases or satisfies the animal, whereas electrical stimulation of other regions caused terror, pain, fear, rage, defense, and escape reactions. Painful or other negative sensations (ie, hunger, thirst, etc) will drive the individual toward behavior that will eliminate or terminate the unpleasant sensation. This behavioral response is instinctive; however, it can be influenced by the cortex. Therefore the present level of activity of the limbic system (ie, mood, anger, rage, etc) can greatly influence the individual's response to pain.

Summary

Following the transmission of a single impulse from a receptor to the brain and back out as a response can facilitate the understanding of the neuroanatomy and physiology of pain. Yet even this simple example becomes complex when one examines the many factors that can alter the impulse as it travels. From the moment the sensory receptor is activated *(transduction)*, the impulse can be altered, such as with peripheral sensitization. Depending on the type of nerve fiber that carries the impulse, different tracts are taken that influence *transmission*. Then as the impulse travels it may be significantly *modulated* before even reaching the cortex. When the cortex finally receives the impulse, *perception* is determined by interaction of the cortex, thalamus, and limbic structures.

The clinician can appreciate the reason for so much variation in pain and suffering between different individuals. As will be discussed in the next chapter, the complexity is far greater than that presented in this chapter.

References

1. Melzack R. Neuropsychological basis of pain measurement. In Kruger L, Liebeskind JC (eds): Advances in Pain Reseach and Therapy, vol 6. New York: Raven Press; 1984: 323–339.

2. Skilling SR, Smullin DH, Larson AA. Extracellular amino acid concentrations in the dorsal spinal cord of freely moving rats following veratridine and nociceptive stimulation. J Neurochem 1988; 51:127–132.

3. Sorkin LS, Westlund KN, Sluks KA, Dougherty PM, Willis WD. Neural changes in acute arthritis in monkeys. IV. Time course of amino acid release into the lumbar dorsal horn. Brain Res Rev 1992; 17:39–50.

4. Seltzer S, Marcus R, Stoch R. Perspectives in the control of chronic pain by nutritional manipulation. Pain 1981; 11:141–148.

5. Basbaum AT. Brainstem control of nociception: The contribution of the monoamines. Pain 1981; 11(suppl 1):231.

6. Beck PW, Handwerker HO. Bradykinin and serotonin effects on various types of cutaneous nerve fibers. Pflugers Arch 1974; 347:209–222.

7. Messing RB, Lytle LD. Serotonin-containing neurons: Their possible role in pain and analgesia. Pain 1977; 4:1–21.

8. Belcher G, Ryall RW, Schaffner R. The differential effects of 5-hydroxytryptamine, noradrenalin, and raphe stimulation on nociceptive and nonnociceptive dorsal horn interneurons in the cat. Brain Res 1978; 151:307–321.

9. Ward NG, Bloom VL, Friedel RO. The effectiveness of tricyclic antidepressants in the treatment of coexisting pain and depression. Pain 1979; 7:331–341.

10. Dubner R. Specialization of nociceptive pathways: Sensory discrimination, sensory modulation, and neural connectivity. In Fields HL, Dubner R, Cervero F (eds): Advances in Pain Research and Therapy, vol 9. New York: Raven Press; 1985: 111–137.

11. Yaksh TL, Hammond DL. Peripheral and central substrates involved in the rostral transmission of nociceptive information. Pain 1982; 13:1–85.

12. Zimmerman M. Peripheral and central nervous mechanisms of nociception, pain, and pain therapy: Facts and hypotheses. In Bonica JJ, Liebeskind JC, Albe-Fessard DG (eds): Advances in Pain Research and Therapy, vol 3. New York: Raven Press; 1979: 3–32.

13. Hosobuchi Y. Elevated CSF level of substance P in arachnoiditis is reduced by systemic administration of morphine. Pain 1981; 11(suppl 1):257.

14. Lembeck F, Donnerer J, Colpaert FC. Increase of substance P in primary afferent nerves during chronic pain. Neuropeptides 1981; 1:175.

15. Yasphal K, Wright DM, Henry JL. Substance P reduces tail-flick latency: Implications for chronic pain syndromes. Pain 1982; 14:155–167.

16. Levine J, Basbaum A. The peripheral nervous system and the inflammatory process. Pain 1987; 31(suppl 4):109.

17. Allen GD. Dental Anesthesia and Analgesia, ed 2. Baltimore: Williams & Wilkins; 1979.

18. Kroening R, Donaldson D. Proposed mechanism of acupuncture. Soc Adv Anesth Dent Digest 1979; 4:28.

19. Watkins LR, Mayer DJ. Organization of endogenous opiate and nonopiate pain control systems. Science 1982; 216:1185–1192.

20. Synder SH. Opiate receptors and internal opiates. Sci Am 1977; 236:44–56.

21. Kosterlitz HW. Interaction of endogenous opioid peptides and their analogs with opiate receptors. In Bonica JJ, Liebeskind JC, Albe-Fessard DG (eds): Advances in Pain Research and Therapy, vol 3. New York: Raven Press; 1979: 377–384.

22. Stacher G, Bauer P, Steinringer H, et al. Effects of the synthetic enkephalin analogue K33–824 on pain threshold and pain tolerance in man. Pain 1979; 7:159–172.

23. Gutstein HB, Bronstein DM, Huda A. Beta endorphin processing and cellular origins in rat spinal cord. Pain 1992; 51:241–247.

24. Von Knorring L, Almay BGL, Johansson F, et al. Pain perception and endorphin levels in cerebrospinal fluid. Pain 1978; 5:359–365.

25. Mayer DJ, Price DD. Central nervous system mechanisms of analgesia. Pain 1976; 2:379–404.

26. Akil H, Liebeskind JC. Monoaminergic mechanisms of stimulation-produced analgesia. Brain Res 1975; 94:279–296.

27. Kosterlitz HW. Opioid peptides and pain: An update. In Bonica JJ, Lindblom U, Iggo A (eds): Advances in Pain Research and Therapy, vol 5. New York: Raven Press; 1983: 199–208.

28. Colt EWD, Wardlaw SL, Frantz AG. The effect of running on plasma endorphin. Life Sci 1981; 28:1637–1640.

29. Levine JD, Gordon NC, Fields HL. The role of endorphins in placebo analgesia. In Bonica JJ, Liebeskind JC, Albe-Fessard DG (eds): Advances in Pain Research and Therapy, vol 3. New York: Raven Press; 1979: 547–551.

30. Grevert P, Albert LH, Goldstein A. Partial antagonism of placebo analgesia by naloxone. Pain 1983; 16:129–143.

31. Barber J, Mayer D. Evaluation of the efficacy and neural mechanism of a hypnotic analgesia procedure in experimental and clinical dental pain. Pain 1977; 4:41–48.

32. Mayer DJ. Endogenous analgesia systems: Neural and behavioral mechanisms. In Bonica JJ, Liebeskind JC, Albe-Fessard DG (eds): Advances in Pain Research and Therapy, vol 3. New York: Raven Press; 1979: 385–410.

33. Mense S, Meyer H. Bradykinin-induced sensitization of high-threshold muscle receptors with slowly conducting afferent fibers. Pain 1981; 11(suppl 1):204.

34. Chahl LA, Iggo A. The effects of bradykinin and prostaglandin E, on rat cutaneous afferent nerve activity. Br J Pharmacol 1977; 59:343–347.

35. Foreman RD, Blair RW, Weber RN. Effects on T3 to T5 primate spinothalamic tract cells of injecting bradykinin into the heart. Pain 1981; 11(suppl 1):212.

36. Keele KD. A physician looks at pain. In Weisenberg M (ed): Pain: Clinical and Experimental Perspectives. St Louis: CV Mosby; 1975: 45–55.

37. Juan H, Lembeck F. Action of peptides and other algesic agents on paravascular pain receptors of the isolated perfused rabbit ear. Naunyn Schmiedeberg Arch Pharmacol 1974; 283:151–164.

38. Armstrong D. Brandykinin, kallidin and kallikrein. In Erdos EG (ed): Handbook of Experimental Pharmacology, vol 25. Berlin: Springer-Verlag; 1970: 434–481.

39. Perl ER. Sensitization of nociceptors and its relation to sensation. In Bonica JJ, Albe-Fessard A (ed): Advances in Pain Research and Therapy, vol 1. New York: Raven Press; 1976: 17–28.

40. Beck PW, Handwerker HO. Bradykinin and serotonin effects on various types of cutaneous nerve fibres. Pflugers Arch 1974; 347:209–222.

41. Higgs GH, Moncada S. Interactions of arachidonate products with other pain mediators. In Bonica JJ, Lindblom U, Iggo A (eds): Advances in Pain Research and Therapy, vol 5. New York: Raven Press; 1983: 617–626.

42. Greenberg S, Palmer GC. Biochemical basis of analgesia: Metabolism, storage, regulation, and actions. Dent Clin North Am 1978; 22:31–46.

43. Pateromichelakis S, Rood JP. Effects of prostaglandin E on A-beta and A-delta mechanoreceptor responses. Pain 1981; 11(suppl 1):203.

44. Ferreira SH. Prostaglandins: Peripheral and central analgesia. In Bonica JJ, Lindblom U, Igga A (eds): Advances in Pain Research and Therapy, vol 5. New York: Raven Press; 1983: 627–634.

45. Bisgaard H, Kristensen JK. Leukotriene B4 produces hyperalgesia in humans. Prostaglandins 1985; 30:791–797.

46. Levine JD, Lau W, Kwiat G, Goetzl EJ. Leukotriene B$_4$ produces hyperalgesia that is dependent on polymorphonuclear leukocytes. Science 1984; 225:743–745.

47. Otsuka M, Konishi S, Yanagisawa M, Tsunoo A, Takagi H. Role of sustance P as a sensory transmitter in spinal cord and sympathetic ganglia. Ciba Found Symp 1982; 91:13–34.

48. LaMotte RH, Thalhammer JG, Robinson CJ. Peripheral neural correlates of magnitude of cutaneous pain and hyperalgesia: A comparison of neural events in monkey with sensory judgments in human. J Neurophysiol 1983; 50:1–26.

49. Wall PD. Mechanisms of acute and chronic pain. In Kruger L, Liebeskind JC (eds): Advances in Pain Research and Therapy, vol 6. New York: Raven Press; 1984: 95–104.

50. DuBrul EL. Sicher's Oral Anatomy, ed 7. St Louis: CV Mosby; 1980: 391–414.

51. Sessle BJ. Anatomy, physiology and pathophysiology of orofacial pain. In Jacobson AL, Donlon WC (eds): Headache and Facial Pain. New York: Raven Press; 1990: 1–24.

52. Bowsher D. Role of the reticular formation in responses to noxious stimulation. Pain 1976; 2:361–378.

4 | The Central Processing of Pain

Now that the normal anatomy and physiology of the peripheral and central nervous systems have been described, a more thorough description of the manner by which pain is processed can be reviewed. Understanding how noxious impulses are regulated by the central nervous system (CNS) is essential for the clinician who wishes to manage pain disorders.

Convergence

It has been known for many years that there are more primary afferent neurons entering the CNS than there are second-order neurons to carry the impulses to the higher centers.[1] It therefore follows that several primary sensory neurons must synapse with a single second-order neuron. The synapsing of several primary afferent neurons with one second-order neuron is known as *convergence.* Activity at the synapse may be a cumulative effect, called *summation.* Such summation may be *spatial* or *temporal.* Intensification of response is known as *facilitation;* suppression of response is called *inhibition.*

Convergence has been well documented in the trigeminal brain stem sensory nuclear complex. Subnucleus oralis and interpolaris receive extensive convergence of orofacial and muscle afferent inputs[2-6] (Fig 4-1). The same convergence has been shown in the subnucleus caudalis. In fact, in a study[7] of the cat brain, almost all of the neurons with temporomandibular joint (TMJ) input received additional afferent input, predominantly from facial skin or intraoral sites. In this same study, 74% of the neurons tested in the subnucleus caudalis showed convergence of tooth pulp and/or hypoglossal nerve afferent inputs. In another study,[8] afferent input from the TMJ and masseter muscle converged on the same second-order neuron in 80% of the nerves that were tested in the subnucleus caudalis. It appears that afferent input from deep structures converges to a greater degree than do afferents from cutaneous structures. Perhaps this is why pain from deep structures is felt as more diffuse and less localized than the more localized pain felt from cutaneous structures. In fact, deep pains are often very difficult for the patient to locate. As will be discussed in the next section, convergence of nociceptive input can lead to a confusing diagnostic clinical presentation.

Fig 4-1 A simplified graphic depiction of convergence of the primary neurons in the nucleus caudalis region of the trigeminal spinal tract nucleus. The neuron representing the ophthalmic division (V_1) and the neuron representing the mandibular division (V_3) of the trigeminal nerve converge on the same second-order neuron. The trigeminal spinal tract nucleus extends caudally to the region of the entrance zone of upper cervical nerves. The second cervical nerve $(C2)$ enters this region of the brain stem and converges on both a cervical input second-order neuron as well as a second-order neuron that is also receiving trigeminal input. (CN) = cranial nerve.

Site of Pain vs Source of Pain

For the clinician to successfully evaluate pain disorders, he or she must appreciate the difference between the site and source of pain. Although these words are often used interchangeably, they have significantly different meanings. The *site of pain* is the location that the patient feels the pain.

The site of pain is easily located by merely asking the patient to point out the region of the body that is painful. The *source of pain* is that area of the body from which the pain actually originates. When the site and the source of pain are in the same location it is called *primary pain*. Primary pains are very common and likely to be the only type of pain familiar to the patient. When one cuts a finger, the area of tissue damage is also the location of the pain. This is an example of primary pain since the site of pain (where it hurts) and the source of pain (where it originates) are in the same location. This type of pain makes sense to the patient and the clinician; therefore, therapy is obvious.

There are pains, however, in which the site of the pain is not in the same location as the source of the pain. This type of pain is called *heterotopic pain*. Heterotopic pains can be quite confusing to both the patient and the clinician. A commonly known heterotopic pain is cardiac pain. When an individual experiences myocardial ischemia, the site of pain is frequently felt in the mandible, shoulder, or radiating down the left arm. The source of pain is the myocardial tissues, yet the site of pain is distant from the site. Heterotopic pains pose a significant problem for the clinician. A basic cardinal rule in therapy is that *treatment must be directed toward the source of pain, not the site of pain.* Treatments directed toward the site of pain will have little to no effect on the pain. The clinician must therefore be able to first recognize heterotopic pains and then differentiate the site from the source of pain. This is basic to orofacial pain therapy since heterotopic pains are extremely common in the head and neck regions. Other common examples of heterotopic pain in the head and neck are frontal and temporal headaches from the neck, and ear and temporomandibular joint pain produced from the sternocleidomastoid muscle. Sooner or later, every dentist has been confronted with a patient who complains of tooth pain but may not present any objective findings. As will be discussed, there are many toothaches that do not arise from the teeth at all.

Each clinician must be prepared to accept the fact that pain, especially from deep sources, is frequently felt in structures that are normal. The clinician must therefore guard against extending treatment to such structures in an attempt to control pain until an accurate diagnosis has been made.

Types of Heterotopic Pains

The term heterotopic pain refers to any pain that is felt in an area other than its true source. Although the terms referred and heterotopic are frequently used interchangeably, a more restricted use of the term referred is advocated. There are three general types of heterotopic pain: *(1)* central pain, *(2)* projected pain, and *(3)* referred pain.

Central Pain

Pain that emanates from structures of the central nervous system is felt peripherally as heterotopic pain. This is especially true of the intracranial structures that are insensitive to pain. When a tumor or other disturbance is present in the central nervous system, the pain is often felt not in the CNS but in peripheral structures. Pain emanating from pain-sensitive intracranial structures on or above the tentorium cerebelli (ie, cerebral vessels) is felt in the peripheral distribution of the trigeminal nerve.

Projected Pain

Projected pain is felt in the peripheral distribution of the same nerve that mediates the primary nociceptive input. Pain due to noxious stimulation of a sensory root or a major nerve trunk is felt in the exact anatomic distribution of that nerve. An example is the radicular pain of posterior root compression. It has been assumed that compression due to herniation of an intervertebral disc produces prolonged firing in the injured sensory fibers. However, acute peripheral nerve compression is usually painless and rarely lasts more than a few seconds. It is likely, therefore, that radicular pain is felt in the peripheral structures through activation of deeper interneurons.[9] The mechanism, however, seems to be different from that of central excitation in that projected pain follows a more precise anatomic pattern relative to the peripheral distribution, while central excitation pain is felt in a reference zone that is only segmentally related to the primary pain source. Projected sensory nerve pain is primarily neurogenous and follows dermatome mapping faithfully. Examples of projected pain include paroxysmal neuralgia, peripheral neuritis, herpes zoster, and postherpetic neuralgia.

It has long been known that noxious stimulation of a motor root or major motor nerve also induces pain, but of a different type and felt in different areas. Rather than the bright, burning, neuropathic pain felt in the dermatome distribution, motor nerve pain is sensed as dull, deep somatic pain diffusely located in the muscles innervated by that nerve. Such pain is now explicable on the basis of afferent neurons that are present in the motor nerves. No doubt, such pain should be classified as projected pain, even though it displays a deep somatic rather than neuropathic quality and follows a motor nerve route rather than a dermatome field. Although the neural mecha-

nisms have not been identified, it is likely that interneurons are involved in a manner similar to that for projected sensory nerve pain. It likewise differs from the heterotopic pain of referred pain.

Projected pains may be accompanied by areas of secondary hyperalgesia that are hypersensitive to stimulation without an appreciable reduction in the local pain threshold. Whatever the mechanism responsible for this phenomenon, it is likely similar to that of secondary hyperalgesia of central hyperexcitability as described in the next section.

Referred Pain

Referred pain is a spontaneous heterotopic pain that is felt in an area innervated by a different nerve from the one that mediates the primary pain. Being spontaneous, referred pain occurs without provocation at the site of pain. It is wholly dependent on the original source of pain. The reason for this dependence is that the original source of nociceptive input produces a *sensitization* of interneurons that is responsible for this type of heterotopic pain. Since the sensitization of interneurons (also called *central excitatory effects*) is very important in understanding heterotopic pains, it is worthy to discuss this phenomena at this time.

Central Sensitization

The diagnostic differentiation between true primary pain and symptoms that occur as secondary effects of that pain is essential. Such manifestations are usually referred to as central excitatory effects on the presumption that they result from hyperexcitability of CNS interneurons.

The neurologic mechanisms involved in the secondary effects of pain are not fully understood. Some researchers think that reflex activity is involved.[10] There seems to be little doubt that convergence of afferent impulses among CNS interneurons takes place.[11] However the factors that control the mechanisms involved have not been elucidated. Sessle et al[12] have shown that, while primary trigeminal neurons normally respond only to stimuli located within their respective receptive fields, at least half the second-order nociceptive (wide dynamic range and nociceptive-specific) neurons are activated by electric stimulation applied outside the normal receptive fields of the corresponding primary neurons. The neurons thus activated are presumed to be those that respond to input from deep structures of the mouth and face. This is taken as evidence that the reference of pain occurs in conjunction with deep pain input rather than a superficial one.[13] It suggests that under certain conditions trigeminal nociceptive interneurons are subject to subliminal stimulation from structures other than those located in the normal receptive fields. Such evidence supports the convergence theory of pain reference. Gross[14] reported that referred pain due to visceral disease followed known dermatomes but referred pain from deep somatic structures did not.

Recent information[15] suggests that the second-order neuron can change with respect to its processing of impulses. It appears that when a second-order neuron receives a constant barrage of nociceptive input, specific receptors sites can be activated that increase the sensitization of that neuron. Some of the receptors that are involved in this sensitization are the N-methyl-D-aspartic acid (NMDA) receptors.[16] Stimulation of these receptors by excitatory amino acids, such as aspartate and glutamate, increase the sensitization of these neurons. This increased sensitization can alter neural impulses as they are processed on the way to the higher centers. When this occurs, even normal neural impulses can be misinterpreted as noxious. This alteration in impulse processing is called *neuroplasticity*. Bonica[17] has reviewed the clinical aspects of central sensitization in depth.

Clinically, sensitization and central excitatory effects are induced by more or less continuous barrages of noxious sensation emanating from deep somatic structures. If the input is not continuous, these secondary effects are less likely to occur. Increased intensity and duration of the deep pain input enhances the secondary effects. Initially these changes in neural sensitization are usual and reversible. With chronicity, however, changes may occur that alter the neuroprocessing more permanently. Permanent alterations can lead to chronic neuropathic pain as discussed in Chapter 17. The symptoms of central sensitization complicate continuous deep somatic pains since they increase with the intensity and duration of the primary pain. Such symptoms can occur in otherwise normal structures; therefore, treatment can be misdirected.

The central excitatory effects produced by deep pain input may involve afferent (sensory) neurons, efferent (motor) neurons, and/or autonomic neurons. Each of these effects will now be discussed.

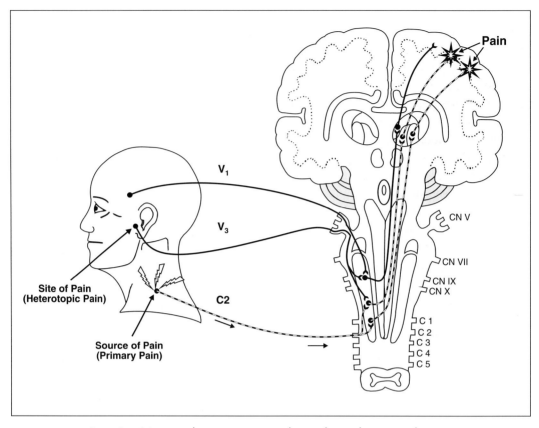

Fig 4-2 Injury to the trapezius muscle results in the tissue damage. Nociception arising in this cervical region is transmitted to the second-order neuron and relayed to the higher centers for interpretation. As this input becomes protracted, note that the adjacent converging neuron is also centrally excited, which relays additional nociception to the higher centers. The sensory cortex now perceives two locations of pain. One area is the trapezius region, which represents a true source of nociception (primary pain). The second area of perceived pain is felt in the temporomandibular joint area, which is only a site of pain, not a source of pain. This pain is heterotopic (referred).

Afferent (Sensory) Neuron Effects

When central excitatory effects are produced in a sensory neuron, the most common clinical finding is pain. The type of pain complaint is either referred pain or secondary hyperalgesia.

Referred Pain. Referred pain due to central sensitization is initially wholly spontaneous as far as the site of pain is concerned. It is not accentuated by provocation of the site where the pain is felt; it is accentuated only by manipulation of the primary pain source (Fig 4-2). It is dependent on continuance of the primary initiating pain: it ceases immediately if the primary pain is arrested or interrupted. Anesthesia of the structure where the referred pain is felt does not arrest the pain.[18] Only by anesthetizing the neural pathway that mediates the primary pain is the referred pain arrested.[19]

It should be noted that although the primary initiating pain is of the deep somatic type, the secondary referred pain may be felt in either deep or superficial structures. This may present a bizarre clinical picture. When reference is felt superficially, it must be differentiated from superficial somatic pain and from projected neuropathic pain. When it is felt deeply, it must be differentiated from other deep somatic pains.

Referred pain does not occur haphazardly but in fact follows three clinical rules. The first rule is that referred pain most frequently occurs within a single nerve root, passing from one branch to another. As an example, a mandibular molar presenting with a source of pain will commonly refer pain to a maxillary molar. In this case, the mandibular branch of the trigeminal nerve is referring pain to the maxillary branch of the same nerve. This is a fairly common occurrence with dental pain. Generally, if the pain is referred to another distribution of the same nerve, it does so in a laminated manner. This lamination follows dermatomes. A dermatome is a sensory root field on the skin where pain is felt when a particular neural segment mediates painful sensation. These have been well charted (Fig 4-3). Each nerve has a corresponding dermatome, but there is considerable overlapping. Humans' upright posture causes some confusion in dermatome arrangement, especially in the extremities. They are better visualized with the subject in the quadruped

position (Fig 4-4). This places them in a more logical metameric arrangement and helps considerably to identify the proper segmental relationships.[20]

Trigeminal lamination patterns are determined by the manner in which the primary afferent neurons enter in the spinal tract nucleus. According to Kunc,[21,22] the location of trigeminal nociceptive terminals within the nucleus caudalis is as follows:

1. The fibers from parts near the sagittal midline of the face terminate highest in the nucleus (cephalad).
2. The fibers from parts located more laterally terminate lowest in the nucleus (caudad).
3. The intermediate fibers terminate intermediately in the nucleus (Fig 4-5). This laminated arrangement of facial innervation appears to coincide with Finneson's metameric arrangement of the dermatomes in the quadruped position.[20]

This grouping of the terminals of the primary trigeminal neurons should influence the location of clinical effects of central excitation, especially with regard to referred pain. It probably accounts for some effects not otherwise readily explained. Kawamura and Nishiyama showed that a molar tooth projects dorsal to a canine and a canine projects dorsal to an incisor, which confirms the vertical lamination just cited.[23]

Simply speaking, this means that incisors refer to incisors, premolars to premolars, and molars to molars on the same side of the mouth. In other words, molars do not refer pain to incisors or incisors to molars.

The second clinical rule is that referred pain in the trigeminal area rarely crosses the midline unless it originates at the midline.

Fig 4-3 Dermal segmentation as represented by Netter and based essentially on the work of Keegan. (From Netter FH. The CIBA Collection of Medical Illustrations. Indianapolis: Curtis Publishing Co; 1953. Used with permission.)

Fig 4-4 The orderly metameric arrangement of dermatomes becomes apparent if we visualize a man in the quadruped position. (From Finneson BE. Diagnosis and Management of Pain Syndromes, ed 2. Philadelphia: WB Saunders Co; 1969. Used with permission.)

For example, pain in the right temporomandibular joint will not likely cross over to the left side of the face nor will right molar pain refer to a left molar. This is not true however, in the cervical region or below. Cervicospinal pain can be referred across the midline, although it normally stays on the same side as the source.

A third clinical rule of referred pain is that if the referred pain is felt outside the nerve that mediates the pain, it is generally felt cephalad to the nerve (upward, toward the head) and not caudally. Clinically this means that deep pain felt in the sacral area may be referred to the lumbar area, as well as lumbar to thoracic, thoracic to cervical, and cervical to trigeminal. Rarely will trigeminal pain refer to the cervical region. Only very intense primary pain causes excitatory effects in a segment caudal to the site of initiating input.[24]

Secondary Hyperalgesia. Hyperalgesia is defined as increased sensitivity to stimulation at the site of pain. Primary hyperalgesia occurs as the result of a lowered pain threshold (sensitization) in the peripheral structures due presumably to the presence of algogenic substances such as bradykinin, potassium, histamine, and serotonin (see

Fig 4-5 Graphic depiction of the spinal trigeminal nucleus and its relationship with incoming sensory input. Note the laminated pattern of innervation from the facial structures into the spinal tract nucleus. These laminated patterns commonly reflect the patterns of referred pain felt in the orofacial structures.

Chapter 3). Secondary hyperalgesia is different. It is an increased response to stimulation at the site of pain in the absence of any local cause.[25] It may occur with or without accompanying referred pain.

Secondary hyperalgesia is also different from referred pain in that it occurs in response to stimulation (provocation) at the site of pain, while referred pain cannot be increased at the site of pain. It is wholly dependent on the source of pain. Both referred pain and secondary hyperalgesia are initiated by deep pain input and remain dependent on the continuance of such input. They differ, however, in that secondary hyperalgesia persists for a while after the primary pain ceases. Thus, analgesic blocking of the primary pain site does not immediately arrest the hyperalgesia as it does with referred pain.

As with referred pain, secondary hyperalgesia may be felt in either superficial or deep structures. Superficial secondary hyperalgesia is felt as sensitive skin, scalp, hair, or gingiva. Deep secondary hyperalgesia is sensed as an area of palpable tenderness, discomfort due to functional manipulation, or hypersensitive or tender teeth.

There are two explanations for the occurrence of secondary hyperalgesia. The first is that related to the sensitization of the second-order neuron. As central sensitization occurs, even normal input can be misinterpreted as noxious.[26,27] Therefore, even input carried by the A-beta and A-delta fibers (nonnoxious) can be felt as pain. When this occurs, even light touch to the face becomes painful. Pain produced by normally nonpainful stimulus is called *allodynia*.

A second explanation for secondary hyperalgesia is a local cause produced by neurogenic inflammation (see Chapter 3). With central sensitization, the primary afferent neuron can create an antidromically produced neurogenic inflammation. In other words, the primary neuron can release excitatory neurotransmitters (ie, substance P) into peripheral sites, increasing the sensitivity of the primary nociceptors. When this occurs, there is usually a small central area of hyperemia indicating some local tissue reaction. In this flare area of an axon reflex, the pain threshold is lowered, thus indicating that this portion of the hyperalgesic area is primary and reflects local tissue change. The entire area of sensitivity, however, extends far beyond the hyperemic zone. The wider area represents true secondary hyperalgesia that is dependent on continuance of primary deep pain impulses.[24] Analgesic blocking of an area of secondary hyperalgesia does in fact decrease the total discomfort, presumably due to its effect on the component of primary hyperalgesia that is present.[28] It does not render the area entirely painless, however, as would be the case with primary hyperalgesia from a local cause.

At a clinical level, superficial secondary hyperalgesia usually presents no great problem because of the obvious lack of local cause. Deep secondary hyperalgesia, however, cannot be distinguished from primary hyperalgesia on the basis of manual palpation or functional manipulation (see Chapter 8). Special diagnostic effort is required to make this judgment, which is important therapeutically. Palpable tenderness or deep discomfort from functional manipulation identifies only a site of pain, not a source of pain. Whether such an identified site of pain is primary hyperalgesia from a local cause such as inflammation or myospasm or a heterotopic manifestation of deep pain input located elsewhere is a judgment that must precede definitive therapy.

Efferent (Motor) Neuron Effects

When central excitatory effects alter the function of an efferent neuron, the influence is felt in the muscle innervated by that neuron. There are two effects that may occur: muscle co-contraction and myofascial trigger points.

A common efferent effect secondary to constant deep pain is a reflex excitation of the muscle slightly modifying its functional activity[29] (Fig 4-6). In the presence of deep pain, the antagonist muscles appear to become activated in an attempt to limit activity of the agonist muscle.[30,31] This phenomenon is called *co-contraction*[32] and has previously been referred to as protective muscle splinting. The exact mechanisms involved will be discussed in later chapters. Suffice to say at this time that deep pains that produce central excitatory effects can influence muscle activity.[33]

71

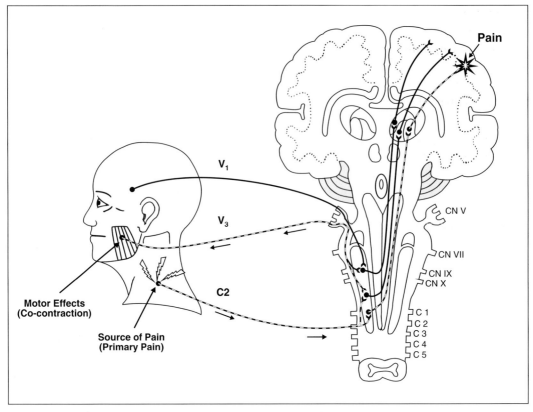

Fig 4-6 Constant afferent nociceptive input can centrally excite efferent (motor) neurons, resulting in co-contraction of associated muscle or the development of myofascial trigger points.

Another motor effect of central excitation is the development of a localized area of hypersensitivity within the muscle tissues. A continuing deep pain input of some intensity may induce a myofascial trigger point mechanism involving a muscle(s) that is segmentally related to the site of primary pain. The masseter and temporalis are the masticatory muscles most frequently affected. The trigger point, in turn, refers pain that is frequently felt at or near the site of the initiating primary pain. The trigger itself, however, is usually silent unless manually palpated; then local muscle pain is felt. Although this mechanism may be initiated

by pain, once trigger points become established, they remain active or latent until eliminated by therapeutic effort.[34] Thus, pain at or near the initial site of primary pain may persist as a continuing or recurrent heterotopic manifestation long after the original pain has ceased. The complexity of such pain problems makes accurate diagnosis more necessary for effective management of the patient's complaint. Myofascial trigger point pain will be discussed in more detail in Chapter 12.

The muscles that are affected by central sensitization are usually those innervated by the same major nerve that mediates the deep pain input, thus establishing a segmental relationship. If the primary pain is mediated by the trigeminal nerve, the muscles most likely to be affected are those innervated by the trigeminal nerve. They are eight in number: the masseter, the temporalis, the medial pterygoid, the lateral pterygoid, the mylohyoid, the anterior belly of the digastric, and the tensor muscles of the soft palate and tympanic membrane.

Autonomic Neuron Effects

Deep somatic pain may induce autonomic effects in an area segmentally related to the site of primary pain. Vasomotor and glandular effects may occur. The symptoms may include temperature and color changes in the skin (flushing, blanching), puffy swelling of the eyelids and other loose cutaneous tissue, injection of the conjunctiva, lacrimation, nasal secretion, and nasal congestion. Such symptoms may simulate allergic rhinitis or maxillary sinusitis.

The autonomic changes induced by deep pain are thought to be central excitatory effects. Their behavior is similar to other such effects and remains dependent on deep pain input. There is a recovery time lag, however, when the primary pain ceases; the autonomic symptoms may persist for a day or so.

It is believed that the secondary effects caused by central sensitization are the result of a barrage of continuous deep nociceptive input entering the CNS. It is felt that these changes are all reversible once the source of deep pain is eliminated. On an acute basis, this is certainly true. However, when the duration is prolonged, these neuroplastic changes may not always be reversible.

When these changes do not revert to normal, neuropathic pains are experienced. These pains will be discussed in Chapter 17.

The Experience of Pain

Until recently, human pain was considered a sensory experience evoked by noxious stimulation of neural structures. The impulses thus generated were thought to be transmitted to the CNS, where they were perceived as pain and reacted to. The reaction was thought to comprise extensive behavior on the part of many body systems. The dominant factors in pain reaction were thought to be on a mentation level such as prior conditioning, evaluative significance of the pain, memory, and emotional response. This perception-reaction hypothesis was originated in the 19th century by Marshall[35] and Strong.[36] It was recognized that great differences in pain reaction were common. Maurice concluded: "The exaggerated reaction is due to psychic factors and is termed psychoneurotic pain."[37] It became popular to think in terms of human discomfort as being organic or psychogenic. Organic pain constituted pain behavior that could be accounted for on the basis of structural conditions. When no structural condition could be found to explain the pain, the clinician labeled it psychogenic pain.

During the second half of the 20th century, there was an increased effort by researchers and clinicians to better understand pain. New experiments and observations gave reason to question the validity of the perception-reaction concept of pain. Thus, the currently held concept of pain modulation evolved.

Fig 4-7 Schematic diagram of the gate control theory of pain mechanisms. L = the large diameter fibers; S = the small diameter fibers. The fibers project to the substantia gelatinosa (SG) and first central transmission (T) cells. The inhibitory effect exerted by SG on the afferent fiber terminals is increased by activity in L fibers and decreased by activity in S fibers. The central control trigger is represented by a line running from the large-fiber system to the central control mechanisms; these mechanisms, in turn, project back to the gate control system. The T cells (second-order neurons) project to the entry cells of the action system. ± = excitation; − = inhibition. (From Melzack R, Wall PD. Pain mechanisms: A new theory. Science 1965; 150:975. Copyright 1965, American Association for the Advancement of Science. Used with permission.)

The Modulation Concept

We now appreciate that pain is much more than noxious stimulation of neural structures. It is more than a systemic reaction to unpleasant signals received by the brain. It is more than a choice between organic and psychogenic. Pain comprises all these features in a unified sensory and emotional experience. The concept of pain modulation is based on documented experimental evidence that neural impulses are altered, changed, or *modulated* as they travel up the neuraxis to the higher centers. Excitatory and inhibitory influences bear on the impulses at various levels in the CNS so that perception and reaction become merely facets of the same mechanism rather than separate components of it.

Whether pain is generated by noxious stimulation of tissues or occurs spontaneously is no longer of great concern. Whether pain is the result of injury or of mentation processes is of little significance. It is more important to consider the various factors that influence the inhibition and

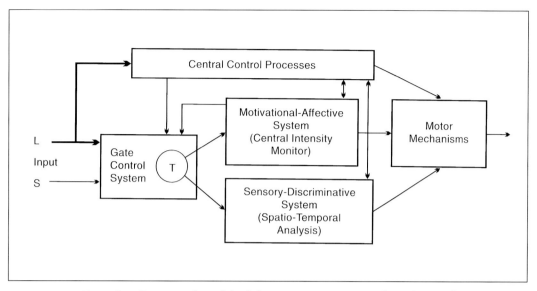

Fig 4-8 Conceptual model of the sensory, motivational, and central control determinants of pain. The output of the T cells of the gate control system projects to the sensory-discriminative system (via neospinothalamic fibers) and the motivational-affective system (via the paramedial ascending system). The central control trigger (comprising the dorsal-column and dorsolateral projection systems) is represented by a line running from the large-fiber system to central control processes; these, in turn, project back to the gate control system and to the sensory-discriminative and motivational-affective systems. All three systems interact with one another and project to the motor system. (From Casey KL, Melzack R. Neural mechanisms of pain: A conceptual model. In Way EL (ed): New Concepts in Pain and its Clinical Management. Philadelphia: FA Davis Co; 1967: 13–31. Used with permission.)

excitation of painful experience. In recent years, worldwide research into pain mechanisms has brought to light much information relative to these factors.

In 1965, Melzack and Wall[38] proposed a new theory to help explain and serve as a model to visualize pain modulation. This they termed the *gate control theory* (Fig 4-7). Although the neurophysiologic mechanisms are still under debate and many uncertainties remain, the theory served to bridge us from the former perception-reaction concept. The gate control theory as ini-

tially presented was subjected to further elaboration (Fig 4-8). This combined the more obvious sensory-discriminative component of pain with a motivational-affective dimension as an integral part of the pain experience on an anatomic and physiologic basis. In 1978, Wall[40] reexamined the gate control theory in light of 13 years of additional neurophysiologic investigation. He confirmed that the substantia gelatinosa did play an important role in organizing the nociceptive input. However, he noted that all nociceptive neurons of the dorsal horn received inhibitory impulses from regions of the brain. He concluded that the theory in its original detail could no longer be sustained, but that the underlying concepts were still valid when restated in a more basic form.

It is now generally agreed that the experience of pain is much more complex than a simple perception-reaction mechanism. Nor is pain variability explicable on the basis of conduction velocity and other structural features as embodied in the gate control theory, although such factors do, no doubt, have an effect. Perl[41] noted that all somatic sensation is subject to modulation by activity descending from rostral levels and, no doubt, by other factors. For example, it is known that fear augments suffering, as does anxiety or the attention that is directed toward discomfort. It has been demonstrated that the pain threshold is lowered by simply increasing the frequency of stimulation without altering its intensity.[42] Also, temperature change is reacted to differently by myelinated and unmyelinated fibers. Within the range of 14°C and 43°C, the firing rate of all myelinated fibers decreased with cooling while the unmyelinated fibers either showed no change or actually increased in firing rate.[43] Ernst et al[44] demonstrated that the repetition of dental stimuli significantly decreased pain sensitivity. All such evidence confirms that pain is more than a measure of noxious stimulation or threat. Indeed, much if not most pain arises in the absence of noxious stimulation or other identifiable local cause.

The concept of modulation is extremely important in understanding the patient's experience of pain. It is based on the premise that neural impulses rising to the higher centers that are termed "painful" can be altered en route. These impulses can be increased or enhanced, which can accentuate the pain experience. The process of increasing the impulse is called *facilitation*. In other conditions the impulses can be reduced or obtunded which will lessen the pain experience. The process of decreasing noxious impulses is called *inhibition*. Pain modulation explains why in some instances a painful experience may occur without any apparent cause while in other instances significant tissue damage may produce no pain at all. Presently much research is being directed toward gaining a better understanding of pain modulation since this may provide valuable insight on therapy.

At this time it is known that pain modulation can occur at various levels of the central nervous system. The following areas of orofacial pain modulation will be discussed in this section: the trigeminal spinal tract nucleus, the reticular formation, the descending inhibitory system, and psychologic modulating factors.

Pain Modulation in the Trigeminal Spinal Tract Nucleus

Melzack and Wall's original paper described how nociceptive impulses could be altered in the dorsal horn of the spinal cord. Since the trigeminal spinal tract nucleus is the brain stem extension of the spinal dorsal horn (see Chapter 2), it is assumed that the same discussion is true for trigeminal nerve input. The gate control theory suggested that both myelinated and unmyelinated primary afferent neurons converge to synapse with both a second-order neuron as well as an interneuron in the substantia gelatinosa (lamina II) (Fig 4-9). Both myelinated and

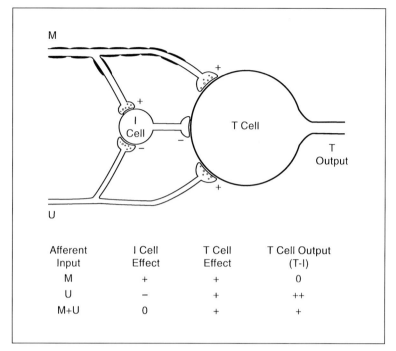

Afferent Input	I Cell Effect	T Cell Effect	T Cell Output (T-I)
M	+	+	0
U	−	+	++
M+U	0	+	+

Fig 4-9 A revised version of the gate control hypothesis. This hypothesis focuses on interactions in the dorsal horn of the spinal cord. *Top:* The four important types of neural element: the unmyelinated, nociceptive primary afferent *(U)*; the myelinated non-nociceptive primary afferent *(M)*; the transmission cell *(T)*, whose activity usually results in the sensation of pain; and inhibitory interneuron *(I)*, which is spontaneously active and whose activity inhibits the T cell, thus reducing perceived pain intensity. The inhibitory interneuron is excited by the myelinated nonnociceptive afferent. The other crucial point is that the unmyelinated nociceptor inhibits the inhibitory interneuron secondarily exciting the T cell. The unmyelinated primary afferent thus has both direct and indirect excitatory effects on the T cell. *Bottom:* The table shows how perceived pain *(T-cell output)* is the result of a balance of input from myelinated *(M)* and unmyelinated *(U)* primary afferents. For example, a stimulus that activates only the M afferents has both a direct excitatory and an indirect inhibitory effect on the T cell. There is no net increase in T cell activity and no pain. A stimulus that activates only the U afferents produces a very large increase in T cell firing because there are both direct and indirect excitatory actions and no inhibition. Most stimuli activate both M and U afferents, producing intermediate levels of pain intensity. (From Fields HL. Pain. New York: McGraw-Hill; 1987: 139. Used with permission.)

unmyelinated primary afferents were proposed to have a direct excitatory effect on the second-order neuron, which they called the transmission cell (T cell). Since these T cells carry nociceptive impulses, we now know that they are either a nociceptive-specific neuron or a wide dynamic range neuron. The substantia gelatinosa neurons were proposed to inhibit transmitter release from both primary afferent neurons, thus inhibiting the impulse carried by the primary afferent neuron. The myelinated afferents were proposed to excite the inhibitory interneurons, which in turn reduce the activity of the pain transmission neuron. This point is supported by the clinical observation that selective stimulation of large diameter myelinated fibers produces analgesia. In contrast, activity of the unmyelinated nociceptive neurons was proposed to inhibit the inhibitory substantia gelatinosa cells, resulting in an enhancement of transmission from the primary afferents to the T cell. The result of this action is to increase the nociceptive impulses sent to the higher centers. This action would therefore increase nociceptive transmission to the higher centers.

Transcutaneous Electrical Nerve Stimulation

The chief product of the gate control theory was the introduction of transcutaneous electrical nerve stimulation (TENS) as a therapeutic modality. The mechanisms involved gave considerable insight into pain modulation. Kane and Taub[45] reviewed the history of local electrical analgesia from the time the early Egyptians used electric fish to minimize pain. They related that, in 1858, Francis used forceps charged with electricity to extract teeth with less pain. The use of electricity to reduce pain has been discovered and rediscovered many times through the years. It lay dormant until resurrected by Wall and Sweet[46] in 1967. In 1975, Long and Hagfors[47] reviewed the resurgent use of electricity in various forms in treating 3,000 patients.

The rationale of TENS is based on the antinociceptive effect of stimulating cutaneous sensory nerves. An interrupted faradic current of very low intensity at a frequency of 50 to 100 Hz is used.[48] The stimulation is usually below what is required to activate A-delta and C nociceptive fibers.[49] No more than a tingling or vibratory sensation should be felt. Although the antinociceptive effect results from stimulation of thick A-beta fibers,[50] stimulation of A-delta and C fibers also yields the same effect as long as it does not reach noxious levels.[51] The effect is immediate and usually disappears rapidly. Pain relief is localized to the segment stimulated.[48] The effect is not reversed by naloxone, thus indicating that it is not dependent upon the release of endorphins[52–57] (which will be discussed later in this section). Both serotonin and dynorphin are released when superficial cutaneous nerves are stimulated. About one-third of all people are nonresponders to TENS.

At a clinical level, the modulating effect of cutaneous stimulation has been known for ages. The almost instinctive act of grabbing, holding, pressing, or rubbing a painful site exemplifies this effect. Many useful pain-reducing remedies are of this category. Massage, analgesic balms, counterirritants, mustard plasters, hot and cold compresses, vibration, hydrotherapy, and vapocoolant therapy are examples.[58,59]

Pain Modulation in the Reticular Formation

As discussed in Chapter 2, the reticular formation is a portion of the brain stem that contains a number of nuclei that can either excite or inhibit the incoming impulses. The reticular formation therefore controls the overall activity of the brain. This region contains a group of neurons that secrete acetylcholine, an excitatory transmitter. Fibers passing through this region of the reticular formation travel to the intralaminar nuclei of the thalamus. The level of activity of the reticular formation is determined to a great extent by the sensory signals that enter this area from the periphery. Pain signals, in particular, increase the activity in this area and strongly excite the brain to attention.[60]

Not only does an excited reticular formation quickly send impulses to the thalamus and cortex but return impulses are also influenced. In other words, impulses leaving the cortex travel down to the thalamus and through this facilitory area. When this area is activated, these descending impulses are enhanced. Therefore, any time the cerebral cortex becomes activated by either thinking or motor processes, reverse signals are sent to the brain stem excitatory area increasing the impulses. This generally provides a positive feedback system that allows any beginning activity in the cerebrum to support still more activity, thus leading to an awake mind.

Activity of the reticular formation is influenced by many brain stem structures as well as incoming impulses. Although many of these influences are not well known, the modulation effect of the reticular formation is likely to be great.

Pain Modulation of the Descending Inhibitory System

In 1983, while studying nerve injuries in rats, Wall and Devor[61] determined that the peripheral receptor is not the only region of the neuron that can initiate afferent impulses. The dorsal root ganglion cells also initiate sensory impulses. These cells initiate a tonic, low-level, spontaneous background discharge that is propagated orthodromically into the root and antidromically into the peripheral nerve. This source of afferent input may account for nociceptive impulses persisting after peripheral anesthesia. More importantly, this ongoing sensory input from the dorsal ganglia (assumed also to be true of the trigeminal gasserian ganglia) participates in the arousal system, which, if not countermanded, would tend to prevent sleep and perhaps even induce a continuous state of pain. The neural mechanism in the brain stem that appears to balance this continuous barrage of sensory input is called the *descending inhibitory system*. A suitable balance between the ongoing sensory barrage and the descending inhibitory system needs to be maintained for normal functional activities, allowing for adequate periods of rest and sleep. Should the balance be tilted in favor of increased excitation, the normal background barrage of sensory input would be facilitated, exciting the reticular formation and increasing the level of brain activity. Spontaneous firing may then occur, leading to ongoing activity.[62] Several neurotransmitters are important in the descending inhibitory system, one of the most important being serotonin. As the relationship between the brain stem descending inhibitory mechanism and the ongoing generation of sensory neural impulses by the dorsal ganglia becomes better understood, a more plausible explanation of the intimate pain-insomnia phenomenon may be forthcoming.

The descending inhibitory system is generally thought to affect all sensory input ascending into the brain stem. The portion of this system that effects nociceptive input has been referred to as the *analgesic system.* The analgesic system consists of three major components; the periaqueductal gray area, the raphe magnus nucleus, and a group of descending neurons that terminate in the substantia gelatinosa of the spinal tract nucleus and dorsal horn (see Chapter 2) (Fig 4-10). Electrical stimulation either in the periaqueductal gray area or in the raphe magnus nucleus can almost completely suppress strong nociceptive impulses. Several different transmitter substances are involved in the analgesia system, especially serotonin and the endorphins.

The discovery of endorphins in 1975 opened a new avenue in pain research. This new knowledge brought considerable insight into the mechanisms of pain modulation. Endorphins were discovered in connection with research seeking an answer to why we have morphine receptors in the CNS. The term endorphin is a contraction of the words endogenous and morphine. There are several endorphins, namely, methionine-enkephalin, leucine-enkephalin, alpha-endorphin, beta endorphin, and gamma-endorphin. The enkephalins and beta endorphin are particularly associated with antinociceptive mechanisms. No doubt these substances have other functions also.[63]

Although what is presently known about the endogenous opioid system may be somewhat hypothetical, it appears that there are three families of peptides that bind to three different opioid receptors in the brain and spinal cord, namely, the mu, the delta, and the kappa receptors. The pro-opiomelanocortin (POMC) family includes beta endorphin and corticotrophin, which bind to mu and delta receptors. The proenkephalin A group includes four metenkephalins, one leuenkephalin, one heptapeptide, one octapeptide, and several large peptides. These opioids bind to all three receptors. The prodynorphin group (proenkephalin B group) includes dynorphin, three leuenkephalins, and several large peptides. These opioids bind to delta and kappa receptors.[64] Endogenous opioids are released during highly threatening circumstances. This has been postulated to indicate that the body is able to defensively minimize the distracting effect of pain to facilitate the coping process. Blood levels of beta endorphin increase following noxious stimulation. Acute and relatively severe pain releases POMC and proenkephalin A peptides in the brain while dynorphin is released in the spinal cord. Although naloxone blocks the effect of the opioid peptides that bind to the receptors in the brain, which is the site of emotional and conscious sensation, it does not seem to block the action of dynorphin, which binds to the kappa receptors in the spinal cord where reflex activity takes place. There is considerable multiplicative interaction between the brain and spinal cord opioid receptors and ligands that make up the endogenous opioid system.[64]

The analgesic system appears to be dominant in the modulating effect of nonpainful cutaneous stimulation. Since direct stimulation of the periaqueductal gray matter (PAG) inhibits nociceptive neurons in the nucleus caudalis and since stimulation of

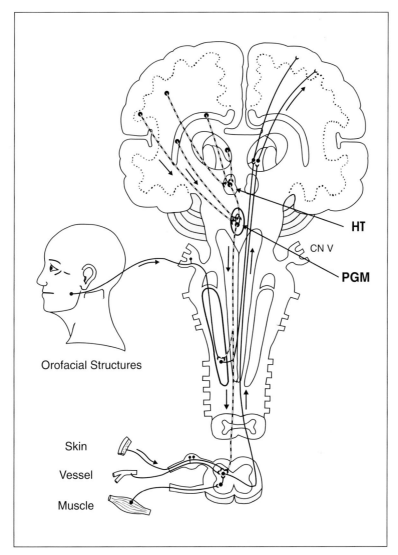

Fig 4-10 A graphic depiction of the descending inhibitory mechanism. Normal afferent input enters the trigeminal spinal tract nucleus from the orofacial structures and the dorsal horn from the rest of the body. The descending inhibitory mechanism *(dashed lines)* descends from the higher centers to the hypothalamus *(HT)* and periaqueductal gray matter *(PGM)*, which then suppresses ascending input. The inhibition of ascending impulses can occur at the region of the periaqueductal gray matter, the raphe magnus nucleus, or at the synapse of the primary afferent in the substantia gelatinosa of the dorsal horn and the trigeminal tract nucleus.

low threshold mechanoreceptors in the peripheral field also inhibits the response of nociceptive specific and wide dynamic range caudalis neurons, it is concluded that pain modulation may result from stimulation of the nonnociceptive peripheral sensory fibers and central regions of the brain.[65] The nonnoxious stimulation of cutaneous afferents activates neurons of the descending inhibitory system, particularly those of the nucleus raphe magnus (NRM) in the brain stem and the PAG in the midbrain.[66] The stimulation of serotoninergic neurons in the NRM releases serotonin, which reduces stimulation-evoked excitation of nociceptive dorsal horn neurons.[67] In other words, the inhibitory effects at the substantia gelatinosa not only occur by local effects of the primary afferent neurons but also by this descending inhibitory mechanism of the analgesic system.

Sensory responses from tooth pulp stimulation are readily suppressed for 250 to 1,000 milliseconds by stimulation of the PAG and NRM.[68] Stimulation of the NRM reduces or abolishes neuronal responses in the subnucleus oralis and caudalis to nociceptive stimulation of the tooth pulp or cornea.[69] Serotonin appears to be the chief neurotransmitter active in this inhibitory mechanism. Stimulation of PAG reduces the aversive reaction to pain.[70]

Thus, this analgesic system can block nociception at the initial entry point as well as at other areas in the brain stem as the nociceptive input ascends.

Modulating Effects of Endorphins

The discovery of endorphins revealed the inherent presence of an endogenous antinociceptive system that normally modulates pain. Like the brain stem descending inhibitory mechanism, this endogenous system likely serves other important body functions. Its pain modulating action may be little more than a spin-off from its other functions. For example, it is known that endorphins play a part in emotional states such as schizophrenia, in matters of addiction, in childbirth,[71] and in sustained physical activities.

Acute pain causes the release of endogenous opioids into the cerebrospinal fluid and into the bloodstream. The action of enkephalin is very short, lasting only a few seconds. The action of beta endorphin in the bloodstream is delayed by several minutes and lasts for longer periods. Although these actions, no doubt, do have some modulating effect on the pain experience, a sustained clinical analgesic effect requires slow but distinctly intermittent repetition of the pain input at a frequency of 1 to 3 Hz. Continuity of input soon nullifies the antinociceptive effect. The action of endorphins is partially, if not completely, arrested by the morphine antagonist naloxone.[72] Therefore, any modulating action that is significantly inhibited or arrested by naloxone is presumed to involve the endorphin antinociceptive system. No doubt, there is interaction between the brain stem descending inhibitory mechanism and the endogenous antinociceptive system. Enkephalin is known to inhibit the activity of thalamic projection neurons at postsynaptic sites.[73] Ward et al[74] reported that serotonin has a role in modulating chronic pain only, while beta endorphin has a role in modulating acute pain only.

Acupuncture and Electroacupuncture

Although acupuncture has been used in Chinese medicine for centuries, it came to public notice in the United States in 1972. Since then, much research has been directed toward this ancient modality of pain control. Needle acupuncture and electroacupuncture, which employs an electric current applied on the surface over acupoints, appear to work in the same general way: both depend on noxious stimulation of specific sites. Both induce the release of beta endorphin into the peripheral circulation.[75-82] Animal studies indicate a similar mechanism.[83] Some investigators believe, however, that acupuncture analgesia involves other mechanisms than the release of endorphin.[84]

Electroacupuncture differs from TENS. This method requires a current of sufficient intensity to cause pain and phasic muscle contractions, but at a very low frequency (2 Hz). The current must also be applied at specific sites where electrical impedance is low and where deeper nociceptors are available to be stimulated.[48] After an active induction period of about 20 to 30 minutes, the profound analgesic effect of acupuncture can be maintained for an hour or so by intermittent stimulation. After about 4 hours, it drops off substantially and is not truly effective again for 18 to 24 hours. When active stimulation is stopped, the residual analgesic effect drops 50% for each 15- to 17-minute interval.[85] Acupuncture nonresponders include about 15% to 20% of the population.

Although unrelated to acupuncture, other deep noxious stimulation such as strong visceral pain may activate a similar antinociceptive effect.[86] Stimulation of the thalamus also exerts a powerful antinociceptive effect, presumably by way of activated raphe neurons.[87] Other antinociceptive amines such as gamma-aminobutyric acid and glycine act as inhibitory neurotransmitters and likely are involved in the mechanism of stimulation-produced analgesia.[88]

TENS verses Acupuncture

Conventional TENS and classic acupuncture are antinociceptive procedures that are mediated by clearly different neural mechanisms. TENS relates to the brain stem analgesic system associated with the descending inhibitory system that releases serotonin, while acupuncture activates the endogenous antinociceptive system that releases endorphins. At the clinical level, however, the two methods of pain control have much in common. Conflicting research reports relative to the action of endorphins in the two methods abound.[89-92]

It is true that very low frequency stimulation (2 Hz) causes the release of enkephalins into the cerebrospinal fluid and beta endorphin into the bloodstream. Stimulation at 15 Hz or more causes the release of serotonin in the brain and dynorphin in the spinal cord, but no enkephalin. Local anesthesia of only the skin arrests TENS but not acupuncture. Only when it anesthetizes the more deeply located nociceptive neurons does it arrest the effect of acupuncture. Naloxone offsets only about half the analgesic effect of acupuncture, which indicates that more than just endorphins are involved.[83] In effectiveness, acupuncture therapy equals the tricyclic antidepressants for the treatment of depression, thus indicating that it does release serotonin into the cerebrospinal fluid in substantial amounts. Taken together, there is adequate evidence that acupuncture at least some of the time activates the brain stem descending inhibitory mechanism as well as the endogenous antinociceptive system. The conclusion that should be drawn is that the acupuncture method stimulates superficial cutaneous nonnociceptive neurons at least some of the time along with the deeper nociceptors located in muscle tissue. Techniques that take this into account should prove superior in clinical value.

Pain Modulation by Psychologic Factors

Some factors that modulate pain fit in a group considered to be psychologic. These factors will be briefly considered here but a more detailed description can be found in Chapter 5. Most psychologic factors are either excitatory factors or inhibitory factors.

Excitatory Modulating Factors. As a rule of thumb, egocentric psychologic conditions that center the subject's attention toward himself or herself have an excitatory effect on pain. This is borne out especially in the matter of attention. Wall determined that the level of pain due to injury was directly related to the degree of attention directed toward the injury at the time.[93,94] This appears to be true for all pains. The more one is absorbed with his suffering, the more intense it becomes.

Expectancy is another important factor.[95] Whether due to memory, anticipation, or prior conditioning, whatever one expects in the way of pain is likely to be what one experiences.[96,97]

The really potent excitatory modulators, however, are anxiety and fear, products of the consequences of the pain experience. Then, as maladaptive behavior ensues, depression and despair flourish, and chronicity associated with the depletion of endorphins sets in.[98] Problems of neuroticism[99] and secondary gain[95,100] that sometimes accompany suffering may further modulate the pain.

Inhibitory Modulating Factors. Generally, outgoing psychologic conditions that direct one's attention to energies away from self have a favorable modulating effect on pain. A feeling of serenity born of confidence and assurance has a marked inhibitory influence. Distraction is particularly inhibitory, as demonstrated by the effect of extraneous sounds,[101] suggestion and hypnosis,[102] mental absorption, and physical activities of different kinds.[103] Overcoming maladaptive behavior by constructively coping with the painful situation has a very favorable modulating influence.

Other Modulating Factors

Other factors relating to the noxious stimulus per se are known to modulate the experience of pain. It appears that factors such as modality, location, intensity, and duration of the physical characteristics of the stimulus itself have bearing on the discomfort that occurs. This implies that the higher centers receive accurate information concerning the stimulus and act on it by way of efferent neural circuits. This phenomenon presupposes the organic presence of bypass circuits in the brain stem that permit direct cerebral evaluation of the impulse before it arrives at the nucleus caudalis. Such circuits involving the lemniscal system have been identified.[104]

Summary

A prerequisite to the perception of orofacial pain sensation is the convergence of peripheral nociceptive impulses, other somatosensory inputs, and especially impulses descending from cortical structures that inhibit the sensory afferents.[105] It should be noted that pain is not a simple conduction of noxious impulses from the receptor through the primary peripheral neuron to synapse in the nucleus caudalis with the secondary medullary neuron, which in turn synapses in a thalamic nucleus with a third neuron that projects to the cerebral cortex where it is sensed and acted on. What is sensed as pain may not necessarily arise from noxious stimulation of peripheral receptors or fibers. Normal ongoing somatosensory input that ordinarily would not be perceived at all, or not at least as painful sensation, may be sensed as pain if certain centrally initiated inhibitory influences are not effective. Conversely, the overactivity of such inhibitory influence may cause the subject not to perceive noxious stimulation as pain that would under other circumstances unquestionably cause pain. Also, the general intensity of suffering relates to the preconditioning experience, attention, attitude, and temperament of the subject. This phenomenon of central pain modulation requires the organic presence of efferent neural circuits extending from the higher centers. Such circuits have been identified.[106] The central inhibitory mechanism is extremely complex.

Not only does a knowledge of modulation of nociceptive impulses help us to better understand pain, it also gives important clues that can be useful in the treatment of people who suffer with pain.

References

1. Ruch TC. Visceral sensation and referred pain. In Fulton JF (ed): A Textbook of Physiology, ed 16. Philadelphia: WB Saunders; 1949: 348–359.

2. Sessle BJ, Greenwood LF. Inputs to trigeminal brain stem neurons from facial, oral, tooth pulp and pharyngolaryngeal tissues: I. Responses to innocuous and noxious stimuli. Brain Res 1976; 117:211–226.

3. Hayashi H, Sumino R, Sessle BJ. Functional organization of trigeminal subnucleus interpolaris: nociceptive and innocuous afferent inputs. Projections to thalamus, cerebellum, and spinal cord, and descending modulation from periaqueductal gray. J Neurophysiol 1984; 51:890–905.

4. Olsen KA, Landgren S, Westberg KG. Location of, and peripheral convergence on, the interneurone in the disynaptic path from the coronal gyrus of the cerebral cortex to the trigeminal motonerones in the cat. Exp Brain Res 1986; 65:83–97.

5. Olsen KA, Westberg KG. Interneutones in the trigeminal motor system. In van Steenberghe D, DeLaat A (eds): Electromyography of Jaw Reflexes in Man. Leuven, Belgium: Leuven University Press; 1989: 19–50.

6. Sessle BJ, Hu JW. Mechanisms of pain arising from articular tissues. Can J Physiol Pharmacol 1991; 69:617–626.

7. Broton JG, Hu JW, Sessle BJ. Effects of temporomandibular joint stimulation on nociceptive and nonnociceptive neurons of the cat's trigeminal subnucleus caudalis (Medullary Dorsal Horn). J Neurophysiol 1988; 59:1575–1589.

8. Kojima Y. Convergence patterns of afferent information from the temporomandibular joint and masseter muscle in the trigeminal subnucleus caudalis. Brain Res Bull 1990; 24:609–616.

9. Howe JF, Loeser JD, Calvin WH. Mechanosensitivity of dorsal root ganglia and chronically injured axons: A physiological basis for the radicular pain of nerve root compression. Pain 1977; 3:25–41.

10. Procacci P, Zoppi M. Pathophysiology and clinical aspects of visceral and referred pain. In Bonica JJ, Lindblom U, Iggo A (eds): Advances in Pain Research and Therapy, vol 5. New York: Raven Press; 1983: 643–658.

11. Milne RJ, Foreman RD, Giesler GJ, et al. Viscerosomatic convergence into primate spinothalamic neurons: An explanation for referral of pelvic visceral pain. In Bonica JJ, Lindblom U, Iggo A (eds): Advances in Pain Research Pain Therapy, vol 5. New York: Raven Press; 1983: 131–137.

12. Sessle BJ, Hu JW, Amano N, et al. Convergence of cutaneous, tooth pulp, visceral, neck and muscle afferents onto nociceptive and nonnociceptive neurons in trigeminal subnucleus caudalis (medullary dorsal horn) and its implications for referred pain. Pain 1986; 27:219–235.

13. Cervero F, Laird JMA, Pozo MA. Selective changes of receptive field properties of spinal nociceptive neurons induced by noxious visceral stimulation in the cat. Pain 1992; 51: 335–342.

14. Gross D. Pain and autonomic nervous system. In Bonica JJ (ed): Advances in Neurology, vol 4. New York: Raven Press; 1974: 93–103.

15. Coderre TJ, Katz J, Vaccarino AL, Melzack R. Contribution of central neuroplasticity to pathological pain: Review of clinical and experimental evidence. Pain 1993; 52:259–285.

16. Woolf CJ, Thompson SWN. The induction and maintenance of central sensitization is dependent on N-methyl-D-aspartic acid receptor activation: Implications for the treatment of post-injury pain hypersensitivity. Pain 1991; 44:293–300.

17. Bonica JJ. The Management of Pain. Philadelphia: Lea & Febiger; 1989.

18. Wolff HG, Hardy JD. On nature of pain. Pain Res 1947; 27:167.

19. Kunkle EC, Kibler RF, Armstead GC, et al. Central sensory excitation and inhibition in response to induced pain. Trans Am Neurol Assoc 1949; 74:64.

20. Finneson BE. Diagnosis and Management of Pain Syndromes, ed 2. Philadelphia: WB Saunders; 1969.

21. Kunc Z. Significance of fresh anatomic data on spinal trigeminal tract for possibility of selective tractotomies. In Knighton RS, Dumke PR (eds): Pain. Boston: Little, Brown; 1966: 351–363.

22. Kunc Z. Significant factors pertaining to the results of trigeminal tractotomy. In Hassler R, Walker AE (eds): Trigeminal Neuralgia. Stuttgart: Georg Thieme Verlag; 1970: 90–100.

23. Kawamura Y, Nishiyama T. Projection of dental afferent impulses to the trigeminal nuclei. Jpn J Physiol 1966; 16:584–597.

24. Wolff HG. Headache and Other Head Pain, ed 2. New York: Oxford University Press; 1963: 35–47.

25. Treede RD, Cole JD. Dissociated secondary hyperalgesia in a subject with a large-fibre sensory neuropathy. Pain 1993; 53:169–174.

26. Cervero F, Meyer RA, Campbell JN. A psychophysical study of secondary hyperalgesia: Evidence of increased pain to input from nociceptors. Pain 1994; 58:21–28.

27. Tal M, Bennett GJ. Extra-territorial pain in rats with a peripheral mononeuropathy: Mechanohyperalgesia and mechano-allodynia in the territory of an uninjured nerve. Pain 1994; 57:375–382.

28. Fields HL. Pain. New York: McGraw-Hill; 1987: 28–40.

29. Broton JG, Sessle BJ. Reflex excitation of masticatory muscles induced by algesic chemicals applied to the temporomandibular joint of the cat. Arch Oral Biol 1988: 37:741.

30. Stohler CS, Wang JS, Veerasarn P. Motor unit behavior in response to experimental muscle pain (abstract 1313). J Dent Res 1990; 69:273.

31. Stohler C, Yamada Y, Ash MM. Antagonistic muscle stiffness and associated reflex behaviour in the pain-dysfunctional state. Helv Odont Acta 1985; 29:2.

32. Lund JP, Donga R, Widmer CG, Stohler CS. The pain-adaptation model: A discussion of the relationship between chronic musculoskeletal pain and motor activity. Can J Pharmacol 1991; 69:683.

33. Carlson CR, Okeson JP, Falace DA, Nitz AJ, Curran SL, Anderson DT. Comparison of psychologic and physiologic functioning between patients with masticatory muscle pain and matched controls. J Orofacial Pain 1993; 7:15–22.

34. Travell JG, Simons DG. Myofascial Pain and Dysfunction. The Trigger Point Manual. Baltimore: Williams & Wilkins; 1983: 5–13.

35. Marshall HR. Pain, Pleasure and Anesthesia. London: Macmillan; 1894.

36. Strong CA. The psychology of pain. Psychol Rev 1895; 2:329–347.

37. Maurice CG. Differential diagnosis of dental pain. J Am Dent Assoc 1955; 50:316.

38. Melzack R, Wall PD. Pain mechanisms: A new theory. Science 1965; 150:971–979.

39. Casey KL, Melzack R. Neural mechanisms of pain: A conceptual model. In Way EL (ed): New Concepts in Pain. Philadelphia: FA Davis; 1967: 13-31.

40. Wall PD. The gate control theory of pain mechanisms: A reexamination and restatement. Brain 1978; 101:1–18.

41. Perl ER. Unraveling the story of pain. In Fields HL, Dubner R, Cervero F (eds): Advances in Pain Research Therapy, vol 9. New York: Raven Press; 1985: 1–29.

42. Virtanen ASJ, Huopaniemi T, Narhi MVO, et al. The effect of temporal parameters on subjective sensation evoked by electrical tooth stimulation. Pain 1987; 30:361–371.

43. Matzner O, Devor M. Contrasting thermal sensitivity of spontaneously active A- and C-fibers in experimental nerve-end neuromas. Pain 1987; 30:373–384.

44. Ernst M, Lee MHM, Dworkin B, et al. Pain perception decrement produced through repeated stimulation. Pain 1986; 26:221–231.

45. Kane K, Taub A. A history of local electrical analgesia. Pain 1975; 1:125–138.

46. Wall PD, Sweet WH. Temporary abolition of pain in man. Science 1967; 155:108–109.

47. Long DM, Hagfors N. Electrical stimulation in the nervous system: The current status of electrical stimulation of the nervous system for relief of pain. Pain 1975; 1:109–123.

48. Andersson SA. Pain control by sensory stimulation. In Bonica JJ, Liebeskind JC, Albe-Fessard DG (eds): Advances in Pain Research and Therapy, vol 3. New York: Raven Press; 1979: 569–585.

49. Swett JE, Law JD. Analgesia with peripheral nerve stimulation: Absence of a peripheral mechanism. Pain 1983; 15:55–70.

50. Zimmerman M. Peripheral and central nervous mechanisms of nociception, pain, and pain therapy: Facts and hypotheses. In Bonica JJ, Liebeskind JC, Albe-Fessard DG (eds): Advances in Pain Research and Therapy, vol 3. New York: Raven Press; 1979: 3–32.

51. Bowsher D. Role of the reticular formation in response to noxious stimulation. Pain 1976; 2:361–378.

52. Sjolund BH, Eriksson MBF. Endorphins and analgesia produced bv peripheral conditioning stimulation. In Bonica JJ, Liebeskind JC, Albe-Fessard DG (eds): Advances in Pain Research and Therapy, vol 3. New York: Raven Press; 1979: 587–592.

53. Walker JB, Katz RL. Nonopioid pathways produce prolonged pain suppression in humans. Pain 1981; 11:141.

54. Long DM, Campbell J, Freeman T. Failure of naloxone to affect chronic pain or stimulation-induced pain relief in man. Pain 1981; 11:111.

55. Pertovaara A, Kemppainen P, Johansson G, et al. Dental analgesia produced by nonpainful, low-frequency stimulation is not influenced by stress or reversed by naloxone. Pain 1982; 13:379–384.

56. Wiler J, Roby A, Boulu P, et al. Comparative effects of electroacupuncture and transcutaneous nerve stimulation on the human blink reflex. Pain 1982; 14:267–278.

57. Freeman TB, Campbell JN, Long DM. Naloxone does not affect pain relief induced by electrical stimulation in man. Pain 1983; 17:189–195.

58. Ellis M. The relief of pain by cooling of the skin. Br Med J 1961; 1:250–252.

59. Steinman JL, Komisaruk BR, Yaksh TL, et al. Spinal cord monoamines modulate the antinociceptive effects of vaginal stimulation in rats. Pain 1983; 16:155–166.

60. Bowsher D. Role of the reticular formation in responses to noxious stimulation. Pain 1976; 2:361–378.

61. Wall PD, Devor M. Sensory afferent impulses originate from dorsal root ganglia as well as from the periphery in normal and nerve injured rats. Pain 1983; 17:321–339.

62. Wall PD. Central control system syndromes: Disorder of sensory systems when the homeostatic set point may be changed. Pain 1987; 31:217.

63. Snyder SH. Opiate receptors and internal opiates. Sci Am 1977; 236:44–56.

64. Kosten TR, Kieber HD. Control of nociception by endogenous opioids. Mediguide Pain 1987; 8:1-5.

65. Fields HL. Pain. New York: McGraw-Hill; 1987: 99–125.

66. Basbaum AT. Brain stem control of nociception: The contribution of the monoamines. Pain 1981; 11:231.

67. Belcher G, Ryall RW, Schaffner R. The differential effects of 5-hydroxytryptamine, noradrenalin, and raphe stimulation on nociceptive and nonnociceptive dorsal horn interneurons in the cat. Brain Res 1978; 151:307–321.

68. Sessle B, Hu JW. Raphe-induced suppression of the jaw-opening reflex and single neurons in trigeminal subnucleus oralis, and influence of naloxone and subnucleus caudalis. Pain 1981; 10:19–36.

69. Lovick TA, Wolstencroft JH. Inhibitory effects of nucleus raphe magnus on neuronal responses in the spinal trigeminal nucleus to nociceptive compared with nonnociceptive inputs. Pain 1979; 7:135–145.

70. Bowsher D. Role of the reticular formation in response to noxious stimulation. Pain 1976; 2:361–378.

71. Goolkasian P, Rimer BA. Pain reactions in pregnant women. Pain 1984; 29:87–95.

72. Seltzer S. Pain Control in Dentistry. Philadelphia: JB Lippincott Co; 1978.

73. Dubner R. Specialization of nociceptive pathways: Sensory discrimination, sensory modulation, and neural connectivity. In Fields HL, Dubner R, Cervero F (eds): Advances in Pain Research and Therapy, vol 9. New York: Raven Press; 1985: 111–137.

74. Ward NB, Bokan JA, Aug J, et al. Differential effects of fenfluramine and dextroamphetamine on acute and chronic pain. In Fields HL, Dubner R, Cervero F (eds): Advances in Pain Research and Therapy, vol 9. New York: Raven Press; 1985: 753–760.

75. Sjolund B, Terenius L, Eriksson M. Increased cerebrospinal fluid levels of endorphins after electroacupuncture. Acta Physiol Scand 1977; 100:382–384.

76. Pomeranz B, Cheng R. Suppression of noxious responses in single neurons of cat spinal cord by electroacupuncture and its reversal by the opiate antagonist naloxone. Exp Neurol 1979; 64:327–341.

77. Cheng RSS, Pomeranz BH. Electroacupuncture analgesia is mediated by stereospecific opiate receptors and is reversed by antagonists of type I receptors. Life Sci 1980; 26:631–638.

78. Salar G, Job I, Mingrino S, et al. Effect of transcutaneous electrotherapy on CSF beta-endorphin content in patients without pain problems. Pain 1981; 10:169–172.

79. Stratton SA. Role of endorphins in pain modulation. J Orthoped Sports Phys Ther 1982; 3:200–205.

80. Kosten TR, Kieber HD. Control of nociception by endogenous opioids. Mediguide Pain 1987; 8:1–5.

81. He L. Involvement of endogenous opioids in acupuncture analgesia. Pain 1987; 31:99-121.

82. Lee JH, Beitz AJ. The distribution of brainstem and spinal cord nuclei associated with different frequencies of electroacupuncture analgesia. Pain 1993; 52:11–28.

83. Han J, Zhou Z, Xuan Y. Acupuncture has an analgesic effect in rabbits. Pain 1983; 15:83–91.

84. Chapman CR, Benedetti C, Colpitts YH, et al. Naloxone fails to reverse pain thresholds elevated by acupuncture: Acupuncture analgesia reconsidered. Pain 1983; 16:13-31.

85. Research Group of Acupuncture Anesthesia, Peking Medical College. Effect of acupuncture on the pain threshold of human skin. Natl Med J Chin 1973; 3:151–157.

86. Kraus E, LeBars L, Besson JM. Behavioral confirmation of diffuse noxious inhibitory controls (DNIC) and evidence for a role of endogenous opiates. Brain Res 1981; 206:495–499.

87. Dickenson A. The inhibitory effects of thalamic stimulation on spinal transmission of nociceptive information in the cat. Pain 1983; 17:213–224.

88. Lovick T, Wolstencroft JH. Actions of GABA, glycine, methionine-enkephalin, and beta endorphin compared with electrical stimulation of nucleus raphe magnus on responses evoked by tooth pulp stimulation in the medial reticular formation in the cat. Pain 1983; 15: 131–144.

89. Boureau F, Luu M, Kisielnicki E. Effects of transcutaneous nerve stimulation (TNS), electrotherapy (ET), and electroacupuncture (EA) on chronic pain: A comparative study. Pain 1981; 11:277.

90. Chapman CR, Colpitts YM, Benedetti C, et al. Evoked potential assessment of acupuncture analgesia: Attempted reversal with naloxone. Pain 1980; 9:183–197.

91. Peets JM, Pomaranz B. Intrathecal or systemic naloxone antagonizes TNS analgesia. Pain 1981; 11:179.

92. Lee JH, Beitz AJ. The distribution of brainstem and spinal cord nuclei associated with different frequencies of electroacupuncture analgesia. Pain 1993; 52:11–28.

93. Wall PD. On the relation of injury to pain. Pain 1979; 6:253–264.

94. Melzack R, Wall PD, Ty TC. Acute pain in an emergency clinic: Latency of onset and descriptor patterns related to different injuries. Pain 1982; 14:33–43.

95. Price DD, Barren JJ, Gracely RH. A psychophysical analysis of experimental factors that selectively influence the affective dimension of pain. Pain 1980; 8:137–149.

96. Dworkin SF, Chen ACN, Schubert M. Expectancy, nitrous oxide (N20) and modification of pain in a clinical setting. Pain 1981; 11:171.

97. Fordyce WE. Behavioral conditioning concepts in chronic pain. In Bonica JJ, Lindblom U, Iggo A (eds): Advances in Pain Research and Therapy, vol 5. New York: Raven Press; 1983: 781–788.

98. Lindblom U, Tegner R. Are the endorphins active in clinical pain states? Narcotic antagonism in chronic pain patients. Pain 1979; 7:65–68.

99. Sternbach RA, Timmermans G. Personality changes associated with reduction of pain. Pain 1975; 1:177–181.

100. Sternbach RA: Varieties of pain games. In Bonica JJ (ed): Advances in Neurology, vol 4. New York: Raven Press; 1974: 423-430.

101. Gardner WJ, Licklider JCR. Auditory analgesia in dental operations. J Am Dent Assoc 1959; 59:1144–1149.

102. Orne MT. Hypnotic methods for managing pain. In Bonica JJ, Lindblom U, Iggo A (eds): Advances in Pain Research and Therapy, vol 5. New York: Raven Press; 1983: 847–856.

103. Szechtman FI, Hershkowitz M, Simantov R. Sexual behavior decreases pain sensitivity and stimulates endogenous opioids in male rats. Eur J Pharmacol 1981; 70:279–285.

104. Darian-Smith I. The neural coding of tactile stimulus parameters in different trigeminal nuclei. In Hassler R, Walker AE (eds): Trigeminal Neuralgia. Stuttgart: Georg Thieme Verlag; 1970: 59-72.

105. Hassler R. Dichotomy of facial pain conduction in the diencephalon. In Hassler R, Walker AE (eds): Trigeminal Neuralgia. Stuttgart: Georg Thieme Verlag; 1970: 123–138.

106. Wiesendanger M, Hammer B, Hepp-Reymond MC. Corticofugal control mechanisms of somatosensory transmission in the spinal trigeminal nucleus of the cat. In Hassler R, Walker AE (eds): Trigeminal Neuralgia. Stuttgart: Georg Thieme Verlag; 1970: 86–89.

Section II

Clinical Considerations of Orofacial Pains

5 | The Psychology of Pain

In the previous chapters, the pathways that carry nociceptive impulses have been mapped out in detail. Factors that influence these incoming and outgoing impulses have also been described (pain modulation). What now needs to be discussed is the effect of nociceptive impulses on the higher brain centers. Remember nociception is not pain until it reaches and is processed by the higher centers. The main higher centers to be considered are the thalamus, cortex, and limbic structures (including the hypothalamus). It is only through interaction of these areas of the brain that the patient begins to give the nociceptive impulses meaning. It is this interpretation provided by these higher centers that separates us from the lower animals. It is at this level that suffering and pain behavior begins.

Factors that Influence the Pain Experience

Once nociceptive impulses reach the higher centers, the patient makes judgment on the pain experience according to at least four factors or conditions: (1) the level of arousal of the brain stem, (2) prior experiences, (3) the emotional state, and (4) certain behavioral traits. Each of these factors will now be discussed.

Level of Arousal of the Brain Stem

As mentioned in Chapter 4, the dorsal root ganglia continuously generate an ongoing barrage of sensory impulses that are poured into the central nervous system (CNS).[1] This constant flow of sensory input can be enhanced by the reticular formation and countered by the descending inhibitory system. This means that there is already a ready source of potentially painful neural impulses at all times just waiting for a decrease in the level of systemic inhibitory influence. When inadequately inhibited, these neural impulses are felt as pain even when there is no local cause. The ongoing neocortical evaluation of our sensibilities may alter the regulating influence of the brain stem descending inhibitory mechanism so that all shades of modulation, excitatory and inhibitory, may occur. In other words, if a nociceptive impulse enters a normally calm, well-functioning brain stem, the impulse may never reach the higher centers and if it did it would not likely initiate a significant response. If, however, the same impulse enters a brain stem with an upregulated reticular formation and little descending inhibition, the impulse could greatly affect higher center response. This is seen clinically in patients who have suffered with pain for a prolonged time. In these individuals, the brain stem is upregulated and even small levels of nociception often produce significant pain responses.

Prior Experiences

Once the nociceptive impulses pass through the brain stem, they move to the thalamus. The thalamus recognizes these sensory impulses as important and directs them to the sensory cortex and limbic structures for interpretation. The cortex is responsible for storing all memory of experiences. It has long been recognized that one's previous pain experience may profoundly influence, if not actually generate, clinical pain. All mammals appear to demonstrate these conditioning effects. Humans are no exception. In fact, humans are subject to autoconditioning, which can greatly affect their response to pain. The repetition of similar circumstances can generate clinical pain like that associated with a former traumatic experience even though no actual noxious stimulation occurs. In lesser ways, prior conditioning exercises can influence a wide variety of acute pain complaints. It perhaps forms the basis for expectancy, which is an important psychologic modulating factor. Prior conditioning, expectancy, and memory may bear on the peculiar tendency of some pain syndromes to cycle, a phenomenon that is very poorly understood. It is

important to recognize such conditions if management is to be effective. It is the cortex that gives meaning and consequence to the painful experience.

Emotional State

When the nociceptive impulses reach the thalamus, they are not only directed to the cortex but also to the limbic structures. It is at these sites that the pain experience is evaluated on an entirely different level; an emotional level. As discussed in Chapter 2, the limbic structures border the cerebrum and diencephalon. These structures contain certain centers or nuclei that are responsible for specific emotions and behaviors. When pain is perceived by the limbic system, certain emotions can be precipitated. Early on these emotions may be fear or rage, which represent protective actions in an attempt to move the individual away from the source of nociception. Later, if the pain experience is prolonged, the emotion may change to a sense of helplessness, sadness, or depression.[2,3] The emotional state of the individual at the time when the pain is initiated can greatly influence the pain experience. If the patient is calm, comfortable, and has a sense of well-being, the pain experience is minimized. If, however, the patient is excited, angry, or agitated, the pain experience is enhanced.

Another significant influencing factor is stress. Stress can be thought of as the individual's response to environmental challenges. These challenges may be physical such as a rapidly approaching automobile while crossing the street. In this situation, the individual responds to the challenge with the alarm or *stress response*. As discussed in Chapter 2, this response is driven by the sympathetic portion of the autonomic nervous system. To rapidly respond to this threat, the sympathetic nervous system quickly increases the blood pressure, blood flow to muscles, and muscle strength. In addition, the sympathetic activity increases certain cellular metabolic functions and generally increases mental activity. These rapid changes in body functions allow the individual to carry out important tasks, for example, quickly crossing the street to avoid an oncoming automobile. This response is called the *fight or flight response*. The body is built to respond to these types of challenges and then return to normal functioning. This response is basic to survival.

Unfortunately there are some challenges or stressors that are not momentary and therefore continue to elicit a fight or flight response over time. These prolonged challenges can impact greatly on functions of the brain stem and higher centers. Many of these challenges are not physical but represent a continued emotional challenge present in an environmental situation. For example, an individual is employed in a position associated with significant responsibilities, deadlines, and unhappy co-workers. Although there does not appear to be any immediate physical threat to the individual, these conditions are likely to significantly increase sympathetic nervous system activity. This type of threat is often referred to as emotional stress. There is a strong relationship between pain and *emotional stress*. Sternbach[4] reported that the greater the stress, the greater the frequency and severity of pain. He stated that stress is a major cause of headaches, backaches, stomach pains, and menstrual pain. The effect of emotional stress on pain, suffering, and pain behavior is enormous and must be considered when evaluating or managing any pain condition.

Carlson et al[5,6] have demonstrated that the major difference between patients with masticatory muscle pain and a control group was the patients' sympathetic response to psychologic stressors. It would appear that these patients with muscle pain have upregulated their sympathetic nervous system so that it reacts more quickly to stressors. This alteration in sympathetic responsiveness is likely to be a significant factor in some chronic pain disorders. The importance of this concept will be discussed in later chapters.

Behavioral Traits

As previously discussed, once nociceptive impulses reach the thalamus they are directed to the cortex and limbic structures for interpretation. Past experiences stored in the cortex as well as the present emotional state influence the pain experience. There is still another dimension to the pain experience that represents direct interaction between the cortex and the limbic structures. This interaction relates to behavior. As mentioned in Chapter 2, the limbic structures contain certain centers of neural activities. Among these centers is the pain/pleasure center that drives the individual toward behaviors that stimulate the pleasure side of the center. These drives are not generally perceived at a conscious level but more as a basic instinct. These instinctive responses result in certain behaviors that present at a clinical level. For example, when an individual experiences chronic pain, behavior will be orientated toward withdrawal from any stimulus that may increase the pain. Often the sufferer will withdraw from life itself and mood alterations such as depression will appear.

Once the limbic system has emotionally labeled the pain and the cortex has given the pain meaning and consequence according to past experiences, the individual reacts with a certain behavior. Some individuals may place significant meaning and emotion on the pain and suffer greatly. Others experiencing the exact same level of pain may place little meaning and emotion and not suffer at all.

The four factors that have just been discussed determine the response of the individual to nociceptive impulses. One can quickly understand that the experience of pain is the result of complex interactions in the higher centers. This helps explain why the experience of pain is as individual as people. These functions separate us from the lower animals. In many lower animals, fast pain is the predominant drive for behavior and is heavily related to reflex responses. In the higher animals, slow pain is common, resulting in intense processing of impulses, which gives the pain meaning and consequence and eventually leads to suffering. We do not have evidence that lower animals suffer.

The influence of the higher centers on nociception is commonly referred to as the *psychologic aspect of pain*. These processes have not been well studied, yet play an extremely important role in clinical pain. Unfortunately it is often used as an excuse or avenue of escape by the inexperienced clinician. In other words, all too often when the clinician finds no somatic reason for pain, the patient is believed to have a psy-chologic problem. I will always remember sitting in a lecture by Dr Welden Bell[7] when he reported that early in his career he saw many patients with psychogenic pains. Yet at the time of his retirement from practice, some 56 years later, he rarely saw psychogenic pains. This was his way of saying that as the clinician becomes more experienced, he or she begins to understand the many possible diagnoses that exist and pain disorders begin to make more sense. The inexperienced clinician will often have the tendency to label unknown pains as psychogenic. This leads to inappropriate patient treatment and can only be improved by educating the clinician.

Psychologic Factors Influence All Pains

Each time nociceptive impulses reach the thalamus, cortex, and limbic structures, psychologic factors influence the processing of pain. The clinician must appreciate that all pains, whether brief or long-term, whether somatic or neuropathic, whether slow or fast are influenced by psychologic factors. Some types of pains are influenced more than others (as will be discussed) but all pains are affected. For the clinician to better understand the patient's pain disorder, one must first begin with an understanding and acknowledgment of the disease model on which he or she is basing therapy. There are two basic medical disease models: the mechanistic model and the biopsychosocial model.

Mechanistic Model versus the Biopsychosocial Model

Most clinicians and also their patients have been trained to believe that all pains arise from somatic disease or structural damage. This concept makes clinical sense and is reinforced when one falls and injuries a knee. The damaged tissue causes pain and once the tissue heals, the pain resolves. This same concept is reinforced in the dental office when a patient reports with a toothache and after the offending tissue (pulp) is removed, the pain is eliminated. This model is known as the *mechanistic model* of disease and implies that when pain is present there is always something wrong with a part of the body (somatic pain). According to this model, all the clinician needs to do to resolve the pain is to find the offending part and repair it. Although this may be appropriate for some somatic pains, it certainly does not represent all pains.

A more accurate way to understand the experience of pain is through the *biopsychosocial model* of disease. This model suggests that the person is a complex unit and that one cannot separate the mind from the body especially when nociception is being experienced. Since nociception enters the CNS from the somatic structures (bio), it passes through the reticular formation and up to the higher centers. The interaction between the higher centers can be thought of as the psychosocial influence on the pain experience. As an example, consider two individuals who both awake one morning with identical pains in the masseter muscles secondary to bruxism. The first individual feels the pain, acknowledges it as soreness from muscle overuse, and goes on with his daily activities. The threat of this pain is

minimum and the consequence insignificant. The other individual, however, awakes, feels the pain but has no appreciation for its origin. In considering this pain, the person remembers an aunt who died 2 years ago from cancer of the jaw. Suddenly the meaning and consequence of this pain becomes enormous. This individual will begin to suffer and the pain behavior will quickly drive him or her to seek care. It is important to recognize that these two individuals are experiencing the same amount of nociception (bio) yet their pain, suffering, and pain behavior (psychosocial) are quite different. It is also important to recognize that the validity of the belief does not influence the amount of pain and suffering. In other words, it does not matter if the individual actually has cancer, if the individual believes he has cancer, the suffering begins. The biopsychosocial model reflects this pain experience and represents the best model for the clinician who manages pain disorders. This model is especially important when one considers chronic pain (as will be discussed).

Figure 5-1 attempts to graphically depict the biopsychosocial model of disease. The "bio" represents the nociceptive input arising from the somatic tissues and the "psychosocial" component arises from interaction between the thalamus, cortex, and limbic structures. The neurotransmission of impulses between all these higher centers is responsible for what we call the psychological aspects of pain. In fact, like all neural functions, psychological factors and moods are based on neurotransmitter activity. Although some cling to the notion that psychological activity somehow operates independently of somatic structures, there is a preponderance of evidence that points to an

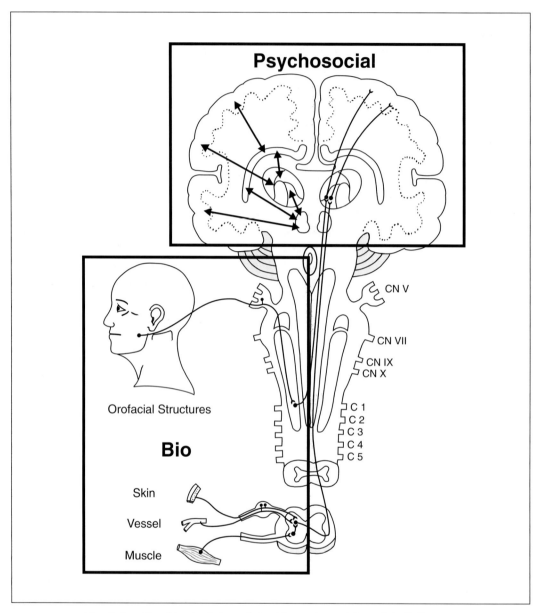

Fig 5-1 Graphic depiction of the biopsychosocial model of disease. The *Bio* is represented by the somatosensory nociceptive input arising in the peripheral structures. The *pyschosocial* factors are represented by the interaction of the thalamus, cortex, hypothalamus, and other limbic structures as the nociceptive input enters the higher centers. No pain is perceived without some influence from the psychosocial factors. *CN* = cranial nerve.

organic neural basis for all such activity. Receptors, neurons, synapses, electric charges, and neurochemicals are the structural elements that underlie all functional activities, psychologic as well as physiologic. Neurochemistry seems to be the key to such mechanisms. One day in a seminar, one of my residents made the following statement: "Psychology is really neurology not yet understood."[8] I believe this was is a very profound statement, revealing great insight. Knowledge of neurotransmitter activity is a key in pain management and, in fact, in all body functions. Additional neurochemicals are being identified almost daily. No doubt, as these mechanisms are better understood, we shall know a great deal more about psychologic behavior and pain.

Acute Pain vs Chronic Pain

Acute pain refers to pains that are of short duration. They are often closely related to somatic tissue changes such as those produced by trauma or disease. Chronic pain refers to pains of long duration and these pains take on a different therapeutic meaning. Most clinicians use the term chronic pain to depict any pain that has lasted longer than 6 months regardless of its origin. Although this is the classic definition perhaps a better concept of chronic pain would be pains that last longer than normal healing time. It is expected that tissue damage will produce nociception and pain but when healing is complete, pain should subside. If pain continues after normal healing time, the origin of the pain is in doubt. One reason for continued pain is the influence of psychologic factors. As pain becomes protracted, a shift in the origin of the pain can be expected from primary somatosensory input to the affective, cognitive, and behavioral origins of pain. As the duration of pain input continues, the level of suffering increases even when the intensity of somatosensory input remains the same. In fact, chronic pain can sustain a high level of discomfort even though the intensity of the somatosensory input may decrease or disappear altogether. It follows that a sustained level of discomfort may remain even after the initiating cause has resolved. With chronicity, all pains, regardless of initial type or origin, seem to take on the clinical characteristics of *psychogenic intensification*. Psychogenic intensification refers to the clinical finding that as pains become chronic, the pain experience can intensify even as the somatosensory input decreases. As such, some chronic orofacial pain disorders display features suggestive of depressive illness. Treatment measures effective for alleviating acute pain may no longer be applicable. As pain becomes chronic, management options shift from local to systemic and central modalities. Pain that initially could be managed on a purely dental level may require extensive and coordinated interdisciplinary therapy when it becomes chronic.

When considering the effects of acute and chronic pains on the biopsychosocial model, one realizes that early in the pain experience the somatosensory input (bio) has the greatest influence on the pain experience. As pain becomes protracted, the influence from the higher centers (psychosocial) will likely predominate (Fig 5-2). As already stated, this has therapeutic significance.

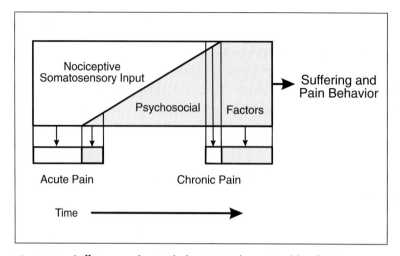

Fig 5-2 Suffering and pain behavior is determined by the interaction of the ascending somatosensory (Bio) input with the input from the thalamus, cortex, and limbic structures (psychosocial factors). The longer the pain is present, the greater the psychosocial factor influence. Acute pain is predominately influenced by somatosensory input. As pain becomes chronic, suffering and pain behavior are more greatly influenced by the psychosocial factors. Understanding this relationship will greatly improve the selection of effective therapy.

Emotional Significance of Orofacial Pains

Historically, considerable emotional significance has been attached to pain in that it was once thought to have a beneficial effect on the person who suffered. In the sense that pain represented a penalty or punishment, it served the purpose of a guilt-canceling device and as such was thought to cleanse the soul.[9] Painful experience therefore has deep religious and moral roots that affect human attitudes even today.

The emotional significance of orofacial pain has important implications, especially in relation to concepts of body image. As therapists, we must never lose sight of the emotional significance of the orofacial structures. The face is the major source of expression, communication, and gratifica-

tion. We depend on these structures for both physical and emotional survival in our environment. We use these structures to express our feelings to others, providing gratification and satisfaction. We also depend on these structures to bring in nutrients that allow the individual to exist. Distortion of this image due to abuse, injury, or surgery may initiate a pain experience that has meaning far beyond somatic tissue damage. It is important for the clinician to keep this in mind when approaching a patient with orofacial pain. If the clinician aggressively approaches the orofacial structures, the patient may feel threatened and the pain experience may heighten. It is best to first establish a rapport and confidence with the patient and then, with a degree of respect, begin to examine the orofacial structures.

100

Depending on past emotional experiences, especially from childhood, one may use pain to gain attention, substitute for other forms of aggression, or express grief.[10] Pain may even be used by the sufferer to receive certain benefits. It commonly excuses one from carrying out an unpleasant task. Headaches have been used frequently as socially acceptable excuses. Pain may serve as a means of avoiding responsibilities, the actual physical pain being the lesser of the two forms of suffering. To be the center of attention may, in some cases, be ego-building.[11] Pain, as with other illness, can be used as a weapon or threat against those over whom the subject would have his way. Thus the victim not only becomes defenseless against his pain-ridden aggressor but frequently is made to suffer with him. When a patient benefits from his or her pain experience, the patient is said to receive *secondary gains*. Secondary gains can have a significant impact on the effectiveness of therapy.[12] Often patients who receive secondary gains will not relinquish their pain even to what appears as appropriate therapies until these beneficial issues are addressed.

Pain may also become a dependable crutch to sustain the subject in a variety of emotional situations. In some instances the patient may not even be aware of this emotional crutch (wholly subconscious). It may be a form of malingering to avoid duty. Sometimes it may even represent justification for addiction to narcotic drugs.

Psychologic Considerations of Orofacial Pains

Orofacial pain disorders can be influenced by a variety of psychologic conditions. Sometimes the psychologic factors directly affect an existing physical condition. For example, a patient may be suffering with masseter muscle pain but reports that the pain is much greater on days when things are not going well at work. The physical condition is the muscle pain but when the psychologic factor of emotional stress is increased, the pain experience is intensified. In this instance, the physical condition is the predominant source of nociception and the psychologic factor is merely a contributor to the pain experience. Other influencing psychologic factors may be anxiety, fear, rage, or depression.[13]

In other patients, these psychologic factors may represent significant mental disorders that may actually be the major contributing factor to the pain condition. For example, there are significant mood disorders and anxiety disorders that may present with certain physical conditions (ie, pain). It is important for the clinician to appreciate this since the therapeutic approach is quite different.

Another mental disorder that needs to be appreciated is somatization. With *somatoform disorders*, an individual may report physical complaints with no evidence of any physical condition. If pain is the chief complaint, the condition is called a *somatoform pain disorder*. Other types of somatoform disorders are conversion disorders and hypochondriasis. Clinicians who are unaware of these disorders will often attempt to treat the patient's physical complaint by directing treatment to the somatic structures associated with the complaint. Since these structures are not the origin of the symptoms, treatment will fail. Other mental disorders that need to be considered are malingering, personality traits or coping style, and maladaptive health behavior. These disorders will be discussed in more detail in later chapters.

References

1. Wall PD, Devor M. Sensory afferent impulses originate from dorsal root ganglia as well as from the periphery in normal and nerve injured rats. Pain 1983; 17:321–339.

2. Chapman CR, Turner JA. Psychological control of acute pain in medical settings. J Pain Symptom Manage 1986; 1:9–20.

3. Magni G, Marchetti M, Moreschi C, Merskey H, Luchini SR. Chronic musculoskeletal pain and depressive symptoms in the National Health and Nutrition Examination. I. Epidemiologic follow-up study. Pain 1993; 53:163–168.

4. Sternbach RA. Pain and "hassles" in the United States: Findings of the Nuprin Pain Report. Pain 1986; 27:69–80.

5. Carlson CR, Okeson JP, Falace DA, Nitz AJ, Curran SL, Anderson DT. Comparison of psychologic and physiologic functioning between patients with masticatory muscle pain and matched controls. J Orofacial Pain 1993; 7:15–22.

6. Curran SL, Carlson CR, Okeson JP. Behavioral and physiological responses to laboratory challenge: Temporomandibular disorder patients vs matched controls. Submitted for review.

7. Bell WE. Personal communication, 1982. Lexington, Ky.

8. Bertrand P. Personal communication, 1993. Lexington, Ky.

9. Bonica JJ. The Management of Pain. Philadelphia: Lea & Febiger; 1953.

10. Pilling LF. Psychosomatic aspects of facial pain. In Alling CC, Mahan PE (eds): Facial Pain, ed 2. Philadelphia: Lea & Febiger; 1977: 213–226.

11. Romano JM, Turner JA, Friedman LS, Bulcroft RA, Jensen MP, Hpos H, Wright SF. Sequential analysis of chronic pain behaviors and spouse responses. J Consul Clin Psych 1992; 60:777–782.

12. Romano JM, Turner JA, Friedman LS, Bulcroft RA, Jensen MP, Hpos H, Wright SF. Sequential analysis of chronic pain behaviors and spouse responses. J Consul Clin Psych 1992; 60:777–782.

13. Magni G, Marchetti M, Moreschi C, Merskey H, Luchini SR. Chronic musculoskeletal pain and depressive symptoms in the National Health and Nutrition Examination. I. Epidemiologic follow-up study. Pain 1993; 53:163–168.

6 | The Genesis of Pain

The genesis of pain is poorly understood, if, indeed, it is understood at all. There was a time when it was generally thought that noxious stimulation, meaning tissue-damaging stimulation, was the chief basis for nociception. It was presumed that pain was some kind of gauge of tissue injury: the greater the pain, the greater the injury that had been sustained. Pain occurring without an initiating antecedent was presumed to be generated by psychic phenomena and therefore was not really pain at all.

As the concept of pain modulation evolved, the question of genesis lost much of its significance. It is now recognized that factors other than noxious stimulation are determinants of discomfort. For example, Wall[1] has shown that pain at the time of injury relates to the attention given; pain later relates to the consequences of the injury and its treatment. Algogenic substances that accompany inflammation incidental to tissue injury require time to develop and therefore are not immediate determinants in the matter of pain from tissue damage per se. So, structural injury from mechanical, chemical, or thermal trauma, as it relates to the genesis of pain, abounds in uncertainty.

Not All Pains Are Alike

The word pain has different meanings to different individuals. Certainly the clinician who attempts to understand and manage pain needs to have a thorough appreciation of the different types of pain that can be encountered. Several types of pains will now be contrasted.

Clinical vs Experimental Pain

Beecher[2] pointed out that pain as presented by patients, so-called clinical or pathologic pain, is different from experimental pain induced and studied in the laboratory. The difference is illustrated in the capacity of morphine to give relief. A large dose of morphine does not significantly alter the brief jabs of experimental pain, while a much smaller dose consistently reduces pain that has meaning to the patient. The difference is also borne out in placebo effects. Beecher determined that the average effectiveness of placebos when dealing with clinical pain was about 35%, whereas it was only 3.2% with experimental pain. Nyquist and Eriksson,[3] in commenting on this problem, said, "We interpret our findings to suggest that clinical and experimental pain are explained by different mechanisms and that direct correlations cannot be drawn between them." Bromm[4] believed that experimental pain was actually a measurement of the sensory-discriminative component only, not the aversive-emotional component displayed in clinical pain.

It is likely that the emotional significance embodied in clinical pain is the real determinant. Indeed, the purpose of the signal detection (sensory decision) theory for determining the effectiveness of analgesic medications is to minimize this bias factor.[5,6]

It should be noted that there is a definite relationship between intensity and duration of pain. The higher the intensity, the shorter the period that can be tolerated by the sufferer. Low-intensity pain can be sustained for up to 7 hours, whereas maximum-intensity pain can be tolerated for no more than a few seconds. The higher the intensity, the more likely it is that the pain will be intermittent. Only low-intensity pain can be protracted. Intractable pain, regardless of the patient's contention to the contrary, must be either periodic or of extremely low intensity. In fact, intractable pain may be little more than an unpleasant or unwanted sensation.[7,8]

Acute vs Chronic Pain

As the duration of pain input continues, the level of suffering increases even though the intensity of the input remains the same. In fact, protracted input may sustain a high level of discomfort although the intensity decreases or disappears altogether. It follows that a sustained level of discomfort may remain even after the initiating cause has resolved. With chronicity, all pains regardless of initial type or origin seem to take on the clinical characteristics of psychologic intensification. As such, some chronic orofacial pain syndromes display features suggestive of depressive illness. Treatment effective for alleviating acute pain may no longer be applicable. As pain becomes chronic, management options shift from local to systemic modalities. Pain that initially could be managed on a purely dental level may require extensive and coordinated interdisciplinary therapy when it becomes chronic.

Primary vs Secondary Pain

The site where pain is felt may or may not identify the location of the source of pain. If the pain does in fact emanate from the structures that hurt, it constitutes a primary nociceptive input. If, however, the true source of pain is located elsewhere, the area of discomfort represents secondary pain. Secondary pains are called *heterotopic pains* and will be discussed in detail in future chapters.

Stimulus-Evoked vs Spontaneous Pain

Most primary somatic pains result from stimulation of neural structures that innervate the site. The actual stimulus may be obscure and positive identification difficult, but the clinical characteristics displayed by stimulus-evoked pain relate to the location, timing, and intensity of such stimulus. Some pains, however, occur spontaneously and do not require a stimulating force. Neuropathic pain may be felt spontaneously along the peripheral distribution of the affected nerve, while heterotopic pains may occur spontaneously as far as the site of pain is concerned.

Somatic vs Neuropathic Pain

Pain emanating from a particular area may result from noxious stimulation of the somatic structures. When this occurs, the nociceptive impulses are being received and transmitted by normal components of the sensory nervous system. Such pain is referred to as *somatic pain.* This type of pain presents clinical characteristics that relate to the effect of stimulation of normal neural structures. Quite a different type of pain, however, may emanate from the same area not from abnormality in the structures in the area but because of abnormality in the neural components that innervate the area. Such pain is termed *neuropathic.* This type of pain presents clinical characteristics that relate to the type and location of the neural abnormality rather than to noxious stimulation as such.

Superficial vs Deep Somatic Pain

Pains emanating from the cutaneous and mucogingival tissues present clinical characteristics that are similar to other exteroceptive sensations. They can be located precisely and relate faithfully to provocation in timing, location, and intensity. In contrast, pains due to stimulation of deeper musculoskeletal and visceral structures resemble other proprioceptive and interoceptive sen-

sations. As such, they are more diffusely felt, are less faithfully responsive to provocation, and frequently initiate secondary effects such as referred pain and muscle spasm activity.

Musculoskeletal vs Visceral Pain

Not all deep somatic pains are alike. Deep somatic pain that emanates from muscles, bones, joints, tendons, ligaments, and soft connective tissue bear a close relationship to the demands of biomechanical function. Such pain also yields a graduated response to noxious stimulation. Visceral structures, however, are innervated by high-threshold receptors so that pain usually is not felt until the threshold level is reached. Such pains therefore do not ordinarily yield a graduated response to noxious stimulation and are less responsive to biomechanical function.

Normal Neural Activities

Central and Peripheral Mechanisms

With the discovery of the normal ongoing barrage of afferent signals generated in the dorsal root ganglia as countered by action of the brain stem descending inhibitory mechanism, a better concept of pain inception and accentuation has developed. It is known that peripheral nerve injury accentuates this generation of impulses.[9] Likewise, it is known that nonpainful sensation conducted by the superficial cutaneous nerves effectively accentuates the inhibitory activity of the descending mechanism and, thus, shifts the balance away from painful sensation experience. There is good reason to presume that most, if not all, exteroceptive sensory input, including that of the special senses, has a similar counterbalancing effect on the dorsal ganglion source of sensory impulses.

The important issue here is that central mechanisms as influenced by peripheral input may be the chief factor in the inception of pain. Indeed, pain may be felt in the absence of noxious stimulation when the descending inhibitory mechanism is deficient, when the ganglionic barrage is accentuated, or both. Likewise, little or no pain may be sensed from otherwise painful causes when the descending mechanism more effectively acts to arrest the passage of impulses to the higher centers. It is known that both peripheral and central influences affect the action of this inhibitory mechanism.[10]

There are many possibilities, both peripheral and central, that may exert an influence on what we feel as pain. We are just beginning to learn the significance of these factors. The antinociceptive action of superficial stimulation (pressure, massage, analgesic balms, vibration, thermal applications, hydrotherapy, counterirritation, transcutaneous electrical nerve stimulation [TENS], etc) is quite well known. The inhibitory effect of distraction, physical activity, and calm serenity as contrasted with the excitatory effect of attention, fear, anxiety, and consequences very likely also involves activity of the descending inhibitory mechanism.

With the discovery of the axon transport system and the antidromic passage of neurotransmitters and other neurochemicals peripherally, a better understanding of the importance of the neurogenic component of inflammation is developing. Since cuta-

neous wheals and localized areas of hyperemia are now known to result from such antidromic activity,[11] the intimate relationship between neural activities and inflammation makes it difficult to decide what part of an inflammatory process generates pain and what part is actually the result of pain.

Inflammatory Pain

The traditional concept of noxious stimulation as the initiating determinant of pain genesis may very well stem from that induced by inflammation. Tissue injury initiates an inflammatory reaction that characteristically induces pain. The symptoms relate to the conditions that prevail such as the kind, extent, and location of injury; the reactivity of the injured structures; the degree of confinement of the inflammatory exudate; and the phase of inflammation.

Inflammatory pain is due chiefly to the action of prostaglandins and bradykinin, substances released by the inflammatory process. They act in conjunction with each other to increase local vasodilation and capillary permeability as well as alter the sensitivity and receptivity of receptors in the area.[12-16] Thus, the pain threshold is lowered so that nociceptors become more sensitive to stimulation, and higher-threshold mechanoreceptors are sensitized to a wider variety of stimuli. As a result, spontaneous primary pain and stimulation-evoked primary hyperalgesia take place. Along with these local effects, there is a prostaglandin-like substance released in the central nervous system (CNS) that sensitizes nociceptive interneurons to mechanical and chemical stimuli and renders neural pathways related to inflammatory pain more sensitive to the action of opiates. This has been called prostaglandin hyperalgesia.[17]

Pain of inflammatory origin may involve different kinds of tissue innervated by receptors with different reactive responses. For example, superficial pain may be inflammatory such as that of dermatitis or gingivitis. Examples of musculoskeletal inflammatory pain are those of myositis and cellulitis. Visceral inflammatory pain may be expressed as that of lymphadenitis or arteritis. Inflammatory neuropathic pain may manifest as neuritis. Many physical ailments are inflammatory, and pain of the inflammatory type is part of the symptom complex.

It should be noted that inflammation due to local tissue injury is a normal immune response that initiates the healing process.[18] The pain generated by inflammation functions to alert the subject to its presence. This type of pain exerts a protective inhibitory influence on biomechanical activty, and it serves to monitor the progress toward recovery of the injured part. Inflammation therefore should be looked on as a protective and beneficial body function. Failure of the immune system to respond appropriately invites disaster. Artificial suppression of the inflammatory process to minimize pain may be counterproductive therapeutically. The recognition of inflammatory pain should alert the examiner to cause-related therapy.

Noninflammatory Pain

It is likely that noninflammatory pain is a much more common source of suffering then inflammatory pain. This concept, however, has certainly not been the traditional approach to explaining pain. Most clinicians have been trained to establish a diagnosis that ends in "itis" (ie, tendonitis, gastritis, otitis, etc). This suggests that the tissue or organ described is inflamed. This is certainly not true of many pain disorders. By this time it is hoped that the reader has an appreciation for the many conditions that exist in the somatic tissues and CNS that may create pain in the absence of inflammation.

It is useful to diagnostically separate inflammatory pains from noninflammatory pains because of their different clinical presentations and courses. As previously stated, true tissue inflammation is a result of an immune response that causes certain changes in local tissues such as reddening, increased temperature, and edema. Inflammation follows a relatively predictable time course, getting worse and then with therapy getting better. Most pains do not show these characteristics, at least not at the clinical level and are therefore considered to be noninflammatory pains. For example, in this text neurogenic inflammation will not be considered in the category of a true inflammatory disorder since it does not seem to present with the obvious clinical symptoms associated with inflammation. It is acknowledged, however, that this separation may not be distinguishable nor appropriate, yet it does offer some diagnostic advantages.

Noninflammatory pain may originate from somatic or neurogenous structures. Some of the more common disorders and features of these two categories will be presented with a more complete description to follow in future chapters.

Somatic Pain

Somatic pains are pains that originate from body structures and may be divided into two main types: superficial and deep. *Superficial somatic pains* have their origin in cutaneous tissues of the skin or the mucogingival tissues of the mouth. These tissues provide information from the environment. *Deep somatic pains* originate from all of the structures that are located deep to the envelope with the exception of the neural structures. Deep somatic structures are either *musculoskeletal structures* or *visceral structures* (the supply system). Within these two categories are some of the most common pains of human suffering; specifically, muscle pains and vascular pains.

Musculoskeletal Pains. Noninflammatory muscle pain is the most common type of somatic pain, and yet it remains very poorly understood. A great deal of mystery continues to shroud myogenous pain in general, which affects doctors and patients alike. Without a good understanding of this pain, one cannot effectively manage the patient's complaints. Muscle pain may frequently occur in relationship to systemic responses. Some pains are a result of a protective response called *co-contraction* (formally called muscle splinting). Co-contraction may result from any alteration in sensory or proprioceptive input. It also may result as a response to deep pain or even the threat of injury. If this condition is protracted, *delay onset muscle soreness* (or local muscle soreness) may result. Another painful muscle condition is myofascial trigger point pain. This type of pain is characterized by localized areas of hypersensitive bands of muscle fibers called trigger points. These trigger points often produce heterotopic pains that predominate the patient's complaints.

Occasionally muscle pain may originate from a CNS-induced contraction of the entire muscle called a myospasm. When muscle pain becomes protracted, myositis may predominate the clinical presentation. True muscle inflammation, however, is rare unless associated with trauma or other injury.

Musculoskeletal pains also includes the articular surfaces of joints and their associated structures. Various types of arthritides can be a source of deep pain. When discussing orofacial pains, the temporomandibular joints become the joints of interest.

Visceral Pains. Visceral pains originate from tissues associated with the supply system. Structures that are of concern in the orofacial region are visceral mucosa (sinus); tooth pulps; and glandular, ocular and auricular structures. The greatest source of orofacial pains from visceral sources, however, come from the vascular tissues. Vascular pain (ie, migraine) was once considered to be the most common pain complaint known to humans[19] and still perhaps ranks second only to myogenous pain. Unfortunately vascular pain continues to be poorly understood by health professionals. Gross[20] has shown that blood vessels are innervated by afferent neurons of both the somatic and visceral nervous systems. Nociceptive impulses arising from vascular structures therefore may be mediated by either or both of these pathways.

It was originally thought that vascular pain was initiated chiefly by dilation of small arteries, which distorts and noxiously stimulates afferent fibers in vascular and perivascular tissues. Vasoconstricting medications, such as ergotamine tartrate, which reduce the dilation and amplitude of pulsation of arteries, decrease the pain. Pressure applied to the carotid artery also diminishes the pain.[7] The presumption, however, that vasodilation is the primary cause of vascular pain is no longer tenable because spontaneous dilation of cranial arteries does not cause pain in healthy subjects. Rather, dilating drugs provide relaxation of arteries, but not pain. Only algogenic substances such as bradykinin and histamine can evoke vasodilation and pain.[21] It is more likely that a neurogenic inflammation within the trigeminal neurovascular complex is responsible for this type of vascular pain (see Chapter 16).

Systemic more than local factors seem to play the major role in the incidence of vascular pain. It occurs in pain patients, so-called hypernoceptors who are thought to have some deficiency in opioid peptides and neurotransmitters of the antinociceptive system.[21] Serotonin deficiency in the CNS has been identified with the incidence of vascular pain.[22–25] Histamine administered to known migraine patients consistently precipitates an attack of pain, while nonmigrainous persons do not react in this way.[26] Patients with vascular pain frequently display a characteristic emotional overlay with personality features of insecurity with tension. This may manifest as inflexibility, conscientiousness, meticulousness, perfectionism, and resentment. Frustration, fatigue, and prostration seem to set the stage for an attack.[7] In the light of serotonin depletion, which also characterizes depressive states,[27] the emotional symptoms and the pain may simply represent different facets of a common problem.[28]

Wolff[29] described four conditions that seemed to contribute to the discomfort of vascular pain: *(1)* dilation of blood vessels, *(2)* local edema of the painful site, *(3)* edema of the vessel wall and perivascular tissue, and *(4)* associated muscle pain (especially in the occipital area). It has been shown that attacks of migraine without aura (see Chapter 16) display accompanying increased electromyographic activity in pericranial muscles.[30,31]

It appears that tension-type headache (commonly associated with myofascial pain) and vascular headache (especially migraine without aura) have much in common.[21,32] The clinical complaint frequently comprises elements of both varieties of pain. It is likely that the systemic factors in these conditions stem from a common cause and the peripheral symptoms may represent little more than different facets of a common problem. The psychologic implications of both conditions therefore are of great importance.

Since vascular pain appears to be originating in the vessel, it is perfectly logical to consider this a type of visceral pain. Recent information, however, does alter our original view of this most common and complex type of pain. It appears that the phenomenon of vascular pain begins with a triggering of a trigeminal neurovascular mechanism. Since the initiating factor appears to be associated with a neurogenic mechanism, the classification of migraine will be discussed in this text under the category of neurovascular pain disorders (see Chapter 16).

Neuropathic Pain

Some clinical pains arise from abnormalities in the neural structures themselves and are therefore called *neuropathic pains.* Neuropathic pains can be confusing to the clinician since the clinical examination may reveal no somatic tissue changes. The clinical examination reveals no reason for the pain condition. The novice clinician is likely to jump to the conclusion that this is a psychogenic pain. Understanding neuropathic pain is fundamental in the management of orofacial pains since it is common in the head and neck. These pains may present as either continuous pain conditions or episodic pain conditions.

Continuous Neuropathic Pains. Continuous neuropathic pain presents as an ongoing, unremitting pain condition. These neuropathic pains fall into one of the following three categories: *(1)* neuritis, *(2)* deafferentation, or *(3)* sympathetically maintained.

Neuritis. Neuritis or neuritic neuralgia is pain manifest as an ongoing, unremitting, burning sensation in the peripheral distribution of the affected nerve.[7,33] The distribution of neuritic pain closely follows dermatomes, which have been described (see Chapter 4). The symptoms depend on the fiber population of the nerve as well as on the kind and degree of involvement of each fiber type. Other sensory, motor, and autonomic symptoms may therefore accompany the complaint of pain.

Like many other clinical pain disorders, the neural mechanism of neuritis is poorly understood. It is usually presumed that an inflammatory condition of the nerve is responsible for the production of nociception impulses. The reason for such inflammation may be obscure. Metabolic and toxic disorders as well as neurovascular phenomena and viral infections are possible etiologic agents.

Herpes zoster is one of the more commonly known types of neuritis. It is generally agreed that the pain of herpes zoster stems from a viral infection of the ganglion, dorsal root, or medullary tract of the involved nerve. The threshold of C fibers is lowered, thus making them more sensitive to nociceptive stimuli. The reactivity of A-delta fibers, however, appears to be partially or completely abolished.[34]

The exact pathogenesis of herpes zoster is not known,[35] but it is caused by herpesvirus varicella.[7,36–38] It is thought that the virus travels to the dorsal root or ganglion during the primary varicella infection where it remains latent within neurons until the immune response of the host falls below a critical level.[39] At that time it becomes activated and fulminates, especially under conditions of local trauma or malignancy or when other therapy utilizes steroids, irradiation, or antimetabolites. Herpes zoster appears to be the unmasking of a latent virus that, when activated, travels along the peripheral nerve to produce active disease. It is thought that chicken pox can be contracted from a patient with herpes zoster, but not vice versa.[40]

Approximately 10% of patients who suffer with herpes zoster seem to progress into a clinical condition known as postherpetic neuralgia.[39,41] Fifty percent of patients with zoster who are over 60 years of age also seem to progress to same condition.[35]

Deafferentation Pains. Crushing or cutting a peripheral nerve induces anesthesia by interrupting the afferent impulses. This loss of afferent input into the central nervous system is called *deafferentation.* Although one might assume that terminating afferent input could only result in anesthesia, clinical case reports reveal that a variety of other symptoms may develop. As strange as it might appear, one of these symptoms may be pain. It is possible, therefore, to have a patient report a painful area of the tissue that is numb (called *anesthesia dolorosa*). The understanding of this condition has greatly curtailed the ablative procedures once performed to eliminate pain.

Being part of a cell, a damaged peripheral sensory axon causes reactions in other peripheral and central cells that are in functional communication with the damaged neuron.[42] Deafferentation pains are initiated within the nervous system and can rarely be significantly altered by the subject's activities or controlled by measures designed to reduce nociceptive stimulation.[43]

Deafferentation can be experimentally demonstrated with capsaicin, the major pungent and irritating component of hot peppers. This substance selectively affects C fibers and depletes these fibers of substance P in the dorsal horn, expanding the sensory receptive field. These effects are quite similar to those of deafferentation due to sectioning a nerve.[44] Capsaicin affects unmyelinated fibers without inducing degeneration.[45] The enzyme fluoride-resistant acid phosphatase disappears from central terminals within a few days, and substance P and cholecystokinin are depleted in the region of spinal cord terminals within 2 weeks.[46] It reduces nociceptive, heat, and nonnociceptive warm responses. However, it does not alter touch, vibration, cold, or nonnociceptive pressure responses.[47] Fitzgerald[48] has reviewed the limitations of assumptions that should be drawn from the local and neonatal use of capsaicin to simulate the effects of mechanical deafferentation.

The neural changes that take place as the result of peripheral deafferentation affect both the peripheral axons and the central terminals. Cutting the nerve peripheral to the dorsal ganglion arrests the afferent barrage of impulses and halts the movement of transport substances. Only limited anatomic degeneration takes place in the central terminals of the afferent fibers.[49] Some sprouts may find their proper neurilemma tubes, and relatively normal reinnervation may ensue. Axon receptor mismatch and alien innervation due to misdirection or collateral sprouting[50] may result in nonsense signals. Sprouts and axons peripheral to the site of damage become sensitive to norepinephrine,[51] which is generated by activity in the sympathetic efferents. They may also become sensitive to acetylcholine.[52] Retrograde shrinkage of axons proximal to the site of damage slows conduction velocity. Degenerative changes in the dorsal ganglion cells and central terminals yield an abnormal, unbalanced input. Sprouting produces an increased number of small fibers proximal to the injury. In the dorsal horn, nearby intact afferents appear to have the ability to excite cells formerly dominated by the cut afferents, and spinal cord cells begin to respond to the nearest intact afferents. Thus, the sensory receptive field is enlarged.[42]

The peripheral effects of deafferentation may be chiefly attributed to alien innervation and mismatch and to sensitization of peripheral axons to autonomic activity. The central effects relate primarily to the loss of C fiber function, which normally maintains organization of the spinal cord with respect to inhibitory mechanisms and the size of receptive fields. Deafferentation therefore markedly reduces normal inhibitory influences and enlarges the receptive fields.[49,53]

The discovery by Wall and Devor[9] that dorsal ganglion cells normally initiate and maintain an ongoing, low-level background barrage of afferent signals may help to elucidate deafferentation phenomena. They observed that this ganglionic source of afferent input is increased considerably in response to peripheral nerve injury. Since the clinical symptoms of deafferentation are masked by the normal sensibility of sufficient regenerated neurons, depending on the extent and manner of such regeneration, there may be some regression of deafferentation symptoms when adequate regeneration takes place.

Deafferentation of peripheral nerves may induce various sensory symptoms, which include paresthesia, dysesthesia, hyperesthesia, hyperalgesia, and spontaneous pain. Symptoms may be felt not only in the region of the initial anesthesia but also in a considerably larger area. Anesthesia dolorosa and phantom pain are examples. Deafferentation effects have been identified following the extraction of succedaneous (not primary) teeth,[54] minor oral surgery,[55] and endodontic therapy.[56] Alling[57] reported that in a national survey dysesthesia of the lingual nerve occurred once in 1,756 patients, with 13% persisting longer than 1 year, while dysesthesia of the inferior alveolar nerve occurred once in 241 patients, with 3.5% persisting 1 year. Goldberg et al[58] reported that, in 500 consecutive procedures in private practice, dysesthesia

occurred in 1.2% of the cases, but only one persisted longer than 6 months. Wofford and Miller[59] reported dysesthesia of 15 inferior alveolar nerves and four lingual nerves following the removal of 576 impacted mandibular third molars. All the dysesthesias except that of one lingual nerve resolved within 6 months. Of 52 inferior alveolar nerves with altered sensation following sagittal ramus osteotomy and mandibular advancement, Upton et al[60] reported that 53.8% returned to normal (meaning that 46.2% did not). Although some phantom pains are deafferentation syndromes,[61] some are not.[62]

When a nerve trunk is sectioned, the regenerating axons may not find their proper neurilemma tubes. They may bundle into a disorganized, random overgrowth of intertwined extraneural and intraneural tissue and Schwann's cells. The neuropathic pain that results is thought to be largely due to ephaptic transfer of neural impulses generated by pressing or stretching the nerve tissue mass,[63] called *traumatic neuroma pain*.

Sympathetically Maintained Pains. There are certain pains that appear to be maintained by efferent activity of the sympathetic nervous system. Evidence of this condition is demonstrated by the clinical observation that a regional blockade of the sympathetic nervous system in certain patients can produce immediate and complete relief of the pain.[64,65] Likewise, electrical stimulation of the sympathetic nervous system in some patients can increase painful conditions.[66] It should be noted that in healthy patients, sympathetic blockade does not reduce pain nor does stimulation of sympathetic neurons produce pain. With this understanding, a group of neuropathic pain conditions were identified as sympathetically maintained pains.

Most sympathetically maintained pains begin with some type of peripheral tissue damage.[67,68] This tissue damage excites the C fibers and nociceptive impulses are carried into the CNS to synapse with a second-order neuron, such as a wide dynamic range (WDR) neuron.[68] During healing, the WDR neuron can become sensitized, which reduces its threshold so that even normal activity of the low threshold, myelinated mechanoreceptors (A-delta and A-beta) can be perceived not as pressure or touch but instead as noxious (ie, hyperalgesia or allo-dynia). The neuroplasticity seen in the WDR neuron can continue to maintain the hyperalgesic state even after healing of the tissue is complete (see Chapter 17).

Normal efferent sympathetic activity results in the release of norepinephrine at the peripheral receptor sites in the target organ. In the cutaneous tissues, this is predominantly the capillaries. In the normal condition this release of norepinephrine does not affect primary sensory neurons. However, if the primary neurons have been sensitized by neuroplastic changes, this release of norepinephrine can excite the A-delta and A-beta receptors, which continue to excite the WDR neurons thus developing a self-maintaining loop. It is thought that even normal sympathetic activity (sympathetic tone) can be responsible for maintaining the pain. Certainly any increase in sympathetic activity would likely increase the pain condition. One can quickly appreciate that increased levels of emotional stress would likely aggravate this condition.

The most common pain described by patients with this condition is one of a burning quality. This condition is called *causalgia*. A general term that is used to describe a specific group of painful disorders initiated by an injury to peripheral tissues and sustained by activity of the sympathetic nervous system is *reflex sympathetic dystrophy* (RSD) (see Chapter 17).

Episodic Neuropathic Pains. Some neuropathic pains have a clinical course that reveal high levels of pain followed by periods of total remission of symptoms. These episodic neuropathic pains fall into two major classes: *(1)* neuralgic pains, and *(2)* neurovascular pains.

Neuralgic Pains. Neuralgic pains are characterized by sudden electric-like volleys of pain that are felt in the exact distribution of the involved nerve. These shock-like pains are called paroxysmal pains and are usually momentary and severe. They are often triggered by relatively mild mechanical stimulation at a site in the peripheral distribution of the same nerve involved in the neuralgia. The pains are often recurrent with no pain experienced between the episodes. Paroxysmal neuralgias are named for the nerve that is affected, for example, trigeminal neuralgia.

Paroxysmal trigeminal neuralgia is one of the most painful conditions known to humans yet it remains an enigma to many health professionals. Trigeminal neuralgia presents in two forms: idiopathic and pathologic. Idiopathic trigeminal neuralgia presents with only the signs and symptoms associated with the paroxysmal pain condition. Clinically idiopathic trigeminal neuralgia reveals one or more trigger sites that seem to elicit the severe momentary pain. When the pain is not present, no other abnormalities can be found. It has been suggested that this condition may be related to an aberrant branch of the superior cerebellar artery looping over the gasserian ganglion producing an unusual arcing of nerve impulses to adjacent fibers.[69] Idiopathic trigeminal neuralgia has also been called tic douloureux.

Pathologic trigeminal neuralgia presents with the same triggering paroxysmal pains but between pain episodes other symptoms may persist. These other symptoms relate to the pathologic condition that is responsible for the condition. For example, if an intracranial tumor is responsible, there maybe a diminished corneal reflex, masseter muscle weakness, facial muscle weakness, or hypoesthesia. Other causes of pathologic trigeminal neuralgia are multiple sclerosis, basilar artery aneurysm, posterior fossa tumor, cerebellopontine angle tumors, and even brain stem diseases from strokes or expanding lesions.[7,37,70-77] When other symptoms are present, the clinician must investigate these potential causes.

It is thought that neuralgic pains are closely associated with demyelination of the nerve fiber. Myelination of peripheral neurons helps to isolate the transmission of impulses in single neurons. Transfer of signals from one neuron to another normally takes place at synapses only. In the absence of neuropathologic change, the transfer of afferent impulses between neurons outside the CNS is unlikely. Kerr,[78] however, has observed demyelination changes in peripheral neurons that make ephaptic transmission of impulses possible. (An *ephapse* is a point of lateral contact, other than a synapse, between nerve fibers across which impulses are conducted directly through the nerve membranes from one fiber to the other.) Experimental demyelination leads to antidromically propagated extraction potentials as well as some postdischarge activity followed by refractory periods.[79] Short-term peripheral nerve compression is usually painless and rarely lasts more than a few seconds.[80,81] Continued compression causes local demyelination without a loss of axonal continuity. Chronic nerve entrapment causes demyelination initially, followed by progressive axonal degeneration. In traumatic neuroma, ephaptic cross-excitation may be a factor in the generation of pain.[82]

The specific etiology of idiopathic trigeminal neuralgia is most consistently with demyelination of axons in the gasserian ganglion, dorsal root, or both (Figs 6-1 and 6-2).[36,77,83] Kerr[83] contended that, since it is unlikely that minor lesions would cause the demyelination seen, an underlying degenerative process aggravated by otherwise negligible mechanical factors probably accounted for the paroxysms of pain. Hypertension and arteriosclerosis appear to have little bearing. An ephaptic response due to progressive degenerative change may be periodically and episodically activated by mechanical vascular influences.[84] This general concept is shared by others.[85] It has been established that the pathogenesis of trigeminal neuralgia is not correlative to endogenous opioids.[86] Destructive lesions of the nerve located within the brain from the entrance of the trigeminal nerve into the pons throughout the numerous sensory circuits to the cortex do not cause paroxysmal neuralgia.[87] Although there is some evidence that the responsible neuropathy is of peripheral rather than central origin,[88] a more central mechanism seems to have the most support.[89]

Fig 6-1 Transverse section through the posterior rootlet of the trigeminal nerve in man that illustrates an area of unusually abundant unmyelinated fibers and several myelinated fibers, × 10,000. (From Kerr FWL. Fine structure and functional characteristics of the primary trigeminal neuron. In Hassler R, Walker AE (eds): Trigeminal Neuralgia, Pathogenesis and Pathophysiology. Stuttgart: Georg Thieme Verlag; 1970. Used with permission.)

Fig 6-2 Proliferative degenerative changes in a myelinated fiber in trigeminal neuralgia, × 10,700. (From Kerr FWL. Pathology of trigeminal neuralgia, light and electron microscopic observations. J Neurosurg 1967; 26:151–156. Used with permission.)

Neurovascular Pains. In the previous section on visceral pains the topic of vascular headache was reviewed. In light of new information regarding the etiology of this type of pain it is difficult to know into which category this pain best fits. Although vascular changes do occur with this pain condition, it is now thought that the etiology lies more with a neurogenic inflammation initiated by some trigeminal neurovascular mechanism. Since the mechanism appears to be associated with neural function, this text will consider migraine headache under the category of neurovascular pains.

Other Causes of Orofacial Pains

Intracranial Pain

Primary intracranial head pain is rare. The parenchyma of the brain including the vessels found within it, most of the dura and pia-arachnoid, the ependymal lining of the ventricles, and the choroid plexuses are not sensitive to pain. The great venous sinuses and their tributaries from the surface of the brain, parts of the dura at the base, the dural arteries, and the cerebral arteries at the base of the brain are sensitive to pain. Stimulation of intracranial pain-sensitive structures on or above the superior surface of the tentorium cerebelli results in pain felt in the trigeminal distribution, whereas stimulation on or below the inferior surface of the tentorium cerebelli results in pain felt in the distribution of the glossopharyngeal and vagus cranial nerves and the upper cervical spinal nerves. Intracranial pain results from the following[7]:

1. Traction on veins that pass from the surface of the brain to the venous sinuses, on the middle meningeal arteries, and on the large arteries at the base of the brain and their main branches.
2. Displacement of the great venous sinuses.
3. Distension and dilation of intracranial arteries.
4. Inflammation of pain-sensitive structures of the head.
5. Pressure by lesions such as tumors on nerves containing afferent pain fibers.

Brain tumors may cause pain by encroachment on pain-sensitive structures or by reason of pressure or weight. Malignant tumors may involve neural structures directly. Brain tumors involving the trigeminal root and ganglion may be divided into four groups[90]:

1. Cerebellopontine angle tumors usually do not cause typical trigeminal neuralgia. Of 44 cases of meningioma, Nguyen et al[91] reported that nine had ipsilateral intermittent sharp lancinating pain somewhat similar to that of trigeminal neuralgia. They reported that the common symptoms associated with the pains were ipsilateral trigeminal nerve deficits, hearing loss, and occasional ipsilateral facial muscle weakness. Hypoesthesia is considerably more common than pain.
2. Middle cranial fossa tumors may cause high-density paroxysms of 10 to 15 minutes' duration. Usually the pain, if any, is a sustained aching and burning sensation associated with areas of hypoesthesia.
3. Extracranial tumors that invade the ganglion from beneath may cause prolonged high-intensity paroxysms of burning pain. Anesthesia also may be the result.
4. Tumors arising from the envelopes of the ganglion cause a neuritic type of pain accompanied by other sensory and motor signs. Usually other nerves are simultaneously involved. Such pain is nonparoxysmal.

Neoplasm Pain

Benign tumors may be quite painless unless they encroach on pain-sensitive structures by their mass or weight and, as such, induce somatic-type discomfort. Malignant neoplasms may induce pain by somatic encroachment as well as by neural involvement.[92] Thus, cancer may induce a chronic structural pain syndrome.

The Concept of Neuroplasticity

In recent years, some extremely important insight has been gained that helps us better understand chronic pain. We now know that there can be changes in the manner by which the second-order neurons process neural impulses entering the central nervous system. As discussed in previous chapters, the primary afferent neuron carries impulses into the CNS to synapse in the nucleus caudalis with the second-order neuron, which carries the impulses to higher centers. The second-order neuron may be a WDR neuron or a nociceptive-specific neuron. If there is continued stimulation of the primary afferent neuron (C fiber), there will also be continued production of excitatory neurotransmitters in the synapse such as substance P,[93] neurokinin A,[94] somatostatin,[95] and calcitonin gene-related peptide.[96] The continued presence of these neurotransmitters can alter the sensitivity of the second-order neuron. This alteration in the neuron is further increased with the release of certain excitatory amino acids such as glutamate and aspartate.[97,98] These amino acids activate the N-methyl-D-aspartic acid (NMDA) receptors located on the second-order neurons.[99] The NMDA receptors are involved in the induction and maintenance of the central sensitization of the dorsal horn neurons. In other words, with continued nociceptive input, the second-order neuron becomes increasingly sensitized, allowing the next impulses to depolarize the neuron even quicker. This change in the processing of second-order neurons is called *central sensitization* or *neuroplasticity.*

As a second-order neuron becomes sensitized, it not only responds quicker to the next impulse but it also responds quicker to the other converging neurons. Therefore the receptive field from where the impulse originates begins to widen or broaden. When the WDR neurons becomes sensitized, the normally nonnoxious impulses carried by the A-delta and B delta fibers can be misinterrupted as nociceptive. This phenomenon may be responsible for certain hyperalgesic and allodynic states. For example, light touch to the face produces an extremely high level of pain.

It is now known that electric stimulation of C fibers located in cutaneous tissues can increase the activity of the dorsal horn neurons, which lasts up to 10 minutes longer then the actual stimulation itself.[100] This is even more dramatic when deep structures are stimulated. When rat muscles are noxiously stimulated, the dorsal horn nocicep

tive neurons remain activated or sensitized for up to 50 minutes after the stimulus has been terminated.[100] The fact that is now becoming evident is that once the NMDA receptors are activated, the processing of impulses by the neuron can change, which may actually result in a permanent sensitization of the neuron. If this neuroplasicity is prolonged or permanent, primary nociceptive input is no longer needed for pain. The clinical findings, therefore, reveal a patient who continues to report pain and suffering yet the examination fails to find any somatic tissue damage that might explain the pain. This, in essence, is chronic pain.

The concept of neuroplasicity has certainly changed the way we evaluate and manage pain. Its ramifications are enormous. For example, if any tissue damage produces neuroplasticity that lasts far longer than the stimulus itself, then the potential for permanent neuroplastic changes is always a risk. If this is true then one could certainly appreciate the need for local anesthetic each and every time tissue is to be surgically injured. In the dental office this is generally the normal procedure. This, however, is not the case in the operating room. When a patient is placed under general anesthesia, the nociceptive impulses created at the surgical site are blocked from reaching the cortex at the brain stem level. Therefore, the C fibers stimulated at the site of the surgical trauma carry the nociceptive impulses into the dorsal horn (or spinal tract nucleus) and excite the second-order neurons. This nociceptive input will sensitize these neurons, creating neuroplasticty even though the anesthetized patient feels no pain. Upon awaking, the patient will likely feel postoperative pain secondary to the sensitized second-order neurons. With this in mind it seems very logical that post-operative pain and perhaps even chronic pain disorders can be minimized by the use of local anesthetic that blocks nociceptive input at the surgical site in conjunction with general anesthetics.[101]

Understanding that neuroplasticity can contribute to any pain condition is basic to pain management. Even a protracted tooth-ache risks a chance of becoming an ongoing pain condition even after the tooth may be extracted. We now realize that pain can no longer be thought of as a simple symptom that resolves with proper management of somatic tissues. Pain can actually be the disease itself. With this in mind, the importance of immediate management of acute pain becomes obvious and relevant.

Other Considerations

Pain may result from numerous causes other than specific inflammatory conditions or other myogenous, vascular, or neuro-pathic phenomena. Pain may occur sponta-neously with no identifiable cause of any kind. It may constitute an integral part of pathologic and pathophysiologic conditions of all types. Alterations in the endogenous antinociceptive mechanisms may occur. A degree or so of elevation in body tempera-ture may induce pain in many structures. The general response to abnormal endo-crine, metabolic, emotional, allergic, or toxic conditions may include a component of pain. Direct noxious stimulation by vari-ous mechanical, thermal, and chemical insults may induce pain. Cutaneous struc-tures are sensitive to all such stimuli. Periosteum is especially reactive to com-pressive force; ligaments and fascia respond to distortion, strain, and traction; tendons and muscle tissue are particularly sensitive to torque and stretching. Glands react espe-cially to pressure, while hollow viscera are sensitive to distension. Some structures are not pain sensitive at all, eg, articular sur-faces of joints and the parenchyma of the brain.

Headache is perhaps the most frequent of all regional pain complaints. Most intermit-tent head pains are heterotopic manifesta-tions. Being secondary in type, most such headaches are not as much a diagnostic concern for the pain itself as for the primary sources of deep somatic pain that initiate them.

Psychologic intensification of pain is a normal modulation phenomenon. If pain is intensified until it continues in the absence of significant peripheral input, a state of pain chronicity becomes evident. The psy-chogenic component of chronic pain syn-dromes of all types becomes a significant management problem. Pains may be due to conversion hysteria or the painful hallucina-tions of schizophrenia.

Some pains result from therapeutic ef-forts. Although such phenomena may relate to the modulating effects of management, there are instances when dental or mastica-tory therapy directly initiates a pain prob-lem. Treatment based on an incorrect or incomplete diagnosis may terminate this way. Therapy applied at the site of hetero-topic pain rather than at the true source may cause injury. Injudicious occlusal grinding may increase the sensitivity of teeth. Alteration of the occlusal relationship may initiate pain involving muscles and temporomandibular joints as well as the teeth and periodontal structures. Any proce-dure (even corrective and otherwise beneficial) that alters the proprioceptive and sensory input may initiate protective co-contraction and if not properly managed, can develop into delay onset muscle soreness or myositis. Overzealous therapy, rapid change in the functional relationship, or unwise selection of treatment may initiate a condition that has a component of pain. Many dental procedures, especially those that involve surgery, entail therapeutic hazards that can result in pain. Accidents happen, complications arise, and unexpected results may follow therapy. Some procedures such as the surgical interruption of nociceptive pathways may generate irreversible sequelae that can offset the possible benefit.

The incidence of iatrogenic pain is sufficient to warrant a high degree of caution on the part of all types of doctors. The ancient maxim "At least do no harm!" should be heeded always.

References

1. Wall PD. On the relation of injury to pain. Pain 1979; 6:253–264.

2. Beecher HK. The use of chemical agents in the control of pain. In Knighton RS, Dumke PR (eds): Pain. Boston: Little, Brown; 1966: 221–239.

3. Nyquist JK, Eriksson MBE. Effects of pain treatment procedures on thermal sensibility in chronic pain patients. Pain 1981; 11(suppl 1):91.

4. Bromm B. Evoked cerebral potential and pain. In Fields HL, Dubner R, Cervero F (eds): Advances in Pain Research and Therapy, vol 9. New York: Raven Press; 1985: 305–329.

5. Chapman CR. An alternative to threshold assessment in the study of human pain. In Bonica JJ (ed): Advances in Neurology, vol 4. New York: Raven Press; 1974: 115–121.

6. Clark WD. Pain sensitivity and the report of pain: An introduction to sensory decision theory. Anesthesiology 1974; 40:272–287.

7. Wolff HG. Headache and Other Head Pain, ed 2. New York: Oxford University Press; 1963: 3–28.

8. Wolff HG, Wolf S. Pain, ed 2. Springfield, Ill: Charles C Thomas; 1958.

9. Wall PD, Devor M. Sensory afferent impulses originate from dorsal root ganglia as well as from the periphery in normal and nerve injured rats. Pain 1983; 17:321–339.

10. Fields HL. Pain. New York: McGraw-Hill; 1987: 59–78.

11. Levine J, Basbaum A. The peripheral nervous system and the inflammatory process. Pain 1987; 31:109.

12. Burgess PR, Perl ER. Cutaneous mechanoreceptors and nociception. In Iggo A (ed): Handbook of Sensory Physiology, vol 2. Heidelberg: Springer Verlag; 1973: 29–78.

13. Beitel RE, Dubner R. The response of unmyelinated (C) polymodal nociceptors to thermal stimuli applied to monkey's face. J Neurophysiol 1976; 39: 1160–1175.

14. Lim RJS. Pain. Annu Rev Physiol 1970; 32: 269–288.

15. Handwerker HO. Influences of algogenic substances and prostaglandins on the discharges of unmyelinated cutaneous nerve fibers identified as nociceptors. In Bonica JJ, Albe-Fessard DG (eds): Advances in Pain Research and Therapy, vol 1. New York: Raven Press; 1976: 41–45.

16. Ahlquist ML, Franzen OG, Edwall LGA, et al. Quality of pain sensations following local application of algogenic agents on the exposed human tooth pulp: A psychophysical and electrophysiological study. In Fields HL, Dubner R, Cervero F (eds): Advances in Pain Research and Therapy, vol 9. New York: Raven Press; 1985: 351–359.

17. Ferreira SH. Prostaglandins: Peripheral and central analgesia. In Bonica JJ, Lindblom U, Iggo A (eds): Advances in Pain Research and Therapy, vol 5. New York: Raven Press; 1983: 627–634.

18. Roitt IM, Brostoff J, Male DK. Immunology. St Louis: CV Mosby; 1985.

19. Bassoe P. Migraine. JAMA 1933; 101:599–605.

20. Gross D. Pain and autonomic nervous system. In Bonica JJ (ed): Advances in Neurology, vol 4. New York: Raven Press; 1974: 93–103.

21. Sicuteri F. Headache as the most common disease of the antinociceptive system: Analogies with morphine abstinence, in Bonica JJ, Liebeskind JC, Albe-Fessard DG (eds): Advances in Pain Research and Therapy, vol 3. New York: Raven Press; 1979: 359–365.

22. Appenzeller O. Headache: Clinical and pathogenetic aspects. In Bonica JJ, Liebeskind JC, Albe-Fessard DG (eds): Advances in Pain Research and Therapy, vol 3. New York: Raven Press; 1979: 345–358.

23. Dvilansky A, Rishpon S, Nathan L, et al. Release of platelet 5-hydroxytryptamine by plasma taken from patients during and between migraine attacks. Pain 1976; 2:315–318.

24. Anthony M, Hinterberger H, Lance JW. Plasma serotonin in migraine and stress. Arch Neurol 1967; 16:544–552.

25. Anthony M, Hinterberger H, Lance JW. The possible relationship of serotonin to the migraine syndrome. Res Clin Studies Headache 1969; 2:29.

26. Krabbe AA, Olesen J. Headache provocation by continuous intravenous infusion of histamine: Clinical results and receptor mechanisms. Pain 1980; 8:253–259.

27. Seltzer S, Marcus R, Stoch R. Perspectives in the control of chronic pain by nutritional manipulation. Pain 1981; 11:141–148.

28. Johansson F, Von Knorring L. A double-blind controlled study of a serotonin uptake inhibitor (zimeldine) versus placebo in chronic pain patients. Pain 1979; 7:69–78.

29. Wolff HG. Headache and Other Head Pain, ed 2. New York: Oxford University Press; 1963: 227–233.

30. Clifford T, Lauritsen M, Bakke M, et al. Electromyography of pericranial muscles during treatment of spontaneous common migraine attacks. Pain 1982; 14:137–147.

31. Bakke M, Tfelt-Hansen P, Olesen J, et al. Action of some pericoronal muscles during provoked attacks of common migraine. Pain 1982; 14:121–135.

32. Oleson J. Clinical and pathophysiological observations in migraine and tension-type headache explained by integration of vascular, supraspinal and myofascial inputs. Pain 1991; 46:125–132.

33. Wolff HG. Headache and Other Head Pain, ed 2. New York: Oxford University Press; 1963: 652–655.

34. Bigelow N, Harrison L, Goodell H, et al. Studies on pain: Quantitative measurements of two pain sensations of the skin with reference to the nature of the hyperalgesia of peripheral neuritis. J Clin Invest 1945; 23:503.

35. Lobato RD, Madrid JL. Clinical and physiopathological mechanisms of postherpetic neuralgia. Clin J Pain 1987; 2:253–257.

36. Sweet WH. Trigeminal neuralgia. In Alling CC, Mahan PE (eds): Facial Pain, ed 2. Philadelphia: Lea & Febiger; 1977: 71–93.

37. Stookey B, Rausohoft J. Trigeminal Neuralgia. Springfield, Ill: Charles C Thomas; 1959.

38. Reuler JB, Chang M. Herpes zoster: Epidemiology, clinical features and management. South Med 1 1984; 77:1149–1156.

39. Oxman MN. Varicella and herpes zoster. In Fitzpatrick TB, Eisen AZ, Wolff K (eds): Dermatology in General Medicine. New York: McGraw-Hill; 1979: 1600–1616.

40. Loeser JD. Herpes zoster and postherpetic neuralgia. Pain 1986; 25:149–164.

41. Reuler JB, Chang M. Herpes zoster: Epidemiology, clinical features and management. South Med J 1984; 77:1149–1156.

42. Wall PD. Changes in damaged nerve and their sensory consequences. In Bonica JJ, Liebeskind JC, Albe-Fessard DG (eds): Advances in Pain Rescarch and Therapy, vol 3. New York: Raven Press; 1979: 39–52.

43. Loeser JD. Definition, etiology, and neurological assessment of pain originating in the nervous system following deafferentation. In Bonica JJ, Lindblom U, Iggo A (eds): Advances in Pain Research and Therapy, vol 5. New York: Raven Press; 1983: 701–711.

44. Wall PD, Fitzgerald M, Gibson SJ. The effect of local sciatic nerve capsaicin and sciatic nerve section on neurophysiological responses and peptide levels in rat lumbar dorsal horn. Pain 1981; 11:202.

45. Nagy JI, Hunt SP, Iversen LL, et al. Effects of capsaicin on dorsal root afferents. In Bonica JJ, Lindblom U, Iggo A (eds): Advances in Pain Research and Therapy, vol 5. New York: Raven Press; 1983: 77–82.

46. Ainsworth A, Hall P, Wall PD, et al. Effects of capsaicin applied locally to adult peripheral nerves: II. Anatomy and enzyme and peptide chemistry of peripheral nerve and spinal cord. Pain 1981; 11:379–388.

47. Buck SH, Miller MS, Burks TF. Specific sensory deficits in adult guinea pigs induced by the putative substance P neurotoxin, capsaicin, and its active analogs. Pain 1981; 11:134.

48. Fitzgerald M. Capsaicin and sensory neurons: A review. Pain 1983; 15:109–130.

49. Wall PD. Alterations in the central nervous system after deafferentation: Connectivity control. In Bonica JJ, Lindblom U, Iggo A (eds): Advances in Pain Research and Therapy, vol 5. New York: Raven Press; 1983: 677–689.

50. Inbal R, Rousso M, Ashur H, et al. Collateral sprouting in skin and sensory recovery after nerve injury in man. Pain 1987; 28:141–154.

51. Ochoa JL, Torebjork E, Marchettini P, et al. Mechanisms of neuropathic pain: Cumulative observations, new experiments, and further speculation. In Fields HL, Dubner R, Cervero F (eds): Advances in Pain Research and Therapy, vol 9. New York: Raven Press; 1985: 431–450.

52. Diamond J. The effect of injecting acetylcholine into normal and regenerating nerves. J Physiol (Lond) 1959; 145:611–629.

53. Wall PD. Mechanisms of acute and chronic pain. In Kruger L, Liebeskind JC (eds): Advances in Pain Research and Therapy, vol 6. New York: Raven Press; 1984: 95–104.

54. Hu JW, Broton JG, Tam L, et al. Dental deafferentation and properties of trigeminal (V) brainstem neurons in kittens and adult cats. Pain 1987; 31:270.

55. Gregg JM. Posttraumatic pain: Experimental trigeminal neuropathy. J Oral Surg 1971; 29:260–267.

56. Gobel S, Binck JM. Degenerative changes in primary trigeminal axons and in neurons in nucleus caudalis following tooth pulp extirpation in the cat. Brain Res 1977; 132:347–354.

57. Alling CC. Dysesthesia of the lingual and inferior alveolar nerves following third molar surgery. J Oral Maxillofac Surg 1986; 44:454–457.

58. Goldberg MH, Nemarich AN, Marco WP. Complications after mandibular third molar surgery: A statistical analysis of 500 consecutive procedures in private practice. J Am Dent Assoc 1985; 111:277–279.

59. Wofford DT, Miller RI. Prospective study of dysesthesia following odontectomy of impacted mandibular third molars. J Oral Maxillofac Surg 1987; 45:15–19.

60. Upton LG, Rajvanakarn M, Hayward JR. Evaluation of the regeneration capacity of the inferior alveolar nerve following surgical trauma. J Oral Maxillofac Surg 1987; 45:212–216.

61. Howe JF. Phantom limb pain: A re-afferentation syndrome. Pain 1983; 15:101–107.

62. Melzack R, Loeser JD. Phantom body pain in paraplegics: Evidence for a central pattern generating mechanism for pain. Pain 1978; 4:195–210.

63. Gregg JM, Walter JR, Driscoll R. Neurosensory studies of trigeminal dysesthesia following peripheral nerve injury. In Bonica JJ, Liebeskind JC, Albe-Fessard DG (eds): Advances in Pain Research and Therapy, vol 3. New York: Raven Press; 1979: 311–315.

64. Livingston WK. Pain Mechanisms. New York: Macmillan; 1943.

65. Bonica JJ. Causalgia and other reflex sympathetic dystrophies. In Bonica JJ, Liebeskind JC, Albe-Fessard DG (eds): Advances in Pain Research and Therapy, vol 3. New York: Raven Press; 1979: 141–166.

66. Walker AE, Nulson F. Electical stimulation of the upper thoracic portion of the sympathetic chain in man. Arch Neurol Psychiatry 1948; 59:559–560.

67. Campbell JN, Raja SN, Meyer RA. Painful sequelae of nerve injury. Pain 1987; 31:334.

68. Roberts W. A hypothesis on the physiolgical basis for causalgia and related pains. Pain 1986, 24:297–311.

69. Jannetta P. Arterial compression of the trigeminal nerve at the pons in patients with trigeminal neuralgia. J Neurosurg 1967; 26:159–162.

70. Rushton JG, Olafson RA. Trigeminal neuralgia associated with multiple sclerosis: A case report. Arch Neurol 1965; 13:383–386.

71. Olafson RA, Rushton JG, Sayre GR. Trigeminal neuralgia in a patient with multiple sclerosis: An autopsy report. J Neurosurg 1966; 24:755–759.

72. Gardner WJ. Trigeminal neuralgia. In Hassler R, Walker AE (eds): Trigeminal Neuralgia. Stuttgart: Georg Thieme Verlag; 1970: 162–165.

73. Friedlander AH, Zeff S. Atypical trigeminal neuralgia in patients with multiple sclerosis. J Oral Surg 1974; 32:301–303.

74. Lazar ML, Greenlee RG Jr, Naarden AL. Facial pain of neuralgic origin mimicking oral pathologic conditions: Some current concepts and treatments. J Am Dent Assoc 1980; 100: 884–888.

75. Parker HL. Trigeminal neuralgia associated with multiple sclerosis. Brain 1928; 51:46–62.

76. Harris W. Rare forms of paroxysmal trigeminal neuralgia and their relationship to disseminated sclerosis. Br Med J 1950; 2:1015–1019.

77. Kerr FWL. Fine structure and functional characteristics of the primary trigeminal neuron. In Hassler R, Walker AE (eds): Trigeminal Neuralgia. Stuttgart: Georg Thieme Verlag; 1970: 11–21.

78. Kerr FWL. Correlated light and electron microscopic observations on the normal trigeminal ganglion and sensory root in man. J Neurosurg 1967; 26:132–137.

79. Burchiel KJ. Abnormal impulse generation in focally demyelinated trigeminal roots. J Neurosurg 1980; 53:674.

80. Howe JF, Loeser JD, Calvin WH. Mechanosensitivity of dorsal root ganglia and chronially injured axons: A physiological basis for the radicular pain of nerve root compression. Pain 1977; 3:25–41.

81. Rosomoff HL. Do herniated disks produce pain? In Fields HL, Dubner R, Cervero F (eds): Advances in Pain Research and Therapy, vol 9. New York: Raven Press; 1985: 457–461.

82. Ochea J, Noorrdenbes W. Pathology and disordered sensation in local nerve lesions: An attempt at correlation. In Bonica JJ, Lieberkind J, Albe-Fessard DG (eds): Advances in Pain Research and Therapy, vol 3. New York: Raven Press; 1979: 67–90.

83. Kerr FWL, Miller RH. The pathology of trigeminal neuralgia: Electron microscopic studies. Arch Neurol 1966; 15:308–309.

84. Kerr FWL. Evidence for a peripheral etiology of trigeminal neuralgia. J Neurosurg 1967; 26: 168–174.

85. Calvin WH, Loeser JD, Howe JF. A neurophysiological theory for the pain mechanism of tic douloureux. Pain 1977; 3:147–154.

86. Salar G, Mangrino S. Trigeminal neuralgia and endorphins. Pain 1981; 11:259.

87. Kaemmerer EF. A review of the etiologic factors in trigeminal neuralgia. In Hassler R, Walker AE (eds): Trigeminal Neuralgia. Stuttgart: Georg Thieme Verlag; 1970: 175–179.

88. Kerr FWL. Peripheral versus central factors in trigeminal neuralgia. In Hassler R, Walker AE (eds): Trigeminal Neuralgia. Stuttgart: Georg Thieme Verlag; 1970: 180–190.

89. Rappaport ZH, Devor M. Trigeminal neuralgia: the role of self-sustaining discharge in the trigeminal ganglion. Pain 1994; 56:127–138.

90. Cushing H. The major trigeminal neuralgias and their surgical treatment. Am Med Sci 1920; 160:157.

91. Nguyen M, Maciewicz R, Bouckoms A, et al. Facial pain symptoms in patients with cerebellopontine angle tumors: A report of 44 cases of cerebellopontine angle meningioma and a review of the literature. Clin J Pain 1986; 2:3–9.

92. Foley KM. The treatment of pain in the patient with cancer. Cancer 1986; 36:194–215.

93. Go VLW, Yaksh TL. Release of substance P from the cat spinal cord. J Physiol 1987: 391:141–167.

94. Duggan AW, Hope PJ, Jarrott B, Schaible HG, Fleetwood-Walker SM. Release, spread and persistence of immunoreactive neurokinin A in the dorsal horn of the cat following noxious cutaneous stimulation. Studies with antibody microprobes. Neuroscience 1990; 35:195–202.

95. Morton CR, Hutchison WD, Hendry IA. Release of immunoreactive somatostatin in the spinal dorsal horn of the cat. Neuropeptides. 1988; 12:189–197.

96. Morton CR, Hutchison WD. Release of sensory neuropeptides in the spinal cord: Studies with calcitonin gene-related peptide and galanin. Neuroscience 1990; 31:807–815.

97. Skilling SR, Smullin DH, Larson AA. Extracellular amino acid concentrations in the dorsal spinal cord of freely moving rats following veratridine and nociceptive stimulation. J Neurochem 1988; 51:127–132.

98. Sorkin LS, Westlund KN, Sluka KA, Doughterty PM, Willis WD. Neural changes in acute arthritis in monkeys. IV. Time course of amino acid release into the lumbar dorsal horn. Brain Res Rec 1992, 17:39–50.

99. Woolf CJ, Thompson SWN. The induction and maintenance of central sensitization is dependent on N-methyl-D-aspartic acid receptor activation: implications for the treatment of post-injury pain hypersensitivity states. Pain 1991; 50:293–299.

100. Cook AJ, Woolf CJ, Wall PD, McMahon SB. Dynamic receptive field plasticity in rat spinal cord dorsal horn following C-primary afferent input. Nature 1987; 325:151–153.

101. Wall PD. The prevention of postoperative pain. Pain 1988; 33:289–290.

7 | Category Classification of Orofacial Pains

This chapter will present a means of assessing the pain complaint and describe a diagnostic road map that will lead the examiner toward an accurate classification of pain disorder, which becomes a valuable diagnostic tool. The more sophisticated the classification, however, the greater the requirement for a good understanding of pain mechanisms and examining techniques.

Pain Diagnosis

Pain diagnosis is by far the most difficult aspect of managing a patient's problem and is also what the therapist does least successfully. In fact, the majority of treatment failures arise directly from misdiagnosis. It is only through proper diagnosis that effective therapy can be selected and instituted. The first prerequisite in classifying pain is a common language with which to communicate intelligibly. Considerable improvement in the meaning of terms used to describe pain has been made in recent years. Some definitions as listed in a standard medical dictionary[1] are not sufficiently precise to prevent ambiguity and misunderstanding.

The International Association for the Study of Pain has taken the lead in defining such terms more precisely.[2,3] A list of definitions as used in this text is located at the front of the book. The reader is encouraged to become familiar with them.

The most elementary classification of pain is that which lists the anatomic locations where pain is felt. An example of such a classification follows:

1. Head and neck pain
2. Thoracic pain
3. Abdominal pain
4. Extremity pain

Subdivisions of head and neck pain include orofacial pains, headaches, and cervical pains. This text will primarily discuss orofacial pains; however, the clinician must have an appreciation for other pain conditions of the head and neck so that proper diagnosis is possible. Other texts should be reviewed for a more complete understanding of headaches and cervical pain disorders.

A simple classification of pain disorders is often used to record the patient's subjective complaint. For example, it might list the complaint as a headache, toothache, chest pain, backache, or leg pain. It should be understood, however, that this type of classification identifies only the site where pain is felt, not the location of its true source. A pain listed as a toothache could be of dental origin and require dental therapy. But it could also be a heterotopic manifestation of some myogenous, vascular, or neuropathic condition that would require treatment at quite a different level. Therefore, such a classification has very little diagnostic value.

More refined pain classifications require additional knowledge of pain behavior and the expenditure of some diagnostic effort. To classify pain by the location of its source requires an understanding of heterotopic pains and entails the need for diagnostic differentiation between primary pain and its secondary effects. Thus, toothache in such a classification might become pulpal pain, periodontal pain, or heterotopic pain when its true site of origin is determined. It should be obvious that this more accurate classification of the patient's complaint implies important therapeutic considerations.

In 1988, the International Headache Society published the first edition of its classification and diagnostic criteria for headache disorders, cranial neuralgias, and facial pain.[4] This classification attempted to separate all headaches according to cause and involved structures. Although this classification has been most useful in unifying international groups, it relies heavily on the clinician's knowledge of the presence of each condition. In this classification (Table 7-1), orofacial pain and temporomandibular disorders fall mostly in section 11, which is listed as "Headache or facial pain associated with disorder of cranium, neck, eyes, nose, sinuses, teeth, mouth, or other facial or cranial structures." Although this section

Table 7-1 Classification of Headache According to International Headache Society*

1. Migraine
   1.1 Migraine without aura
   1.2 Migraine with aura
2. Tension-Type Headache
3. Cluster Headache and Chronic Paroxysmal Hemicrania
4. Miscellaneous Headaches Unassociated with Structural Lesion
5. Headache Associated with Head Trauma
6. Headache Associated with Vascular Disorders
7. Headache Associated with Nonvascular Intracranial Disorder
8. Headache Associated with Substances or their Withdrawal
9. Headache Associated with Noncephalic Infection
10. Headache Associated with Metabolic Disorder
11. Headache or Facial Pain Associated with Disorder of Cranium, Neck, Eyes, Ears, Nose, Sinuses, Teeth, Mouth, or other Facial or Cranial Structures
12. Cranial Neuralgias, Nerve Trunk Pain, and Deafferentation Pain
13. Headache not Classifiable

*From Headache Classification Committee of the International Headache Society. Classification and diagnosis criteria for headache disorders, cranial neuralgia, and facial pain. Cephalalgia 1988; 8:1–96.

sounds conclusive it does not describe orofacial pains of neuropathic source or that which is referred from nonmasticatory structures. This classification also fails to consider the psychologic aspect of the pain condition.

An understanding of the genesis of pain can add more refinement to a pain classification. The previous chapters in this text have described in detail how nociceptive input from different tissues of the body can produce pain. An important concept presented was that the clinical characteristics of the pain can be useful in identifying the tissues or structures that are responsible for the pain. A reasonable classification for pain disorders, therefore, would be based on the structures that are responsible for producing the nociceptive input (the true origin of the pain). However, even this type of classification does not consider the psychologic factors that may influence or even cause the pain disorder. For the clinician to fully classify the pain disorder, he or she must consider both the somatosensory input and the psychosocial input. A complete pain classification must assess the pain condition on two levels or axes. One axis represents the physical factors that are responsible for the nociceptive input and the other axis represents the psychologic factors that influence the pain experience. In this text, *Axis I* will depict the physical factors and *Axis II* will depict the psychologic factors. In evaluating any pain disorder both axes must be considered. Once both axes have been considered, a diagnosis can be established and proper therapy selected. Therapy that addresses only one axis will likely fail if the other axis is a major contributor to the pain disorder.

As previously discussed, some pain disorders are influenced by one axis more than the other. For example, acute pains are commonly related more to Axis I factors than Axis II factors. Therefore acute pains often respond well to therapies directed toward the somatosensory input. Chronic pains, however, often have significant Axis II factors and therefore therapies directed only to somatosensory inputs will likely fail. This concept is essential to successful management of pain.

Axis I (Physical Conditions)

Axis I represents the physical conditions that are responsible for the initiation of nociceptive impulses. These conditions can be classified according to the tissues that produce the nociception. The following is a list of orofacial structures that comprise the basis for a classification of orofacial pains:

1. Cutaneous and mucogingival pains
2. Mucosal pains of the pharynx, nose, and paranasal sinuses
3. Pains of dental origin
4. Pains of the musculoskeletal structures of the mouth and face
5. Pains of the visceral structures of the mouth and face
6. Pains of the neural structures of the mouth and face

Axis II (Psychologic Conditions)

Axis II represents the psychologic conditions that can either produce or influence the pain experience. The American Psychiatric Association has developed a comprehensive classification for mental disorders.[5] Only the categories that may be associated with pain will be discussed in this text. For a more complete review of all mental disorders, the clinician should review this document. Mental disorders that need to be considered as Axis II factors are:

1. Anxiety disorders
2. Mood disorders
3. Somatoform disorders
4. Other conditions, such as psychologic factors affecting a medical condition

Categories of Orofacial Pains

For the clinician to begin classifying orofacial pain disorders, he or she must first be able to differentiate the signs and symptoms associated with each category. In this section, physical and psychologic factors will be separated and identified. This begins the process called diagnosis and represents the most important process for the successful management of pain. Without proper diagnosis, appropriate therapy cannot be selected.

Reliable pain classification needs to be based on the symptoms. This requires an understanding of the clinical characteristics displayed by the different categories of pain. It is on the basis of the subjective and objective symptoms of the nociceptive condition under examination that proper identification is made. If one fully appreciates the concept of pain modulation, understands and can differentiate primary from secondary pain, has some knowledge of pain genesis, can identify the categories of pain by their clinical characteristics, and appreciates psychologic factors, a truly sophisticated and useful classification of orofacial pains is possible. As concepts have evolved in recent years, this pain classification has undergone considerable metamorphosis. It represents a logical classification for orofacial pains that conforms well to current knowledge of nociceptive mechanisms and psychologic factors. Table 7-2 outlines these classification categories.

Axis I Categories (Physical Conditions)

The various tissues of the body make up the physical conditions that are responsible for nociceptive input that can eventually produce pain. These tissues can be divided into two broad categories: somatic and neurogenous. Neurogenous tissues are those tissues that comprise the communication system while somatic tissues refer to all other body tissues. The somatic structures are the envelope, the musculoskeletal system, the supply system, and the special sensory organs. The manner by which each system communicates with the neurologic system is perceived differently by the brain and brain stem. Therefore each type of somatic tissue can be differentiated from the other somatic tissues by unique clinical characteristics. Understanding these characteristics is essential to diagnosis.

Somatic Pain. Somatic pains occur in response to the stimulation of normal neural receptors. Local conditions such as inflammation increase the receptivity of the neural structures so that stimulation becomes more evident. Reduced central inhibitory control of the passage of peripheral impulses to the higher centers also causes less intense peripheral stimulation to become more noxious. The degree of pain therefore does not necessarily relate to the intensity of the stimulus.

The neural structures involved in such pain reception and transmission are presumed to be normal, and the sensation serves to warn, alert, or inform the patient about such noxious stimulation. The conscious sensation of pain under such conditions is an added component to the voluminous sensory input the brain receives constantly, and it serves the purpose of preparing the patient for the appropriate response. Afferent neurons of both the peripheral (somatic) and autonomic (vis-

Table 7-2 Orofacial Pain Classification

Axis I (Physical Conditions)

I. Somatic pain
  A. Superficial somatic pain
    1. Cutaneous pain
    2. Mucogingival pain
  B. Deep somatic pain
    1. Musculoskeletal pain
      a. Muscle pain
        i. Protective co-contraction
        ii. Delay onset muscle soreness
        iii. Myofascial pain
        iv. Myospasm
        v. Myositis
      b. Temporomandibular joint pain
        i. Ligamentous pain
        ii. Retrodiscal pain
        iii. Capsular pain
        iv. Arthritic pain
      c. Osseous and periosteal pain
      d. Soft connective tissue pain
      e. Periodontal dental pain
    2. Visceral pain
      a. Pulpal dental pain
      b. Vascular pain
        i. Arteritis
        ii. Carotidynia
      c. Neurovascular pain
        i. Migraine with aura
        ii. Migraine without aura
        iii. Cluster headache
        iv. Paroxysmal Hemicrania
        v. Neurovascular variants
      d. Visceral mucosal pain
      e. Glandular, ocular, and auricular pain
II. Neuropathic pain
  A. Episodic neuropathic pain
    1. Paroxysmal neuralgia
      a. Trigeminal neuralgia
      b. Glossopharyngeal neuralgia

      c. Geniculate neuralgia
      d. Superior laryngeal neuralgia
      e. Nervous intermedius
    2. Neurovascular pain (see visceral pain)
  B. Continuous neuropathic pains
    1. Neuritis
      a. Peripheral neuritis
      b. Herpes zoster
      c. Postherpatic neuralgia
    2. Deafferentation pain
      a. Neuroma
      b. Atypical odontalgia
    3. Sympathetically maintained pain

Axis II (Psychologic Conditions)

I. Mood disorders
  A. Depressive disorders
  B. Bipolar disorders
  C. Mood disorders due to a medical condition
II. Anxiety disorders
  A. Generalized anxiety disorders
  B. Posttraumatic stress disorders
  C. Anxiety disorders due to a medical condition
III. Somatoform disorders
  A. Undifferentiated somatoform disorders
  B. Conversion disorders
  C. Pain disorders
  D. Hypochondriasis
IV. Other conditions
  A. Malingering
  B. Psychologic factors affecting a medical condition
    1. Personality traits or coping style
    2. Maladaptive health behavior
    3. Stress-related physiologic response
  C. Any other mental disorders not mentioned in this classification

ceral) nervous systems participate in this mechanism.

The clinical characteristics of pain that originates in superficial structures are distinctly different from those of deep origin. It is by these differences that the two types of somatic pain are distinguished.

Superficial Somatic Pain. The external surface of the body is richly innervated with receptors and sensory fibers of different types. These constantly feed information to the somatosensory cortex concerning the organism's environment. Not only does such sensation establish full conscious contact between the organism and its surroundings, it also furnishes the impetus for involuntary reflex activity. Superficial sensation serves a protective function so the organism may react appropriately to the constant and varied environmental threat to its well-being, comfort, and survival.

The sensory system provides input at conscious levels that allow precise definition of the physical characteristics of the stimulus including its modality, location, duration, and intensity. Pain emanating from these superficial structures presents characteristics at a conscious level of the definition of the physical properties of the noxious stimulus. These qualities are inherent in superficial somatic pain and furnish the examiner a means of identifying it.

Superficial pains have a bright, stimulating quality.[6-8] This probably results from the alarm reaction that such discomfort tends to create. As part of the environmental threat, superficial pain causes the patient to react in such a way to escape such threat (fight or flight response). The more severe the superficial pain, the more pronounced this stimulating quality becomes.

Superficial pains can be correctly located by the patient so that he is aware precisely of where he or she hurts. The patient is able to describe the location of the pain with anatomic accuracy.

Since the source of superficial pain is noxious stimulation of the very structures that hurt, the location of the pain clearly identifies where to look for its cause: the site of pain and site of origin are identical. In fact, if the cause of the pain is not immediately evident or reasonably explicable, the diagnosis of superficial pain should be questioned.

Since superficial somatic pain is due to a lowered pain threshold and since the site of pain and the location of its true source are the same, the discomfort that results from provocation at the site of pain relates faithfully to the stimulus. This means that the reaction is immediate, it is proportional to the intensity of the stimulus, it lasts as long as the stimulus, and there is no reference of pain to other normal structures. Superficial pain responds faithfully to provocation. Effects of central sensitization such as referred pain, secondary hyperalgesia, local autonomic effects, and secondary muscle co-contraction are not observed.

Since superficial pain emanates from the surface tissue, application of a topical anesthetic interrupts the pain. It should be noted that neither neuropathic pain felt in superficial tissues nor pain referred from deeper structures to the surface is arrested by the application of topical local anesthesia.

Two types of superficial orofacial pain are recognized; namely, cutaneous pain and mucogingival pain.

To summarize, the following clinical characteristics are displayed by superficial somatic pain: the pain has a bright, stimulating quality; subjective localization of the pain is excellent and anatomically accurate; the site of pain identifies the correct location of its source; response to provocation at the site of pain is faithful in incidence, intensity, and location; and the application of a topical anesthetic at the site of pain temporarily arrests it.

Deep Somatic Pain. Sensory innervation of the deeper structures of the body supplies the somatosensory cortex with a constant inflow of information monitoring all the internal functioning of the body. No doubt the information has a certain precision of definition as to the physical characteristics of the stimulus including its modality, location, duration, and intensity, but this information is normally below conscious levels unless volition brings it to the attention of the subject. Functions that require precise definition of the physical characteristics of the stimulus, such as the action of skeletal muscles, are attended by some conscious sensation that is fairly precise for location. Most functions that operate at an involuntary level, such as the action of smooth muscle, are attended by sensations that remain below conscious levels unless unusual conditions prevail such as distension, pressure, sustained hyperemia, or inflammation.[9] In such cases, the conscious sensation usually is that of diffusely located and poorly defined discomfort or pain.

Deep pain has a dull, depressing quality,[6–8] sometimes causing a sickening sensation of nausea. The background sensation may be punctuated by momentary lancinating pains that the patient describes as stimulating and exciting. Such lancinating pain is usually initiated by sudden traction, distension, or distortion of deep tissues.

The depressing effect of pain arising in deeper body structures and mediated by either deep somatic or visceral afferent fibers is likely to be a manifestation of withdrawal reaction. In contrast to the alarm effect from an environmental threat as witnessed in superficial pain, the usual reaction to discomfort emanating from deeper structures is to prepare the subject for conservation and recovery. Therefore, a decrease in somatic skeletal activity occurs in favor of increased visceral function. The characteristic quality of deep pain is that the discomfort induces a depressing effect leading to inactivity and withdrawal, sometimes accompanied by lassitude, depression, weakness, or lowered blood pressure.[10]

Deep pain is less accurately localized by the patient. Some pains of deep origin, such as those from skeletal muscle or from the periodontal ligament, are fairly localizable. However, such localizing sensation is considerably less accurate and the ability of the patient to describe the painful site anatomically less certain than that with superficial pain. The area where pain is sensed is usually larger than the site from which it arises. Many deep pains, such as those emanating from the dental pulp or from blood vessels, are hardly localizable, and the patient's anatomic description of where he or she feels the pain may be diffuse indeed. Some deep pains manifest effects of central sensitization so that the pain may be referred to otherwise normal structures, and the descriptive location of the pain is nonanatomic.

Because of the variable and inconsistent localization of deep pain, the site of pain may not indicate the true origin. This applies especially to pains that occur spontaneously or in response to normal function. Pain provoked by manual palpation and manipulation more accurately identifies its true location, and this diagnostic maneuver often can be useful to isolate otherwise vague and diffusely located pain sites. Muscle and organ pains especially show this trait. It is true that the site of some deep pains may clearly identify the origin, but even then it is considerably less precise and dependable than with superficial pain. Although some deep pains are felt in sites much larger than the true source of pain, others may be felt in entirely normal structures. Since these variables are characteristic of deep pain, it behooves the examiner to take measures that prove the location of the pain source and not to depend on the site of pain for this information.

Deep pain may not be proportional to the stimulus. Although some deep pains (usually those with better localization) respond rather faithfully to a stimulus, the response is not as faithful as that with superficial pain. In contrast, some deep pains manifest little relationship between stimulus and response, and others cannot be provoked by manual palpation or the demands of function. Although the lack of faithful response to provocation is characteristic of deep pain (sometimes greater, sometimes less than the intensity of provocation would suggest), true summation effects are not seen. Therefore, triggering of intense pain by light touch or superficial movement is not characteristic of deep pain disorders.

One of the most important identifying clinical characteristics of deep pain is its tendency to display effects caused by central sensitization or hyperexcitability.[6,7] Deep pain input tends to provoke referred pains, secondary hyperalgesia, localized autonomic effects, and secondary muscle co-

contraction. This tendency relates to the continuity, severity, and duration of the deep pain input. When diagnostic evidence of such central excitatory effects is observed, a deep pain disorder must be suspected and a serious diagnostic search made for the primary pain source. Great care must be exercised not to confuse secondary pain effects, which may actually be the patient's clinical complaint, with the primary pain syndrome, which may be silent and therefore nonsymptomatic to the patient. It is the manifestation of such secondary effects that creates much of the diffuse variability and spreading effect of some deep pains. Certainly, these effects are largely responsible for the confusion that surrounds many deep pain disorders and the therapeutic failure that sometimes occurs.

Deep pain usually is not arrested by the application of a topical anesthetic except when it arises from visceral mucosa such as the nasal mucosa in so-called sinus headache. Analgesic blocking of the nerve that mediates the primary painful impulses usually arrests deep pain, and this technique is useful diagnostically in localizing the source of such pains. Vascular pains, however, may not respond well to ordinary analgesic blocking.

To summarize, the following clinical characteristics are displayed by deep somatic pain: the pain has a dull, depressing quality; subjective localization of the pain is variable and somewhat diffuse; the site of pain may or may not identify the correct location of its true source; response to provocation at the site of pain is fairly faithful in incidence and intensity but not in location; and secondary central excitatory effects frequently accompany the deep pain.

There are two distinct types of deep somatic pain, namely, musculoskeletal pain and visceral pain. Musculoskeletal pain involves the action of receptors that respond to varying degrees of stimulation. Such pain therefore yields a graduated response to stimulation. Musculoskeletal pain relates intimately to biomechanical function. It can be localized to the degree that such a sense of localization is required in the course of normal functioning. Musculoskeletal pain is further subdivided into muscle pain, temporomandibular joint pain, osseous and periosteal pain, soft connective tissue pain, and dental pain of periodontal origin. Muscle pains include protective co-contraction, delayed onset muscle soreness, myofascial pain, myospasm, and myositis. Temporomandibular joint pain includes ligamentous pain, retrodiscal pain, capsular pain, and arthritic pain.

Visceral pain involves the action of high-threshold receptors of the interoceptive type. Such pain is not usually felt until the threshold is reached. Unless inflammatory, it does not present a graduated response to stimulation. It has little or no relationship to biomechanical function and is poorly localized by the subject. Visceral pain is further subdivided into neurovascular pain; vascular pain; dental pain of pulpal origin; visceral mucosal pain; and glandular, ocular, and auricular pain. Neurovascular pains are common and can be subdivided into migraine with aura; migraine without aura; cluster headache; paroxsymal hemicrania; and neurovascular variants.

Neuropathic Pain. Neuropathic pains are those that are generated within the nervous system itself.[11] Stimulation of receptors and nerve fibers is therefore unnecessary. Stimulation may cause summation effects so that the evoked response may be wholly disproportionate to the stimulus. A common clinical characteristic of neuropathic pain is the lack of any obvious source of the nociception. Since the pain originates in the neural structures, the somatic structures appear normal. Therefore, heterotopic pain is usually present. Neuropathic pains are commonly associated with other neurologic symptoms such as burning, hyperalgesia, dysesthesia, and even sometimes anesthesia. Neuropathic pain can present as either episodic pain or continuous pain. Since this characteristic is useful for classifying neuropathic pains, it will be used in this text.

Episodic Neuropathic Pains. Episodic neuropathic pains are characterized by periods of very intense pains followed by total remission. These pains may last from seconds to hours depending on the type. Usually, the individual is able to localize the site of pain quite well. The site, however, does not identify the correct source, since many of these pains are projected heterotopic pains. Response to provocation at the site of pain is unfaithful. Since these pains will demonstrate periods of total remission, secondary symptoms associated with central excitatory effects are not usually seen. Episodic neuropathic pains are classified into neuralgic pains or neurovascular pains.

Neuralgic pains are characterized by a bright, stimulating, burning quality that simulates superficial somatic pain from which it must be differentiated. These pains are said to be paroxysmal and therefore the name paroxysmal neuralgia. The pain is extremely intense but rarely lasts more than 20 to 30 seconds. Between episodes the individual will not experience pain. Neuralgic pains are categorized according to the affected nerve; for example, trigeminal neuralgia. Other neuralgias are glossopharyngeal neuralgia, geniculate neuralgia, superior laryngeal neuralgia, and intermedius neuralgia.

Neurovascular pains are characterized by periods of intense, debilitating, pulsating pain that typically last from 6 to 8 hours. These pains have already been classified under the visceral pain category. They are mentioned here because of recent studies that have demonstrated that their etiology is likely to begin with a neuromechanism. Neurovascular pains will be discussed under the category of visceral pains since their clinical characteristics are more typical of visceral pains.

Continuous Neuropathic Pains. Continuous neuropathic pains result from interference with the normal transmission of afferent impulses by primary sensory neurons. Many of these pains are felt as a persistent, ongoing, unremitting, burning sensation. These pains may have some fluctuation in intensity but no periods of total remission. These will often show an enlargement of the receptive field and diminished central inhibitory activity. They occur from a variety of conditions, but trauma or some other form of damage to the neuron is common. Continuous neuropathic pains are classified into one of three categories: neuritis, deafferentation pains or sympathetically maintained pains. The neuritic neuropathic pains (neuritis) are subdivided into three types: peripheral neuritis, herpes zoster and postherpatic neuralgia. Deafferentation pains are subdivided into traumatic neuralgia and atypical odontalgia.

Axis II Categories (Psychologic Conditions)

As previously stated, psychologic conditions influence all pains. These conditions have their greatest effects on chronic pains. The longer a patient suffers, the greater the influence of these factors. All clinicians treating pain disorders must be familiar with certain important psychologic factors so that when indicated, these conditions can be properly addressed.

Psychologic intensification of pain may proceed until the suffering is wholly disproportionate to the peripheral nociceptive input. Although the original pain complaint may have displayed the usual clinical characteristics of somatic or neuropathic pain, as psychologic intensification converts it into a chronic pain disorder, the clinical symptoms take on identifying features. Such pain lacks an adequate source of input that is anatomically related to the site of pain. It may be felt in multiple and sometimes changeable locations. Pain bilaterally may become evident in the absence of bilateral sources of noxious input. The complaint may display unusual or unexpected responses to therapy. It may respond too quickly or too slowly. It may respond in an exaggerated way or with unusual side effects or complications. The response may be followed by a relapse without organic justification, or the condition may remain refractory in spite of otherwise effective therapy. Pains that are greatly influenced by psychologic factors may display variability in location, intensity, or temporal behavior without a reasonable, identifiable organic cause.

To summarize, the following clinical characteristics are common to pain conditions that are greatly influenced by psychologic factors: the site of pain lacks an adequate, anatomically related source of nociceptive input; and its clinical behavior and responsiveness to reasonable therapy is unusual, unexpected, and nonphysiologic.

The psychologic influence of orofacial pains can be categorized into certain identifiable mental disorders.[12] Although there are numerous disorders, the clinician needs to be familiar with the following common mental disorders since these can greatly influence the individual's pain experience: mood disorders, anxiety disorders, somatoform disorders, and another category that includes many other mental conditions or psychologic factors that affect the outcome of a medical condition.

Each of these major categories can be separated into subcategories. Mood disorders are divided into the depressive disorders, bipolar disorders, and a general category in which the mood disorder is due to a medical condition.

Anxiety disorders are subdivided into the generalized anxiety disorders, posttraumatic stress disorders, and anxiety disorders that are due to a medical condition.

Somatoform disorders are a group of disorders that are characterized by physical symptoms suggesting a physical disorder for which there are no demonstrable organic findings of known physiologic mechanisms. Strong positive evidence that the symptoms are linked to psychologic factors or conflicts is important. The somatoform disorders are subdivided into undifferentiated somatoform disorders, conversion disorders, pain disorders, and hypochondriasis.

The last category is a broad group of mental disorders that may be related to pain conditions. This category includes malingering, psychologic factors affecting a medical condition, such as certain personality traits, coping styles, maladaptive health behavior, and stress-related physiologic responses.

Each category in Axis I and Axis II conditions will be presented in detail in later chapters along with treatment strategies.

References

1. Dorland's Illustrated Medical Dictionary, ed 26. Philadelphia: WB Saunders; 1981.
2. Merskey H. Pain terms: A list with definitions and notes on usage. Pain 1979; 6:249–252.
3. Merskey H. Pain terms: A supplementary note. Pain 1982; 14:205–206.
4. Headache Classification Committee of the International Headache Society. Classification and diagnosis criteria for headache disorders, cranial neuralgia, and facial pain. Cephalalgia 1988; 8 (suppl 7):1–96.
5. Diagnostic and Statistical Manual of Mental Disorders (DSM-IV), ed 4. Washington, DC: The American Psychiatric Association; 1994.
6. Bonica JJ. The Management of Pain. Philadelphia: Lea & Febiger, 1990; 161-169.
7. Wolff HG. Headache and Other Head Pain, ed 2. New York: Oxford University Press; 1963: 25–31.
8. Procacci P, Zoppi M, Maresea M. Experimental pain in man. Pain 1979; 6:123–140.
9. Wolff HG. Headache and Other Head Pain, ed 2. New York: Oxford University Press; 1963: 31–39.
10. Dellow PG, Morgan NJ. Trigeminal nerve inputs and central blood pressure change in the rat. Arch Oral Biol 1969; 14:295.
11. Bowsher D. A camel is a horse designed by a committee. J Pain Symptom Manage 1987; 2:237–239.
12. Diagnostic and Statistical Manual of Mental Disorders (DSM-IV), ed 4. Washington, DC: The American Psychiatric Association; 1994.

8

Principles of Pain Diagnosis

Everyday, patients seek care for the reduction or elimination of pain. Nothing is more satisfying to the clinician then the successful elimination of the patient's pain. This elimination is usually the result of some form of therapeutic intervention. Both the patient and clinician therefore tend to focus on the importance of the therapy. The most important part of managing pain, however, is in understanding the problem and establishing a proper diagnosis. It is only through proper diagnosis that the appropriate therapy can be selected. Diagnosis is not easy. Too often it is overlooked or deemphasized and yet success cannot be achieved without it. This chapter will describe the necessary components for diagnosis.

The objective of diagnosis is to accurately identify the what, where, how, and why of the patient's complaint. Pain diagnosis is complicated by some very difficult problems. Pain is a dynamic changing experience that embraces sensation, emotion, and reaction. Nociception is predominantly subjective in nature, while objective pain behavior reflects consequences as much as cause. Complex pain modulation phenomena individualize every painful experience.

These characteristics of pain make the diagnosis and management of obscure pains a sobering and sometimes humbling experience for even the most astute clinician.

One difficulty that many clinicians face is his or her mechanistic approach to disease. We are often very cause-oriented. The why in diagnosis, important as it is, may become a stumbling block when dealing with obscure pain, for there may be no cause at all. Understanding that all pains are not somatic is basic to diagnosis. Neuropathic pains and psychologic factors are not always obvious on examination. The clinician must be cognitive of the biopsychosocial model of disease. On the other hand, if the condition seems related to an actual stimulus of somatic structures, then identification of the cause is essential for proper management.

Another difficulty to which we must be aware is the temptation to assume that the symptoms of which the patient complains represent the real problem that needs to be investigated and managed. Pain behavior consists of audible and visible signals exhibited by the patient that indicate his suffering. These signals have filtered down through a chain of modulating influences, not the least of which are the consequences that attend the whole experience. Thus, the complaint as manifest by suffering may bear little relevance to the real underlying problem. Yet it is the suffering itself that the patient presents for treatment.

Diagnosing a pain complaint consists essentially of three major steps:

1. Accurately identifying the location of the structure from which the pain emanates.
2. Establishing the correct pain category that is represented in the condition under investigation. This is a matter of recognizing the clinical characteristics that are displayed. Establishing the proper pain category is dependent on a good understanding of the genesis and mechanisms of pain.
3. Choosing the particular pain disorder that correctly accounts for the incidence and behavior of the patient's pain problem. This requires familiarity with the clinical symptoms displayed by pain disorders that occur in the orofacial region.

Evaluating the Pain Condition

When a patient reports with pain, information must be gathered so that the clinician can determine the proper pain diagnosis. This information is gathered in two forms: the history and the clinical examination. The data collected in the history and clinical examination must be thorough enough to determine not only the physical factors that contribute to the pain disorders but also the psychologic factors. The main objective of the history and the clinical examination is to locate the true source of the pain that relates to the patient's chief complaint.

All pain complaints merit an interview with the patient to determine the significance of the complaint. Some pains are easy to identify and require little diagnostic effort. In these instances an elaborate evaluation may not be needed. Other pains require significant evaluation effort by the clinician. These pains require a very detailed orofacial pain history and examination. Determining the need for a thorough history and examination is determined by the preliminary interview.

Preliminary Interview

The initial contact with the patient and his problem is extremely important. Unless satisfactory professional rapport can be immediately established, it may be wise to refer the patient before becoming further involved. The rapport on which proper communication must rest requires sincere effort by both patient and doctor. The patient must be willing to honestly and accurately divulge the information the doctor needs. He or she must do so cooperatively and with a sincere desire to obtain relief from the complaint. If his or her intentions and objectives are anything less than this, not only will valuable time and effort be wasted, but the chances are that more harm than good will result.

The doctor must feel confident of his or her own competence in the identification and management of pain problems. Any lack of confidence will quickly be sensed by the patient and can destroy the chances of a satisfactory patient-doctor relationship. Moreover, it would be professionally dishonest for a doctor to pursue any course of action for which he or she felt unprepared. Competence, honesty, patience, and an earnest desire by the therapist to serve his or her patient are the minimal prerequisites for establishing a satisfactory professional rapport.

At the preliminary interview, sufficient data should be collected to help determine the future course of the examining procedure. Some overall idea of the location, inception, duration, and clinical behavior of the complaint should be obtained. Plans should then be made to either continue the examination, refer the patient to another doctor, or plan for consultations as indicated. Very simple pain problems such as mucogingival pain of local origin, localized pain due to obvious dental cause, and some cases of typical trigeminal neuralgia may be solved without further examination. More obscure pain complaints justify a carefully planned diagnostic procedure.

It is important to evaluate the patient's pain in terms of what it means to him or her. This is accomplished by obtaining specific and meaningful descriptors from the patient that accurately describe his or her complaint. Many patients may not have at their disposal an adequate means of communicating such exact information. In his McGill Pain Questionnaire, Melzack[1-4] arranged descriptive adjectives in several groups. Each series of words is arranged in an order of increasing intensity. The patient can be instructed to select one word in each series, the word that best describes the complaint. The first group is composed of sensory descriptors that help describe what the discomfort feels like to the patient:

1. Temporal: flicking, quivering, pulsing, throbbing, beating, pounding
2. Spatial: jumping, flashing, shooting
3. Punctate pressure: pricking, boring, drilling, stabbing, lancinating
4. Incisive pressure: sharp, cutting, lacerating
5. Constrictive pressure: pinching, pressing, gnawing, cramping, crushing
6. Traction pressure: tugging, pulling, wrenching
7. Thermal: hot, burning, scalding, searing
8. Brightness: tingling, itchy, smarting, stinging
9. Dullness: dull, sore, hurting, aching, heavy
10. Miscellaneous: tender, taut, rasping, splitting

The second group consists of affective descriptors that yield information about how the patient is reacting to the pain:

1. Tension: tiring, exhausting
2. Autonomic: sickening, suffocating
3. Fear: fearful, frightful, terrifying
4. Punishment: punishing, grueling, cruel, vicious, killing
5. Miscellaneous: wretched, blinding

The third group is a series of evaluative descriptors that tend to classify the intensity of pain: annoying, troublesome, miserable, intense, unbearable.

A fourth group of general descriptors has been added to the questionnaire:

1. Spreading, radiating, penetrating, piercing
2. Tight, numb, drawing, squeezing, tearing
3. Cool, cold, freezing
4. Nagging, nauseating, agonizing, dreadful, torturing

Patients who cannot verbalize the description of their complaint may find these descriptors useful.

When the clinician identifies a complex pain complaint a more through evaluation should be accomplished. This evaluation is composed of two major components: the history and the clinical examination. Information gained during the history and examination should allow the clinician to place the pain complaint in the proper pain category so that effective therapy may be selected. Establishing the proper diagnosis is the most important task accomplished by the clinician and should never be underemphasized. It is the basis for successful pain management.

The history is an investigation of all aspects of the pain complaint. It should assess the present location of the pain complaint, the time it began, and a detailed description of the pain as initially felt. An evaluation of the early characteristics of the complaint may give valuable clues to its identification prior to modification. Information concerning the duration and clinical course of the complaint with special reference to efforts at treatment is valuable. The general physical and emotional background for the complaint should be noted as well as the influence of prior trauma, infection, or systemic illness. All medications currently in use should be listed.

The examination should gather information from clinical, radiographic, and laboratory procedures relative to the oral cavity, masticatory system, and regional musculature. Special information derived from diagnostic analgesic blocking, the effect of diagnostic drugs, and trial therapy may also be helpful.

History for Orofacial Pain

An accurate history is the most important aspect in the diagnosis obscure pain. It is far more important than the examination. If the clinician will carefully listen, the patient will report the precise pain problem that exists. The patient may use nonmedical terms but, nevertheless, the information should allow the clinician to establish a differential diagnosis. The examination can then be used to further clarify the proper pain category or disorder. Much thought should therefore be given to the skillful interviewing of the patient.

History-taking can be accomplished in one of two forms: oral or written. An oral history provides some advantages over the written history in that it allows the clinician to meet the patient and establish important rapport. It also allows the patient to express his feelings and experiences in his or her own words. The clinician can often gain insight regarding the patient's feelings concerning experiences, anger, fear, hostility, and disability. Oral history-taking allows the clinician to gain information in a logical sequence, asking appropriate questions as needed. The major disadvantage of the oral history is that it relies heavily on the clinician's ability to remember all aspects of the history so that no important information is missed. A written history form can eliminate this concern. With a written history form all important aspects can be included and the patient can fill the form out leisurely in advance of the appointment. Although this type of history is certainly more reliably complete, it may be frustrating to the patient when the questions do not adequately allow him or her to depict the problem.

In many offices, both types of histories are used. The written form is completed in advance of the appointment. This is reviewed by the clinician before actually meeting the patient. Then when the patient is seated, the clinician allows the patient to verbalize the pain complaint while establishing the important doctor/patient rapport. Any confusing items observed in the written history can then be clarified.

Table 8-1 outlines the important features that should be included in a thorough orofacial pain history.

The Chief Complaint

A good starting point in history-taking is to obtain an accurate description of the patient's chief complaint. This should first be taken in the patient's own words and then restated in technical language as indicated. If the patient has more than one pain complaint, they should all be noted and when possible placed in a list according to their significance to the patient. Each complaint needs to be evaluated according to each factor listed in the history outline. Once this has been accomplished, each pain complaint should be assessed as to its relationship to any of the other complaints. Some complaints may be secondary to another complaint while others may be independent. Determining these relationships is basic to management.

Location of Pain. The patient's ability to locate the pain with accuracy is diagnostic. The examiner, however, should always guard against assuming that the site of pain necessarily identifies the true source of pain: the structure from which the pain actually emanates. The patient's description of

Table 8-1 Features to Include in an Orofacial Pain History

I. The chief complaint (perhaps more than one)
  A. Location of pain
  B. Onset of Pain
    1. Associated with other factors
    2. Progression
  C. Characteristics of pain
    1. Quality of pain
    2. Behavior of pain
      a. Temporal
      b. Frequency
      c. Duration
    3. Intensity
    4. Concomitant symptoms
    5. Flow of the pain
  D. Aggravating and alleviating factors
    1. Physical modalities
    2. Function and parafunction
    3. Sleep disturbances
    4. Medications
    5. Emotional stress
  E. Past consultation and/or treatments
  F. Relationship to other complaints
II. Past medical history
III. Review of systems
IV. Psychologic assessment

the location of his or her complaint identifies only the site of pain. It is the examiner's responsibility to determine whether it is also the true source of the pain. Sometimes, what appears to be adequate cause at the site of pain may mislead both patient and doctor, such as visible superficial herpetic lesions or deep tenderness to manual palpation or functional manipulation.

It can be very helpful to provide the patient with a drawing of the head and neck and ask him or her to outline the location of the pain (Fig 8-1). This allows the patient to reflect in his or her own way any and all of the pain sites. The patient can also draw

Fig 8-1 Asking the patient to draw the location of the pain and any patterns of referral on a drawing of the head and neck can be very helpful. 1a reveals how a patient with masticatory muscle pain described her pain. Note the broad areas of pain and the radiating patterns of referral. 1b depicts how a patient experiencing TMJ pain describes the location of her pain. 1c reveals the location of the pain felt by a patient suffering with myofascial pain in the cervical region with referral to the head as headache.

8-1a

8-1b

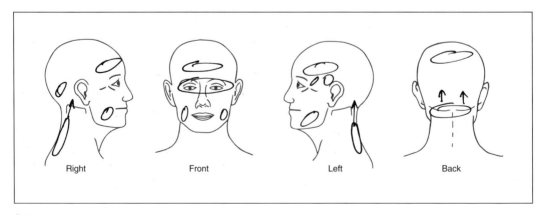

8-1c

arrows revealing any patterns of pain referral. These drawings can give the clinician significant insight regarding the location and even the type of pain the patient is experiencing.

Onset of the Pain. It is important to assess any circumstances that were associated with the initial onset of the pain complaint. These circumstances can give great insight as to etiology. For example, in some instances the pain complaint began immediately following a motor vehicle accident. Trauma is a frequent cause of a pain condition and not only gives insight as to etiology but also enlightens the examiner to other considerations such as other injuries, related emotional trauma, and possible litigation. The onset of some pain conditions are associated with systemic illnesses, or jaw function, or may even be wholly spontaneous. It is important that the patient present the circumstances associated with the initial onset in chronologic order so that proper relationships can be evaluated.

It is equally important to ask the patient what he or she feels caused the pain condition. This may provide great insight into the patient's view of his or her pain. In many instances, the patient knows precisely what caused the condition. Even if the patient is confused as to cause, the examiner may gain valuable information that is useful in management. For example, this question may reveal anger associated with blame for the pain condition. It is important to know if the patient believes the pain has been caused by mistreatment or another practitioner. This type of anger may greatly impact on future treatment outcome.

Characteristics of the Pain. The characteristics of the pain need to be precisely described by the patient as to its quality, behavior, intensity, concomitant symptoms, and manner of flow.

Quality of the Pain. The quality of pain should be classified according to how it makes the patient feel. This classification is usually termed bright or dull. When pain has a stimulating or exciting effect on the patient it is classified as bright. When the pain has a depressing effect that causes the patient to withdraw to some extent, it is classified as dull. It is important that such judgment be wholly independent of pain intensity, variability, temporal characteristics, or any accompanying lancinating exacerbations that may punctuate the basic underlying painful sensation.

Further evaluation of the quality of pain should be made to classify it as pricking, itching, stinging, burning, aching, or pulsating. Many pains, of course, require more than a single designation. Bright, tingling pain is classified as a pricking sensation, especially when mild and stimulating. Superficial discomfort that does not reach pain threshold intensity may be described as itching. As intensity increases, it may take on a pricking, stinging, aching, or burning quality. Deep discomfort that does not reach pain threshold intensity may be described as a vague, diffuse sensation of pressure, warmth, or tenderness. As intensity increases, the pain may take on a sore, aching, throbbing, or burning quality. When the discomfort has an irritating, hot, raw, caustic quality, it is usually described as burning. Most pains have an aching quality. Some noticeably increase with each heart beat and are described as pulsating or throbbing.

Behavior of the Pain. The behavior of the pain should be evaluated according to frequency or temporal behavior as well as its duration and localizability.

Temporal behavior reflects the frequency of the pain as well as the periods between episodes of the pain. If the suffering distinctly comes and goes, leaving pain-free intervals of noticeable duration, it is classified as *intermittent.* If such pain-free intervals do not occur, it is classified as *continuous.* Intermittency should not be confused with variability in which there may be alternate periods of high and low level discomfort. Intermittent pain implies the occurrence of true intermissions or pain-free periods during which comfort is complete. This temporal behavior should not be confused with the effect of medications that induce periods of comfort by analgesic action. When episodes of pain, whether continuous or intermittent, are separated by an extended period of freedom from discomfort only to be followed by another similar episode of pain, the syndrome is said to be *recurrent.*

The *duration* of individual pains in an episode is an important descriptive feature that aids in pain identification. A pain is said to be *momentary* if its duration can be expressed in seconds. Longer lasting pains are classified in minutes, hours, or a day. A pain that continues from one day to the next is said to be *protracted.*

The *localization behavior* of the pain should be included in its description. If the patient is able to define the pain to an exact anatomic location, it is classified as *localized pain.* If such description is less well defined and somewhat vague and variable anatomically, it is termed diffuse pain. Rapidly changing pain is classified as *radiating.* A momentary cutting exacerbation is usually described as *lancinating.* More gradually changing pain is described as *spreading,* and if it progressively involves adjacent anatomic areas, the pain is called *enlarging.* If it changes from one location to another, the complaint is described as *migrating.* Referred pain and secondary hyperalgesia are clinical expressions of secondary pain.

Intensity of the Pain. The intensity of pain should be established by distinguishing between mild and severe pain. This can be based on how the patient appears to react to his suffering. Mild pain is associated with pain that is described by the patient but there is no display of visible physical reactions. Severe pain are associated with significant reactions of the patient to provocation of the painful area. One of the best methods of assessing the intensity of the pain is with a visual analog scale. The patient is presented with a line that has "no pain" written on one end and "the most possible pain experienced" written on the other end. The patient is then asked to place a mark on the location of the line that best describes his or her pain today. A scale of 0 to 5 or 0 to 10 can be used to assess the intensity of the pain, zero being no pain and 10 being the most pain possible. This scale is not only helpful for the initial assessment of pain but is also useful at follow-up appointments to evaluate the success or failure of therapies.

Concomitant Symptoms. All concomitant symptoms such as sensory, motor, or autonomic effects that accompany the pain should be included. Sensations such as hyperesthesia, hypoesthesia, anesthesia, paresthesia, or dysesthesia should be mentioned. Any concomitant change in the special senses affecting vision, hearing, smell, or taste should be noted. Motor changes expressed as muscular weakness, muscular contractions, or actual spasm should be recognized. Various localized autonomic symptoms should be observed and described. Ocular symptoms may include lacrimation, injection of the conjunctivae, pupillary changes, and edema of the lids. Nasal symptoms include nasal secretion and congestion. Cutaneous symptoms comprise skin temperature, color, sweating, and piloerection. Gastric symptoms include nausea and indigestion.

Manner of Flow of Pain. The manner of flow yields important information by determining whether the individual pains are steady or paroxysmal. A flowing type of pain, even though variable in intensity or distinctly intermittent, is described as *steady.* Such pain is to be distinguished from *paroxysmal* pain, which characteristically consists of sudden volleys or jabs. The volleys may vary considerably in both intensity and duration. When they occur frequently, the pain may become nearly continuous.

Aggravating and Alleviating Factors

Effect of Functional Activities. The effect of functional activities should be observed and described. Common biomechanical functions include such activities as movement of the face, jaw, or tongue and the effects of swallowing, head position, and body position. The effect of activities such as talking, chewing, yawning, brushing the teeth, shaving, washing the face, turning the head, stooping over, or lying down should be noted. The effect of emotional stress, fatigue, and time of day also should be recorded.

It may be triggered by minor superficial stimulation such as touch or movement of the skin, lips, face, tongue, or throat. When pain is triggered by such activities, one must distinguish between stimulation of overlying tissues that are only incidentally stimulated and the result of functioning of the joints and muscles themselves. The former is true triggering while the latter is pain induction. This distinction can usually be made by stabilizing the joints and muscles with a bite block to prevent their movement while the other structures are stimulated or moved. If uncertainty exists, the distinction can be made more positively by utilizing local anesthesia. Topical anesthesia of the throat effectively arrests triggering in the glossopharyngeal nerve distribution. Mandibular block anesthesia stops triggering from the lower lip and tongue. Infraorbital anesthesia arrests triggering from the upper lip and maxillary skin. None of these procedures prevents the induction of true masticatory pain.

Parafunctional activities should also be assessed. The patient should be questioned regarding bruxism, clenching, or any other oral habit. One should remember that often these activities occur at subconscious levels and reporting may not be accurate with the reporting.

Effect of Physical Modalities. The patient should be questioned regarding the effectiveness of hot or cold on the pain condition. The patient should be asked if other modalities such as massage or transcutaneous electrical nerve stimulation therapy have been tried and if so what were the results. The results of such therapies may shed light of the type and therapeutic responsiveness of the pain condition.

Medications. The patient should review all past and present medications taken for the pain condition. Dosages should be reported along with the frequency taken and effectiveness in altering the chief complaint. It is also helpful to know who prescribed these medications since their input may also shed light on the pain condition.

Emotional Stress. As previously discussed, emotional stress can be a major contributing factor to the pain condition. In some instances, however, emotional stress may not be a major factor but instead an aggravating factor. When this is present, patients will report that although their pain is present at all times it seems to be accentuated during times of increased stress. It is important for both the clinician and the patient to recognize this relationship.

Sleep Quality. There appears to be a relationship between some pain conditions and the quality of the patient's sleep.[5-8] It is important, therefore, that quality of sleep be reviewed. Patients who report poor-quality sleep should be questioned regarding the relationship of this finding with the pain condition. Particular notice should taken when the patient reports waking during the night in pain or when the pain actually wakes the patient.

Litigation. During the interview, it is important to inquire if the patient is involved in any form of ligation related to the pain complaint. This information may help the clinician better appreciate all conditions surrounding the pain. The presence of litigation does not directly imply secondary gains, but this condition may be present.

Past Consultations and Treatments. During the interview, all previous consultations and treatments should be thoroughly discussed and reviewed. This information is extremely important so that repetition of tests and therapies is avoided. If information is incomplete or unclear the previous treating clinician should be contacted and appropriate information requested. Clinical notes from previous treating clinicians can be extremely helping in planning future treatments.

When a patient reports previous treatments such as an occlusal appliance, the patient should be asked to bring the appliance to the evaluation appointment. The previous success of this treatment should be reported and the appliance evaluated. This evaluation may shed light on future treatment considerations.

Relationship to Other Pain Complaints. As previously discussed, some patients may report more than one pain complaint. When more than one complaint is reported, the clinician needs to evaluate each aspect of each complaint separately. Once each complaint is evaluated according to all the previously mentioned criteria, the relationship of one complaint to the others should be ascertained. Sometimes a pain complaint may actually be secondary to another complaint. In these instances effective management of the primary pain complaint will likely also resolve the secondary pain complaint. In other instances one complaint may be totally independent of another complaint. When this exists, individual therapy may need to be directed to each complaint.

Identifying the relationship between these complaints is essential and best determined by the history.

Medical History

Since pain can be a symptom related to many physical illnesses and disorders, it is essential that the past and present medical condition be carefully evaluated. Any past serious illnesses, hospitalizations, operations, medications, or other significant treatments should be discussed in light of the present pain complaint. When indicated, treating physicians should be contacted for additional information. It may also be appropriate to discuss your suggested treatment with the patient's physician when significant health problems are present.

Review of Systems

A complete history should also include appropriate questions concerning the present status of the patient's general body systems. Questions should investigate the present health status of the following systems: cardiovascular (including lungs), digestive, renal, liver, as well as the peripheral and central nervous systems. Any abnormalities should be noted and any relationship with the pain complaint should be determined.

Psychologic Assessment

As pain becomes more chronic, psychologic factors relating to the pain complaint become more common. Routine psychologic evaluation may not be necessary with acute pain; however, with chronic pain it becomes essential. It may be difficult for the general practitioner to confidently evaluate psychologic factors. For this reason, patients with chronic pain are best evaluated and managed by a multidisciplinary approach.

There are a variety of measuring tools that can be used to assess the psychologic status of the patient. Turk and Rudy[9] have developed the Multidimensional Pain Inventory (MPI). This scale evaluates three pain profiles: adaptive coping, interpersonal distress, and dysfunctional chronic pain. Dysfunctional chronic pain is a profile of severe pain, functional disability, psychologic impairment, and low perceived life control.

Another useful tool is the Symptom Check List 90 (SCL-90).[10] This evaluation provides both a depression scale and a scale measuring the severity of nonspecific physical symptoms (the somatization subscale). Assessment of these factors is essential when evaluating the patient who has chronic pain.

Often the general practitioner may not have immediate access to psychologic evaluation support. In this instance, the practitioner may elect to use IMPATH[11] or the TMJ Scale.[12,13] These two scales have been developed for use in the private dental practice to assist in evaluating clinical and certain psychologic factors associated with orofacial pains. Although these scales are helpful, they are not as complete as the previously mentioned psychologic tests and certainly do not replace evaluation by a clinical psychologist.

As discussed in Chapters 6 and 7, there are a number of psychologic conditions that can contribute to or actual be responsible for the pain disorder. One category of psychologic conditions is the *somatoform disorders*. These disorders are characterized by complaints of physical symptoms for which there are no demonstrable organic findings or known physical mechanisms. When pain is the chief complaint, this disorder is called a *somatoform pain disorder*.[14] Another type of somatoform disorder is a *conversion disorder*. The essential feature of this disorder is an alteration or loss of physical functioning that suggests a physical disorder, but instead of the presence of an actual physical disorder the symptoms are an apparent expression of a psychologic conflict or need. The symptoms are not intentionally produced, yet they cannot be explained by any physical disorder or known pathophysiologic mechanism. A third type of somatoform disorder is hypochondriasis. The essential feature of this disorder is preoccupation with the fear of having, or the belief that one has, a serious disease, based on the patient's interpretation of physical signs or symptoms as evidence of physical illness.

Psychologic assessment is also important in identifying other mental disorders such as mood disorders (ie, depression) and anxiety disorders. There is also a broad category that includes psychologic factors that are affecting a physical condition. In this category, the psychologic factor may not be significant enough to warrant its own disorder but in fact does affect an existing condition. This category may likely be the most common psychologic condition associated with chronic orofacial pain disorders.

Psychologic assessment is an essential part of the orofacial pain history. The manner by which it is performed will vary according to the expertise of the clinician. As pain disorders become more chronic, it is best for the clinician to rely on a trained clinical psychologist or psychiatrist for this evaluation.

Summary of History

Once the history has been obtained, the clinician should be able to accurately and completely describe the pain condition. For example, a typical narrative description of trigeminal neuralgia involving the right mandibular division of the trigeminal nerve would be as follows:

A 1-year history of severe pain in the right mandibular dental and alveolar process area spontaneously triggered by light touch and movement of lower lip. The complaint is described as recurrent episodes of bright burning pain that occur intermittently in repeated paroxysms lasting a few seconds each time and felt in the same precise anatomic location with little or no variation from time to time. No secondary pains are noticed. The paroxysms are excited by all functional activities that cause minor stimulation of the lower lip. The pains are accompanied by contraction of facial muscles, but no other concomitant neurologic effects are seen. The pain is not relieved or prevented by any medications. The patient does not present any significant psychologic conditions, although does admit the pain has increased his general anxiety level secondary to not knowing when the next pain will strike.

Orofacial Pain
Clinical Examination

An effective examination form helps the doctor obtain essential data with the least expenditure of time and effort. Making sure that such data are complete is an important step in the identification of pain. An examination form should be as simple and flexible as possible to be readily adaptable to the many different pain problems that present themselves.

The purpose of the clinical examination is to identify any variations from normal health and function of the orofacial structures. The examination should include an assessment of nonmasticatory structures, such as the neurologic status as well as evaluation of the eyes, ears, and neck. If abnormal findings are identified, an immediate referral to the appropriate specialty is indicated. The examination should also include an assessment of the masticatory structures.

Locating the Source of Pain

Although the history is important in identifying the site of pain, it is the examination that is most helpful in locating the true source of the pain. The clinician should always be suspicious of heterotopic pains since they are so common in the orofacial structures. Remember, for therapy to be effective, it must be directed toward the source of pain not the site. This, of course, is no problem if the pain is primary pain since both the site and source are in the same location. If, however, the pain is referred, this presents an interesting twist.

When referred pains are present, the clinician may often have a tendency to direct therapy to the site of pain as directed by the patient. Of course this type of therapy will fail since it will not affect the cause of the pain. The astute pain clinician will always be suspicious of referred pain and will always clinically confirm the source of the pain.

Primary pains can be differentiated from referred pains by their characteristics during local provocation (Fig 8-2a). Remember, referred pains are wholly dependent on the original source of the pain. Therefore, when a source of pain is located during an examination, palpation of the source will not only increase the pain at the source but will also likely increase the pain at the referred site (Fig 8-2b). If palpation of the site of pain does not increase the pain, one should be suspicions of a referred site of pain. If the information gained during the examination is not complete enough to identify the pain, then selective local anesthetic blocking of selected tissues may be needed. Local anesthetic blocking of the site of pain will not decrease the pain since it does not interrupt the true source of the pain (Fig 8-2c). On the other hand, when the source of pain is anesthetically blocked (Fig 8-2d), the pain will be reduced not only at the source but also at the site. When the clinician is confused regarding the true source of the pain, local anesthetic blocking should be used. In some instances it may be the only way to locate the true source of pain. Pain therapists need to be familiar with the various local anesthetic blocks used in the head and neck. These injections will be discussed later in this chapter.

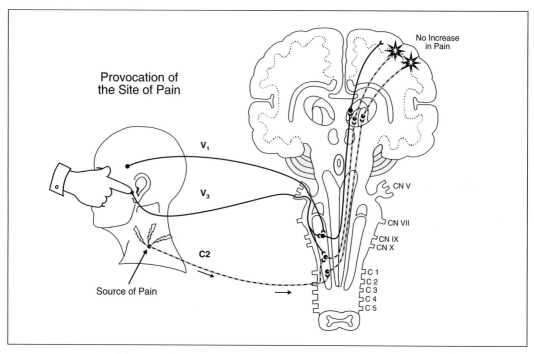

8-2a   Provocation of the site of pain does not increase the pain.

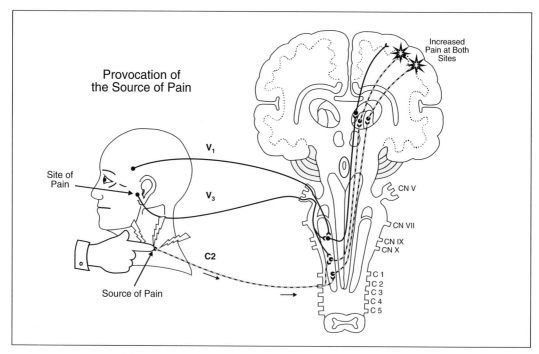

8-2b   Provocation of the source of pain increases the pain at the source and may also increase the pain at the site.

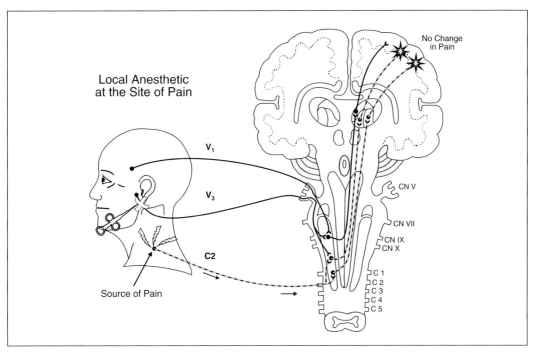

8-2c   Local anesthesia at the site of pain fails to reduce the pain.

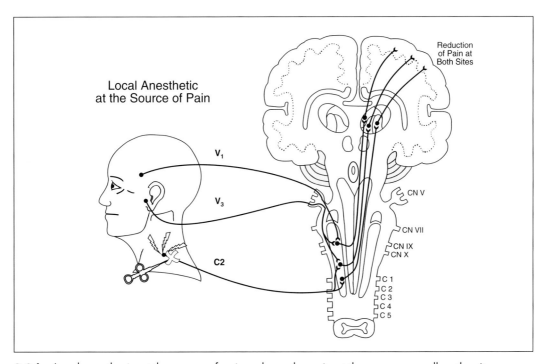

8-2d   Local anesthesia at the source of pain reduces the pain at the source as well as the site.

The following four rules summarize the examination techniques used to differentiate primary pain from referred pain: local provocation of the site of pain does not increase the pain; local provocation at the source of pain increases the pain not only at the source, but also increases the pain at the site; local anesthetic blocking of the site of pain does not decrease the pain; and local anesthetic blocking of the source of the pain decreases the pain at the source as well as the site.

An orofacial pain examination should thoroughly evaluate all structures of the orofacial region. Table 8-2 summarizes a comprehensive examination.

General Examination

Vital Signs. For the clinician to become well acquainted with the patient, vital signs should be taken. Although this information may not always be helpful in making a diagnosis, in some instances it may prove to be a major contributor to the pain. Certain headaches may be associated with hypertension. Systemic infections are often associated with elevated body temperature. Increased breathing rates are often associated with an upregulation of the sympathetic nervous system. Therefore, blood pressure, pulse rate, respiration rate, and body temperature should be assessed especially when the pain condition is obscure.

Cranial Nerve Evaluation. The 12 cranial nerves supply sensory information to and motor impulses from the brain. Any gross problem relating to their function must be identified so abnormal conditions can be immediately and appropriately addressed.

Table 8-2 Summary of a Comprehensive Clinical Examination

I. General examination
  A. Vital signs
    1. Blood pressure
    2. Pulse rate
    3. Respiration rate
    4. Temperature
  B. Cranial nerve evaluation
  C. Eye evaluation
  D. Ear evaluation
  E. Cervical evaluation
  F. Balance and coordination
II. Muscle examination
  A. Palpation
    1. Pain and tenderness
    2. Trigger points and pain referral
III. Masticatory evaluation
  A. Range of mandibular movement
    1. Measurements
    2. Pain
  B. Temporomandibular joint evaluation
    1. Pain
    2. Dysfunction
  C. Oral structures
    1. The mucogingival tissues
    2. The teeth
    3. The periodontia
    4. The occlusion
IV. Other diagnostic tests
  A. Imaging
  B. Laboratory tests
  C. Psychologic provocation tests

The orofacial pain therapist does not need to be trained as a neurologist. In fact, a cranial nerve examination does not need to be a complex evaluation. Any clinician who regularly evaluates pain problems can test the gross function of the cranial nerves to evaluate for any neuropathic disorders. Each nerve can be assessed by using the following simple evaluation procedures.

Fig 8-3 Checking the patient's visual field (optic nerve): With the patient looking forward, the examiner's fingers are brought around to the front from behind. The initial position at which the fingers are seen marks the extent of the visual field. Right and left fields should be very similar.

Fig 8-4 Checking the patient's extraocular muscles: Without moving the patient's head the examiner asks him or her to follow the finger as it makes an X in front of the patient. Any variation in right or left eye movement is noted.

Olfactory Nerve. The first cranial nerve has sensory fibers originating in the mucous membrane of the nasal cavity and provides the sensation of smell. It is tested by asking the patient to detect differences between the odors of peppermint, vanilla, and chocolate. (It is helpful to have these available in the office for testing.) It must also be determined whether or not the patient's nose is obstructed. This can be done by asking the patient to exhale nasally onto a mirror. Fogging of the mirror from both nostrils denotes adequate air flow.

Optic Nerve. The second cranial nerve, also sensory, with fibers originating in the retina, provides for sight. It is tested by having the patient cover one eye and read a few sentences. The other eye is checked in the same manner. The visual field is assessed by standing behind the patient and slowly bringing your fingers from behind around into view (Fig 8-3). The patient should report when the fingers first appear. There normally will be no variation between when they are seen on the right and on the left.

Oculomotor, Trochlear, and Abducent Nerves. The third, fourth, and sixth cranial nerves, supplying motor fibers to the extraocular muscles, are tested by having the patient follow your finger as you make an X (Fig 8-4). Both eyes should move smoothly and similarly as they follow your finger. The pupils should be of equal size and rounded and should react to light by constricting. The accommodation reflex is tested by having the patient change focus from a distant to a near object. The pupils should constrict as the object (your finger) approaches the patient's face. Not only should they both constrict to direct light, but each should also constrict to light directed in the other eye (consensual light reflex) (Fig 8-5).

Fig 8-5 Constriction of the pupil can be seen when light is directed toward the eye. The opposite pupil should also constrict, demonstrating the consensual light reflex.

Fig 8-6 Cotton tip applicators can be used to compare light touch discrimination between the right and left maxillary branches of the trigeminal nerve. The ophthalmic and mandibular branches are also tested.

Trigeminal Nerve. The fifth cranial nerve is both sensory (from the face, scalp, nose, and mouth) and motor (to the muscles of mastication). Sensory input is tested by lightly stroking the face with a cotton tip bilaterally in three regions: forehead, cheek, and lower jaw (Fig 8-6). This will give a rough idea of the function of the ophthalmic, maxillary, and mandibular branches of the trigeminal. The patient should describe similar sensations on each side. The trigeminal nerve also contains sensory fibers from the cornea. The corneal reflexes can be tested by observing the patient's blink in response to light touch on the cornea with a sterile cotton pledget or tissue. Gross motor input is tested by having the patient clench while you feel both masseter and temporal muscles. The muscles should contract equally bilaterally.

Fig 8-7 Gross hearing can be evaluated by rubbing a strand of hair between the finger and thumb near the patient's ear and noting any difference between right and left hearing sensitivities.

Facial Nerve. The seventh cranial nerve also is sensory and motor. The sensory component, supplying taste sensations from the anterior portion of the tongue, is tested by asking the patient to distinguish between sugar and salt using just the tip of the tongue. The motor component, which innervates the muscles of facial expression, is tested by asking the patient to raise both eyebrows, smile, and show the lower teeth. During these movements, any bilateral differences are recorded.

Acoustic Nerve. Also called *vestibulocochlear,* the eighth cranial nerve supplies the senses of balance and hearing. The patient should be questioned regarding any recent changes in upright posture or in hearing, especially if they were associated with the problem that initiated the office visit. If there is a question regarding balance, ask the patient to walk heel-to-toe along a straight line. Gross hearing can be evaluated by rubbing a strand of hair between your first finger and thumb near the patient's ear and noting any difference between right and left sensitivities (Fig 8-7).

Glossopharyngeal and Vagus Nerves. The ninth and tenth cranial nerves are tested together because they both supply fibers to the back of the throat. The patient is asked to say "ah" and the soft palate is observed for symmetric elevations. The gag reflex is tested by touching each side of the pharynx.

Accessory Nerve. The spinal accessory nerve is the eleventh cranial nerve and it supplies fibers to the trapezius and sternocleidomastoid muscles. The trapezius muscle is tested by asking the patient to shrug the shoulders against resistance. The sternocleidomastoid muscle is tested by having the patient look first to the right and then to the left against resistance. Note any differences in muscle strength.

Hypoglossal Nerve. The twelfth cranial nerve supplies motor fibers to the tongue. To test it, ask the patient to protrude the tongue and note any uncontrolled or consistent lateral deviation. The strength of the tongue can also be evaluated by having the patient push laterally against a tongue blade.

Parasympathetic functioning of the oculomotor (third cranial) nerve has already been checked by testing pupillary accommodation to light. That of the facial (seventh cranial) and glossopharyngeal (ninth cranial) nerves can be checked by lacrimation and salivation. The parasympathetic functioning of the vagus (tenth cranial) nerve can be checked by testing the carotid sinus reflex by which the heart rate is reduced in response to pressure on the internal carotid artery at the level of the cricoid cartilage. A deficit in cranial sympathetic functioning is recognized by the presence of Horner's syndrome, which presents with narrowing of the palpebral fissure, ptosis of the upper lid, elevation of the lower lid, constriction of the pupil, and facial anhidrosis.

Superficial reflexes: The corneal reflex has already been tested by closure of the eyelids in response to irritation of the cornea by touching with a sterile cotton applicator. It involves afferent impulses transmitted by the trigeminal (fifth cranial) nerve and efferent motor impulses via the facial (seventh cranial) nerve. The palatal reflex is involuntary swallowing in response to stimulation of the soft palate. It involves afferent impulses transmitted by the trigeminal (fifth cranial) and glossopharyngeal (ninth cranial) nerves and efferent motor impulses via the glossopharyngeal (ninth cranial) and vagus (tenth cranial) nerves. The pharyngeal or gag reflex is contraction of the constrictor muscle of the pharynx that is elicited by touching the posterior wall of the pharynx. It involves afferent impulses transmitted by the glossopharyngeal (ninth cranial) nerve and efferent motor impulses via the glossopharyngeal (ninth cranial) and vagus (tenth cranial) nerves.

As previously stated, any abnormalities found during the cranial nerve examination should be viewed as important and should be assessed as to their relationship to the pain condition. The purpose of this evaluation is to determine with certainty whether referral to a neurologist is essential and justified. When one or more of the following conditions are observed, immediate neurologic consultation is indicated:

1. Unexplained areas of facial hypoesthesia
2. Loss of normal corneal reflex
3. Unexplained persistent muscular weakness
4. Simultaneous involvement of otherwise unrelated nerve trunks

Eye Evaluation. The patient is questioned regarding his or her vision and any recent changes, especially any associated with the reason for seeking treatment. As in the cranial nerve examination, simple techniques will be sufficient in testing gross vision. The patient's left eye is covered and he or she is asked to read a few sentences from a paper. The other eye is then similarly examined. Any diplopia or blurred vision is noted as well as whether this relates to the pain problem. Pain felt in or around the eyes is noted as is whether or not reading affects it. Reddening of the conjunctivae should be recorded along with any tearing or swelling of the eyelids.

Ear Evaluation. Ear pain is a common source of facial pain and needs to identified so that proper therapy can be instituted. The proximity of the ear to the temporomandibular joint (TMJ) and muscles of mastication as well as their common trigeminal innervation creates a frequent condition for referral of pain. Any clinician who treats orofacial pains should become proficient at examining the ear for gross pathologic conditions. Hearing should be checked as in the eighth cranial nerve examination. Infection of the external auditory meatus (otitis externa) can be identified by simply pushing inward on the tragus. If this causes significant pain, there could be an external ear infection and the patient should be immediately referred to an otolaryngologist. An otoscope will be necessary to visualize the tympanic membrane for inflammation, perforations, or fluid.

Remember the clinician's role is to identify the source of pain. When ear disease is suspected, the patient should be referred to an otolaryngologist for a more thorough evaluation and appropriate treatment. On the other hand, normal findings from an otologic examination may be taken as encouragement to continue to search for the true source of pain or dysfunction.

Cervical Evaluation. As described in Chapter 4, cervicospinal pain and dysfunction can be referred to the orofacial structures. Since this is a frequent occurrence, it is important to evaluate the neck for pain or movement difficulties. A simple screening examination for craniocervical disorders is easily accomplished. The mobility of the neck is examined for range and symptoms. The patient is asked to look first to the right and then to the left (Fig 8-8a). There should be at least 70 degrees of rotation in each direction.[15] Next, the patient is asked to look up as far as possible (extension) (Fig 8-8b) and then down as far as possible (flexion) (Fig 8-8c). The head should normally extend back about 60 degrees and flex down 45 degrees.[15]

Finally, the patient is asked to bend the neck to the right and left (Fig 8-8d). This should be possible to approximately 40 degrees each way.[15]

Any pain is recorded and any limitation of movement carefully investigated to determine whether its source is a muscular or a vertebral problem. When patients with limited range of movement can be passively stretched to a greater range, the source is usually muscular. Patients with vertebral problems cannot normally be stretched to a greater range. If the clinician suspects that the patient has a craniocervical disorder, proper referral for a more complete cervicospinal evaluation may be indicated. This is very important, since craniocervical disorders can be closely associated with some orofacial pain disorder symptoms.[16]

Balance and Coordination. Each patient should be asked if he or she is experiencing any problems with balance or coordination. If there is a positive response, a few simple tests can help determine the significance of these complaints. The patient is asked to close his or her eyes and attempt to touch a finger to the nose. This is repeated with both hands. This can give the clinician some appreciation of the patient's proprioceptive abilities. The patient can also be asked to walk along a straight line on the floor with the toe of one shoe touching the heel of the other. Significant balancing problems can be quickly identified. The presence of a balance or coordination problem should be assessed as to its relationship with the pain disorder. Proper referral may be indicated.

Muscle Examination

There is no pain associated with the normal function or palpation of a healthy muscle. In contrast, a frequent clinical sign of compromised muscle tissue is pain. The condition that brings about compromise or unhealthy muscle tissue may be physical abuse or trauma such as overstretching or receiving a blow to the muscle tissue itself. Often muscles become compromised through increased activity. As the number and duration of contractions increase, so also do the physiologic needs of the muscle tissues. Increased muscle tonicity or hyperactivity, however, may decrease blood flow to the muscle tissues, lowering the inflow of nutrient substances needed for normal cell function while accumulating metabolic waste products. This accumulation of metabolic wastes and of other algogenic substances can cause muscle pain.[17]

The degree and location of muscle pain and tenderness are identified during direct palpation of the muscle.

8-8a

8-8b

8-8c

8-8d

Fig 8-8 Examination for craniocervical disorders: The patient is asked to *(a)* look to the extreme left and then extreme right, *(b)* look upward fully, *(c)* look downward fully, and *(d)* bend the neck to the right and left. Normal ranges are listed in the text. Any pain or restriction in normal range is noted.

Palpation. A widely accepted method of determining muscle tenderness and pain is by digital palpation.[18–20] A healthy muscle does not elicit sensations of tenderness or pain when palpated. Deformation of compromised muscle tissue by palpation can elicit pain.[21] Therefore, if a patient reports discomfort during palpation of a specific muscle, it can be deduced that the muscle tissue is a source of pain.

Pressure algometry has become a useful adjunct in evaluating muscle tenderness and myofascial trigger point sensitivity.[22–27] The pressure algometer provides objective quantitative documentation of myalgia.[28]

Palpation of the muscle is accomplished mainly by the palmar surface of the middle finger, with the index finger and forefinger testing the adjacent areas. Soft but firm pressure is applied to the designated muscles, the fingers compressing the adjacent tissues in a small circular motion. A single firm thrust of 1 or 2 seconds' duration is usually better than several light thrusts. During palpation, the patient is asked whether it hurts or is just uncomfortable.

For the muscle palpation examination to be most helpful, the degree of discomfort is ascertained and recorded. This is often a difficult task. Pain is subjective and is perceived and expressed quite differently from patient to patient. Yet the degree of discomfort in the structure can be important in recognizing the patient's pain problem as well as an excellent method of evaluating treatment effects. An attempt is made, therefore, not only to identify the affected muscles but also to classify the degree of pain in each. When a muscle is palpated, the patient's response is placed in one of four categories.[29,30] A zero (0) is recorded when the muscle is palpated and there is no pain or tenderness reported by the patient. A number 1 is recorded if the patient responds that the palpation is uncomfortable (tenderness or soreness). A number 2 is recorded if the patient experiences definite discomfort or pain. A number 3 is recorded if the patient shows evasive action or eye tearing or verbalizes a desire not to have the area palpated again. The pain or tenderness of each muscle is recorded on an examination form, which will assist diagnosis and later be used in the evaluation and assessment of treatment progress.

A routine orofacial muscle examination includes *palpation* of the following muscles or muscle groups: temporalis, masseter, sternocleidomastoid, and posterior cervical (eg, the splenius capitis and trapezius). For increased efficiency of the examination, both right and left muscles are palpated simultaneously. The technique of palpating each muscle will be described.

Temporalis. The temporalis muscle is divided into three functional areas; therefore, each area is independently palpated. The *anterior* region is palpated above the zygomatic arch and anterior to the TMJ (Fig 8-9a). Fibers of this region run essentially in a vertical direction. The *middle* region is palpated directly above the TMJ and superior to the zygomatic arch (Fig 8-9b). Fibers in this region run in an oblique direction across the lateral aspect of the skull. The *posterior* region is palpated above and behind the ear (Fig 8-9c). These fibers run in an essentially horizontal direction. If uncertainty arises regarding the proper finger placement, the patient is asked to clench the teeth together. The temporalis will contract and the fibers should be felt beneath the fingertips. It is helpful to be positioned

8-9a

Fig 8-9 Palpation of *(a)* the anterior, *(b)* the middle, and *(c)* the posterior regions of the temporal muscles.

8-9b

8-9c

behind the patient and to use the right and left hands to palpate respective muscle areas simultaneously. During palpation of each area, the patient is asked whether it hurts or is just uncomfortable and the response is classified as 0, 1, 2, or 3, according to the previously described criteria.

When evaluating the temporalis muscle, it is important also to palpate its tendon. The fibers of temporalis muscle extend inferiorly to converge into a distinct tendon that attaches to the coronoid process of the mandible. It is common for some TMJ disorders to produce a temporalis tendonitis, which can create pain in the body of the

muscle as well as referred pain behind the adjacent eye (retro-orbital pain). The tendon of the temporalis is palpated by placing the finger of one hand intraorally on the anterior border of the ramus and the finger of the other hand extraorally on the same area (Fig 8-10). The intraoral finger is moved up the anterior border of the ramus until the coronoid process and the tendon are palpated. The patient is asked to report any discomfort or pain.

Masseter. The masseter is palpated bilaterally at its superior and inferior attachments. First, the fingers are placed on each zygo-

a

Fig 8-10 Palpation of the tendon of the temporalis. *(a)* Proper hand and head position. The fingers of both hands (one intraorally, the other extraorally) move simultaneously up the anterior border of the ramus until the coronoid process and the attachment of the tendon of the temporalis are felt. *(b)* Proper intraoral finger placement.

b

a

b

Fig 8-11 *(a)* Palpation of the deep masseters at their superior attachment to the zygomatic arches. *(b)* Palpation of the superficial masseters near the lower border of the mandible.

matic arch (just anterior to the TMJ). They are then dropped down slightly to the portion of the masseter attached to the zygomatic arch, just anterior to the joint (Fig 8-11a). Once this portion (the deep masseter) has been palpated, the fingers drop to the inferior attachment on the inferior border of the ramus. The area of palpation is directly above the attachment of the body of the masseter (ie, the superficial masseter) (Fig 8-11b). The patient's response is recorded.

Sternocleidomastoid. Although the sternocleidomastoid (SCM) does not function di-

Fig 8-12 Palpation of the sternocleidomastoid muscles. The full length of this muscle should be palpated from its attachment to the mastoid process down to the clavicle.

Fig 8-13 Palpation of muscular attachments in the occipital region of the neck. The fingers should then be brought inferiorly down the cervical spine area to examine these muscles for pain or tenderness.

rectly in moving the mandible, it is specifically mentioned because it often becomes symptomatic with TM disorders and it is easily palpated. The palpation is done bilaterally near its insertion on the outer surface of the mastoid fossa behind the ear. The entire length of the muscle is palpated, down to its origin near the clavicle (Fig 8-12). The patient is asked to report any discomfort during the procedure. Also, any trigger points found in this muscle are noted since they are frequent sources of referred pain to the temporal, joint, and ear area.

Posterior cervical muscles. The posterior cervical muscles (trapezius, longissimus [capitis and cervicis], splenius [capitis and cervicis], and levator scapulae) are the major muscles responsible for cervical function. They originate at the posterior occipital area and extend inferiorly along the cervicospinal region. Because they are layered over each other, they are sometimes difficult to identify individually.

In palpating these muscles, the examiner's fingers slip behind the patient's head. Those

of the right hand palpate the right occipital area, and those of the left hand the left, at the origins of the muscles. The patient is questioned regarding any discomfort. The fingers move down the length of the neck muscles through the cervical, and any patient discomfort is recorded (Fig 8-13). It is important to be aware of trigger points in these muscles, since they are a common source of frontal headache.

The *splenius capitis* is palpated for general pain or tenderness as well as for trigger points. Its attachment to the skull is a small depression just posterior to the attachment of the SCM (Fig 8-14). Palpation is begun at this point and moves inferiorly as the muscle blends into the other neck muscles. Any pain, tenderness, or trigger points are recorded.

The *trapezius* is an extremely large muscle of the back, shoulder, and neck that (like the SCM and the splenius) does not directly affect jaw function but is a common source of headache pain and is easily palpated. The major purpose of its palpation is not to evaluate shoulder function but to search for active trigger points that may be producing referred pain. The trapezius commonly has trigger points that refer pain to the face. In fact, when facial pain is the patient's chief complaint this muscle should always be investigated. The upper part is palpated from behind the SCM, inferolaterally to the shoulder (Fig 8-15), and any trigger points are recorded.

There are three muscles that are basic to jaw movement but impossible to palpate. These muscles are the inferior lateral pterygoid, superior lateral pterygoid, and medial pterygoid. The inferior and superior lateral pterygoids reside deep within the skull, originating on the lateral wing of the sphenoid bone and the maxillary tuberosity and inserting on the neck of the mandibular condyle and the TMJ capsule. The medial pterygoid has a similar origin, but it extends downward and laterally to insert on the medial surface of the angle of the mandible. All three muscles receive their innervation from the mandibular branch of the trigeminal nerve.

Since these muscles cannot be palpated, they are best evaluated with functional manipulation. Functional manipulation is based on the concept that a painful muscle will not only be tender to palpation but will also be painful to contraction and/or stretching of the muscle. For example, a painful inferior lateral pterygoid muscle will produce increased pain when the patient is asked to push the mandible forward against resistance. If pain is increased during resisted protrusion of the mandible, the inferior lateral pterygoid muscle should be suspected as a source of pain. A more detailed description of functional manipulation can be found in other texts.[31]

Fig 8-14   The splenius capitis is palpated at its attachment to the skull just posterior to the sternocleidomastoideus.

Fig 8-15   The trapezius is palpated as it ascends into the neck structures.

Trigger Points and Pain Referral. A thorough muscle palpation examination should identify not only generalized muscle tenderness and pain but also the small hypersensitive trigger points associated with myofascial pain. As stated in Chapter 4, trigger points act as sources of deep pain input that can produce central excitatory effects. It is important that these areas be identified and recorded. To locate trigger points, the examiner palpates the entire body of each muscle. Generalized muscle pain may not exist in a muscle with trigger points. In recording examination findings, it is important to differentiate between generalized muscle pain and trigger point pain since the diagnosis and treatment are often different.

Trigger points are clinically identified as specific hypersensitive areas within the muscle tissue. Often a small firm tight band of muscle tissue can often be felt. Active trigger points represent a source of deep pain and can therefore produce referred pain.[32] When referred (heterotopic) pain is detected, one should remember that it is wholly dependent on the conditions of the trigger points (the source of the pain). This means that if active referring trigger points are provoked, the referred pain will usually be increased, which becomes a significant diagnostic observation in relating pain complaints to their source. For example, when a patient's chief complaint is headache, careful palpation of the aforementioned neck muscles for trigger points will demonstrate its source. When a trigger point is located, applying pressure to it will usually increase the headache (referred) pain.

The specific pattern of referred pain from various trigger point locations has been outlined by Travell and Simons.[33] An understanding of these common referral sites may help the clinician attempting to diagnose an orofacial pain problem. Anesthetic blocking of the trigger point often eliminates the referred headache pain and thus becomes a helpful diagnostic tool.

Masticatory Evaluation

Since the masticatory structures can be a significant source of orofacial pain, the ex-amination must include a thorough evaluation of these structures for pain and dysfunction. The following criteria have been found useful and dependable for accurate identification and localization of masticatory pain sources[34]:

1. The pain should relate directly and logically to the movements and functioning of the mandible incidental to mastication.
2. Tenderness in the masticatory muscles or the temporomandibular joints should be discernible by manual palpation or functional manipulation.
3. Analgesic blocking of a tender muscle or joint should confirm the presence and precise location of such pain.

An examination of masticatory structures should include evaluation of the range of mandibular movement, temporomandibular joints, and the oral structures.

Range of Mandibular Movement. The normal range of mouth opening when measured interincisally is between 53 and 58 mm.[35] Even a 6-year-old child can normally open a maximum 40 mm or more.[36] Since muscle symptoms are often accentuated during function, it is common for patients to present with a restricted pattern of movement. The patient is asked to open slowly until pain is first felt. At that point, the distance between the incisal edges of the maxillary and mandibular anterior teeth is measured. This is the maximum comfortable opening. The patient is next asked to open maximally. This is recorded as the maximum opening. In the absence of pain, the maximum comfortable opening and maximum opening are the same.

A restricted mandibular opening is con-

a

b

Fig 8-16 (a) Measuring the comfortable and maximum mouth opening by using a millimeter ruler from incisal edge of the mandibular incisor to the maxillary incisor. (b) Checking the end feel. Gentle but steady pressure is placed on the incisors for approximately 5 to 6 seconds. Increased mouth opening indicates a soft end feel (usually associated with a masticatory muscle disorder).

sidered to be any distance less than 40 mm. Only 1.2% of young adults open less then 40 mm.[37] One must remember however, that 15% of the healthy elderly population open less then 40 mm.[37] Less then 40 mm of mouth opening therefore, seems to represent a reasonable point to designate restriction but one should always consider the patient's age and body size. This distance is measured by observing the incisal edge of the mandibular central incisor traveling away from its position at maximum intercuspation (Fig 8-16a). If a person has a 5-mm vertical overlap of the anterior teeth and the maximum interincisal distance is 57 mm, the mandible has actually moved 62 mm in opening. In people who have extreme deep bites these measurements must be considered when determining normal range of movement.

The path taken by the midline of the mandible during maximum opening should also be observed. In the healthy masticatory system, there is no alteration in the straight opening pathway. Any alterations in opening are recorded. There are two types of alteration that can occur: deviations and deflections. A *deviation* is any shift of the jaw midline during opening that disappears with continued opening (a return to midline) (Fig 8-17a). It is usually due to a disc derangement in one or both joints and is a result of the condylar movement necessary to get past the disc during translation. Once the condyle has overcome this interference, the straight midline path is resumed. A *deflection* is any shift of the midline to one side that becomes greater with opening and does not disappear at maximum opening (does not return to midline) (Fig 8-17b). It is due to restricted movement in one joint. The source of the restriction varies and must be investigated.

Restricted movements of the mandible are caused by either extracapsular or intracapsular sources. The former are generally the muscles and therefore relate to a muscle disorder. The latter are generally associated

Fig 8-17 Alterations in the opening pathway. *(a)* Deviation. The opening pathway is altered but returns to a normal midline relationship at maximum opening. *(b)* Deflection. The opening pathway is shifted to one side and becomes greater with opening. At maximum opening, the midline is deflected to its greatest distance. (From Okeson JP. Management of Temporomandibular Disorders and Occlusion, ed 3. St Louis: Mosby Year Book; 1993: 251. Used with permission.)

with disc-condyle function and the surrounding ligaments and thus are usually related to a disc derangement disorder.

Extracapsular and intracapsular restrictions present different characteristics.

Extracapsular restrictions typically occur with elevator muscle spasms and pain. These muscles tend to restrict translation and thus limit opening. Pain in the elevator muscles, however, does not restrict lateral and protrusive movements. Therefore with this type of restriction normal eccentric movements are present but opening movement is restricted, primarily because of pain. The point of restriction can range anywhere from 0 to 40 mm interincisally. It is common with this type of restriction for the patient to be able to increase opening slowly, but the pain is intensified (soft end feel).

Extracapsular restrictions often create a deflection of the incisal path during opening. The direction of the deflection depends on the location of the muscle that causes the restriction. If the restricting muscle is lateral to the joint (as with the masseter), the deflection during opening will be to the ipsilateral side. If the muscle is medial (as with the medial pterygoid), the deflection will be to the contralateral side.

Intracapsular restrictions typically present a different pattern. A disc derangement disorder such as a disc dislocation (see Chapter 13) very decisively restricts translation of that joint. Typically the restriction is in only one joint and limits mandibular opening in that joint primarily to rotation (25- to 30-mm interincisally). At this point, further movement is restricted not because of pain but because of structural resistance in the joint. When intracapsular restrictions are present, deflection of the incisal path during opening is always to the ipsilateral (affected) side.

Pain produced during mouth opening commonly occurs from either a muscle disorder or a joint disorder. When limited mouth opening is present, the clinician needs to pursue the reason for the restriction. Testing the end feel can be helpful. The end feel describes the characteristics of the joint when an attempt is made to increase mouth opening passively[38] by gently placing downward force on the lower incisors with the fingers to increase the interincisal distance (see Fig 8-16b). This force should be light but steady. If the end feel is soft, increased opening can be achieved but it must be done slowly. A soft end feel suggests muscle-induced restriction.[39] If no increase in opening can be achieved, the end feel is said to be hard. Hard end feels are likely associated with intracapsular sources, such as a disc dislocation.[40]

Temporomandibular Joint Evaluation. The temporomandibular joints should be examined for any signs or symptoms associated with pain and dysfunction. Radiography as well as other imaging techniques can also be useful and will be discussed.

Pain or tenderness of the TMJs is determined by digital palpation of the joints when the mandible is stationary and during dynamic movement. The fingertips are placed over the lateral aspects of both joint areas simultaneously. If uncertainty exists regarding the proper position of the fingers, the patient is asked to open and close a few times. The fingertips should feel the lateral poles of the condyles passing downward and forward across the articular eminences. Once the position of the fingers over the joints has been verified, the patient relaxes and medial force is applied to the joint areas (Fig 8-18a). The patient is asked to report any symptoms and they are recorded with the same numerical code as used for the muscles. Once the symptoms are recorded in a static position, the patient opens and closes and any symptoms associated with this movement are recorded (Fig 8-18b). As the patient opens maximally, the fingers should be rotated slightly posteriorly to apply force to the posterior aspect of the condyle (Fig 8-18c). Posterior capsulitis and retrodiscitis are clinically evaluated in this manner.

To evaluate the temporomandibular joint effectively, one must have a sound understanding of the anatomy in the region. When the fingers are placed properly over the lateral poles of the condyles and the patient is asked to clench, very little to no movement is felt. However, if the fingers are misplaced only 1 cm anterior to the lateral pole and the patient is asked to clench, the deep portion of the masseter can be felt contracting. This very slight difference in positioning of the fingers may influence the examiner's interpretation regarding the origin of the pain. It is important to be aware also that a portion of the parotid gland extends to the region of the joint and parotid symptoms can arise from this area. The examiner must be astute in identifying whether the symptoms are originating from joint, muscle, or gland. The basis of treatment will be determined by this evaluation.

Dysfunction of the TMJs can be separated into two types: joint sounds and joint restrictions. Joint sounds can be generally divided into either clicks or crepitation. A

Fig 8-18 Palpation of the TMJ. *(a)* Lateral aspect of the joint with the mouth closed. *(b)* Lateral aspect of the joint during opening and closing. *(c)* With the mouth fully open, the finger is moved behind the condyle to palpate the posterior aspect of the joint.

8-18a

8-18b

8-18c

click is a single sound of short duration. If it is relatively loud, it is sometimes referred to as a pop. Crepitation is a multiple gravel-like sound described as grating and complicated.[41] Crepitation is most commonly associated with osteoarthritic changes of the articular surfaces of the joint.[42]

Joint sounds can be perceived by placing the fingertips over the lateral surfaces of the joint and having the patient open and close. Often they may be felt by the fingertips. A more careful examination can be performed by placing a stethoscope over the joint area. Not only will the character of any joint sounds be recorded (clicking or crepitation), but also the degree of mandibular opening associated with the sound. In addi-

tion, it is equally important to note whether the sound occurs during opening or closing or can be heard during both these movements (ie, a reciprocal click; see Chapter 13).

The presence or absence of joint sounds gives insight regarding disc position. One should be aware however, that the absence of sounds does not always mean normal disc position. In one study,[43] 15% of silent, asymptomatic joints where found to have disc displacements on arthrograms. Information received during examination of the joints must be evaluated with respect to all other examination findings.

The dynamic movements of the mandible are observed for any irregularities or restrictions. The characteristics of intracapsular restrictions have already been described in connection with the muscle examination. Any mandibular movements that either are restricted or have unusual pathway characteristics are recorded. Their relationship to pain should also be noted.

Oral Structures. The gingiva and entire oral mucosa should be tested by touch, pinprick, and manual palpation to identify areas of abnormal sensibility. Visual inspection of the superficial mucogingival tissues of the mouth and throat is done to identify hyperemia, inflammation, abrasion, ulceration, neoplasm, or other abnormality.

No doubt, pains around the mouth and face stem most frequently from local dental causes, and a thorough examination of the teeth is an indispensable part of the orofacial examination. Odontogenous pains have the propensity to simulate many other pain disorders, and a very careful examination is needed to attain a correct differential diagnosis.

The teeth, especially on the side in question, should be examined individually to obtain the following data:

1. Sensitivity or tenderness without provocation
2. Sensitivity or tenderness due to occlusal function
3. Sensitivity to touch, percussion, or probing with a dental explorer
4. Tenderness from pressure directed down the long axis of the tooth
5. Tenderness from pressure exerted laterally on the tooth
6. Response to thermal shock (Warmth may be applied via a heated instrument; chilling may be done by applying ethyl chloride on a cotton applicator. The tooth should be isolated with celluloid strips, especially when adjacent metallic fillings are present or when covered with an artificial dental crown.)
7. Response to electric pulp tester (Each tooth should be isolated with celluloid strips, especially when adjacent metallic fillings are present. Care should be taken to differentiate between pulpal and gingival responses.[44])
8. Radiographic evidence of pathologic change
9. Evidence of occlusal trauma
10. Evidence to justify direct exploration of the tooth

The periodontal condition, especially in the region of the pain, should be carefully evaluated. Gingival tissue color and surface texture should be noted. A periodontal probe should be used to identify any loss of gingival attachment or pocketing that might be associated with the pain. The tooth should be percussed apically and laterally to determine any relationship to the pain. Radiographs should be taken to help identify any changes in the alveolar bone support for the teeth.

For many years, the dental profession placed significant emphasis on the occlusal contact pattern of the teeth and pain in the orofacial structures. In more recent years, the significance of this relationship has been questioned. A review of the literature can be found in other texts.[45] Although the controversy continues, the relationship is likely to be associated with occlusal conditions that create significant orthopedic instability between the mandible and the cranium.

It is important for the clinician to assess the occlusal relationship between the mandible and the maxilla when masticatory pains are present. This can be accomplished by placing the mandible in its most orthopedically stable relationship with the cranium and observing the occlusion of the teeth. A simple method of finding the stable joint position utilizes a bilateral manual manipulation technique.[46] It begins with the patient lying back with the chin pointed upward. Lifting the chin upward places the head in an easier position to locate the condyles near the superior anterior position, which is the most stable relationship of the condyle in the fossa. The four fingers of each hand are placed on the lower border of the mandible. It is important that the fingers be located on the bone and not in the soft tissues of the neck. Next, both thumbs are placed over the symphysis of the chin so they touch each other. When the hands are in this position, the mandible is guided by upward force placed on its lower border and angle with the fingers while at the same time the thumbs press downward and backward on the chin (Fig 8-19). The overall force on the mandible is directed so that the condyles will be seated in their most superoanterior position braced against the posterior slopes of the eminences. Firm but gentle force is needed to guide the mandible to not elicit any protective reflexes.

The mandible is positioned with a gentle arcing until it freely rotates around the stable joint position. This arcing consists of short movements of 2 to 4 mm. Once the mandible can be slightly rotated in an opening and closing position, force is firmly applied by the fingers to seat the condyles in their most superoanterior position. The mouth is slowly closed with the condyles in this position and the occlusal contacts of the teeth are observed. If orthopedic stabil-

ity is present, the teeth should occlude in their maximum intercuspation with no slide. If orthopedic stability is not present, a significant shift will occur as the teeth are brought into intercuspal position. Only shifts of 2 mm or more should be considered a significant finding since smaller shifts seem to be within most tolerance levels. The clinician should remember that the presence of a significant shift does not in itself represent an etiology for orofacial pain. Many patients with significant shifts have no pain symptoms. The clinician must evaluate this information with all of the other information gained from the history and examination to attain a diagnosis.

Other Diagnostic Tests

Imaging. Various types of imaging techniques can be used to gain additional insight regarding the health and function of the masticatory structures. When painful symptoms arise from the orofacial structures, radiographs of the teeth, sinuses, and temporomandibular joints can be helpful. Radiographs of the TMJs will provide information regarding the morphologic characteristics of the bony components of the joint, and certain functional relationships between the condyle and the fossa.

When a radiographic examination of the temporomandibular joints is needed to confirm the clinical diagnosis, the following criteria should be met if the radiographic method is to yield maximal results:

1. It should clearly depict the subarticular osseous surfaces of the joint with the least distortion and superimposition of other osseous structures.

8-19a

8-19b

8-19c

8-19d

8-19e

Fig 8-19 *(a)* Successfully guiding the mandible into its most stable relationship with the fossae be-gins with having the patient recline and directing the chin upward. *(b* and *c)* The four fingers of each hand are placed along the lower border of the mandible. They should be positioned on the bone and not in the soft tissues of the neck. *(d* and *e) The* thumbs meet over the symphysis of the chin. Once the hands are properly positioned, gentle force is placed downward on the chin with upward and forward force applied to the angle of the mandible. This allows the condyles to be seated into a superior ante-rior position in the fossae.

2. It should permit the patient to be examined in a comfortable, erect sitting position that does not inhibit mandibular movements.

3. It should permit radiography to be performed by the examiner or under his or her direct supervision with standard dental X-ray equipment.

4. It should permit obtaining a series of radiographs in different mandibular positions with sufficient precision so that they can be exactly superimposed for reading. This requires a film holder of some type so that the entire series of one joint can be accomplished with no movement or change of position of the tube, patient, or film between exposures.

Common radiographs of the TMJs are the transcranial view, the transpharyngeal view, the anteroposterior view, and the panoramic view (Fig 8-20). When additional information is needed, tomography can be helpful. When soft tissue imaging is needed, arthrography or magnetic resonance imaging (MRI) may be useful. Periapical and bitewing radiographs are appropriate to assess dental and periodontal conditions while a Water's view is helpful for evaluating sinus disease.

Unfortunately, neither the articular disc nor the actual articular surfaces are seen radiographically. Only the subarticular bone and the intervening space are seen on the radiograph. Also, usually the central articulating relationship of these subarticular osseous structures is not recorded (except by the tomographic method). Rather, what is seen on the radiograph is the lateral contour of the joint. This interarticular space may not accurately represent the true thickness of the articular disc. If actual osseous disease is observed on the flat plate, tomographic visualization is the best technique for accurate evaluation. The usual open and closed views of the joint give some information about joint structure and the extent of condylar movement as restricted by all factors (intracapsular and extracapsular), but more usable information comes from a series of radiographs as previously indicated.

Another type of image that may have some usefulness in identifying sites of pain is thermography. The crystals change color in response to temperature gradients, presumably due to altered blood flow in superficial structures.[47-49] This altered blood flow is likely related to sympathetic activity and therefore may have some usefulness in identifying certain neuropathic pains.

Laboratory Tests. When the clinician is suspicious of significant medical problems, medical laboratory testing may be needed to confirm a diagnosis. This is especially true for arthritides such as rheumatoid arthritis, psoriatic arthritis, and hyperuricemia. Blood studies may also be helpful in ruling out systemic infections or other systemic conditions such as diabetes.

The following are indications for a medical consultation:

1. Obvious illness, as indicated by the patient's appearance and behavior and by the medical history questionnaire.

2. The presence of obscure illness, as indicated by the medical history questionnaire.

3. Evidence obtained during the history interview that the pain complaint may primarily relate to physical or emotional illness.

Fig 8-20 Examples of several types of radiographs that can be useful in evaluating the temporomandibular joints. *(a)* Panoramic view, an excellent screening radiograph of the orofacial structures. *(b)* Transcranial view, closed and opened view. *(c)* Transpharyngeal view, note osteophyte. *(d)* Tomographic view, closed and opened view.

8-20a

8-20b

8-20c

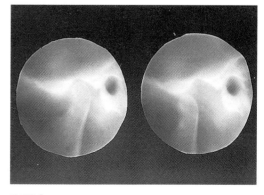

8-20d

4. Evidence obtained during the clinical examination that systemic factors may be present and need investigating.
5. Determination that the pain disorder does not stem from orofacial structures.
6. Indication that the pain disorder coexists with or is aggravated by some systemic condition that should be approached at a medical level.

Psychologic Provocation Tests. If during the examination the clinician becomes suspicious of significant psychologic factors, certain provocation tests may be helpful. One such test is to evaluate how the patient responds to an attempt to induce pain purely by suggestion. This may be done by pressing firmly on the painful site and strongly suggesting to the patient that he will feel the pain simultaneously in the corresponding site on the opposite normal side. If he does in fact complain of similar pain on the opposite side, the emotional overlay is probably great. Or the reverse may be tried. This consists of attempting to relieve the pain purely by suggestion. The examiner presses firmly at the corresponding site on the opposite normal side and strongly suggests that by doing so the patient will sense relief of pain at the site in question. If the pain is thus substantially relieved by this maneuver, significant psychologic factors are likely to be present.

Another testing device is trial placebo therapy, even though this method has not been looked on with favor by some investigators.[50] It should be remembered that a normal placebo effect may account for up to 40% of the effectiveness of any form of treatment, especially in emotionally tense individuals.[51] Therefore, to evaluate placebo

therapy, the results up to this percentage must be discounted. Testing can be done by prescribing a definite plan of treatment utilizing only placebo medications and suggesting to the patient that definite benefit will occur at a specified time. If such benefit occurs according to the specified time schedule and the benefit is substantially greater than 40%, it may be presumed that the purely psychologic element is important.

Establishing the Pain Category

Once the history and examination have been completed, the clinician should have a significant understanding of the patient's pain complaint. The next step in diagnosis is to place the pain complaint into the proper pain category. This can only be accomplished if the clinician has a complete understanding of all the possibilities. When one appreciates that different pain categories are characterized by different symptoms, diagnosis becomes more simplified. The pain classification in Figure 8-21 can be used as a road map to direct the clinician to an accurate diagnosis. Remember, it is only through proper diagnosis that appropriate therapy can be selected.

Establishing the proper category may be accomplished by answering the following six questions:

Is the Pain Chronic or Acute?

As previously described, pain may be considered chronic if it continues after normal healing time. The classic definition of chronic pain is pain that has lasted longer than 6 months. The important diagnostic

Classification of Orofacial Pains

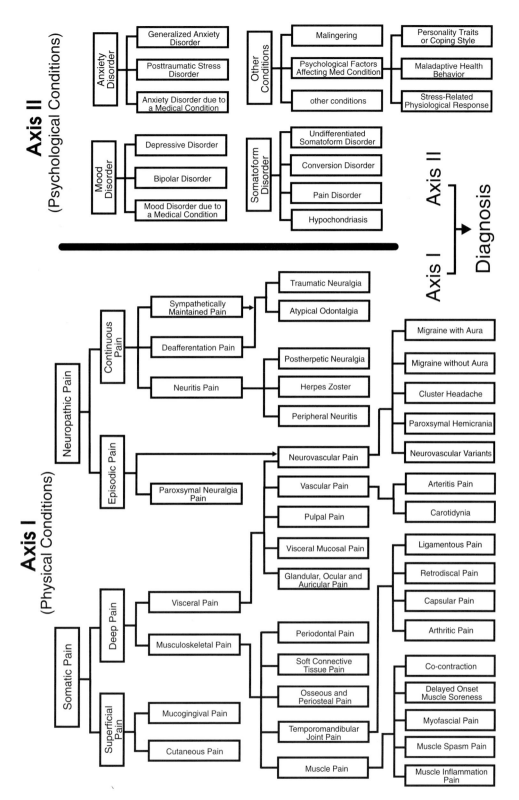

Fig 8-21 Pain classification chart used as a diagnostic roadmap.

consideration is that the longer pain is present, the greater the possibility of significant psychologic factors. As stated earlier, all pains have to some degree a psychologic component (Axis II). It is important to identify early those patients who may have a significant Axis II diagnosis since these conditions are managed differently than the Axis I disorders. If the patient is experiencing chronic pain, some Axis II disorders are almost always present even if it is only the category *Psychologic Factors Affecting a Medical Condition.*

The following clinical evidence should provide the clinician with suspicion that significant psychologic factors may be associated with the chronic pain condition:

1. Progressive inadequacy of local cause
2. Progressive nonphysiologic behavior of the pain
3. Withdrawal from normal daily activities
4. Progressive emotional and/or physical deterioration
5. Mood changes (depression)
6. Evidence of significant anxiety
7. Significant alterations in sleep patterns
8. Preoccupation or obsession with the pain condition

Is the Pain Neuropathic or Somatic?

Assuming that Axis II factors are not dominant features of the patient's complaint, the next diagnostic issue is whether the pain stems from somatic structures supplied by normal neural elements (somatic pain) or from abnormal neural structures (neuropathic pain). Recognition of evidence of neuropathic pain therefore is of prime importance.

Neuropathic pains include the following clinical characteristics:

1. Burning-type pains that are spontaneous, triggered, or ongoing and unremitting
2. Pains that occur disproportionately to the stimulus
3. Pains that are accompanied by other neurologic symptoms
4. Pains that are initiated or accentuated by efferent sympathetic activity in the area

Neuropathic orofacial pains are classified as either episodic pains or continuous pains. Episodic pains are pains that will appear for a time and then completely resolve. There are two categories of episodic pains, neuralgic pains or neurovascular pains. Continuous neuropathic pains are present constantly, although they may fluctuate between mild and severe. There are three categories of continuous neuropathic pains, neuritis, deafferentation pains, and sympathetically maintained pains (Fig 8-22).

Is the Pain Primary or Secondary?

Assuming that evidence of neuropathic pain is absent in the patient's complaint, the next diagnostic issue is whether the problem is a true primary pain or a secondary manifestation such as referred pain or secondary hyperalgesia. Since there is no definitive treatment for secondary pains other than identifying and managing the primary source, it is of prime importance that secondary pains be clearly recognized and primary pain sources be identified.

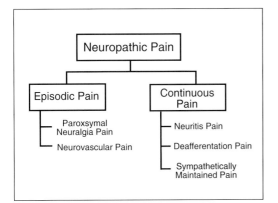

Fig 8-22 The major categories of neuropathic pain disorders.

Differentiating secondary pain from primary pain is accomplished by the rules described earlier in this chapter. Secondary pains are not increased by local provocation unless it is a site of secondary hyperalgesia. Secondary pains are not arrested by anesthesia at the site of pain. Secondary pain that is felt superficially as a touchy or sensitive area (secondary hyperalgesia) is not arrested by a topical anesthetic applied where the pain is felt. Secondary pain that is felt more deeply as an area of palpable tenderness is not arrested by analgesic blocking of that area.

Primary pain is present when local provocation of the site of pain increases the pain. Primary pains are arrested by local anesthesia at the site of pain. Primary somatic pain emanating from superficial skin or the mucogingiva is arrested by a topical anesthetic applied at the site of pain. Primary somatic pain emanating from musculoskeletal or visceral structures and felt as tenderness to manual palpation or functional manipulation is arrested by analgesic blocking of that area.

Is the Pain Superficial or Deep?

Assuming that the patient's complaint is positively identified as a primary somatic pain and not due to reference or secondary hyperalgesia, the next diagnostic issue is whether it stems from superficial or deep somatic structures (Fig 8-23).

Superficial somatic pain displays the following clinical characteristics by which it can be recognized:

1. The pain is a bright, stimulating sensation that is precisely located by the patient.
2. Response to local provocation is faithful in location, duration, and intensity.
3. The pain remains clean-cut without secondary manifestations such as reference, secondary hyperalgesia, autonomic symptoms, and/or muscle effects.
4. The pain is arrested by topical anesthesia at the site of pain.

Deep somatic pain displays the following clinical characteristics by which it can be recognized:

1. The pain is a duller, more depressing sensation that is less precisely located by the patient.
2. Response to local provocation is less faithful, especially with regard to location and size.
3. The pain frequently and expectantly exhibits secondary manifestations such as referred pain, secondary hyperalgesia, autonomic symptoms, and/or muscle effects.
4. The pain is arrested by analgesic blocking of the site of pain.

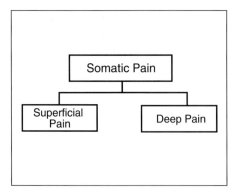

Fig 8-23 The major categories of somatic pain.

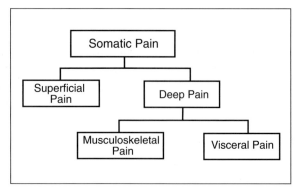

Fig 8-24 The major categories of deep somatic pain.

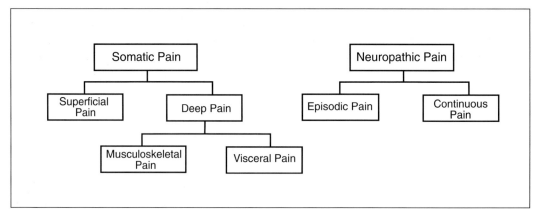

Fig 8-25 Pain classification chart used to help identify the proper category represented by the patient's pain complaint.

Is the Pain Musculoskeletal or Visceral?

Assuming that the primary pain that represents the patient's complaint originates from deep somatic structures, the next diagnostic issue is whether it is of musculoskeletal or visceral origin (Fig 8-24).

Musculoskeletal structures are primarily engaged in biomechanical function, and pain from such structures as muscles, bone, joints, ligaments (including periodontal ligaments), and soft connective tissue exhibits two characteristic clinical features: it relates intimately to biomechanical function; and response to provocation is a gradient reaction that is proportionate to the stimulus.

Visceral structures are primarily engaged in metabolic rather than biomechanical functions, and pain from such structures as blood vessels, glands, viscera, and tooth pulps exhibits two characteristic clinical features: it occurs irrelevant to biomechanical function; and it is relatively nonresponsive to local provocation until a threshold level is reached.

This series of questions should clearly establish the category of the patient's pain complaint (Fig 8-25) and place the examiner in an excellent position to attain a final diagnosis.

Is the Pain Inflammatory?

There is one more question that may be useful therapeutically as well as diagnostically. This question relates to whether or not the pain disorder is associated with an inflammatory condition. Whether superficial somatic, deep somatic, or neuropathic, primary pain that is inflammatory should be recognized because it needs cause-related therapy that requires a diagnostic search for the cause.

Inflammatory pain can usually be recognized by clinical features:

1. Concomitant signs of inflammation such as swelling, redness, heat, and dysfunction are present.
2. The pain reflects the type, intensity, location, and phase of inflammatory reaction.
3. The pain follows an inflammatory time frame. This means that it requires time to develop, plateau, and resolve.

Choosing the Correct Pain Disorder

Once the patient's pain complaint has been placed in the proper category, the clinician needs to select the precise diagnosis from within that category. This requires accurate knowledge of the clinical symptoms and behavior of all such pain disorders. The clini-cian's knowledge of the many possible orofacial pain disorders is of great importance. Remember, a clinician can never diagnose a condition that he or she has never heard about. The most important pain disorders in each category will be discussed in the third section of this book.

Confirmation of the Clinical Diagnosis

Before undertaking definitive therapy, confirmation of the clinical diagnosis is advisable. There are four methods that can help confirm the diagnosis: diagnostic analgesic blocking, utilization of diagnostic drugs, consultations, and trial therapy.

Diagnostic Analgesic Blocking

The value of local anesthetic injections and application of topical anesthetics to identify and localize pain cannot be overemphasized. It is essential when differentiating primary from secondary pains. It is equally useful to identify the pathways that mediate peripheral pain and to localize pain sources. The examiner should therefore become skilled in the use of this valuable diagnostic tool by using not only the routine injections common to dental practice but also infraorbital, pterygopalatine canal, second-division, third-division, auriculotemporal and cervical plexus blocks.[52] Skillful analgesic blocking of muscles of the masticatory system (Figs 8-26 to 8-29) and maxillofacial region as well as anesthetizing the temporomandibular joint proper are especially useful in the diagnoses of masticatory pains

Fig 8-26 Drawing to illustrate a technique for extraoral injection of the masseter muscle. The needle enters the muscle at the anterior border about midbody and is passed through the muscle at several angles and depths to reach the deep and superficial layers. With each pass of the needle, after aspirating it, the solution is slowly deposited as the needle is withdrawn. (From Bell WE. Management of masticatory pain. In Alling CC, Mahan PE [eds]. Facial Pain, ed 2. Philadelphia: Lea & Febiger; 1977: 188. Used with permission.)

Fig 8-27 Drawing to illustrate a technique for injecting the temporalis muscle. The needle penetrates the muscle at several points *(X)* just above the zygomatic arch to reach most of the fibers. With each penetration, after aspiration of the needle, the solution is slowly deposited. (From Bell WE. Management of masticatory pain. In Alling CC, Mahan PE [eds]: Facial Pain, ed 2. Philadelphia: Lea & Febiger; 1977: 188. Used with permission.)

and nonmasticatory myofascial pain disorders. Although the area is outside the scope of dental practice, the examiner should be familiar with the indications for analgesic blocking of the stellate ganglion for the diagnosis of face and head pains that are mediated by the afferent sympathetic pathways or that are dependent on sympathetic efferent activity.[53] An anesthesiologist or neurologist should be consulted to perform this injection.

When any injection is to be performed the following fundamental rules for local anesthesia should always be observed:

1. The clinician should have a sound knowledge of the anatomy of all structures to be injected.
2. The clinician should have a sound knowledge of the pharmacology of all solutions that will be used.

Fig 8-28 Drawing to illustrate a technique for extraoral injection of the lateral pterygoid muscle. After the needle is carefully passed through the mandibular sigmoid notch, it is directed slightly upward and inward to a total depth of 35 to 40 mm. After aspiration of the needle, the solution is slowly deposited. Motor fibers of the facial nerve also may be anesthetized. (From Bell WE. Management of masticatory pain. In Alling CC, Mahan PE [eds]: Facial Pain, ed 2. Philadelphia: Lea & Febiger; 1977: 188. Used with permission.)

Fig 8-29 Drawing to illustrate a technique for extraoral injection of the medial pterygoid muscle. After the needle is carefully passed through the mandibular sigmoid notch, it is directed boldly downward and inward to a total depth of about 40 mm. After aspiration of the needle, the solution is slowly deposited. Motor fibers of the facial nerve may also be anesthetized. (From Bell WE. Management of masticatory pain. In Alling CC, Mahan PE [eds]: Facial Pain, ed 2. Philadelphia: Lea & Febiger; 1977: 188. Used with permission.)

3. The clinician should avoid any injection into inflamed or diseased tissues.

4. The clinician should maintain strict asepsis at all times.

5. The clinician should always aspirate before injecting the solution to be sure the needle is not in a blood vessel.

Since prolongation of the anesthetic effect is unimportant diagnostically, the use of short-acting drugs is desirable. Usually one without a vasoconstricting agent is best. Good anesthesia for skeletal muscle requires a nonvasoconstricting solution due to the vasodilating effect of epinephrine-like substances on such tissue. This reverse effect on muscle tissue is sometimes forgotten and may account for the transient anesthesia of poor quality sometimes obtained

179

when muscles are injected for diagnostic purposes.

It has been demonstrated that local anesthetics have a measure of myotoxicity. Procaine appears to be the least myotoxic of the local anesthetics in common use.[54] Mild inflammatory reactions follow the injection of 1% and 2% procaine hydrochloride as well as isotonic sodium chloride.[55] Single injections of either procaine or isotonic saline cause no muscle necrosis.[56] The longer-acting and stronger anesthetics induce more severe inflammation and occasional coagulation necrosis of muscle tissue.[33] Regeneration takes place in about 7 days. Solutions containing epinephrine cause greater muscle damage.[57] To minimize the danger of muscle damage in analgesic blocking for both diagnostic and therapeutic purposes, low concentrations of procaine are advisable, and such injections should be spaced at least 7 days apart. Since procaine is not available in dental carpules, the dentist may select 2% lidocaine without any vasoconstrictor. The diagnostic use of local anesthetics on muscles should be curtailed to actual need. It should be noted that, despite some myotoxicity, the diagnostic and therapeutic use of local anesthesia in the management of myogenous pain disorders is clinically justified. Many diagnostic procedures and therapeutic modalities are attended by some risk. Note the destructive effects of radiation in radiography. All anesthetics and most medications are toxic to some degree. The inherent risks therefore must be weighed against the benefits derived. Reasonable judgment should be exercised in the application of all procedures that entail a measure of risk to the patient.

Diagnostic Drugs

Since at least part of the discomfort of vascular and neurovascular pain disorders seems to derive from the dilation and amplitude of pulsation of the blood vessels involved, the diagnostic use of medications that temporarily constrict blood vessels may help confirm the diagnosis. For this purpose, ergotamine tartrate is used and administered as 0.5 to 1 mg of drug injected intramuscularly or 2 mg via a sublingual tablet. The drug constricts the cranial blood vessels and decreases the amplitude of pulsation. Relief of pain relates only to that portion that comes from distended vessels and does not affect concomitant pain due to neurogenic inflammation, edema of the vessels, or to pain of muscle origin. The effect therefore is only partial and relates especially to pain that has a throbbing quality. The temporary benefit occurs within 30 to 45 minutes and may last for an hour or longer. A single intramuscular injection usually suffices for testing purposes. If the sublingual route is used, a second tablet should be placed beneath the tongue if no response is noticed within 30 minutes. Neither mode of administration should be repeated within a 24-hour period. Treatment with the drug is contraindicated with peripheral vascular disease, coronary heart disease, hypertension, impaired hepatic or renal function, sepsis, and pregnancy. Side effects may include paresthesia of the fingers and toes, muscle pain and weakness in the extremities, precordial distress, transient tachycardia or bradycardia, nausea, and vomiting. Ordinarily such side effects are not seen from a single testing dose unless the patient is hypersensitive to the drug or a specific contraindication is violated. Intravenous infusion of histamine is known to precipitate a headache only in patients with migraine.[58] This substance may become a useful test for neurovascular pain disorders.

Confirmation of pain due to myocardial ischemia is usually accomplished by using a testing dose of nitroglycerin beneath the tongue. The drug relaxes smooth muscle principally in the smaller blood vessels and therefore dilates the arterioles, especially in the coronary circulation. Treatment with the drug is contraindicated in early myocardial infarction, severe anemia, glaucoma, increased intracranial pressure, and idiosyncrasy. Occasionally, it causes a transient headache. An overdose may cause flushing, headaches, tachycardia, and vertigo.

Confirmation of acute muscle spasm can sometimes be accomplished by testing with methocarbamol. One 10-mL ampule is used intravenously at an injection rate that does not exceed 3-mL/min. It is specifically contraindicated in patients with renal disease, pregnant women, children under 12 years of age, patients with epilepsy, and hypersensitive patients. Adverse reactions include vertigo, hypotension, syncope, drowsiness, gastrointestinal upset, metallic taste, thrombophlebitis, sloughing at the injection site, anaphylaxis, allergy, various autonomic effects, muscular incoordination, and fever. A high rate of injection and alcoholism increase the incidence of these symptoms. Convulsive seizures have been reported. It goes without saying that this type of medication should be used with caution, and the examiner must be prepared to properly manage any adverse reaction. The more potent intravenous muscle relaxant succinylcholine chloride should be used only when apparatus for assisted or controlled respiration with oxygen is available and only by persons skilled in the use of such apparatus.

Consultations

There are occasions when pain problems require medical, otolaryngologic, orthopedic, neurologic, rheumatologic, or psychologic consultation for proper identification of the pain disorder. It requires judgment, therefore, on the part of the examiner to guide the patient through the examining procedure that will arrive at a firm diagnosis in the most direct, time-saving, and economic manner. Elaborate diagnostic and consultative procedures should not be routine. Yet if the problem justifies it, every avenue of exploration should be used to attain at a confirmed working diagnosis.

Trial Therapy

A short period of trial therapy is a good means of confirming a diagnosis, provided the examiner is familiar with the effectiveness of placebo therapy. This is particularly true with patients who have significant Axis II diagnoses. These factors must be taken into account when evaluating the results of trial therapy. One form of trial therapy is the use of phenytoin (Dilantin) to help confirm a doubtful diagnosis of paroxysmal neuralgia. This medication has no analgesic action and therefore does not relieve pain per se. If relief well beyond the 40% maximum placebo effect is obtained with this medication within a few days, it is presumptive evidence that the disorder in question is in fact paroxysmal neuralgia. One should guard against assuming that absence of ef-

181

fect from this drug excludes neuralgia. This would be a serious error since not all such neuralgias respond to this medication. Its exact mode of action is not known.

Trial therapy with a medication that constricts the cranial arteries can do much to confirm a diagnosis of neurovascular pain. One of the many ergotamine tartrate preparations available may be utilized for this purpose. If the drug used does in fact diminish the pain, especially the throbbing component, even though some muscle pain and tender edematous vessels still cause discomfort, it is highly suggestive that a neurovascular pain disorder exists.

Trial therapy for muscular pains is useful to help confirm the diagnosis. This includes the use of vapocoolants, analgesic blocking of painful muscles, controlled physical therapy, and the use of muscle relaxants. If definite benefit accrues from such therapy, a firm diagnosis of muscle pain becomes justified.

Temporomandibular arthralgia suspected to be due to hyperuricemia can be subjected to a period of trial therapy consisting of colchicine if the condition is an acute attack or colchicine combined with a uricosuric agent such as probenecid in subacute and chronic conditions. Such medications should be given under medical supervision. If the arthralgia responds favorably to such therapy, the diagnosis should stand confirmed, and further medical care would be in order.

Multiple Categories of Pain

In managing pain problems around the mouth and face, one should avoid assuming that the complaint necessarily consists of a single category of pain. There are many occasions when two or more types of pain may be represented, and when this is true, the diagnostic identification of the different categories may be complex indeed. An early indication of this complication may come with the series of questions that constitute the second step of making the diagnosis. Difficulty in obtaining clear answers to these questions should alert the examiner to this possibility. Management difficulties also are likely to follow.

References

1. Melzack R. The McGill pain questionnaire: Major properties and scoring methods. Pain 1975; 1:277–299.

2. Grushka M, Sessle BJ. Applicability of the McGill pain questionnaire to the differentiation of "toothache" pain. Pain 1984; 19:49.

3. Corson JA, Schneider MJ. The Dartmouth pain questonnaire: An adjunct to the McGill pain questionnaire. Pain 1984; 19:59.

4. Melzack R. The short-form McGill pain questionnaire. Pain 1987; 30:191–197.

5. Moldofsky H, Scarisbrick P. Induction of neurasthenic musculoskeletal pain syndrome by selective sleep deprivation. Psychsom Med 1976; 38:35–44.

6. Moldofsky H, Scarisbrick P, England R, Smythe H. Musculoskeletal symptoms and non-REM sleep disturbance in patients with "fibrositis" and healthy subjects. Psychosom Med 1986; 37:341–351.

7. Moldofsky H, Tullis C, Lue FA. Sleep related myoclonus in rheumatic pain modulation disorder (fibrosis syndrome). J Rheumatol 1986; 13:614–617.

8. Molony RR, MacPeck DM, Schiffman PL, et al. Sleep, sleep apnea, and the fibromyalgia syndrome. J Rheumatol 1986; 13:797–800.

9. Turk DC, Rudy TE. Toward a comprehensive assessment of chronic pain patients: A multiaxial approach. Behav Res Ther 1987; 25:237–249.

10. Derogatis LR. SCL-90-R: Administration, Scoring and Procedures Manual-II for the Revised Version. Towson, Md: Clinical Psychometric Research; 1977.

11. Fricton J, Nelson A, Monsein M. IMPATH: Microcomputer assessment of behavioral and psychosocial factors in craniomandibular disorders. J Craniomand Pract 1987; 5:372–381.

12. Levitt SR, McKinney MW, Lundeen TF. The TMJ scale cross-validation and reliability studies. J Craniomand Pract 1988; 6:17–25.

13. Levitt SR. Predictive value of the TMJ scale in detecting clinically significant symptoms of temporomandibular disorders. J Craniomandibular Disord Facial Oral Pain 1990; 4:177–185.

14. Diagnostic and Statistical Manual of Mental Disorders (DSM-IV), ed 4. Washington, DC: The American Psychiatric Association; 1994:458–462.

15. Clark GT. Examining temporomandibular disorder patients for craniocervical dysfunction. J Craniomand Pract 1984; 2:55–63.

16. Clark GT, Green EM, Dornan MR, Flack VF. Craniocervical dysfunction levels in a patient sample from a temporomandibular joint clinic. J Am Dent Assoc 1987;115:251–256.

17. Keele KD. A physician looks at pain. In Weisenberg M (ed): Pain: Clinical and Experimental Perspectives. St Louis: CV Mosby; 1975: 45–52.

18. Mahan PE, Alling CC. Facial Pain, ed 3. Malvern, Pa: Lea & Febiger; 1991: 145–151.

19. Okeson JP. Management of Temporomandibular Disorders and Occlusion, ed 3. St Louis: Mosby Year Book; 1993: 239–251.

20. McNeill C. Temporomandibular Disorders, Guidlines for Classification, Assessment, and Management. Chicago: Quintessence; 1993: 64–65.

21. Frost HM. Musculoskeletal pains. In Alling CC, Mahan PE (eds): Facial Pain, ed 2. Philadelphia: Lea & Febiger; 1977: 140.

22. Reeves JL, Jaeger B, Graff-Radford SB. Reliability of the pressure algometer as a measure of myofascial trigger point sensitivity. Pain 1986; 24:313–321.

23. Jensen K, Andersen HO, Olesen J, et al. Pressure-pain threshold in human temporal region. Evaluation of a new pressure algometer. Pain 1986; 25:313–323.

24. Fischer AA. Instruments for pain diagnosis in clinical practice: Pressure algometers for measurement of pain sensitivity and documentation for tender spots; tissue compliance meter for objective quantitative recording of muscle spasm. Pain 1987(suppl 4); 31:292.

25. Schiffman E, Fricton J, Haley D, et al. A pressure algometer for MPS: Reliability and validity. Pain 1987(suppl 4); 31:291.

26. Fischer AA. Pressure algometry over normal muscles: Standard values, validity, and reproducibility of pressure threshold. Pain 1987; 30:115–126.

27. Fischer AA. Pressure threshold measurement for diagnosis of myofascial pain and evaluation of treatment results. Clin J Pain 1987; 2:207–214.

28. Jaeger B, Reeves JL. Quantification of changes in myofascial trigger point sensitivity with the pressure algometer following passive stretch. Pain 1986; 27:203–210.

29. Moody PM, Calhoun TC, Okeson JP, Kemper JT. Stress-pain relationships in MPD syndrome patients and non-MPD syndrome patients. J Prosthet Dent 1981; 45:84–88.

30. Okeson JP, Kemper JT, Moody PM. A study of the use of occlusion splints in the treatment of acute and chronic patients with craniomandibular disorders. J Prosthet Dent 1982; 48:708–712.

31. Okeson JP. Management of Temporomandibular Disorders and Occlusion, ed 3. St Louis: Mosby Year Book; 1993: 245–248.

32. Travell J, Rinzler SH. The myofascial genesis of pain. Postgrad Med J 1952; 11:425.

33. Travell JG, Simons DG. Myofascial Pain and Dysfunction. The Trigger Point Manual. Baltimore: Williams & Wilkins; 1983: 165–332.

34. Bell WE. Management of temporomandibular joint problems. In Goldman HM, Gilmore HW, Royer R, et al (eds): Current Therapy in Dentistry, vol 4. St Louis: CV Mosby; 1970: 398–415.

35. Agerberg G. Maximal mandibular movement in young men and women. Swed Dent J 1974; 67:81–100.

36. Solberg W. Occlusion-related pathosis and its clinical evaluation. In: Clarke, JW. Clinical Dentistry. New York: Harper & Row; 1976: 1–29.

37. Bitlar G, Atchison K, Bibb C, Pullinger A. Range of jaw opening in a elderly non-patient population (abstract 1225). J Dent Res 1991; 70:419.

38. McCarroll RS, Hesse JR, Naeije M, et al. Mandibular border positions and their relationship with peripheral joint mobility. J Oral Rehabil 1987;14:125.

39. Hesse J, Naeije M, Hansson TL. Craniomandibular stiffness toward maximum mouth opening in healthy subjects: A clinical and experimental investigation, J Craniomandib Disord Facial Oral Pain 1990; 4:257–266.

40. Okeson JP. Management of Temporomandibular Disorders and Occlusion, ed 3. St Louis: Mosby Year Book; 1993: 192–214.

41. Burch JG. History and clinical examination. In: The President's Conference on the Examination, Diagnosis, and Management of Temporomandibular Disorders. Chicago: American Dental Association; 1983: 51–56.

42. Bezuur JN, Habets LLMH, Jimenez Lopez V, Naeije M, Hansson TL. The recognition of craniomandibular disorders, a comparison between clinical and radiographic findings in eighty-nine subjects. J Oral Rehabil 1988: 15: 215–222.

43. Westesson PL, Eriksson L, Kurita K. Reliability of a negative clinical temporomandibular joint examination: Prevalence of disk displacement in asymtomatic temporomandibular joints, Oral Surg Oral Med Oral Pathol 1989; 68:551–554.

44. Mumford JM. Toothache and Orofacial Pain, ed 2. Edinburgh: Churchill Livingstone; 1976: 265–279.

45. Okeson JP. Management of Temporomandibular Disorders and Occlusion, ed 3. St Louis: Mosby Year Book; 1993: 149–177.

46. Okeson JP. Management of Temporomandibular Disorders and Occlusion, ed 3. St Louis: Mosby Year Book; 1993: 262–266.

47. Thomas PS, Chen L, Frederickson BE, et al. Liquid-crystal thermography: A noninvasive technique to document treatment results in patients with low back syndrome. In Fields HL, Dubner R, Cervero F (eds): Advances in Pain Research and Therapy, vol 9. New York: Raven Press; 1985: 403–407.

48. Hobbins WB. Differential diagnosis of somatic pain by thermography. Pain 1987; 31:293.

49. Ochoa JL, Torebjork E, Marchettini P, et al. Mechanisms of neuropathic pain: Cumulative observations, new experiments, and further speculation. In Fields HL, Dubner R, Cervero F (eds): Advances in Pain Research and Therapy, vol 9. New York: Raven Press; 1985: 431–450.

50. Keats AS. Use of analgesics at bedside. In Way EL (ed): New Concepts in Pain. Philadelphia: FA Davis; 1967: 143–154.

51. Beecher HK. The use of chemical agents in the control of pain. In Knighton RS, Dumke PR (eds): Pain. Boston: Little, Brown; 1966: 221–239.

52. Mahan PE, Alling CC. Facial Pain, ed 3. Philadelphia: Lea & Febiger; 1991: 72–94.

53. Bonica JJ. The Management of Pain, ed 2. Philadelphia: Lea & Febiger; 1990: 1931–1944.

54. Travell JG, Simons DG. Myofascial Pain and Dysfunction. Baltimore: Williams & Wilkins; 1983: 74–86.

55. Pizzolato P, Mannheimer W. Histopathologic Effects of Local Anesthetic Drugs and Related Substances. Springfield, Ill: Charles C Thomas; 1961.

56. Burke GW Jr, Fedison JR, Jones CR. Muscle degeneration produced by local anesthesia. Va Dent J 1972; 49:33.

57. Yagiela JA, Benoit PW, Buoncristiani RD, et al. Comparison of myotoxic effects of lidocaine with epinephrine in rats and humans. Anesth Analg 1981; 60:471–480.

58. Krabbe AA, Olesen J. Headache provocation by continuous intravenous infusion of histamine: Clinical results and receptor mechanisms. Pain 1980; 8:253–259.

9 | General Considerations in Managing Orofacial Pains

The conditions that generate pain are susceptible to modification. The treatment of people who suffer pain entails the manipulation of those factors that initiate and accentuate pain, and/or the institution of means and methods by which patients can better cope with their complaint. The conditions that we may set out to manipulate, therefore, comprise on the one hand factors such as the elimination of causative noxious stimuli, the interruption of nociceptive circuits, and the enhancement of our natural mechanisms of pain inhibition. On the other hand, we may elect to direct the main attention toward the patient rather than his or her problem in an effort to help that person contend more successfully with the disease. Sternbach[1] has shown that, whereas pain in acute pain is a symptom of disease, pain in chronic pain is the disease itself. Instantly, it should be obvious that pain management is a complex undertaking. Unfortunately, we are just beginning to learn the rules of the game. This much we do know: it is the patient's body that does the healing, not the doctor. The most that we can do is provide favorable conditions for healing. Our patients must understand that it is they, not we, who determine the final outcome of therapy. Healing is an activity that only the patients can do. We cannot do it for them.

The first step in the treatment of any condition is accurate and complete diagnostic evaluation of what the problem is, what structures are involved, and what conditions account for it. The diagnosis of pain is not a naming process. It is an understanding of pain genesis, of modulating conditions, of inhibitory and excitatory mechanisms, of secondary effects, of accompanying symptoms, and of physical and emotional reactions that occur in human beings as distinct individuals. Every patient who presents a pain complaint has a problem that is peculiar to him or her. Yet we as dentists are trained as therapists more than as diagnosticians. We are conditioned to treat, and our patients are conditioned to expect decisive and effective treatment from us. We are more mouth-oriented than patient-oriented. We do well as long as everything is obvious; when we face obscure problems, our conditioning may fail us. Therefore, when we meet an obscure pain complaint, we need to call forth all our best diagnostic capabilities.

It is essential at the very outset to decide whether we are dealing with an acute pain or a chronic pain. We must decide whether the behavioral characteristics suggest somatic or neuropathic pain; whether the pain emanates from superficial or deep structures; whether the pain is primary or secondary. To skip these ABCs is to invite failure. Very early we need to decide whether the complaint appears to be stimulus-evoked. Will our therapy be directed toward the elimination of a source of noxious stimulation? Will it use techniques that manipulate modulating influences? Will it entail the management of neuropathic pain sources? Will it employ the use of systemic medications? Will psychotherapy likely be utilized? A decision is needed: "Is this a problem that I can handle alone, or do I need help? What kind of help? Who?" Ultimate success or failure may well rest on such early decisions. They should form the overall guidelines for managing the problem at hand. Each case should be individualized. We are not dealing so much with different kinds of problems as with different kinds of people. Genuine caring on the part of the clinician is the one indispensable attribute necessary for good pain management.[2]

Cause-Related Therapy

Many patients who experience orofacial pain have an organic structural cause that is responsible. The main thrust of therapy for such complaints is to identify the cause and eliminate it. The extent to which one achieves this will determine his or her success in the management of the pain problem. The cause of pain emanating from somatic structures is thought to be due chiefly, if not exclusively, to the action of algogenic substances such as bradykinin, histamine,

serotonin, potassium, and phosphates.[3] The cause of neuropathic pain is less well understood.

Somatic Pain

Much somatic pain results from trauma, intrinsic injury, infections, and disease that induce inflammatory reactions. The variety of traumatic conditions as to the type of agent as well as the extent and location of injury is nearly endless. Inflammatory conditions reactive to abusive use, intrinsic strains, microtraumas, bacterial/fungal/viral infections, pathologic lesions, and biomechanical dysfunctions are almost without number. At a dental level, inflammatory conditions of the teeth, the supporting structures, and the mucogingival tissues as well as dysfunctional and inflammatory conditions of the temporomandibular joints and masticatory musculature are common. It is known that ischemia liberates bradykinin[4]; that hemolyzed red blood cells in muscle tissue liberate potassium ions; and that phosphates, histamine, and serotonin are liberated from blood platelets.[3] Some of the visceral somatic structures elicit pain without such evident cause. Vascular pain involves more than simple vasodilation; it is likely that algogenic substances are involved.

There are occasions when the somatic condition that generates pain is refractory to therapy, and the complaint persists as chronic structural pain. Cancer presents this problem. Some masticatory pains such as inflammatory arthritis may also fall into this category.

Neuropathic Pain

The matter of eliminating the cause of neuropathic pain presents problems. A traumatic neuroma in accessible scar tissue can be excised. Some benefit may come from anti-inflammatory therapy for inflammatory neuritis pain, and symptomatic neuralgia may respond to neurosurgical elimination of the neuropathy. But on the whole, pains due to idiopathic neuralgia and deafferentation cannot be managed with cause-related therapy. These therapies will be discussed in Chapter 17.

Pain Related to Psychologic Disorders

When Axis II diagnoses predominate the pain complaint, an entirely different treatment strategy is often indicated. Any therapies that alter somatic or neurogenous structures should be avoided. Therapy should be directed toward the factors or conditions that relate to the specific psychologic disorder. Sometimes pharmacologic agents or physical therapy modalities may be helpful but they should not be used as a substitute for proper psychotherapy. Psychotherapies are best provided by trained personnel and referral may be indicated if these professionals are not immediately available (see Chapter 18).

Therapeutic Modalities

Table 9-1 outlines the many different approaches that should be considered when managing orofacial pain disorders. The relevance of each modality is determined by the specific diagnosis. Each modality will be reviewed in this chapter. The specific use of these modalities will be discussed in the chapters that review each orofacial pain disorder.

Table 9-1 Modalities for Managing Orofacial Pain Disorders

I. Pharmacologic therapy
  A. Analgesic agents
    1. Non-narcotic agents
    2. Narcotic agents
    3. Adjuvant analgesics
  B. Anesthetic agents
    1. Topical anesthetic
    2. Injectable local anesthetic
  C. Anti-inflammatory agents
  D. Muscle relaxants
  E. Antidepressants
  F. Antianxiety agents
  G. Vasoactive agents
  H. Norepinephrine blockers
  I. Antimicrobial agents
  J. Antiviral agents
  K. Antihistamine agents
  L. Anticonvulsive agents
  M. Neurolytic agents
  N. Uricosuric agents
  O. Dietary considerations
II. Physical therapy
  A. Modalities
    1. Sensory stimulation
    2. Ultrasound
    3. Electrogalvanic stimulation (EGS)
    4. Deep heat
  B. Manual techniques
    1. Massage
    2. Spray and stretch techniques
    3. Exercise
    4. Physical activity
III. Psychological therapy
  A. Counseling
  B. Behavioral modification training
    1. Stress reduction training
    2. Relaxation training

Pharmacologic Therapy

Although analgesics are the drugs most frequently used in the treatment of patients in pain, several other classes of pharmaceutical agents are useful for palliative and cause-related therapy. Some drugs bind to known *receptors*, which are cellular components with which the natural body chemicals (*ligands*) interact to produce physiological responses. Some drugs (*agonists*) mimic rather closely the action of the natural substances. Others prevent those actions (*antagonists* or blocking agents). For example, morphine (agonist) binds to certain receptors (mu and kappa) in the central nervous system (CNS) that normally interact with the natural endorphins (ligands); this interaction is prevented by naloxone (antagonist or blocking agent).

Some drugs act by neutralizing the effect of certain enzymes, thus producing a physiologic effect indirectly. The antidepressant drugs, monoamine oxidase (MAO) inhibitors, act to increase the concentration of serotonin, dopamine, and norepinephrine in the cerebrospinal fluid (CSF) by reducing their natural breakdown through an inhibitory action on the enzyme MAO. Aspirin produces an anti-inflammatory effect by inhibiting the action of the enzyme cyclo-oxygenase, which normally metabolizes arachidonic acid into prostaglandins as the result of local tissue injury. Other drugs act in still different ways, and the action of many is not known.

Since drugs induce both intentional (primary) and unintentional (secondary) effects, the selection of the best drug in a given situation requires careful consideration of the various effects that may occur. When two or more drugs are ingested, their possible interactions should be understood. Some combinations are clearly incompatible; some drugs potentiate the action of others; some act synergistically. To properly gauge dosage, one should be familiar with the estimated half-life of the medication being used, especially if a sustained effect is desired. A drug's half-life is the time necessary for the plasma concentration to decrease by 50%. A relatively steady blood level can usually be achieved after five doses are administered at periods that correspond to the drug's half-life.[5]

Medications of different kinds play an important role in the treatment of patients with pain. Their proper use is a major concern. It is the clinician's responsibility to be adequately familiar with the drug being administered and with the patient who is receiving it so that safety and effectiveness are ensured. Individualization is necessary.

Many things need to be known about a medication: indications and contraindications for its use, drug incompatibilities, modes of administration, safe and toxic dosage, side effects, and possible complications. The clinician should be prepared to recognize and effectively deal with such things as sensitivity to the drug, undesirable side effects, toxicity, idiosyncrasy, anaphylaxis, or other untoward reactions to its use. He or she should know about the possibility of potentiation of other medications being used, synergisms, dependence, and the probability of addiction.

Adequate medical supervision and emergency care should always be available if needed. All these responsibilities rest firmly on the prescribing doctor, and they cannot be abrogated. If one is not prepared to accept these responsibilities, he or she should place the medicinal treatment of his or her patient in the hands of someone who is.

Analgesic Agents. Medications that reduce pain are an important class of drugs useful in pain control. As a general rule, the objective of analgesics should not be to eliminate pain altogether. Pain has some value in monitoring progress in the patient's condition. It helps guide the patient when his actions are excessive or abusive. The objective of analgesics should be to make the pain tolerable. The American Pain Society[6] classified analgesic drugs into three groups: non-narcotic analgesics, narcotic analgesics, and adjuvant analgesics.

Non-narcotic Analgesics. The non-narcotic analgesics include aspirin and the non-steroidal anti-inflammatory drugs (NSAIDs), which have four major actions: analgesic, antipyretic, antiplatelet, and anti-inflammatory. They differ from narcotic analgesics in that they presumably prevent the formation of prostaglandin E by inhibitory action on the enzyme cyclo-oxygenase; they do not produce tolerance, physical dependence, or addiction; and they have a ceiling effect whereby increasing the dosage beyond peak limits does not increase the analgesic effect even though it may affect the duration. Representative of such analgesics are aspirin, fenoprofen, and ibuprofen, which have relatively short half-lives, and diflunisal and naproxen, which have relatively longer half-lives and therefore are longer acting.

Also included in the non-narcotic group are acetaminophen, which has no antiplatelet or anti-inflammatory action, and choline magnesium trisalicylate, which lacks antiplatelet action.[6] The non-narcotic analgesics are general-purpose medications indicated for use in the treatment of mild-to-moderate pain and chronic cancer pain.

Aspirin and the NSAIDs prolong bleeding time and therefore are contraindicated with anticoagulant therapy and other coagulation deficiency conditions. It is thought that the antiplatelet action is beneficial to those at risk for cardiac attacks. Gastric irritation is a common side effect of these drugs. The effect of acetaminophen is approximately equipotent to that of aspirin.

As previously mentioned, aspirin-like drugs strongly inhibit the action of cyclooxygenase, thus interfering with the biosynthesis of prostaglandins from arachidonic acid that occurs as part of an inflammatory process.[7-9] The resulting decreased concentration of prostaglandins in inflamed tissue coincides with the alleviation of pain.[10,11] This helps explain the anti-inflammatory effect of the drug and no doubt has some bearing on its analgesic action. It does not, however, fully explain the analgesic action of aspirin.[12] Age-related changes modify the response to aspirin. A higher incidence of drug reaction occurs in the aged. Some caution is indicated, therefore, in the use of aspirin in geriatric patients.[13]

Narcotic Analgesics. Morphine-like drugs act through CNS receptors to induce a peripheral analgesic effect.[14,15] They depress nociceptive neurons while stimulating nonnociceptive cells.[16] Both aspirin and morphine inhibit the release of bradykinin, but aspirin inhibits its release regardless of the type of noxious stimulus, while morphine inhibits its release when mediated by neural mechanisms.[17] There is evidence that part of morphine-induced analgesia is contributed indirectly by the release of endogenous opioid peptides.[18] There is also some evidence that opiates exert an inhibitory influence on substance P release.[19] There is no hard evidence that the addition of codeine to NSAIDs yields any measurable increase in analgesic effect.[20] As with all drug therapy, it is the responsibility of the prescribing doctor to know the proper dosage, indications, contraindications, incompatibilities, and signs of toxicity and/or side effects of medications he or she prescribes. The prescribing doctor should be prepared to cope with any ill effects that his or her therapy may induce.

Narcotic analgesics comprise three classes of drugs: morphine-like agonists, mixed agonists-antagonists, and partial agonists. Included among the morphine-like agonists are codeine, oxycodone, meperidine, propoxyphene, morphine, hydromorphine, methadone, levorphanol, oxymorphone, and heroin. Representative of the mixed agonist-antagonist drugs are pentazocine, nalbuphene, and butorphanol. Buprenorphine is a partial agonist drug.

Narcotics are useful in managing severe acute pain and chronic cancer pain but are generally contraindicated in the management of chronic orofacial pain disorders. They cause constipation; therefore, stool softeners and laxatives should be administered. The clinician should carefully individualize the selection of drug, the mode of administration, and the dosage. Narcotics are best administered on a regular time schedule rather than as needed to minimize unnecessary pain periods that may require increased dosage attendant with overmedication and increased toxicity. Side effects should be recognized and treated appropriately. The clinician should be watchful for tolerance, physical dependence, and/or addiction (psychologic dependence). Tolerance means that larger doses are required to obtain a satisfactory analgesic effect. Physical dependence means that withdrawal symptoms accompany abstinence. Addiction means compulsive craving for the drug and the need to use it for effects other than the relief of pain.

Adjuvant Analgesics. The drugs listed as adjuvant analgesics are those that enhance the analgesic effect of other medications or have independent analgesic activity in certain situations. These include tricyclic antidepressants,[21] antihistamines, caffeine, dextroamphetamine, steroids, phenothiazines, and anticonvulsants.

Anesthetic Agents. Local anesthetics have an essential role in pain management both diagnostically and therapeutically. Anesthetic agents can be used either topically or within the tissues by injection.

Topical Anesthetic. Topical anesthetics may be used as solutions, sprays, ointments, or lozenges. Water-soluble ointments containing a topical anesthetic and a germicide are useful for managing dental alveolitis.

Analgesic balms are agents that give soothing, palliative relief of inflammatory pain of both superficial and deep somatic categories when applied topically to exposed or ulcerated tissue. Aloe vera juice is an ancient remedy for superficially generated inflammatory pain. It is an ingredient of compound benzoin tincture. Balsam of Peru, eugenol, and guaiacol are other well-known balms. Applied in various forms as liquid, ointment, or cement-like or adhesive dressings, analgesic balms are extremely useful in the palliative control of pain emanating from exposed or ulcerated cutaneous and mucogingival tissues, exposed dentin, and acute alveolitis.

Injectable Local Anesthetic. A variety of injectable local anesthetics are available in different concentrations, with and without a vasoconstricting agent. Long-acting local anesthetics such as bupivacaine hydrochloride (Marcaine) are useful even though they entail a higher risk of toxicity. Proper dosage, correct technique, adequate precautions, and readiness for emergencies are essential to the safety and effectiveness of all local anesthetics. Resuscitative equipment, oxygen, and other resuscitative drugs should be instantly available, and adequate training in their proper use is necessary. Extreme caution is required when vasopressor agents are used in patients receiving MAO inhibitors or antidepressants of the triptyline or imipramine types because severe prolonged hypertension may result. Since most untoward reactions with local anesthetics follow accidental intravascular injection, aspiration prior to injecting any medication is an absolute necessity.

The local injection of 0.02% morphine sulfate around peripheral nerves has been reported to yield a level of local anesthesia that is equal to that of bupivacaine in onset, profundity, and duration.[22] This small dose of 1 mg or less did not produce systemic opiate effects.

The use of local anesthesia to control surgical pain and diagnostically to identify nociceptive pathways and primary sources of pain is common. The therapeutic use of analgesic blocking is less well known. Four facets of this modality of pain control are useful at a clinical level (*1*) to arrest primary pain input, (*2*) to interrupt pain cycling, (*3*) to resolve myofascial trigger point activity, and (*4*) to induce a sympathetic blockade.

Arresting Primary Pain Input. Primary deep pain input is an important factor, not only in initiating heterotopic pains and secondary muscle effects but also in perpetuating them. For example, the pain of local muscle soreness by its own central excitation tends to perpetuate cycling muscle pain (see Chapter 12). To arrest cyclic muscle pain by analgesic blocking has marked therapeutic value; it shuts off this perpetuating influence. This can be done by anesthetizing the muscle itself. Since myotoxicity of local anesthetics may restrict the choice of agent to short-acting anesthetics of low potency, it is preferable to block the nociceptive pathway rather than the muscle proper. Long-acting potent anesthetics can then be used with relative impunity; thus, the benefits of arresting the deep pain input can be extended.

Interrupting Pain Cycling. On the basis of clinical evidence, a cycling mechanism appears to complicate several pain disorders that occur in the orofacial region. When such cycling is effectively interrupted by local anesthetic blockage of nociceptive impulses at the primary source or somewhere along its mediating pathway, remission of pain may significantly outlast the period of anesthesia. It is thought that this prolonged relief may be the result of a decrease in the sensitization of the second-order neuron after the nociceptive input is terminated. Such remission indicates that a therapeutic effect has been achieved. When such an effect can be obtained with a short-acting anesthetic, a still greater therapeutic effect usually results from the use of a longer-acting drug.

Repeated analgesic blocking of the pathway that subserves the peripheral receptors that trigger trigeminal neuralgia may induce an extended period of remission. Analgesic blocking of the primary source of pain input may effectively arrest some myofascial trigger point pains in the facial region. Myospasm of masticatory muscles can be influenced favorably if not completely resolved by one or more analgesic blocks of the nociceptive pathway that subserves the muscle.

Trigger Point Therapy. It is well known that the injection of a short-acting, aqueous local anesthetic of low myotoxicity at a myofascial trigger point located in muscle tissue effectively resolves the referred pain phenomena that characterize myofascial pain syndromes.[23] Kraus[24] believed that such therapy is required when the trigger point is located in a muscle tendon.

Sympathetic Blockade. The diagnostic analgesic blocking of afferent sympathetic pathways to identify pain mediated by such neurons is well known. The stellate ganglion block is usually used for afferent sympathetic routes from the head.[25] Analgesic blocking at the same site also arrests the efferent sympathetic impulses and constitutes an ipsilateral sympathetic blockade as far as the orofacial region is concerned. It is reported that daily stellate ganglion analgesic blocking is as effective as guanethidine for the treatment of reflex sympathetic dystrophy.[26] Thompson[27] reported that half of his 120 cases of causalgia were relieved by repeated sympathetic analgesic blocks. Procacci et al[28] reported that, in 11 of their 30 subjects with reflex sympathetic dystrophy of the limbs, a significant increase in cutaneous pain threshold developed after analgesic blocking of the sympathetic ganglia on the affected side. Wetchler and Wyman[29] reported that all 23 of their patients with acute herpes zoster of the ophthalmic nerve had excellent pain relief and freedom from cutaneous scarring by treatment with daily analgesic blocks of the stellate ganglion. Three of this group, however, complained of postherpetic neuralgia at the 6-month follow-up.

The three pain disorders for which analgesic blocking of the stellate ganglion appears to be specifically indicated are *(1)* sympathetic-maintained deafferentation pains such as reflex sympathetic dystrophy,[30–32] *(2)* herpes zoster,[33–35] and *(3)* postherpetic neuralgia.[36] With both reflex sympathetic dystrophy and acute herpes zoster, early treatment appears to be the key to success. For postherpetic neuralgia, Milligan and Nash[36] reported that 75% of their patients were helped if sympathetic blockade was performed within the first year.

Anti-inflammatory Agents. In addition to the anti-inflammatory analgesics, there are several similar nonsteroidal medications that are used chiefly for their anti-inflammatory effect. They are mildly analgesic and antipyretic. The specific action of all such medications is not known. The therapeutic effect appears to relate to the inhibition of prostaglandin biosynthesis. All such drugs should be used with caution, especially when protracted therapy is needed. Good medical supervision is appropriate. These agents do not alter the course of disease; they only suppress the symptoms of inflammation; hence their usefulness in the management of inflammatory pain.

Corticosteroids exert apotent anti-inflammatory effect, presumably by acting to inhibit prostaglandin biosynthesis. However, in addition they cause profound and varied metabolic effects and modify the body's immune responses to diverse stimuli. They are eminently useful medications but require considerable care in administration. Extended use should be under close medical supervision. Their suppressive effect on inflammation may mask infection. They are contraindicated for systemic fungal and herpes simplex infections. Corticosteroid ointments are available in different strengths and with different bases. They are useful for topical application of the drug.

Devor et al[37,38] reported that locally applied corticosteroid rapidly and effectively arrested the pain from damaged nerve fibers in experimental neuromas. They suggested that it acts directly on the membrane rather than as an anti-inflammatory action.

Muscle Relaxants. Medications that tend to relax skeletal muscle have some value especially in the management of myogenous pains. If prescribed in sufficient dosage to induce real muscle relaxation, however, the patient cannot remain ambulatory or safely continue his usual activities. The potent relaxants such as succinylcholine chloride should be restricted to hospitalized patients and administered under expert supervision. The intravenous (IV) use of methocarbamol also requires special care. Some muscle relaxants are anticholinergic; therefore, physical symptoms incidental to that action may occur. There are also some incompatibilities with which the prescribing doctor should be familiar. Although the use of muscle relaxants with fully ambulatory patients has some value, if no more than placebo effect, the actual amount of relaxation achieved is equivocal.

Antidepressant Agents. Some patients with neurovascular pain and patients with chronic pain who verbalize reactive depression may respond to the judicious use of antidepressant medications. The tricyclic antidepressants increase the availability of serotonin and norepinephrine in the CSF. The dimethylated tricyclic drugs make serotonin proportionately more available and induce some sedative effect. They are useful in treating agitated depression. The monomethylated tricyclics make norepinephrine proportionately more available and induce some CNS stimulation. They are used more for retardant depression.[39]

Recently tricyclic antidepressants have been used for a variety of chronic pain conditions.[40-42] It has been demonstrated that a low dose of amitriptyline (10 mg) just before sleep can have an analgesic effect on chronic pain after several weeks of use.[43-46] This clinical effect is not related to any antidepressive action since antidepressive dosages are from 10 to 20 times higher. Although tricyclic antidepressants increase the available serotonin in the CSF, they may not have inherent analgesic properties. In healthy subjects, they have no greater effect on pain than does placebo.[47] Ward et al[48] reported that all moderately to severely depressed individuals complained also of pain, headache being the most frequent complaint. Patients who obtained minimal antidepressant effect from tricyclic agents also obtained minimal analgesic effect.

The MAO inhibitors increase the available serotonin, norepinephrine, and dopamine in the CSF by inhibiting their breakdown. They potentiate the action of sympathomimetic substances and may induce a hypertensive crisis. The use of all antidepressant agents should be under adequate medical supervision.

Serotoninergic antidepressant medications are useful in the management of some chronic pain disorders.[49,50] Antidepressant therapy, however, is not effective for deafferentation dysesthesia.[51] Amitriptyline has a pain-relieving action in postherpetic neuralgia that is not primarily linked with its serotoninergic and antidepressant effect.[52] Although amitriptyline has a beneficial effect on some chronic pains, it does not appear to have the same positive effect on acute pain.[53] It has been reported that subanalgesic doses of antidepressant drugs potentiate the action of morphine.[54,55]

Caution should be exercised in the administration of tricyclic antidepressants, especially in patients with a history of cardiac disease. A potentially serious outcome may accompany overdosing as well as combinations with other drugs such as antihistamines, beta blockers, calcium channel blockers, and anticonvulsants.[56] It is well that such medications be administered with medical supervision and consent.

Antianxiety Agents. Numerous sedative and tranquilizing medications are available, some of which have muscle relaxant action as well. The major tranquilizers such as the phenothiazines are very useful in pain control by reducing the modulating effects of anxiety and apprehension. They are not addictive. They may display some objectionable side effects, however, and therefore require careful monitoring. Extrapyramidal effects are not uncommon. Protracted use has caused tardive dyskinesia.

The minor tranquilizers such as meprobamate and diazepam have the advantage of fewer side effects. Their muscle relaxant action is also useful. But they present a serious potential for drug tolerance and for dependence if not outright addiction. Abuse of such drugs is common. When utilized in pain control, they should be prescribed for limited periods only. When protracted use is needed, different drugs should be used periodically so that neither dependence nor tolerance is permitted to occur. Tranquilizers appear to exert some potentiating effect on narcotic analgesics.[57]

Vasoactive Agents. Neurovascular pain disorders may be favorably influenced by the alpha-adrenergic blocking action of ergotamine tartrate, which causes a stimulating effect on the smooth muscle of peripheral and cranial blood vessels. It is available in several different preparations, with and without the addition of caffeine. The caffeine enhances this vasoconstricting effect without increasing the dosage. Its effect appears to be greatest on the pulsatile component of neurovascular pain. The drug has several contraindications, including peripheral vascular and coronary heart disease, hypertension, and pregnancy.

Coronary vasodilators may be useful in some coronary complaints but have little application in orofacial pain syndromes.

Beta-adrenergic blocking agents that decrease vasodilator responses to beta-adrenergic receptor stimulants may have value in neurovascular pain disorders even though the mechanism for the antimigraine effect has not been established. The successful use of beta blockers in the treatment of phantom limb pain has also been reported.[58] Somatostatin has been reported to inhibit the effect of the release of substance P from peripheral sensory nerve terminals. Since substance P induces effects that resemble some of the symptoms of neurovascular pain disorders such as cluster headache, the use of somatostatin has been investigated as a possible treatment modality. It is reported to be as effective as ergotamine tartrate in the treatment of cluster headache.[59]

Serotonin receptors have been strongly implicated in the mechanism of migraine headache. Many of the drugs that are effective in migraine are believed to affect one or more of the various serotonin receptors. Methysergide, cyproheptadine, and dihydroergotamine (DHE) interact with the 5-HT_2 receptor. Sumatriptan and also DHE interact at the $5HT_{1a}$ and 5-HT_{1d} receptors.[60,61]

Norepinephrine Blockers. In lieu of analgesic blocking of the stellate ganglion for the control of sympathetically maintained pains around the orofacial region, the norepinephrine blocking agent guanethidine has been used. It appears to block the uptake of norepinephrine by sensitized deafferented axons. The clinical benefit outlasts the pharmacologic actions.[62,63] Bonelli et al[26] reported that IV guanethidine every 4 days for four times was equal in effectiveness to daily stellate ganglion analgesic blocks for 8 days. In a controlled, randomized, double-blind crossover study of 12 patients with reflex sympathetic dystrophy, Lief et al[64] reported that weekly IV injections of guanethidine or reserpine achieved equally significant short-term pain relief. Levine and Basbaum[65] reported that both guanethidine- and reserpine-induced sympathectomy decreased the severity of joint inflammation and pain, especially in rheumatoid arthritis.

Antimicrobial Agents. A variety of antibiotic and other antimicrobial drugs for both topical and systemic administration is available. The choice depends on the type of organism represented in the infection. Culturing and susceptibility testing to identify the best suited drug are good practice. The antinociceptive benefit of such agents relates to the resolution of infection that causes pain.

Antiviral Agents. Acyclovir and vidarabine are effective drugs for treating infections caused by the herpes simplex virus (HSV-1, HSV-2).[66] Acyclovir appears to be the more effective of the two. They may be administered topically,[67] orally, or IV. They appear to be more effective in the treatment of primary infections than recurrent episodes.[68] The Journal of the American Dental Association reported an experimental herpes vaccine that proved effective in animal studies for both HSV-1 and HSV-2.[69] Acyclovir and vidarabine are also effective against the varicella-zoster virus that causes herpes zoster.[70–72]

Antihistamine Agents. Antihistamines counteract the vasodilating action of histamine by blocking certain histamine receptors. Many antihistamine preparations are available. They may be useful in allergic responses and in some neurovascular pain disorders. A direct analgesic effect has been reported for several antihistamines (diphenhydramine, hydroxyzine, orphenadrine, pyrilamine).[73]

Anticonvulsive Agents. Phenytoin (Dilantin) is an anticonvulsant and cardiac depressant that also has the capability of suppressing the pain of paroxysmal neuralgia in about 20% of the cases.[74] There is wide interpatient variability, and the dosage must be individualized. Extended use of this medication should be under medical supervision.

A considerably more effective drug, but also more toxic, is carbamazapine (Tegretol). Pretreatment blood studies are necessary, and careful monitoring at regular intervals during treatment is essential for patient safety. Active medical supervision is prerequisite to its use. It is an anticonvulsant that appears to be specific for suppression of paroxysmal neuralgia. There are a number of contraindications and drug incompatibilities with which one must be familiar before prescribing. When tolerated, however, this medication gives surprising benefit in about 70% of trigeminal and glossopharyngeal neuralgias.[74]

Neurolytic Agents. The most common neurolytic drug used to destroy peripheral nerves is 95% ethyl alcohol. Sometimes phenol is added. Although it is an effective neurolytic, its denervating effect does not preclude regeneration of the peripheral axons and therefore provides only long-term temporary relief. The hazards of neuritis, extensive local fibrosis, and deafferentation effects restrict its use in modern practice.

The successful use of glycerol (0.30 mL) injected into the retrogasserian space for the treatment of trigeminal neuralgia has been reported.[75] About 90% of the patients remained pain-free after one or two injections. About 60% noticed slight numbness, but otherwise there were no significant sensory effects. No dysesthesia or anesthesia dolorosa was observed. It is thought that glycerol acts on demyelinated axons assumed to be involved in the triggering mechanism of neuralgia.

Uricosuric Agents. Antihyperuricemic agents are needed in the treatment of hyperuricemia involving the temporomandibular joints. Although its specific action is unknown, colchicine suppresses acute attacks

of gout and relieves the pain that such attacks generate. For the treatment of chronic gouty arthritis, probenecid is useful. It is a uricosuric and renal tubule blocking agent that inhibits the reabsorption of urates in the tubules of the kidney. By thus increasing the excretion of uric acid, the serum urate level is lowered. It may induce exacerbations of acute gout, however, and should not be used until the acute symptoms are controlled with colchicine. A combination of the two medications is useful in treating chronic gouty arthritis that is complicated by occasional recurrent attacks of acute gout.

Dietary Considerations. The possibility of dietary manipulation to influence a number of physical complaints including pain has come under serious investigation in recent years. The chief relationship between diet and pain appears to be with L-tryptophan, which converts into serotonin. Brain and spinal cord serotoninergic neurons are actively involved in nociceptive responses as well as in the analgesic effects of opiates. On the basis of pharmacologic, surgical, electrophysiologic, and dietary manipulative data, it is evident that increased activity of serotonin interneurons is associated with analgesia and enhanced drug potency.[76] Hosobuchi et al[77] reported that, when patients with chronic pain who were unable to obtain pain relief from 30 mg of IV morphine in divided doses due to drug tolerance were placed on diets supplemented with 4 g of L-tryptophan a day for several weeks, they were able to achieve significant pain relief from opiates. They were also able to lead more active lives even while reducing their daily opiate intake. Seltzer et al[78,79] reported significant elevation of pain tolerance with dietary supplementation of L-tryptophan. Cheng and Pomeranz[80] reported that naloxone-reversible analgesia induced by electroacupuncture was significantly increased when dietary D-phenylalanine and D-leucine were added.

The synthesis of brain serotonin is dependent on the disposition of plasma tryptophan, 90% of which is bound to albumin and must compete with other amino acids at the blood-brain barrier.[81] It is estimated that only about 2% of plasma tryptophan is hydroxylated by tryptophan hydroxylase to form the precursor to serotonin.[82] This conversion requires the presence of adequate vitamin B6.[83] Brady et al[84] reported that in a double-blind study the ten patients with chronic pain included in their study obtained a measure of relief by taking 4 g daily of L-tryptophan with a low-protein, low-fat, high-carbohydrate dict for 8 weeks. Seltzer et al[85] reported a reduction in clinical pain and elevated pain tolerance for randomly selected patients with chronic maxillofacial pain as the result of 4 weeks of tryptophan supplement therapy.

The use of tryptophan and other amino acids as a dietary supplement appears to be a valid approach to otherwise refractory chronic pain problems. Several conditions appear to be required for effective results:

1. Adequate dosage: 4 g/day
2. Low-protein, low-fat, high-carbohydrate diet
3. Adequate vitamin B6 intake: 10–25 mg/day
4. Four weeks or more of continuous therapy

The dietary considerations in pain therapy, especially for neurovascular and chronic pain disorders, open new vistas. As more is learned about the role of neurotransmitters and protein fractions such as glutamic acid, substance P, glycine, gamma-aminobutyric acid (GABA), cholecystokinin, and somatostatin, a variety of dietary manipulations and additional medicinal forms of therapy likely will become available.[86] The dietary approach would not be expected to influence the management of acute pain complaints, however, because of the time factor. Like other nutritional approaches to disease, it usually requires several weeks for the effects of dietary therapy to become apparent clinically.

Physical Therapy

Modalities. Physical therapy modalities refer to those treatments that utilize an instrument, device or agent to accomplish the desired effect. These are sensory stimulation, ultrasound, electrogalvanic stimulation (EGS), and deep heat.

Sensory Stimulation. Sensory stimulation can be divided into several categories according to the tissue and mode of stimulation: cutaneous, transcutaneous, and percutaneous.

Cutaneous Stimulation. Although the stimulation of skin has been used to obtain relief from pain since ancient times, it has only been during the past few decades that some understanding of the mechanism involved has come to light, and with it a revival of many old remedies. The effect occurs through stimulation of thick myelinated cutaneous afferents, A-beta neurons chiefly. Whether other inhibitory mechanisms are involved remains to be determined.

There are many forms of cutaneous stimulation that effectively attenuate pain. Perhaps the oldest and most natural is pressing or rubbing the skin over the site of injury. Superficial massage is an important means of reducing pain. It is enhanced by adding a stimulating substance such as alcohol or menthol ointment.

Counterirritation is an age-old pain remedy.[87] Mustard plasters can still be remembered by many. It is well known that mild stimulation of nociceptors also increases pain-inhibitory mechanisms. A mixture of aconite and iodine has been used for this purpose by dentists. Presently, vapocoolant therapy is important in myofascial trigger point pain. Initially thought to be effective through its local anesthetic action, it is now recognized that the vapocoolant mildly stimulates the cutaneous nociceptors as well as the thicker A-beta fibers. Thus, the body's pain inhibitory system is activated. As long ago as 1902, ethyl chloride was sprayed on the eardrum to alleviate the pain of otitis media.[88] Kraus[89] introduced the use of ethyl chloride spray for the treatment of painful motion in 1941. Travell advocated its use for the treatment of somatic trigger areas in 1949[90] and for treating skeletal myospasms in 1952.[91] Schwartz[92] applied it for the treatment of painful mandibular movement in 1954.

Intermittency is an essential element in vapocoolant therapy and probably is the reason why it is more effective than other forms of thermal therapy. Thick afferents adapt quickly to stimulation and therefore are more reactive to gradient changes. The application of heat and cold to obtund pain is very old. It has long been known to be more effective when the heat and cold are applied alternately for brief periods. Infra-red heat is another form of cutaneous stimulation.

An old pain remedy that has recently reentered the experimental laboratory is the use of mechanical vibration to relieve pain. It has been reported that at least one-third of patients obtain complete relief from dental pain with this method, and the period of relief outlasts the stimulation by several hours.[93-96] Mechanical vibration also enhances the effect of transcutaneous electrical stimulation in about half the subjects.[97] Lundeberg[98] reported that, in a study of 267 patients with chronic neuropathic or musculoskeletal pain treated with vibratory stimulation, 59% achieved more than 50% relief.

Hydrotherapy is another form of cutaneous stimulation, especially for neck and back pains of muscle origin. Agitated circulating bath water has a therapeutic effect, and a brisk stream of shower water directed against the neck and back gives considerable relief. On the whole, cutaneous stimulation as a therapeutic tool for the management of pain has not been fully utilized.

Transcutaneous Stimulation. In ancient times, electric fish are said to have been used to relieve pain.[99] During the past century there have been several attempts to utilize electrical stimulation for this purpose. The method was resurrected by Wall and Sweet[100] in 1967 as the result of the gate control theory verbalized by Melzack and Wall[101] 2 years earlier. Soon, transcutaneous electrical nerve stimulation (TENS) became a popular form of pain control. The units employed a low-intensity faradic current at high frequency (50 to 100 Hz) applied to the skin through electrodes attached by conduction paste. No discomfort was felt. It was remarkably effective in relieving pains of various types. It was innocuous except for an occasional rash from the conduction paste. Being portable, the mechanism could be worn and used by subjects at will.

In 1972 the American public became aware of traditional Chinese acupuncture methods through media coverage. This initiated a wave of nociceptive research to explain this miracle from the Orient. It was not until the discovery of the endogenous antinociceptive system in 1975 that a plausible explanation for acupuncture became available. Research into electroacupuncture (EA) on a worldwide scale established a relationship between it and the newly discovered endorphins. Although some confusion still exists and conflicting reports appear, the following summarizes the present understanding of transcutaneous stimulation methods.[102,103]

TENS utilizes a high-frequency (50 to 100 Hz) but very low-intensity electric current. It is used to stimulate the nonnociceptive A-beta cutaneous afferents that activate the descending pain inhibitory mechanism without involving the opioid peptides.[104,105] It may be felt as a tingling or vibratory sensation with no phasic muscle contraction; some minor tonic contraction may occur in nearby muscles. Its action is immediate, is generally restricted to the segment that is stimulated, and induces little or no aftereffects. Therapeutic benefit is negligible. It does not depend on skin location where impedance is low, but if applied at such sites (acupoints), an EA effect may result. The analgesic effect ranges from 50% to 70%.[106,107]

Electroacupuncture utilizes a low-frequency (2 Hz) but high-intensity electric current. It is applied at specific cutaneous sites, the so-called acupoints. It is used to stimulate the muscle nociceptors (group III

and group IV afferents), which in turn activate the endogenous antinociceptive system. Phasic muscle contraction and pulsing muscle pain are required. The antinociceptive effect is not immediate but requires an induction period of 15 to 20 minutes. Some therapeutic effect may result. The analgesia may be either segmental or general. The segmental relief of pain is thought to involve the CSF enkephalin level, while the general effects appear to involve the action of beta endorphin secreted by the pituitary gland into the bloodstream.[108]

Antinociception of the teeth and mouth occurs segmentally by applying EA at the intraorbital acupoint; more general effects come from the HoKu acupoint located between the thumb and index finger. Best results are obtained by simultaneously using both acupoints bilaterally.

A comparison of the two methods of transcutaneous sensory stimulation on a clinical level indicates that both are effective if properly applied and yield satisfactory relief from pain in 50% to 70% of the subjects. The antinociceptive mechanism that is involved in either case is of more academic than clinical value. The two techniques have much in common and often overlap. It seems to matter little whether they are used separately or conjointly.[109–113] Cold laser (helium-neon) stimulation at acupoints is as effective as EA and has the advantage of being practically painless.[114–116]

Although Sweet[117] did not find transcutaneous sensory stimulation useful in the management of tic douloureux, Melzack[118] reported significant relief from peripheral nerve injury pain, phantom limb pain, shoulder-arm pain, and low-back pain. Sodipo[119] reported acupuncture to be beneficial in 60% of patients with chronic pain. It has been reported useful in the management of tension headache.[120] It can also effect mood changes that resemble those of opioids.[121]

Percutaneous Stimulation. Percutaneous stimulation is done by electrodes that penetrate the skin. Such methods have been used by neurosurgeons for many years. Subcutaneous nerve stimulation (SCNS) by an electric current produces prolonged analgesia that is not reversible by naloxone, which indicates that it does not recruit the opioid peptides. Tolerance is not developed, and it can be administered with other analgesic medications, including narcotics.[122,123]

Lawrence[124] introduced a new form of percutaneous stimulation. It is electric stimulation of the periosteum by insulated needles. He used 9 to 12 V at 100 to 300 Hz for 45 minutes. He kept the stimulation intensity at a level just perceived by the subject. He reported results subjectively superior to EA and TENS for the relief of chronic pain.

Ultrasound. Ultrasound is a method of producing an increase in the temperature at the interface of the tissues and therefore affects deeper tissues than does surface heat.[125] Not only does ultrasound increase the blood flow in deep tissues, it also seems to separate collagen fibers. This improves the flexibility and extensibility of connective tissues.[126] It has been suggested[127,128] that surface heat and ultrasound be used together especially when treating posttrauma patients.

Ultrasound has also been used[129] to administer drugs through the skin, by a process known as *phonopheresis.* For example, 10% hydrocortisone cream is applied to an inflamed joint and the ultrasound transducer is then directed at the joint. The effects of salicylates and other topical anesthetics can also be enhanced in this manner.

Electrogalvanic Stimulation. Electrogalvanic stimulation (EGS)[130,131] utilizes the principle that electrical stimulation of a muscle causes it to contract. A rhythmic electrical impulse is applied to the muscle, creating repeated involuntary contractions and relaxations. The intensity and frequency of these can be varied according to the desired effect, and they will help to break up myospasms as well as increase blood flow to the muscles. Both effects lead to a reduction of pain in compromised muscle tissues. Muscle pulsing has been reported to yield favorable results with the myofascial pain-dysfunction syndrome.[132]

Deep Heat Therapy. Physical therapy in the form of penetrating heat has value in treating patients with pain. Diathermy and ultrasound are used for this purpose. The judicious use of deep heat is beneficial in treating inflammatory pain. Although it has been used to help relieve myospasm activity, its effects are equivocal. It is reported to be a useful adjunct in the treatment of myofascial trigger point pain.[23]

Manual Techniques

Massage. As just stated, mild stimulation of cutaneous sensory nerves exerts an inhibitory influence on pain.[133] Thus, gentle massage of the tissues overlying a painful area can often reduce pain perception. The patient can be taught gentle self-massage techniques and is encouraged to do this as needed for reduction of pain. The technique is often helpful.

Deep massage can be even more helpful in reducing pain and reestablishing normal muscle function than gentle massage. Deep massage, however, must be provided by another individual such as a physical therapist. Deep massage can assist in mobilizing tissues, increasing blood flow to the area and eliminating trigger points.[134] It is often most effective when it follows 10 to 15 minutes of preparing the tissues with deep moist heat. The deep heat tends to relax the muscle tissues, decreasing pain and enhancing the effectiveness of the deep massage.

Spray and Stretch Techniques. The primary physical therapeutic technique for the treatment of myofascial trigger points is so-called spray and stretch.[135] A mixture of fluorocarbons is used as the vapocoolant (Fluori-Methane, Gebauer Chemical). A spring-capped bottle with a calibrated nozzle that delivers a fine stream is needed. While the muscle is moderately stretched just short of pain, the vapocoolant is applied by using parallel sweeps in one direction, traveling toward the reference area. The nozzle is held 15 to 18 inches away from the skin, and the stream is directed at an acute angle of about 30 degrees. The sweeps are made at the rate of about 4 in/s. After two or three sweeps, the muscle should be rewarmed. At the end of the treatment, moist heat should be applied and range-of-motion exercises instituted. The best results are obtained by first spraying, then stretching, using care not to stretch to the point of pain, and then spraying again. It is thought that the vapocoolant modulates the pain so that more manipulation is possible without discomfort. It should be noted that painfully stretching a muscle with myofascial triggers may induce a muscle spasm. Other forms of physical therapy applicable to the treatment of myofascial trigger points include ischemic compression, deep massage and kneading, and ultra-sound. Ischemic compression is done by applying 20 to 30 lb of pressure at the trigger site for 1 minute while the muscle is stretched just short of pain.[134]

Exercise. Forceful contraction of antagonist muscles causes reflex relaxation of an agonist muscle. This principle of reciprocal inhibition is useful in the treatment of masticatory myospasms.[136] For example, a spastic elevator muscle is relaxed by exercises that open the mouth against resistance. Retruding the protruded mandible against resistance tends to relax a spastic inferior lateral pterygoid muscle.

It has been reported that stimulation of muscle proprioceptors tends to normalize excessive electromyographic (EMG) activity in painful spastic skeletal muscles.[137] When using this principle, resumption and maintenance of normal muscular activity in masticatory muscles is beneficial as long as pain is not generated by the activity.

For a muscle to maintain its normal resting length, occasional stimulation of the inverse stretch reflex is necessary. This is accomplished by occasionally stretching the muscle. An immobilized muscle not only loses its strength by disuse atrophy, it also shortens due to myostatic contracture.[138] Exercises that stimulate both the muscle spindles (contraction) and the Golgi tendon organs (stretching) are therefore needed to maintain normality of muscles. So-called functional manipulation is useful physical therapy. Exercise elevates the pain threshold.[139,140]

Physical Activity. In patients with chronic pain, the maintenance of physical activity is an important part of therapy. Patients tend to withdraw and take to their beds. Fordyce et al[141] found that, during periods when the pain is increased, extending exercises to the limit of patient tolerance was significantly beneficial: the more exercises performed, the fewer the pain behaviors displayed. The maintenance of physical activity kept the body in better condition and reduced time in bed.

Psychologic Therapy

Psychologic therapies are orientated toward minimizing the Axis II factors that either influence or create the pain disorder. These therapies can be generally categorized into two types: counseling or behavioral modification training.

Counseling. As previously discussed, all pain disorders are influenced to some degree by psychologic factors. The therapist should always keep this in mind when first managing a pain condition. The first therapy that should be offered to the patient is education. Educating the patient to his or her pain condition can have marked therapeutic value. Many patients experiencing pain have an increased level of anxiety, emotional stress and depression secondary to the pain itself. Often much of this distress can be reduced by proper education. The following five factors should be included when initially discussing the pain condition with the patient.

Provide a Definitive Diagnosis. Most patients would like to know exactly what is causing their pain. Understanding the source of pain is often the beginning of the healing process. The clinician should inform the patient, as precisely as possible, of the exact cause of the pain. Since pain complaints are often complex, this may be a difficult task. When a specific diagnosis is impossible on the first visit, the patient should be at least informed as to the general type and category of pain he is experiencing. Several high probable diagnoses should be explained with a more specific diagnosis to come with additional tests. The circumstance that should be avoided is the clinician leaving the patient with the idea that he does not know the reason for the pain. If this occurs, the patient will likely think the worst and anxiety and emotional stress levels will increase the pain experience. Remember, attention and consequence are two major factors in pain and suffering. Both attention and consequence increase when the source of pain is unknown.

If the clinician has no clue as to the source of the pain, it is his or her obligation to immediately refer the patient to the proper medical or dental professionals who can help with the diagnosis. Time is of essence in addressing pain and suffering.

Provide Assurance. Life-threatening disorders that present as orofacial pains are rare but certainly can exist. It is important to immediately identify and refer patients with these disorders (ie, neoplasia) to proper specialists. Most orofacial pains, however, are not life-threatening. This is especially true of the musculoskeletal disorders of the masticatory system known collectively as temporomandibular disorders. Once the clinician has properly ruled out significant life-threatening disorders, he or she should provide assurance to the patient that the disorder is benign and in many cases quite common. It is important that the patient know the significance of the condition so that

202

proper attention can be placed. Often when a patient learns that the pain is not coming from cancer but instead a muscle cramp, the pain experience may greatly reduce.

The excitatory influence of attention directed toward the complaint can be countered by distraction, by directing the mind toward more positive thinking, and by a good measure of physical activity. Pleasurable sensations derived from suggested diversive activities can be used to counter the painful experience.

Explain the Problem in Appropriate Terms. Most patients want to know exactly where their pain comes from, how it started, and how it can be treated. This information will usually reduce anxiety and emotional stress associated with the pain as well as provide them with realistic consequences for the pain. In general, therefore, this explanation can reduce suffering. The clinician should be careful to use terminology to which the patient can relate and understand. When appropriate, drawings or models can be helpful.

Apprehension concerning the consequential damage and the expectancy of future threat to the patient's well-being cause psychologic intensification of the painful experience. This can be reversed by an open discussion of the realistic consequences that exist and the true expectancy that the particular problem holds for the patient. The patient should be made to understand that there may be little relationship between the level of discomfort and the true significance of its cause.

Do Not Deny the Patient's Pain. As mentioned in Chapter 1, pain is a very individual experience. A condition that may be quite painful to one individual may not be very painful to another. The clinician should always keep this in mind when talking with patients. There is absolutely no benefit to denying the patient's pain. In fact this behavior can be quite devastating to the patient. The clinician should always be supportive of the patient and provide proper explanation for the pain. In those conditions in which psychologic factors are predominant (Axis II), the psychologic factors should be properly introduced so that it does not appear that the clinician is suggesting that the patient is crazy. In some instances, this may be difficult, but it is essential for proper management. It may be helpful to emphasize the physical conditions first and than discuss how the psychologic factors can greatly enhance these conditions. A warm, caring attitude by the clinician is imperative.

Provide Realistic Expectations. Most patients who seek treatment for a pain condition want, and expect, complete relief from their pain along with return to normal function. These expectations may not be realistic and the patient needs to be aware of this fact when beginning treatment. Once the pain disorder has been explained to the patient, realistic expectations for the treatment should be present. It is often helpful to explain the natural course of the disorder to the patient. It is necessary, therefore, that the clinician know the natural course of the disorder, which may not always be apparent. For example, in the past, many TM disorders have been thought to be progressive, yet recent studies have not supported this concept.[142] As always, the clinician's knowledge of the disorder is basic to treatment and proper expectations.

203

The patient should be aware that the symptoms of a pain condition often follow a cyclic course. It is common, therefore, to experience both decreases and increases in the pain during treatment. When the patient is told this before treatment begins, recurrence of pain is better tolerated and accepted.

These five factors should be considered with all patients who present with pain regardless of the specific conditions. When significant psychologic factors have been identified, however, specific counseling may be indicated. Some formal psychotherapy is needed in many Axis II disorders such as significant depression, anxiety, or emotional stress. Many somatoform disorders require psychiatric consultation. A small percentage of temporomandibular disorders that are refractory to nonsurgical therapy may need psychotherapy rather than more aggressive surgical treatment.[143] In most Axis II disorders local peripheral therapy, including surgery, should be restricted to a secondary role in management. The chief therapeutic effort should be systemic, psychologic, or both.

Fordyce[144] considered that some pains are behavioral and for the most part learned. To a considerable degree, pain is controlled by consequences in the environment. The modification of such consequences may be needed for pain management to be effective. Pain behavior may be unlearned by manipulation of consequences such as withdrawing positive reinforcers and by rewarding better behavior. Such contingency management usually requires full knowledge and cooperation, not only of the patient but also of all those in close personal contact with him or her. This includes family members, doctors, nurses, therapists, and aids.[145]

Since pain behavior is learned, it can be unlearned. Illness behavior should simply be ignored while wellness behavior should be rewarded by attention and tender loving care. Severe pain can be made tolerable by replacing the suffering with something better to do, like doing something that benefits others. The patient should be encouraged to engage in activities that direct one's attention away from self. Coping with pain is a matter of attitude: "After all, it is only pain. I not only can live peaceably with it, I can overcome it!"[141]

Melzack[146] pointed out the importance of coping strategies in chronic pain because some pains may last a lifetime. The objective in such cases is not to abolish the pain but to make it bearable. Melzack trained his subjects to reach a meditational state, thus gaining the benefits of distraction, response to suggestion, relaxation, and the development of voluntary control over the pain. Strong suggestion is essential to psychologic approaches for pain management.

Sternbach[147] assumed that pain behavior was acquired and therefore modifiable. Subjective improvement followed behavioral improvement. He utilized social modeling, conditioning, and cognitive forms of therapy.

Roberts[148] focused therapy not on nociceptive sources or the alteration of an emotional state but directly on patient behavior. His objective was to rehabilitate the patient rather than to alleviate the pain. He avoided all strategies that focus on pain per se; eg, analgesics, electrical stimulation, analgesic blocking, and biofeedback training.

A more detailed description of therapies for each Axis II disorder will be presented in Chapter 18.

Behavioral Modification Training. Often patients can significantly alter their pain experiences by modifying certain aspects of their routine daily activities. These modifications should be encouraged since they provide the patient an active role in treatment. Patients who can influence their own symptoms gain a great psychologic edge over those who cannot. These activities reduce the feelings of helplessness and hopelessness that too often accompany chronic pain conditions. Two types of behavioral modifications are stress reduction training and relaxation training.

Stress Reduction Training. Many persons who have orofacial pain and/or functional disturbance of the masticatory system are not aware of the possible relationship between their problem and emotional stress. It would be surprising to think any differently, since their symptoms arise from structures in the masticatory system. Therefore when a patient comes to the clinician with pain symptoms, the first treatment is to educate that person regarding the relationship of emotional stress and anxiety to the problem. An awareness of this relationship must be created before any treatment begins. It is common for the patients to deny the presence of high levels of emotional stress in their life. One must be sure, therefore, that the patient is aware that stress is a common everyday experience and not a neurotic or psychotic disorder.

Emotional stress can also be controlled to some extent voluntarily. Once the stressors are identified, the patient is encouraged, when possible, to avoid them. For example, if stress is increased by driving through heavy traffic, alternate routes should be developed to avoid major traffic areas. When

stress is caused by specific encounters at work, these should be avoided.

It is obvious that all stressors cannot and should not be avoided. Some stressors are positive and help motivate the individual toward particular goals. As Hans Selye[149] has stated, complete freedom from stress is death. When negative stressors cannot be completely avoided, the frequency and duration of exposure to them should be reduced.

Patients should be encouraged when possible to remove themselves from stressors and substitute other activities that they enjoy—such as allowing more time for sports, hobbies, or recreational activities. For some patients this may include some quiet time alone. It should be an enjoyable time and an opportunity to forget their stressors. Such activities are considered to be external stress-releasing mechanisms and to lead to an overall reduction of emotional stress experienced by the patient.

Regular exercise may also be an active external stress-releasing mechanism. It is encouraged for patients who find it enjoyable. Obviously it will not be suitable for all patients, and general body condition and health must always be considered before advising patients to initiate an active exercise program.

Relaxation Training. Training the patient in the art of relaxation can be a great benefit in several ways. First, it requires regular quiet periods of time away from the stressors. The training sessions are in themselves a type of relaxation therapy. Second, it aids in reducing the level of activity of the autonomic nervous system that is often upregulated in the patient with pain.[150] This training should be oriented toward reducing muscle activity, slowing breathing rate, lowering blood pressure and decreasing skin temperature.

Training a patient to relax effectively can be accomplished with several techniques. One that has been well researched is progressive relaxation. Most of these techniques used in dentistry are modifications of Jacobson's method,[151] developed in 1968. The patient tenses the muscles and then relaxes them until the relaxed state can be felt and maintained. The patient is instructed to concentrate on relaxing the peripheral areas (hands and feet) and to move progressively centrally to the abdomen, chest, and face. Results can be enhanced by having the patient relax, preferably by lying down,[152] in a quiet comfortable environment with the eyes closed. The relaxation procedures are slowly explained in a calm and soothing voice. An audiotape of the procedures can be developed to aid in the technique. The patient listens to the tape at the training session in the office and then, after understanding what is to be accomplished, takes the tape home with instructions to listen at least once a day to become proficient at relaxing the muscles. As proficiency increases, the muscle symptoms will decrease.

This technique has been demonstrated to be effective in several studies.[153-162] It would appear to be best accomplished by well-trained therapists during frequent visits to help and encourage proper relaxation habits. Although it is not harmful to send the patient home to learn the technique alone, it is less likely that good results will be achieved by simple explanations of the relaxation procedures.[163] Also the best results are achieved over months of training and not just a week or two.

Another form of progressive relaxation utilizes a reverse approach. Instead of asking the patient to contract the muscle and then relax, the muscles are passively stretched and then relaxed.[164-166] It appears that this technique is also effective in teaching progressive relaxation and has one major inherent advantage over the Jacboson technique. Patients with muscle pain disorders often produce pain when asked to contract their muscles. This increase in pain makes relaxation more difficult. In contrast, gently stretching the muscle seems to assist in relaxation. Many patients with pain find this technique more suitable then the Jacboson technique.

Progressive relaxation techniques are the most common method of promoting relaxation. Other training methods also encourage relaxation but are used to a lesser degree. Self-hypnosis,[167] meditation, yoga,[168] and even music[169] can all promote relaxation and may help reduce levels of emotional stress. They likewise are best learned and applied with help from a trained therapist.

Hypnotherapy can be a useful antinociceptive method provided the pain is not due to psychoneurosis. Some suffering is too valuable to the patient to be given up; personality disintegration may follow the sudden withdrawal of pain.[170] Some form of psychiatric screening therefore should precede the use of hypnosis in the management of a pain problem.

The effectiveness of hypnosis depends largely on the susceptibility of the subject to suggestion. A direct-induction technique may be quite satisfactory in highly susceptible subjects. Indirect induction, however, is equally effective and is superior in less susceptible individuals.[171] Hypnosis is clinically effective for a large number of patients presenting with symptoms of severe pain of organic origin.[172] Almost all patients derive some benefit through the placebo effect and relaxation. Some well-hypnotized individuals can block high-intensity pain of organic origin. Chronic pain usually requires behavioral modification also.[173] Hypnotherapy is especially useful in the management of pain associated with burns.[174]

Although the issue is still unsettled, there is some evidence that long-term reduction of pain by hypnotherapy involves endorphins.[175]

Although the relaxation of muscles would appear to be a simple procedure, often it is not. Patients, especially those experiencing pain, frequently find it difficult to learn to relax their muscles effectively. They can sometimes benefit from immediate feedback regarding the success or failure of their efforts.

One method of achieving this is with biofeedback, a technique that assists the patient in regulating bodily functions that are generally controlled unconsciously. It has been used to help patients alter such functions as blood pressure, blood flow, and brain wave activity as well as muscle relaxation. It is accomplished by electromyographically monitoring the state of contraction or relaxation of the muscles through surface electrodes placed over the muscles to be monitored. Among facial muscles, the masseter is often selected. When full body relaxation is the goal, the frontalis muscle is commonly monitored. The electrodes are connected to a monitoring system that lets the patient see the spontaneous electrical activity in the muscles being assessed. The monitor provides feedback by way of a scale or a digital readout or sometimes even a light bar mechanism. Most biofeedback units also give auditory feedback, which is beneficial for patients who relax best with

their eyes closed. When a patient tenses the muscles, high readings appear on the scale or an elevated tone is heard. When the muscles are relaxed, these signals are lowered. The patient attempts to lower the readings or the tone. This can be achieved by any relaxation technique, but progressive relaxation is encouraged since it is easily accomplished at a later date when the biofeedback instrument is not available. Once the patient can achieve low levels of activity in the muscles, the next instruction is to become familiar with the sense or feeling of relaxation. When this has been accomplished and low levels of muscle activity have been adequately sensed, the patient can be more effective in regaining this state at a later time even without the aid of the biofeedback instrument and is encouraged to work toward achieving this goal. A progressive relaxation tape can aid in the training.[176]

Several studies report the usefulness of relaxation training in the management of headaches.[177-181] Sternbach[182] stated that biofeedback could not be expected to help unless the clinical condition presented symptoms of peripheral vasomotor origin. In other words, he questioned the use of biofeedback in the management of certain neurovascular pains such as migraine. Turner and Chapman[183] reported that, although biofeedback may be helpful with some headaches and some temporomandibular joint pain, it was not helpful in chronic pain. Sherman et al[184] reported substantial benefit from muscle relaxation training in the treatment of phantom limb. Half of their patients obtained virtually complete relief from pain. Large and Lamb[185] reported that a significant correlation existed between subjective pain levels and surface EMG activity and that EMG feedback was superior to other methods of relaxation, but not in reducing the subjective pain level. Nouwen[186] reduced the EMG activity significantly in paraspinal muscles with EMG feedback training, but it did not reduce the pain. Brooke and Stenn[187] reported on 174 patients with myofascial pain who were randomly treated with physical therapy, occlusal splinting, biofeedback, and relaxation training without biofeedback. The biofeedback-assisted relaxation was reported to be as effective as either physiotherapy or occlusal splinting, but it was no more effective than relaxation training without the feedback assistance.

Relaxation training with or without the aid of biofeedback training appears to have merit in the overall management of masticatory problems in that it does reduce EMG activity. Its actual value in reduction of pain, however, is equivocal. Relaxation of muscles seems to be accomplished more readily with biofeedback techniques.

For many years it has been clinically obvious that occlusal disengagement induced a substantial beneficial effect on the discomfort of temporomandibular disorders. This constituted the treatment used by Costen when he inserted thin cork wedges between the teeth. Disengagement sets the occlusion at rest and does for the masticatory system what restricted function does for other musculoskeletal systems. It constitutes a form of relaxation.

Occlusal disengagement can be accomplished in several ways: (1) by voluntarily leaving the teeth apart or ajar, (2) by a variety of simple habit-training devices such as a thin pat of chewing gum between the molar teeth, (3) by the use of muscle relaxing medications, and (4) by interocclusal appliances.

Christensen et al[188] showed that voluntary isometric contraction of elevator masticatory muscles induced pain and muscle fatigue. The pain seemed not to be due to cumulative EMG activity alone because delay in pain was achieved by elongating the elevator muscles with an occlusal appliance. Solberg and coworkers[189] showed that occlusal appliances significantly decreased the nocturnal EMG activity of bruxism. Kemper and Okeson[190] showed that patients with a TM disorder complained of frequent headaches more than twice as often as a control group and the frequency of such headaches was cut in half by occlusal appliances. Referring again to the work of Brooke and Stenn,[187] it may well be assumed that much of the benefit of occlusal appliances derives from muscular relaxation.

Occlusal appliances may be classified according to their intended function as stabilization or muscle relaxation appliances, and mandibular repositioning appliances. Stabilization appliances are particularly useful in the management of masticatory muscle pain. These appliances tend to normalize sensory and proprioceptive impulses generated by the occlusal condition, thus shut off the afferent input that initiates muscle co-contraction and aggravates muscle pain conditions. Mandibular repositioning appliances are used to improve the condyle-disc relationship associated with some painful intracapsular disorders.

This chapter has presented some general considerations in the management of orofacial pain. The remainder of this text will focus on each of the major pain categories, presenting information on diagnosis and present specific treatment suggestions.

References

1. Sternbach RA. Chronic pain as a disease entity. Triangle 1981; 20:27–32.

2. Degenaar JJ. Some philosophical considerations in pain. Pain 1979; 7:281–304.

3. Keele KD. A physician looks at pain. In Weisenberg M (ed): Pain: Clinical and Experimental Perspectives. St Louis: CV Mosby; 1975: 45–52.

4. Foreman RD, Blair RW, Weber RN. Effects on T3 to T5 primate spinothalamic tract cells of injecting bradykinin into the heart. Pain 1981; 11:212.

5. Becker D. Scientific principles of drug use in dental practice. Part 1: Clinical pharmacokinetics. Compend Contin Educ Dent 1988; 9:46–52.

6. Payne R, Max M, Inturrisi C, et al. Principles of Analgesic Use in the Treatment of Acute Pain and Chronic Cancer Pain. Washington, DC: American Pain Society; 1987.

7. Crossley HL, Bergman SA, Wynn RL. Nonsteroid anti-inflammatory agents in relieving dental pain: A review. J Am Dent Assoc 1983; 106:61–64.

8. Sheridan P. Flurbiprofen as an alternative pain suppressor to standard analgesic therapy. J Am Dent Assoc 1986; 113:671.

9. Guilbaud G, Iggo A, Tegner R. Sensory changes in joint-capsule receptors of arthritic rats: Effect of aspirin. In Fields HL, Dubner R, Cervero F (eds): Advances in Pain Research and Therapy, vol 9. New York: Raven Press; 1985: 81–89.

10. Granstrom E. Biochemistry of the prostaglandins, thromboxanes, and leukotrienes. In Bonica JJ, Lindblom U, Iggo A (eds): Advances in Pain Research and Therapy, vol 5. New York: Raven Press; 1983: 605–615.

11. Higgs GA, Moncada S. Interaction of arachidonate products with other pain mediators. In Bonica JJ, Lindblom U, Iggo A (eds): Advances in Pain Research and Therapy, vol 5. New York: Raven Press; 1983: 617–626.

12. Hunskaar S, Berge 0, Hale K. Dissociation between antinociceptive and anti-inflammatory effects of acetyl salicylic acid and indomethacin in the formalin test. Pain 1986; 25:125–132.

13. Baskin SI, Smith L, Hoey LA, et al. Age-associated changes of responses to acetyl salicylic acid. Pain 1981; 11:1–8.

14. Ferreira SH. Prostaglandins: Peripheral and central analgesia. In Bonica JJ, Lindblom U, Iggo A (eds): Advances in Pain Research and Therapy, vol 5. New York: Raven Press; 1983: 627–634.

15. Boas RA, Holford NHG, Villiger JW. Clinical pharmacology of opiate analgesia. In Fields HL, Dubner R, Cervero F (eds): Advances in Pain Research and Therapy, vol 9. New York: Raven Press; 1985: 695–708.

16. Belcher G, Ryall RW. Differential excitatory and inhibitory effects of opiates on nociceptive and nonnociceptive neurons in the spinal cord of the cat. Brain Res 1978; 45:303–314.

17. Inoki R, Hayashi T, Kudo T, et al. Effects of opium and morphine on the release of a bradykinin-like substance into the subcutaneous perfusate of the rat paw. Pain 1978; 5:53–63.

18. Schlon H, Bentley GA. The possibility that a component of morphine induced analgesia is contributed indirectly via the release of endogenous opioids. Pain 1980; 9:73–84.

19. Tamsen A, Sakurada T, Wahlstrom A, et al. Postoperative demand for analgesics in relation to individual levels of endorphins and substance P in cerebrospinal fluid. Pain 1982; 13:171–183.

20. McQuay HJ, Carroll D, Watts PG, et al. Does adding small doses of codeine increase pain relief after third molar surgery? Clin J Pain 1987; 2:197–201.

21. Sharav Y, Singer E, Schmidt E, et al. The analgesic effect of amitriptyline on chronic facial pain. Pain 1987; 31:199–209.

22. Mays KS, Schnapp M, Lipman JJ, et al. Pain relief after peripheral perineural injection of morphine. Pain 1981; 11:120.

23. Travell JG, Simons DG. Myofascial Pain and Dysfunction. Baltimore: Williams & Wilkins; 1983: 74–86.

24. Kraus H. Clinical Treatment of Back and Neck Pain. New York: McGrawHill International; 1970: 74–86.

25. Bonica JJ. The Management of Pain, ed 2. Philadelphia: Lea & Febiger; 1990: 1931–1944.

26. Bonelli S, Conoscente F, Movilia PG, et al. Regional intravenous guanethidine vs. stellate ganglion block in reflex sympathetic dystrophies: A randomized trial. Pain 1983; 16: 297–307.

27. Thompson JE. The diagnosis and management of posttraumatic pain syndromes (causalgia). Aust NZ J Surg 1979; 49:299–304.

28. Procacci P, Francini F, Zoppi M, et al. Cutaneous pain threshold changes after sympathetic block in reflex dystrophies. Pain 1975; 1:167–175.

29. Wetchler BV, Wyman TM. The role of stellate ganglion block in the treatment of acute herpes zoster ophthalmicus. Pain 1981; 11 (suppl 1):120.

30. Loh L, Nathan PW, Schott GD. Pain due to the lesions of central nervous system removed by sympathetic block. Br Med J 1981; 282: 1026–1028.

31. Wang JK, Johnson KA, Ilstrup DM. Sympathetic blocks for reflex sympathetic dystrophy. Pain 1985; 23:13–17.

32. Payne R. Neuropathic pain syndromes, with special reference to causalgia and reflex sympathetic dystrophy. Clin J Pain 1986; 2:59–73.

33. Tenicela R, Lovasik D, Eaglstein W. Treatment of herpes zoster with sympathetic blocks. Clin J Pain 1985; 1:63–67.

34. Dan K, Higa K, Noda B. Nerve block for herpetic pain. In Fields HL, Dubner R, Cervero F (eds): Advances in Pain Research and Therapy, vol 9. New York: Raven Press; 1985: 831–838.

35. Yanagida H, Suwa K, Corssen G. The role of sympathetic blockade in terminating acute herpes zoster and preventing postherpetic neuralgia. Pain 1987; 31 (suppl 4):205.

36. Milligan NS, Nash TP. Treatment of postherpetic neuralgia. A review of 77 consecutive cases. Pain 1985; 23:381–386.

37. Devor M, Govrin-Lippman R, Raber P. Corticosteroids suppress ectopic neural discharge originating in experimental neuromas. Pain 1985; 22:127–137.

38. Devor M, Govrin-Lippmann R, Raber P. Corticosteroids reduce neuroma hyperexcitability. In Fields HL, Dubner R, Cervero F (eds): Advances in Pain Research and Therapy, vol 9. New York: Raven Press; 1985: 451–455.

39. Allen GD. Dental Anesthesia and Analgesia, ed 3. Baltimore: Williams & Wilkins; 1984: 9–18.

40. Kreisberg MK. Tricyclic antidepressants: Analgesic effect and indications in orofacial pain. J Crainomandib Disord Facial Pain 1988; 2:171–177.

41. Lascelles RG. Atypical facial pain and depression. Br J Psychiatry, 1966; 112:651–659.

42. Brown RS, Bottomley WK. The utilization and mechanism of action of tricyclic antidepressants in the treatment of chronic facial pain: A review of the literature. Anesth Prog 1990; 37:223–239.

43. Sharau Y, Singer E, Schmidt E, et al. The analgesic effect of amitriptyline on chronic facial pain. Pain 1987; 31:199–209.

44. Fields HL. Pain II: New approaches to management. Ann Neurol 1981; 9:101–106.

45. Spiegel K, Kalb R, Pasternak GW. Analgesic activity of tricyclic antidepressants. Ann Neurol 1983; 13:462–465.

46. Zitman FG, Linssen AC, Edelbrock PM, Stijnen T. Low dose amitriptyline in chronic pain. 1990; 42:35–42.

47. Chapman CR, Butler SH. Effects of doxepin on perception of laboratory induced pain in man. Pain 1978; 5:253–262.

48. Ward NG, Bloom VL, Friedel RO. The effectiveness of tricyclic antidepressants in the treatment of coexisting pain and depression. Pain 1979; 7:331–341.

49. Feinmann C. Pain relief by antidepressants: Possible modes of action. Pain 1985; 23:1–8.

50. Hameroff SR, Cork RC, Weiss JL, et al. Doxepin effects in chronic pain and depression: A controlled study. In Fields HL, Dubner R, Cervero F (eds): Advances in Pain Research and Therapy, vol 9. New York: Raven Press; 1985: 761–771.

51. Davidoff G, Guarracini M, Roth E, et al. Trazodone hydrochloride in the treatment of dysesthetic pain in traumatic myelopathy: A randomized, double-blind, placebo-controlled study. Pain 1987; 29:151–161.

52. Watson CPN, Evans R. A comparative trial of amitriptyline and zimelidine in postherpetic neuralgia. Pain 1985; 23:387–394.

53. Kerrick JM, Fine PG, Lipman AG, Love G. Low-dose amitriptyline as an adjunct to opioids for postoperative orthopedic pain: A placebo-controlled trial. Pain 1993; 52:325–330.

54. Taiwo YO, Fabian A, Pazoles CJ, et al. Potentiation of morphine antinociception by monoamine reuptake inhibitors in the rat spinal cord. Pain 1985; 21:329–337.

55. Levine JD, Gordon NC, Smith R, et al. Desipramine enhances opiate postoperative analgesia. Pain 1986; 27:45–49.

56. Roose SP, Galsman AH, Giardina EGU, et al. Tricyclic antidepressants in depressed patients with cardiac disease. Arch Gen Psychiatry 1987; 44:273–275.

57. Morichi R, Pepeu G. A study of the influence of hydroxyzine and diazepam on morphine antinociception in the rat. Pain 1979; 7:173–180.

58. Marsland AR, Weekes JWN, Atkinson RL, et al. Phantom limb pain: A case for beta blockers? Pain 1982; 12:295–297.

59. Sicuteri F, Geppetti P, Marabini S, et al. Pain relief by somatostatin in attacks of cluster headache. Pain 1984; 18:359–365.

60. Buzzi MG, Moskowitz MA. The antimigraine drug sumatriptan (GR43175) selectively blocks neurogenic plasma extravasation from blood vessels in dura mater. Br J Pharmacol 1990; 99:202–206.

61. Saper JR, Silberstien S, Gordon CD, Hamel RL. Handbook of Headache Management. Baltimore: Williams & Wilkins; 1993: 21–22.

62. Noordenbos W. Sensory findings in painful traumatic nerve lesions. In Bonica JJ, Liebeskind JC, Albe-Fessard DG (eds): Advances in Pain Research and Therapy, vol 3. New York: Raven Press; 1979: 91–101.

63. Hannington-Kiff JG. Hyperadrenergic-effected limb causaigia: Relief by pharmacologic norepinephrine blockade. Am Heart J 1982; 103: 152–153.

64. Lief PA, Reisman R, Rocca A, et al. IV regional guanethidine vs. reserpine for pain relief in reflex sympathetic dvstrophy (RSD): A controlled, randomized, double-blind, cross-over study. Pain 1987; 31:205.

65. Levine J, Basbaum A. The peripheral nervous system and the inflammatory process. Pain 1987; 31 (suppl 4):109.

66. Corey L, Spear PG. Infections with herpes simplex viruses. N Engl J Med 1986; 314:749–757.

67. Rowe NH, Shipman C Jr, Drach JC. Herpes simplex virus disease: Implications for dental personnel. J Am Dent Assoc 1984; 108:381.

68. Raborn GW, McGaw WT, Grace M, et al. Oral acyclovir and herpes labialis: A randomized, double-blind, placebo-controlled study. J Am Dent Assoc 1987; 115:38–42.

69. Johnson S. Advances in Dental Research. J Am Dent Assoc 1985; 111:796.

70. Reuler JB, Chang M. Herpes zoster: Epidemiology, clinical features and management. South Med J 1984; 77:1149–1156.

71. Sklar SH. Herpes zoster, the treatment and prevention of neuralgia with adenosine monophosphate. JAMA 1985; 253:1426–1430.

72. Shepp DH, Dandliker PS, Meyer JD. Treatment of varicella-zoster virus infection in severely immunocompromised patients. N Engl J Med 1986; 314:208–212.

73. Rumore MM, Schlichting DA. Clinical efficiency of antihistamines as analgesics. Pain 1986; 25:7–22.

74. Loeser JD. The management of tic douloureux. Pain 1977; 3:155–162.

75. Hakanson S. Retrogasserian glycerol injection as a treatment of tic douloureux. In Bonica JJ, Lindblom U, Iggo A (eds): Advances in Pain Research and Therapy, vol 5. New York: Raven Press; 1983: 927–933.

76. Messing RB, Lytle LD. Serotonin-containing neurons: Their possible role in pain and analgesia. Pain 1977; 4:1–21.

77. Hosobuchi Y, Lamb S, Bascom D. Tryptophan loading may reverse tolerance to opiate analgesics in humans: A preliminary report. Pain 1980; 9:161–169.

78. Seltzer S, Marcus R, Stoch R. Perspectives in the control of chronic pain by nutritional manipulation. Pain 1981; 11:141–148.

79. Seltzer S, Stoch R, Marcus R, et al. Alteration of human pain thresholds by nutritional manipulation and L-tryptophan supplementation. Pain 1982; 13:385–393.

80. Cheng RSS, Pomeranz B. A combined treatment with D-amino acids and electroacupuncture produces a greater analgesia than either treatment alone; naloxone reverses these effects. Pain 1980; 8:231–236.

81. Fernstrom JD, Wurtman RJ. Brain serotonin content: Physiological regulations of plasma neutral amino acids. Science 1972; 178:414–416.

82. Van Woert MV, Rosenbaum D. L-5-hydroxytryptophan therapy in myoclonus. In Fahn S (ed): Advances in Neurology, vol 26. New York: Raven Press; 1979: 107–115.

83. Shealy CN. Vitamin B6 and other vitamin levels in chronic pain patients. Clin J Pain 1987; 2:203–204.

84. Brady JP, Cheatle MD, Ball WA. A trial of L-tryptophan in chronic pain syndrome. Clin J Pain 1987; 3:39–43.

85. Seltzer S, Dewart D, Pollack RL, et al. The effects of dietary tryptophan on chronic maxillofacial pain and experimental pain tolerance. J Psychiatr Res 1982; 17:181–186.

86. Yaksh TL, Hammond DL. Peripheral and central substrates involved in the rostral transmission of nociceptive information. Pain 1982; 13:1–85.

87. Gammon GD, Starr I Jr. Studies on the relief of pain bv counterirritation. J Clin Invest 1941; 20:13–20.

88. Politzer A. A Textbook of Diseases of the Ear, ed 4. Philadelphia: Lea Brothers; 1902.

89. Kraus H. The use of surface anesthesia in the treatment of painful motion. JAMA 1941; 116:2582–2583.

90. Travell J. Basis for the multiple uses of local block of somatic trigger areas. Miss Valley Med J 1949; 71:13.

91. Travell J. Ethyl chloride spray for painful muscle spasm. Arch Phys Med 1952; 33:291–298.

92. Schwartz LL. Ethyl chloride treatment of limited painful mandibular movement. J Am Dent Assoc 1954; 48:497.

93. Ottoson D, Ekblom A, Hansson P. Vibratory stimulation for the relief of pain of dental origin. Pain 1981; 10:37–45.

94. Lundeberg T, Ottoson D, Hakansson S, et al. Vibratory stimulation for the control of intractable chronic orofacial pain. In Bonica JJ, Lindblom U, Iggo A (eds): Advances in Pain Research and Therapy, vol 5. New York: Raven Press; 1983: 555–561.

95. Pantaleo T, Duranti R, Bellini F. Effects of vibratory stimulation on muscular pain threshold and blink response in human subjects. Pain 1986; 24:239–250.

96. Sherer CL, Cielland JA, O'Sullivan P, et al. The effect of two sites of high frequency vibration on cutaneous pain threshold. Pain 1986; 25:133–138.

97. Hansson P, Ekblom A. Transcutaneous electrical nerve stimulation (TENS) as compared to placebo TENS for the relief of acute orofacial pain. Pain 1983; 15:157–165.

98. Lundeberg T. Long-term results of vibratory stimulation as a pain relieving measure for chronic pain. Pain 1984; 20:13–23.

99. Kane K, Taub A. A history of local electrical analgesia. Pain 1975; 1:125–138.

100. Wall PD, Sweet WH. Temporary abolition of pain in man. Science 1967;155:108–109.

101. Melzack R, Wall PD. Pain mechanisms: A new theory. Science 1965; 150:971–979.

102. Anderson SA. Pain control by sensory stimulation. In Bonica JJ, Liebeskind JC, Albe-Fessard DG (eds): Advances in Pain Research and Therapy, vol 3. New York: Raven Press; 1979: 569–585.

103. Facchinetti F, Sandrini G, Petraglia F, et al. Concomitant increase in nociceptive flexion reflex threshold and plasma opioids following transcutaneous nerve stimulation. Pain 1984; 19:295–303.

104. Hansson P, Ekblom A, Thomsson M, et al. Influence of naloxone on relief of acute orofacial pain by transcutaneous electric nerve stimulation (TENS) or vibration. Pain 1986; 24:323–329.

105. Honig S, Zeale P, Mason A, et al. High-frequency transcutaneous electrical nerve stimulation: Lack of correlation with serum beta-endorphin levels and failure of analgesic reversal with naloxone. Clin J Pain 1987; 2:215–217.

106. Augustinsson L, Bohlin P, Bundsen P, et al. Pain relief during delivery by transcutaneous electrical nerve stimulation. Pain 1977; 4:59–65.

107. Mannheimer C, Carlsson C. The analgesic effect of transcutaneous electrical nerve stimulation (TNS) in patients with rheumatoid arthritis: A comparative study of different pulse patterns. Pain 1979; 6:329–334.

108. Peets JM, Pomeranz B. Acupuncture-like transcutaneous electrical nerve stimulation analgesia is influenced bv spinal cord endorphins but not serotonin: An intrathecal pharmacological study. In Fields HL, Dubner R, Cervero F (eds): Advances in Pain Research and Therapy, vol 9. New York: Raven Press; 1985: 519–525.

109. Fox EJ, Melzack R. Transcutaneous electrical stimulation and acupuncture: Comparison of treatment for low-back pain. Pain 1976; 2:141–148.

110. Eriksson MBE, Sjolund BH, Nielzen S. Long-term results of peripheral conditioning stimulation as an analgesic measure in chronic pain. Pain 1979; 6:335–347.

111. Willer JC, Boureau F, Luu M. Differential effects of electroacupuncture (EA) and transcutaneous nerve stimulation (TNS) on nociceptive component (R2) of the blink reflex in man. Pain 1981; 11 (suppl 1):280.

112. Sodipo OA. Transcutaneous electrical nerve stimulation (TENS) and acupuncture: Comparison of therapy for low-back pain. Pain 1981; 11 (suppl 1):277.

113. Chapman CR, Colpitts YM, Benedetti C, et al. Evoked potential assessment of acupunctural analgesia: Attempted reversal with naloxone. Pain 1980; 9:183–197.

114. Bischko JJ. Use of laser beam in acupuncture. Int J Acupuncture Electro Ther Res 1980; 5:29.

115. Barnes JF. Electronic acupuncture and cold laser therapy as adjunct to pain treatment. J Craniomand Pract 1984; 2:148–152.

116. Waker J,Akharrjec LK, Cooney MM. Laser therapy for pain of trigeminal neuralgia. Pain 1987; 31 (suppl 4):85.

117. Sweet WH. Some current problems in pain research and therapy. Pain 1981; 10:297–309.

118. Melzack R. Prolonged relief of pain by brief, intense transcutaneous somatic stimulation. Pain 1975; 1:357–373.

119. Sodipo JOA. Therapeutic acupuncture for chronic pain. Pain 1979; 7:359–365.

120. Ahonen E, Hakumaki M, Mahlanaki S, et al. Acupuncture and physiotherapy in the treatment of myogenic headache patients: Pain relief and EMG activity. In Bonica JJ, Lindblom U, Iggo A (eds): Advances in Pain Research and Therapy, vol 5. New York: Raven Press; 1983: 571–576.

121. Toyama PM, Heyder C. Acupuncture-induced mood changes reversed by narcotic antagonist naloxone. Pain 1981; 11 (suppl 1):279.

122. Walker JB, Katz RL. Nonopioid pathways suppress pain in humans. Pain 1981; 11:347–354.

123. Cottingham B, Phillips PD, Davies GK, et al. The effect of subcutaneous nerve stimulation (SCNS) on pain associated with osteoarthritis of the hip. Pain 1985; 22:243–248.

124. Lawrence RM. Stimulation of the periosteum of the bone for chronic pain reduction. Pain 1981; 11 (suppl 1):112.

125. Esposito CJ, Veal SJ, Farman AG. Alleviation of myofascial pain with ultrasound therapy. J Prosthet Dent 1984; 51:106–110.

126. Griffin JE, Karselis TC. Physical Agents for Physical Therapists, ed 2. Springfield, Ill; Charles C Thomas; 1982: 279–312.

127. Mahan PE. Temporomandibular joint dysfunction: Physiological and clinical aspects in occlusions, in research, and in form and function. Proceedings of a symposium, 1975: 112.

128. Kahn J. Iontophoresis and ultrasound for postsurgical temporomandibular tissues and paresthesis. Phys Ther 1980; 60:307–308.

129. Kleinkort JA, Wood F. Phonopheresis with one percent versus ten percent hydrocortisone. Phys Ther 1985; 55:1320.

130. Jankelson B, Swain CW. Physiological aspects of masticatory muscle stimulation: the Myomonitor. Quintessence Int 1972; 3(12): 57–62.

131. Murphy GJ. Electrical physical therapy in treating TMJ patients. J Craniomand Pract 1983; 1:67–73.

132. Wessberg GA, Carroll WL, Dinham R, et al. Transcutaneous electrical stimulation as an adjunct in the management of myofascial pain-dysfunction syndrome. J Prosthet Dent 1981; 45:307–314.

133. Wall PD. The gate-control theory of pain mechanisms: A reexamination and restatement. Brain 1978; 101:1.

134. Travell JG, Simons DG. Myofascial pain and dysfunction. The trigger point manual. Baltimore: Williams & Wilkins; 1983: 87–88.

135. Travell JG, Simons DG. Myofascial pain and dysfunction. The trigger point manual. Baltimore: Williams & Wilkins ; 1983: 63–74.

136. Schwartz L. Disorders of the Temporomandibular Joint. Philadelphia: WB Saunders; 1959.

137. De Steno CV. The pathophysiology of TMJ dysfunction and related pain. In Gelb H (ed): Clinical Management of Head, Neck and TMJ Pain and Dysfunction. Philadelphia: WB Saunders; 1977: 1–31.

138. Bechtol CO. Muscle physiology. In American Academy of Orthopedic Surgeons: International Course Lectures, vol 5. St Louis: CV Mosby; 1948.

139. Kemppainen P, Pertovaara A, Huopaniemi T, et al. Modification of dental pain and cutaneous thermal sensitivity by physical exercise in man. Brain Res 1986; 360:33–40.

140. Kemppainen P, Pertovaara A. The contribution of experimental stress to the modulation of dental pain threshold in man. Pain 1987; 31 (suppl 4):414.

141. Fordyce W, McMahon R, Rainwater G, et al. Pain complaint-exercise performance relationship in chronic pain. Pain 1981; 10:311–321.

142. Okeson JP. Management of Temporomandibular Disorders and Occlusion, ed 3. St Louis: Mosby-Year Book;1993: 403–417.

143. Speculund B, Goss AN, Hughes A, et al. Temporomandibular joint dysfunction: Pain and illness behavior. Pain 1983; 17:139–150.

144. Fordyce WE. Pain viewed as learned behavior. In Bonica JJ (ed): Advances in Neurology, vol 4. New York: Raven Press; 1974: 415–422.

145. Fordyce WE. Treating chronic pain by contingency management, in Bonica JJ (ed): Advances in Neurology, vol 4. New York: Raven Press; 1974: 583–589.

146. Melzack R. Psychological concepts and methods for the control of pain. In Bonica JJ (ed): Advances in Neurology, vol 4. New York: Raven Press; 1974: 275–280.

147. Sternbach RA. Fundamentals of psychological methods in chronic pain. In Bonica JJ, Lindblom U, Iggo A (eds): Advances in Pain Research and Therapy, vol 5. New York: Raven Press; 1983: 777–780.

148. Roberts AA. Contingency management methods in the treatment of chronic pain. In Bonica JJ, Lindblom U, Iggo A (eds): Advances in Pain Research and Therapy, vol 5. New York: Raven Press; 1983: 789–794.

149. Selye H. Stress without Distress. Philadelphia: JB Lippincott; 1974: 32.

150. Carlson CR, Okeson JP, Falace DA, Nitz AJ, Curran SL, Anderson DT. Comparison of psychologic and physiologic functioning between patients with masticatory muscle pain and matched controls. J Orofacial Pain 1993; 7:15–22.

151. Jacobson E. Progressive Relaxation. Chicago: The University of Chicago Press; 1968.

152. Moller E, Sheik-Ol-Eslan A, Lous I. Deliberate relaxation of the temporal and masseter muscles in subjects with functional disorders of the chewing apparatus. Scand J Dent Res 1971; 79:478–482.

153. Gessel AH, Alderman MM. Management of myofascial pain dysfunction syndrome of the temporomandibular joint by tension control training. Psychosomatics 1971; 12:302–330.

154. Goldberg G. The psychological, physiological, and hypnotic approach to bruxism in the treatment of periodontal disease. J Am Soc Psychosom Dent Med 1973; 20:75–91.

155. Reading A, Raw M. The treatment of mandibular dysfunction pain. Br Dent J 1976; 140:201–202.

156. Blanchard F, et al. Behavioral treatment of 250 chronic headache patients: A clinical replication series. Behav Ther 1985; 16:308–327.

157. Larsson B, Melin L. Chronic headaches in adolescents: treatment in a school setting with relaxation training as compared with information contact and self-registration. Pain 1986; 25:325–336.

158. Dahlstrom L, Carlsson SG. Treatment of mandibular dysfunction: the clinical usefulness of biofeedback in relation to splint therapy. J Oral Rehabil 1984; 11:277–284.

159. Lacroix J, Clarke MA, Bock JC, Doxey NC. Muscle-contraction headaches in multiple-pain patients. Treatment under worsening baseline conditions. Arch Phys Med Rehabil 1986; 67:14–18.

160. Hijzen TH, Slangen JL, Van Houweligen HC. Subjective clinical and EMG effect of biofeedback and splint treatment. J Oral Rehabil 1986; 13:529–539.

161. Raft D, Toomey T, Gregg JM. Behavior modification and haloperidol in chronic facial pain. South Med J 1979; 72:155–159.

162. Erlandson PM, Poppen R. Electromyographic biofeedback and rest position training of masticatory muscles in myofascial pain-dysfunction patients. J Prosthet Dent 1989; 62:335–338.

163. Okeson JP, Moody PM, Kemper JT, Haley JV. Evaluation of occlusal splint therapy and relaxation procedures in patients with temporomandibular disorders. J Am Dent Assoc 1983; 107:420–424.

164. Carlson CR, VenTrella MA, Sturgis ET. Relaxation training through muscle stretching procedures: A pilot case. J Behav Ther Exp Psychiatry 1987; 18:121–126.

165. Carlson CR, Collin FL, Nitz AJ, et al. Muscle stretching as an alternative relaxation training procedure. J Behav Ther Exp Psychiatry 1990; 21:29–38.

166. Carlson CR, Okeson JP, Falace DA et al. Stretch-based relaxation and the reduction of EMG activity among masticatory muscle pain patients. J Craniomandib Disord Facial Pain 1991; 5:205–212.

167. Manns A, Zuazola RV, Sirhan R, Quiroz M, Rocabado M. Relationship between the tonic elevator mandibular activity and the vertical dimension during the states of vigilance and hypnosis. J Craniomand Pract 1990; 8:163–170.

168. Kabat-Zinn J, Lipworth L, Burney R, et al. Four-year follow-up of a meditation based program for the self-regulation of chronic pain: Treatment outcomes and compliance. Clin J Pain 1987; 2:159–173.

169. Bailey LM. Music therapy in pain management. J Pain Symptom Manag 1986; 1:25–28.

170. Pilling LF. Psychosomatic aspects of facial pain. In Alling CC, Mahan PE (eds): Facial Pain, ed 2. Philadelphia: Lea & Febiger; 1977: 213–226.

171. Fricton JR. The effects of direct and indirect hypnotic suggestion for analgesia in high and low susceptible subjects. Pain 1981; 11 (suppl 1):175.

172. Hilgard ER. The alleviation of pain by hypnosis. Pain 1975; 1:213–231.

173. Orne MT. Hypnotic methods for managing pain. In Bonica JJ, Lindblom U, Iggo A (eds): Advances in Pain Research and Therapy, vol 5. New York: Raven Press; 1983: 847–856.

174. Toomey TC, Larkin D. Trance as a pain control strategy for the nurse in the burn unit setting. Pain 1981; 11 (suppl 1):113.

175. Finer B, Terenius L. Endorphin involvements during hypnotic analgesia in chronic pain patients. Pain 1981; 11 (suppl 1):27.

176. Gale EN. Behavioral management of MPD. In The President's Conference on the Examination, Diagnosis, and Management of Temporomandibular Disorders. Chicago: American Dental Association; 1983: 161–173.

177. Chapman CR, Turner JA. Psychological control of acute pain in medical settings. J Pain Symptom Manag 1986; 1:9–20.

178. Egan KJ, Betrus P. Psychological functioning in five pain syndromes: Tension headache, backache, migraine, and temporomandibular and gastrointestinal pain syndromes. Clin J Pain 1987; 2:233–238.

179. Chapman SL. A review and clinical perspective on the use of EMG and thermal biofeedback for chronic headaches. Pain 1986; 27:1–43.

180. Schwartz MS. Biofeedback and stress management in the treatment of headache. J Craniomandib Disord Facial Oral Pain 1987; 1:41–45.

181. Jessup BA, Neufeld RWJ, Merskey H. Biofeedback therapy for headache and other pain: An evaluative review. Pain 1979; 7:225–270.

182. Sternbach RA. Letter to the editor. Pain 1980; 9:111.

183. Turner JA, Chapman CR. Psychological intervention for chronic pain: A critical review. 1. Relaxation training and biofeedback. Pain 1982; 12:1–21.

184. Sherman RA, Gall N, Gormly J. Treatment of phantom limb pain with muscular relaxation training to disrupt the pain-anxiety-tension cycle. Pain 1979; 6:47–55.

185. Large RG, Lamb AM. Electromyographic (EMG) feedback in chronic musculoskeletal pain: A controlled trial. Pain 1983; 17:167–177.

186. Nouwen A. EMG biofeedback used to reduce standing levels of paraspinal muscle tension in chronic low back pain. Pain 1983; 17:353–360.

187. Brooke RI, Stenn PG. Myofascial pain-dysfunction syndrome: How effective is biofeedback-assisted relaxation training? In Bonica JJ, Lindblom U, Iggo A (eds): Advances in Pain Research and Therapy, vol 5. New York: Raven Press; 1983: 809–812.

188. Christensen LV, Mohamed SE, Harrison JD. Delayed onset of masseter muscle pain in experimental tooth clenching. J Prosthet Dent 1982; 48:579–584.

189. Solberg WK, Clark GT, Rugh JD. Nocturnal electromyographic evaluation of bruxing patients undergoing short-term splint therapy. J Oral Rehabil 1975; 2:215–223.

190. Kemper JT Jr, Okeson JP. Craniomandibular disorders and headaches. J Prosthet Dent 1983; 49:702–705.

Section III

Clinical Pain Syndromes

In the orofacial region, primary somatic pain of the superficial type emanates from the skin of the lips, face, outer nares, and outer external auditory canal and from the mucogingival tissues of the oral cavity proper (Fig 10-1). Pains from these structures display clinical features that distinguish them from primary deep somatic pains and from secondary heterotopic manifestations of somatic and neuropathic pain disorders.

Behavior of Cutaneous and Mucogingival Pain

The following are clinical characteristics of superficial somatic pain:

1. The pain has a bright, stimulating quality.
2. Subjective localization of the pain is excellent and anatomically accurate.
3. The site of pain identifies the correct location of its source.
4. Response to provocation at the site of pain is faithful in incidence, intensity, and location.
5. The application of a topical anesthetic at the site of pain temporarily arrests it.

Types of Cutaneous and Mucogingival Pain

There are a variety of pains that originate from the cutaneous and mucogingival tissues of the face and oral structures. Many of these conditions are specifically identified by the tissues that are affected. In this chapter, these pains will be simply divided into two categories according to the tissues affected: cutaneous pains and mucogingival pains.

Cutaneous Pains of the Face

Cutaneous pain is usually described as an itching, pricking, raw, stinging, burning sensation depending chiefly on the intensity of the complaint. Stimulation-evoked pain is initially felt as a fast, sharp, pricking pain. Since this is prevented by A fiber blocking, it is presumed that the initial sensation is mediated by A-delta nociceptive neurons.[1] The initial pricking sensation is followed by a slightly delayed, less sharp, less precisely localized, burning pain that quite assuredly is mediated by C-fiber nociceptive units.

Since the pain is precisely felt at the location of the initiating cause, little diagnostic

Classification of Orofacial Pains

Axis II
(Psychological Conditions)

Anxiety Disorder
- Generalized Anxiety Disorder
- Posttraumatic Stress Disorder
- Anxiety Disorder due to a Medical Condition

Other Conditions
- Malingering
- Psychological Factors Affecting Med Condition
  - Personality Traits or Coping Style
  - Maladaptive Health Behavior
  - Stress-Related Physiological Response
- other conditions

Mood Disorder
- Depressive Disorder
- Bipolar Disorder
- Mood Disorder due to a Medical Condition

Somatoform Disorder
- Undifferentiated Somatoform Disorder
- Conversion Disorder
- Pain Disorder
- Hypochondriasis

Axis II
Axis I
Diagnosis

Axis I
(Physical Conditions)

Somatic Pain

Neuropathic Pain

Continuous Pain
- Sympathetically Maintained Pain
  - Traumatic Neuralgia
  - Atypical Odontalgia
- Deafferentation Pain
- Neuritis Pain
  - Postherpetic Neuralgia
  - Herpes Zoster
  - Peripheral Neuritis

Episodic Pain
- Paroxsymal Neuralgia Pain
  - Neurovascular Pain
    - Migraine with Aura
    - Migraine without Aura
    - Cluster Headache
    - Paroxsymal Hemicrania
    - Neurovascular Variants
  - Vascular Pain
    - Arteritis Pain
    - Carotidynia
  - Pulpal Pain
  - Visceral Mucosal Pain
  - Glandular, Ocular and Auricular Pain

Deep Pain

Visceral Pain

Musculoskeletal Pain
- Periodontal Pain
- Soft Connective Tissue Pain
- Osseous and Periosteal Pain
- Temporomandibular Joint Pain
  - Ligamentous Pain
  - Retrodiscal Pain
  - Capsular Pain
  - Arthritic Pain
- Muscle Pain
  - Co-contraction
  - Delayed Onset Muscle Soreness
  - Myofascial Pain
  - Muscle Spasm Pain
  - Muscle Inflammation Pain

Superficial Pain
- Mucogingival Pain
- Cutaneous Pain

Fig 10-1 Pain classification chart highlighted to show the relationship of superficial somatic pains to other orofacial pain disorders.

effort is needed to determine its origin. When the cause of the cutaneous pain is not immediately evident, the examiner should question whether the complaint might be heterotopic, such as referred pain from other deep pain input or as projected pain of neuropathic etiology.[2-4] A topical anesthetic applied at the site of pain temporarily arrests superficial somatic pain. It should be noted, however, that the irritating effect of the medication, when first applied, may initially increase the discomfort.

Caution should be exercised in assuming that a visible lesion at or near the site of pain necessarily represents the primary initiating cause. It may or may not be so. For example, the lesions of herpes zoster stem from a neural disorder and are not the cause of the peripheral pain. Again, one should not assume that the complaint does not emanate from cutaneous structures simply because the etiology is obscure. Subtle forms of noxious stimulation that cause itching and stinging may be encountered. When such confusing situations arise, the use of topical anesthesia to confirm the diagnosis is indicated.

Mucogingival Pains of the Mouth

There may be some question about classifying mucogingival pains in the same category with pains of cutaneous origin. They are not identical in behavior. For example, mucogingival discrimination of painful sensation does not include the familiar pricking-burning pattern of cutaneous pain. Also, the number of thick fibers innervating the oral mucosa is negligible compared with that of the skin. However, palatal mucosa senses both itch and tickle, and all oral tissues feel stinging and burning sensations. Muco-

gingival pains have a bright stimulating quality, are easily localized, and identify an adequate local cause. These pains respond faithfully to provocation at the site of pain, do not present central excitatory effects, and are arrested by the application of a topical anesthetic at the site of pain. They therefore present the characteristics of superficial somatic pain by which identification can be made. The true site of origin of such pain is less evident than that for cutaneous pain only because of the added difficulty of intraoral examination and failure on the part of the examiner to fully appreciate the implications of oral functioning.

The oral tissues are fragile and easily injured by rubbing against the teeth, tongue, cheeks, and each other during normal use. They are subjected to countless insults from foods, beverages, burns, tobacco, alcohol, toothpastes, mouthrinses, medications, dental defects, dental restorations, dental appliances, objects held in the mouth, habits of clenching the teeth, and unusual functional demands and many more. The oral tissues are reactive to systemic disorders and diseases. The saliva, which normally acts as the oral lubricant, is especially responsive to the effects of emotional stress, physical disorders, and diseases as well as many medications now in common use. The identification of the cause of pain from these tissues is obviously more difficult than for cutaneous pains, but it should be within the capability of the knowledgeable dental examiner. As with cutaneous pain, when the cause of pain felt in the mucogingival tissues is not immediately evident, the examiner must differentiate between primary pain of mucogingival origin and projected or referred pain that stems from neurogenous or deep somatic sources.

221

Mucogingival pains are usually described as distinct raw, stinging, or burning sensations. Pains arising from the lining tissues of the oral cavity can be precisely located by the patient. Such pain may be generalized throughout the mouth when the cause widely affects the mucogingival tissues, or it may be isolated if the hyperalgesic area is small. In either case the patient can precisely locate the discomfort. The location changes only as the underlying cause varies. This precision of localization may become less accurate in the deeper recesses of the oral cavity.

The location of pain accurately identifies its source. The pain arises from primary hyperalgesia due to local cause such as the irritating effect of foods, liquids, mouthrinses, dentifrices, and medications. It may be due to the abrasive effect of excessive rubbing of the tongue and cheeks, and this effect may be compounded when the quality and quantity of saliva do not afford adequate lubricative protection to the moving tissues. When the salivary deficit is great, normal functioning may become traumatic to the oral tissues. Localized hyperalgesia may occur from numerous causes such as trauma; infection by bacterial, fungal, or viral agents; allergy; and neoplasia. Frequently, one may identify objective signs of hyperemia, inflammation, vesiculation, ulceration, or some other pathosis at the site of pain.

Primary hyperalgesia of the oral lining tissues may show no objective signs, and mucogingival tissues may appear entirely normal. Hyperalgesia may occur with no clinical signs of other tissue change. It is in such instances that the examiner should carefully consider a salivary deficit as the possible cause.

There is a precise, accurate, and propor-tional relationship between any noxious stimulation and the resulting discomfort. When no stimulus is applied, little or no discomfort occurs. When the stimulus is increased, the discomfort increases accordingly without summation effects. The pain faithfully reflects the degree of hyperalgesia and the intensity of the stimulus.

Ordinarily, central excitatory effects are not seen as a result of mucogingival pain, even when severe and continuous. Referred pains, secondary hyperalgesias, and the development of secondary painful muscle co-contraction do not occur. This gives the pain a constancy and sameness that is characteristic.

Since pain of mucogingival origin is an expression of primary hyperalgesia of the tissues that hurt, application of a topical anesthetic to those tissues arrests the pain due to action of the medication on the receptors and pain fibers in the mucogingival tissues. This is an important point of differentiation from referred pain of superficial type and neuritic pain, neither of which is arrested by the application of topical anesthesia.

Mucogingival pains may result from trauma, allergic responses, local infections, systemic conditions, or may present as burning mouth syndromes. Each of these categories will be discussed.

Trauma. Generalized surface injuries cause mucogingival pains, but the etiology is usually so evident that no diagnostic problem is presented. Other signs are present or promptly become apparent, such as hyperemia, inflammation, vesiculation, or ulceration. Such traumatic effects may have mechanical, thermal, or chemical causes such as scalding with hot foods or liquids (Fig

10-2), excessive smoking or other use of to-bacco, abrasions from toothbrushes and other objects, chemical burns (Fig 10-3), ac-cidents as a result of dental treatment, or the use of harmful medications by the pa-tient. Examples of the latter are aspirin burns and injuries produced by toothache remedies.

Traumatic abrasions and decubital ulcer-ations are common secondary to poorly fitting dental appliances (Fig 10-4). Exo-stoses and bony prominences are especially vulnerable to injury, and when severely traumatized, full-thickness mucogingival ul-cers may develop and cause exposure and surface devitalization of the underlying cor-tical bone. Such lesions are slow to heal and cause pain with deep somatic characteristics in addition to the expected superficial so-matic variety. Whenever the periosteal and osseous structures become involved, pains of mixed quality should be expected. This is true not only of the full-thickness ulcers but also of gingival lesions that involve the deeper periodontal structures. Examples of such lesions are acutely inflamed periodon-tal pockets and superficial infections that spread as cellulitis. Pains of mixed quality are less likely to be arrested by application of a topical anesthetic. They frequently pre-sent secondary symptoms of central sensiti-zation.

Allergic Responses. Various allergic re-sponses, including stomatitis medicamentosa and stomatitis venenata, may produce rather generalized mucogingival pain, the cause of which may at times be obscure. These condi-tions are usually accompanied by objective signs of tissue change, and the cause may be established by careful history-taking. Stomatitis venenata presents with lesions of the oral mucosa that result from contact with ordinarily innocuous substances such as denture materials, dentifrices, mouth-rinses, lozenges, lipsticks, topical medica-tions, foods, and flavoring materials (Figs 10-5 and 10-6). Sometimes desquamation of the protective surface layers of epithelium occurs and reveals the deeper vascular bed. When the shedding is extensive, the term desquamative stomatitis may be applicable.

Stomatitis medicamentosa is an allergic reaction to systemic medications such as antibiotics, sulfonamides, aminopyrine, qui-nine, arsphenamine, phenolphthalein, bar-biturates, mercurials, salicylates, and birth control pills. Some cases of erythema multi-forme (Fig 10-7) as well as variants de-scribed as Stevens-Johnson syndrome, Behcet's syndrome, and ectodermosis ero-siva pluriorificialis may represent allergic responses of this type.

Other allergens may cause oral manifesta-tions accompanied by superficial mucogin-gival pain. At times, such manifestations may require consultation with an allergist. From the standpoint of pain diagnosis, such conditions should be distinguished from lo-calized autonomic effects that result from central excitation. The key to diagnosis re-lates to one's knowledge of the neuroanat-omy of the visceral nervous system. Sys-temic allergic responses do not follow neuroanatomic patterns and therefore are observed bilaterally and diffusely, whereas localized autonomic effects relate to the anatomic distribution of the neurons in-volved and are predominantly unilateral.

Local Infections. Widespread local infec-tions of the mucogingival tissues cause gen-eralized superficial somatic pain. Usually the accompanying local signs of inflamma-

Fig 10-2 Ulcer on palatal tissues secondary to a pizza burn. (Courtesy of Dr John F. Johnson, US Navy.)

Fig 10-3 Aspirin burn secondary to the placement of an aspirin tablet in the buccal mucosa. (Courtesy of Dr John F. Johnson, US Navy.)

Fig 10-4 Decubital ulcer due to pressure from a denture.

Fig 10-5 Stomatitis venenata due to contact with denture base material. Note that tissue reaction conforms to the shape of the denture base.

Fig 10-6 Stomatitis venenata due to contact with a dentifrice to which the patient was sensitive.

Fig 10-7 Stomatitis medicamentosa expressed clinically as erythema multiforme due to ingestion of a laxative medicine that contained phenolphthalein.

225

Fig 10-8 Acute necrotizing ulcerative gingivitis (Vincent's infection).

Fig 10-9 Fungal infection of the oral mucosa.

tion and ulceration make the cause of pain obvious. Examples of this are fulminating acute necrotizing ulcerative gingivitis (Vincent's infection) and fungal infections (Figs 10-8, 10-9).

Systemic Conditions. Systemic disease may cause oral manifestations that affect the mucogingival tissues and induce generalized superficial somatic pain. Included are nutritional deficiencies, intoxications, exanthematous diseases, anemia and other blood dyscrasias, pellagra, diabetes mellitus, pem-

phigus, and infections. Even pregnancy and general debilitation can affect mucogingival tissues (Fig 10-10). These conditions exhibit objective signs of congestion so that discoloration and swelling are evident. Such effects frequently occur at sites where other local irritation is present such as trauma, malocclusion, gingivitis, and periodontal involvement.

Most isolated pains emanating from the oral mucogingival tissues present no diagnostic problem because they are usually associated with local lesions that are clinically evident subjectively and objectively. Two such common disorders are recurrent aphthous stomatitis and herpes simplex infection. Both of these conditions are characterized by recurrent, painful, superficial oral ulcers that persist 8 to 14 days. They are both associated with a tender regional lymphadenopathy and heal spontaneously, usually without sequelae. There are differences between these conditions and therefore each will be briefly discussed.

Recurrent aphthous stomatitis is the most common ulcerative disease of the oral cavity, accounting for 90% of all ulcers seen in dental practice and affecting nearly 20% of the general population.[5] Aphthous stomatitis appears as an erythematous macula or papilla that undergoes central blanching followed by necrosis and ulceration (Fig 10-11). The ulcers most commonly occur on nonkeratinized, freely movable mucosa, such as the lips, buccal mucosa, tongue, mucobuccal fold, floor of the mouth, or soft palate. They usually occur singly but on occasion several occur simultaneously. As already mentioned, the ulcers will occur, resolve, and then recur.

The etiology of recurrent aphthous stomatitis is still unknown. Studies suggest that the disorder is an immunopathic process that involves cell-mediated cytolytic activity that leads to decreased tissue integrity.[6,7] Precipitating factors include certain foods (ie, gluten-containing foods, acidic foods, and juices), trauma, stress, hormones, nutritional deficiencies, and chemicals in oral hygiene products (Fig 10-12).[8–11]

Since the etiology is unknown, there is no known cure for recurrent aphthous ulcers, however, in most cases the disease can be controlled to the satisfaction of the patient. The patient should be educated about the natural course of the disease and its self-limiting nature. The patient should be told of the noncommunicability of the disease and the benefits of avoiding any precipitant factors when they are known. During the pain episode topical anesthetic may be helpful. Topical steroid preparations may also be useful.[12]

Herpes simplex infects nearly a half a million people each year in the United States.[13] The initial or primary infection usually occurs early in life, between the ages of 1 and 10 years. Young adults, ages 15 to 25 years old, make up the second most commonly infected group with 45% of the college students being infected.[14] Herpes simplex infection presents as a cluster of small discrete gray or white vesicles without a red erythematous halo. The vesicles quickly rupture, forming small punctuate ulcers 1 mm or less in diameter. Unlike recurrent aphthous ulcers, herpes simplex usually presents as several small ulcers clustered in a localized area. The lesions are usually found on fixed keratinized mucosa such as tightly bound periosteum, hard palate, gingiva, and alveolar ridge.

Herpes simplex infection is caused by the herpesvirus. There are seven known herpesviruses, two of which are known to occur only in humans: HSV-1 and HSV-2. Both of these viruses produce epithelial disease, enter a latent state, and reactivate to produce recurrent disease. HSV-1 classically is associated with infection of the orofacial complex, whereas HSV-2 predominantly causes genital infections. Both are natural infections occurring in humans with equal involvement of both sexes and all races; HSV-1 has affinity for cells of neuroectodermal origin.

Transmission occurs by direct personal

Fig 10-10 Gingivitis that became acute during the third month of pregnancy and persisted 5 weeks postpartum.

Fig 10-11 Several aphthous ulcers located on the buccal mucosa of the lower lip. (Courtesy of Dr John F. Johnson, US Navy.)

Fig 10-12 A very larger aphthous ulcer that developed following trauma to the tongue. (Courtesy of Dr John F. Johnson, US Navy.)

contact with infected secretions at mucosal surfaces or abraded skin. The most common portal of entry for HSV-1 is the oral mucosa. The virus binds to the epithelial cell membrane and than penetrates the cell by fusion with the plasma membrane.[15] The virus than affects cellular DNA synthesis, producing balloon degeneration, chromatin condensation, multinucleated giant cell formation, and eventually the lesions.[16,17]

The initial herpes simplex infection may be asymptomatic. It may occur in children and young adults as a pharyngitis or gingivostomatitis. The lesions may be accompanied by fever, malaise, irritability, inability to eat, regional lymphadenopathy, and myalgia. The infection in infants and small children may be unrecognized.

After the initial episode, the virus can travel to the sensory nerve ganglia and persist within the nucleus in a nonreplicating, nonlytic (latent) state. The trigeminal ganglia is the most common site of the latent HSV-1 virus. Recurrent herpes simplex is the result of a reactivitation of the virus in the same site of the originally infected nerve. An estimated 98 million cases of recurrent herpes simplex occur in the United States each year.[18] It has been estimated that 35% to 40% of the people that harbor the HSV-1 virus will have recurrent episodes.[19]

The first symptoms of recurrent herpes simplex may be felt as the prodromal symptoms of tingling, throbbing, itching, and burning at the infected site beginning 12 to 24 hours before the lesions erupt. Once the lesions form and erupt, diagnosis becomes obvious. In immunosuppressed patients, recurrent HSV-1 infections may penetrate deeply and disseminate widely.[20]

Treatment of herpes simplex is often determined by the severity of the symptoms.

The initial case of herpes simplex can be very painful and widespread, thus demanding treatment. Supportive and palliative care and anti-infective treatments are the basis of managing the primary HSV-1 infection. Bed rest and isolation are important for limiting transmission and speeding healing. Adequate hydration and nutrition are essential, particularly in small children. Symptoms may be alleviated with topical anesthetics agents, including diphenhydramine. Specific antiviral therapy, such as acycloguanosine, may be helpful in minimizing the severity and duration of the primary infection. Salicylates, nonsteroidal anti-inflammatory drugs, and acetaminophen may be useful in reducing pain and/or fever. Salicylates should be avoided in children to minimize the risk of Reye's syndrome.

Recurrent herpes simplex may be precipitated by harsh outdoor elements, stress, menses, trauma, and possibly diet. Therefore, prophylactic measures are the best method of managing the recurrence. Once the recurrence has occurred, topical measures, similar to the primary treatments, may be helpful.

Burning Mouth Syndrome. The complaint of burning mouth, burning tongue, or *glossodynia* is common and is usually described as a steady, continuous though variable, typical superficial somatic pain. Very frequently, the oral examination reveals a clean hygienic mouth with little objective evidence of pathosis of any kind. A distinguishing characteristic of this condition is the fact that the location of the pain corresponds to areas of greatest movement, thus revealing the cause as the abrasive effect of the tissues rubbing against themselves and the teeth.

Pain location depends on which tissues are being rubbed and where. At times, hyperemia may be observed as well as inflammation and ulceration. Secondary infection of the irritated tissues may complicate the symptom picture. There is a tendency for the complaint to be better and worse in a cyclic pattern, presumably because of the inhibitory effect of pain on functional movements, which permits some regression of the complaint, only to be followed by an exacerbation from increased rubbing when the discomfort eases.

The tip of the tongue or one side of the tongue may be involved. The inner surface of the lips is also a common site. Although the gingiva proper is more resistant to such irritation, localized burning gingival pain may occur.

All oral irritants increase the patient's discomfort. This includes especially highly spiced foods, hot liquids, carbonated drinks, strong coffee and tea, certain juices, dentifrices, mouthrinses, and medications. Sometimes mastication becomes so painful that nutritional difficulties arise.

The condition of glossodynia and burning mouth seems to be poorly understood. Much of it is iatrogenic from medications. Anxiety and emotional tension frequently induce or aggravate the condition. It is especially common in women of menopausal age.[21] The condition frequently accompanies increased tongue and mouth movements due to oral consciousness following dental treatment. Although dentures normally require more lubrication from saliva than do natural teeth, they may at times depress salivary flow due to the apprehension and resentment that their presence induces in some individuals. Thus, a normally difficult situation may become compounded by the emotional problems that accompany it.

Xerostomia, or so-called dry mouth syndrome, accompanies burning mouth and is thought to be important etiologically. Grad et al[22] identified many medications that induce xerostomia. These included certain antispasmodics, antidepressants, antipsychotics, skeletal muscle relaxants, parkinsonism medications, antiarrhythmic drugs, antihistamines, appetite suppressants, anticonvulsants, anxiolytics, diuretics, and antihypertensives. This has been found to be especially important in the elderly.[23] Fox et al[24] found that, although xerostomia most commonly was associated with salivary gland dysfunction, it may be an early symptom of several morbid systemic conditions including dry gland disease, polyglandular failure syndrome, autoimmune exocrinopathy such as Sjögren's syndrome, systemic lupus erythematosus, primary biliary cirrhosis, and autoimmune hemolytic anemia.

Although psychogenesis is thought to be important in burning mouth syndrome,[25] recent investigation has failed to indicate significant relevance.[26,27] In a review of 98 cases of burning mouth syndrome, Gorsky et al[28] reported that 75% were women, that dentures and medications predominated, and that glossitis was the only mucosal lesion of significance. It is thought that diminished salivary function due to aging; radiation therapy; mouth breathing from nasal obstruction and other causes; and sustained periods of anxiety, resentment, and/or apprehension may contribute to the condition. Diabetes mellitus and anemia appear to have etiologic importance. Quinn[29] reported that tongue-thrusting predominated in patients with glossodynia.

The diagnostic key to this problem is the application of topical anesthetic to the painful site. Its penetration is too limited to appreciably affect pain sources situated more deeply in the tissues. Heterotopic pains are not affected. Therefore, if application of a topical anesthetic promptly and effectively arrests the pain and induces numbness, the condition truly represents primary hyperalgesia. The diagnosis is confirmed by analgesic lozenges. It should be noted that some neuralgias are triggered by stimulation of the oral and pharyngeal mucosa and such triggering may be temporarily arrested by the application of a topical anesthetic. This phenomenon should never be confused with the problem under consideration because of the clinical difference in the two complaints.

Differential Diagnosis

The clinician should always remember that pain felt in the cutaneous or mucogingival tissues may be heterotopic. The decisive diagnostic evidence that the complaint is heterotopic is the failure of an effective topical anesthetic to arrest the pain even though surface anesthesia is attained. Therapeutic considerations require that the type and source of such heterotopic pain be identified.

Referred pain and/or secondary hyperalgesia induced as a central excitatory effect of deep somatic pain may involve the skin or the oral mucogingival structures. Spontaneous referred pain usually is readily recognized. Stimulus-evoked secondary hyperalgesia, however, can be difficult to identify. The key to diagnosis in either case is to become suspicious that the problem is that of

a secondary effect of deep pain input located elsewhere.

The diagnostic criteria of this phenomenon relate to identifying the primary pain source. Analgesic blocking or the application of a topical anesthetic at the site where heterotopic pain is felt does not arrest the pain even though some altered sensation from the local anesthesia may be felt.

Referred pains and areas of hypersensitivity in the mucogingival tissues may occur as a direct result of other deep pain sources such as toothache, earache, sinusitis, temporomandibular arthralgia, myogenous pains, and neurovascular pains. Frequently, other central excitatory effects such as local autonomic signs and secondary painful muscle effects may be identified as well.

Following are a few differential diagnoses that should be considered when superficial somatic cutaneous or mucogingival pains are suspected:

Heterotopic neuropathic pains may project superficially and present with clinical features that simulate superficial somatic pain. Although these neuropathic pains have not yet been discussed (see Chapter 17), the differentiation between the two categories of pain is necessary.

Paroxysmal neuralgia may be triggered by stimulation of cutaneous or mucogingival receptors in the peripheral distribution of the same nerve that mediates the pain. In trigeminal neuralgia, the sites of such triggering are predominantly cutaneous, being located especially in the lips. Mucogingival triggering, however, sometimes occurs, the tongue being a frequent site. Glossopharyngeal trigger sites are located in the pharyngeal mucosa, and pain is induced by swallowing, talking, and chewing. The clinical criterion for identifying mucosal triggering of paroxysmal neuralgia has to do with the summation effects displayed: the triggering provokes pain that is wholly disproportionate to the stimulus. Analgesic blocking of the peripheral receptors of the affected nerve prevents the triggering effect of superficial stimulation. Topical anesthesia of mucosal trigger sites such as those of glossopharyngeal neuralgia also prevents the paroxysms of pain.

Deafferentation pain may become a complication sequential to trauma, surgery, tooth extraction, or tooth pulp extirpation. The best differential criterion is a history of injury. The pain complaint may be accompanied by paresthesia, dysesthesia, anesthesia, hyperesthesia, or hyperalgesia in an area larger than that innervated by the injured nerve. The symptoms may be accentuated by efferent sympathetic activity involving vasomotor and glandular function. The pain may be arrested temporarily by analgesic blocking of the stellate ganglion.

Traumatic neuralgia or a neuroma is characterized by its location relative to prior injury or surgery and by the specific induction of pain due to compressing or stretching the tissue involved. Topical anesthesia does nothing. Injection, however, of a drop or so of local anesthetic into the site of pain completely arrests it.

Neuritis that involves cutaneous and mucogingival structures may be difficult to recognize because of the similarity to superficial somatic pain. One clinical criterion for identifying this neuropathic pain is its ongoing, persistent, unremitting character. It is not dependent on superficial stimulation even though such stimulation accentuates the discomfort. A more important criterion, however, is the presence of other neural effects (such as paresthesia, hypoesthesia,

anesthesia, and paralysis) that may accompany the neuritic pain. Neuritis of the facial nerve is characterized by paralysis of facial muscles. Analgesic blocking central to the site of neuropathy arrests the pain.

Herpes zoster can be particularly difficult to distinguish from superficial somatic pain unless the typical lesions are present also. Cutaneous herpetic lesions are usually recognized because they occur in the neuroanatomic peripheral distribution of the affected nerve exactly where the pain is felt. The intraoral mucosal lesions of trigeminal and geniculate herpes zoster, however, may be confused with aphthous ulcers. As such, the lesions may be thought to cause the pain. When herpetic lesions are absent, go unnoticed, or are misdiagnosed, leaving only the persistent neuritic pain, diagnosis may be extremely difficult. Perhaps the best criterion is that analgesic blocking does not arrest the pain. If the condition persists more than a few weeks, a diagnosis of postherpetic neuralgia is indicated.

The primary superficial somatic pains felt in the cutaneous and mucogingival tissues of the orofacial area need to be distinguished from the following:

1. Heterotopic referred pains, projected pains, secondary hyperalgesias, and autonomic effects that occur secondary to deep somatic pain and neuropathic pains
2. Systemic illness
3. Heterotopic pains of central origin
4. Pains related to psychologic conditions

Therapeutic Options

For the management of primary superficial somatic pains arising from the cutaneous and mucogingival tissues of the orofacial area, the following are therapeutic options (see Chapter 9):

1. Analgesics for palliative relief and counseling
2. Cause-related therapy
   a. Identification and treatment of etiologic factors and contributing conditions present
   b. Elimination of all oral irritants
   c. Restriction of oral function within reasonable limits
   d. Antibiotics and antimicrobials, topical and systemic
   e. Antiviral agents, especially for initial episodes[20]
   f. For xerostomia: elimination or reduction of saliva-depressing drugs; chewing paraffin or gum to stimulate salivary flow; saliva substitutes; and electric stimulation of saliva.
3. Pharmacologic therapy
   a. Topical anesthetics (liquid, ointment, lozenge)
   b. Analgesic balms
   c. Anti-inflammatory agents
4. Medical consultation

References

1. Ochea JL, Torebjork HE. Pain from skin and muscle. Pain 1981; 11:87.

2. Bonica JJ. The Management of Pain, ed 2. Philadelphia: Lea & Febiger; 1990: 169–174.

3. Wolff HG. Headache and Other Head Pain, ed 2. New York: Oxford University Press; 1963: 35–46.

4. Fields HL. Pain. New York: McGraw-Hill; 1987: 79–97.

5. Savage NW. Oral ulceration: Assessment and treatment of commonly encountered oral ulcerative disease. Aust Fam Physician 1988; 17: 247–250.

6. Dolby AE. Recurrent aphthous ulceration: Effect of sera and peripheral blood lymphocytes upon oral epthelial culture cells. Immunology 1969; 17:709–714.

7. Rogers RS, Movius DL, Pierre R. Lymphocyte-epithelial cell interactions in oral mucosal inflammatory disease. J Invest Dermatol 1976; 67:599–602.

8. Wright A, Ryan FP, Willingham SE, et al. Food allergy or intolerance in severe recurrent aphthous ulceration of the mouth. Br Med J 1986; 292:1237–1238.

9. Nolan A, Lamey PJ, Milligan KA, Forsyth A. Recurrent aphthous ulceration and food sensitivity. J Oral Pathol Med 1991; 20:473–475.

10. Ferguson MM, Carter J, Boyle P. An epidemiological study of factors associated with recurrent aphthae in women. J Oral Med 1984; 39:212–217.

11. Wray D, Ferguson JM, Hutcheon AW, Dagg JH. Nutritional deficiencies in recurrent aphthae. J Oral Pathol 1978; 7:418–423.

12. Miller C. Diagnosis and management of acute disorders of the oral mucosa. In Falace DA (ed): Emergency Dental Care. Philadelphia: Lea & Febiger; 1994: 304–306.

13. Ades AE, Peckhan CS, Dale FE et al. Prevalence of antibodies to herpes simplex virus types 1 and 2 in pregnant women, and estimated rates of infection. J Epidemiol Community Health 1989; 43:53–60.

14. Gibson JJ, Hornung CA, Alexander GR, et al. A cross-sectional study of herpes simplex virus types 1 and 2 in college students: Occurrence and determinants of infection. J Infect Dis 1990; 162:306–312.

15. Spear PG. Glycoproteins specified by herpes simplex virus. In Roizman B, ed: The Herpesviruses, vol 3. New York: Plenum Press; 1983: 315–356.

16. Darlington RW, Moss H. Herpesvirus envelopment. J Virol 1968; 2:48–55.

17. Rapp F. Virus replication. In Stringfellow DA (ed): Virology: A Scope Publication. Kalamazoo, Mich: Upjohn; 1983: 21.

18. Spruance SL, Overall JC, Kern ER, et al. The natural history of recurrent herpes simplex labialis: Complications for antiviral thearpy. N Engl J Med 1977; 197:69–75.

19. Young SK, Rowe NH, Buchanan RA. A clinical study for the control of facial mucocutaneous herpes virus infections: I. Characterization of natural history in a professional school population. Oral Surg Oral Med Oral Pathol 1976; 41:498–507.

20. Corey L, Spear PG. Infection with herpes simplex viruses. N Engl J Med 1986; 314:749–757.

21. Grushka M, Sessle BJ. Burning mouth syndrome: A historical review. Clin J Pain 1987; 3:245–252.

22. Grad H, Grushka M, Yanover L. Drug-induced xerostomia: The effects and treatments. J Can Dent Assoc 1985; 51:296–300.

23. Binnie W, Wright JM. Oral mucosa disease in the elderly. In Cohen B, Thomson H (eds): Dental Care for the Elderly. London: William Heinemann Medical Books; 1986: 40–81.

24. Fox PC, Vander Van PF, Sonies BC, et al. Xerostomia: Evaluation of a symptom with increasing significance. J Am Dent Assoc 1985; 110:519–523.

25. Zegarelli DJ. Burning mouth: An analysis of 57 patients. Oral Surg Oral Med Oral Pathol 1984; 58:34–38.

26. Grushka M, Sessle BJ, Miller R. Pain and personality profiles in burning mouth syndrome. Pain 1987; 28:155–167.

27. Grushka M, Sessle BJ, Howley TP. Psychophysical assessment of tactile, pain, and thermal sensory function in burning mouth syndrome. Pain 1987; 28:169–184.

28. Gorsky M, Silverman S Jr, Chinn H. Burning mouth syndrome: Review of 98 cases. J Oral Med 1987; 42:7–9.

29. Quinn JH. Glossodynia. J Am Dent Assoc 1965; 70:1418–1421.

30. Weiss WW, Brenman HS, Katz P, et al. Use of an electric stimulator for the treatment of dry mouth. J Oral Maxillofac Surg 1986; 44:845–850.

11

Pains of Dental Origin

In a recent survey of 45,711 American households, Lipton et al[1] found that nearly 22% of the general population had experienced at least one of five types of orofacial pain in the previous 6 months. The most common type of orofacial pain was toothache, which was reported by 12.2% of the population. Because toothache is so common, it is essential for the clinician who is managing orofacial pain to have a thorough understanding of its clinical presentation. Once proper diagnosis is established, treatment for pains of dental origin are usually quite reliable.

The teeth are unique structures in that they are visceral tissues that function as part of the musculoskeletal system. This, perhaps, helps to explain some of the enigmatic behavior of dental pain. Tooth pulps serve as isolated organs, each an individual in its own right. The sensory capabilities of dental pulpal tissue are like those of other visceral structures as well as pulpal pain is like that of other visceral pains. The connection of the teeth to the bone, however, is a true joint and therefore constitutes a musculoskeletal structure. This fibrous joint, called the *periodontal ligament*, is constructed in such a manner as to convert masticatory

pressure into traction on the alveolar bone. These joints, termed *gomphosis*, are structurally similar to other fibrous joints in which tractive forces predominate. The mechanoreceptors in periodontal ligaments are similar to those of other fibrous joints, although they differ considerably from the proprioceptors of synovial joint ligaments, tendons, and muscles.[2] Their nerve cell bodies are located in the mesencephalon along with the other masticatory proprioceptors. They serve to inhibit the action of elevator muscles, which constitutes the driving force of masticatory function.[3-5] The uniqueness of teeth and their alveolar attachment is that visceral structures function as an integral segment of the musculoskeletal system. The sensory behavior, including dental pain, constitutes a mixture of visceral and musculoskeletal characteristics (Fig 11-1).

While facial sensory input is represented almost exclusively in the subnucleus caudalis, nociceptive signals from the oral cavity have double representation in the subnucleus oralis and caudalis.[6] Periodontal afferent fibers terminate in the rostrally located main sensory trigeminal nucleus. The tooth pulp afferents, however, terminate there as well as in all three subnuclei of the

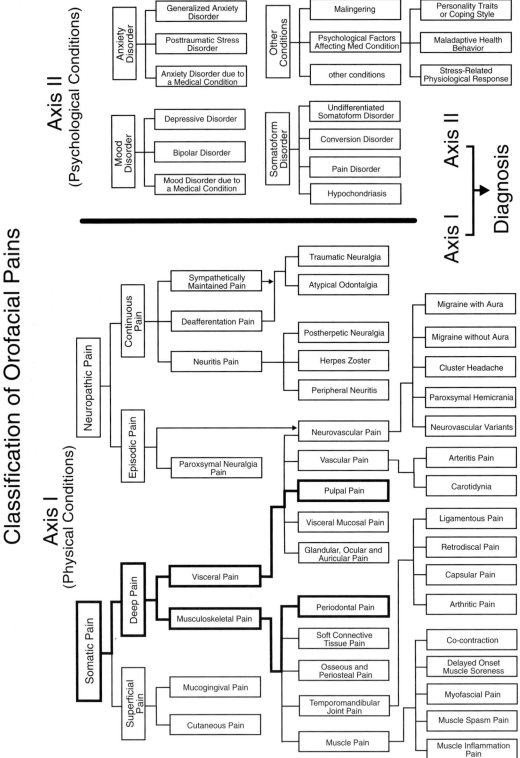

Fig 11-1 Pain classification chart highlighted to show the relationship of pulpal dental pain to other visceral pains and of periodontal dental pain to other musculoskeletal pains.

spinal tract of the trigeminal nucleus complex.[7]

Dentin sensibility is mediated by way of the pulpal nerves. The intradental neural mechanism of this innervation is not yet known. Several theories have been offered: (1) the odontoblast-receptor theory, (2) the direct nerve ending theory, and (3) the hydrodynamic theory.[8] It is known that many if not all nociceptive impulses from human dental pulps are conducted to the trigeminal nucleus by way of sympathetic visceral afferents that leave the head and reach the spinal cord through elements of the cervical sympathetic chain and upper thoracic spinal nerves.[9]

The unique innervation of teeth is pointed out by the report of two patients with cancer who had undergone trigeminal trachotomy along with rhizotomy of the ninth and tenth cranial nerves and of several cervical spinal nerves to control intractable face pain. Both patients displayed analgesia or hypalgesia throughout the cutaneous trigeminal distribution; yet they continued to maintain normal sensory response to dental pulp stimulation.[10]

The sensory capabilities of the dental pulp are predominantly but not exclusively nociceptive.[11] The dental pulp also senses thermal stimuli and tingling.[12] It has been determined that, under specially controlled circumstances, pulpal receptors may give rise to nonnociceptive impulses that have some sensory function other than the mediation of painful sensation.[13] It is thought that nonpain sensations of the pulp are mediated by a distinct population of afferents that are not nociceptive.[14] The pulp contains both fast and slowly conducting neurons.[15] There is conclusive evidence for the presence of a significant C-fiber population in tooth pulps that can be activated by electrical stimulation.[16] The innervation density of the dental pulp is calculated to be about 15 times that of skin.[17] The mediation of sensory impulses from the dental pulp to the subnucleus caudalis as well as to the more rostrally located subnucleus oralis has been confirmed.[18,19]

The teeth are united to the alveolar bone by fibrous joints, the periodontal ligaments comprising the flexible, fibrous portions. The collagenous fibers that connect the cementum to the alveolar cortex are arranged in an oblique fashion to convert the pressures entailed in masticatory strokes into traction forces on the bone. The sensory receptors include free nerve endings and mechanoreceptors. When stimulated by pressure on the tooth, the mechanoreceptors exert inhibitory influence on masticatory elevator muscle action.[20,21] It should be noted that sensory innervation of the teeth is strictly ipsilateral.[22] Except for pain emanating from midface structures, sensory manifestations from the oral cavity are not expressed contralaterally or bilaterally.

Behavior of Dental Pains

It should be recognized that dental pains are extremely versatile and have the propensity to mimic nearly any pain disorder. The degree of such pain may vary from mild tenderness to unbearable intensity. Dental pain may be spontaneous or it may be induced in various ways. It can be intermittent, with periods between attacks that are wholly pain-free. It may be continuous but punctuated by lancinating exacerbations that radiate throughout the face and head. *The extreme variability of toothache is such that a good rule for any examiner is to consider all pains about the mouth and face to be of dental origin until proved otherwise.* An adequate dental examination is the essential first step in the management of all pain disorders involving the teeth, mouth, and face.

Despite such variability, pains of dental origin present clinical features that categorize them as deep somatic pain. It is on the basis of these features that the examiner is able to clinically classify such pains.

Quality of Pain

The basic background discomfort of odontogenous pain is a dull, depressing quality characteristic of all pain that emanates from deep body structures. This feature should not be confused with pain intensity or its temporal behavior.

Dental pain is usually described as an aching sensation, sometimes throbbing. When mild, it may be felt only as a tenderness or soreness. When severe, it may have a burning quality. The basic background aching pain may be punctuated by momentary repeated lancinating pains that radiate widely. Such effects are not true paroxysms but short sudden exacerbations of otherwise steady pain. Dental pains may occur spontaneously or be induced by a variety of stimuli such as thermal changes, contact with sweets and other foods and liquids, or by touch or pressure. Dental pains may be momentary or protracted. They may be continuous or intermittent.

Localization

Pain arising solely from the dental pulp is very poorly localizable by the patient. It frequently is difficult for him or her to determine whether the offending tooth is mandibular or maxillary, much less which tooth is involved. The pain is felt diffusely in the teeth, jaws, face, and head.

Pain arising from the periodontal structures, however, is quite readily localizable by the patient, especially when the offending tooth is touched or pressed. This feature may be in addition to otherwise widespread diffuse pain throughout the jaws and face and may require diagnostic manipulation. It is not unusual for the patient to question the validity of this means of locating the offending tooth when he or she feels the pain so diffusely elsewhere. In fact, the patient may be mistaken as to which tooth is being pressed by the examiner. Yet, localization from periodontal receptors is accurate enough to make this a dependable means of diagnosis.

Localization of odontogenous pain depends on whether the pain emanates solely from pulpal sources, periodontal sources, or both.

Relationship of Dental Pain to Initiating Stimulus

The relationship between dental pain and noxious stimulation is accurate in that summation effects are not observed. Since pulpal receptors answer all noxious stimulation as pain, there may be considerable variation in threshold level for different types of stimulation such as thermal, electric, and mechanical. Subthreshold stimulation is painless. The apparent delay between application of the irritant and pain reaction is not central summation as seen in neuralgia, but rather the time required for the stimulation to reach threshold level.

Although accurate, the relationship between stimulus and pain reaction is not necessarily proportional. A moderate stimulus may induce pain that is disproportionate to it. Thus, the discomfort incurred does not indicate the seriousness of its cause.

Types of Dental Pains

Dental pains may have their origin in the dental pulps or the periodontal structures. These two categories will be discussed separately since their clinical presentations are different.

Dental Pains of Pulpal Origin

The visceral character of pulpal pain is displayed particularly in its clinical behavior. The pain is of the threshold type, as compared with the graduated response exhibited by musculoskeletal pain. No response occurs until the threshold level is reached. Pulpal pain responds to noxious stimulation that is unrelated to ordinary masticatory movements. It responds to impact, shock, thermal and chemical irritants, and direct exploration, but not to ordinary masticatory function. The pain is nearly nonlocalizable by the subject.

Pulpal pains may be classified as acute, chronic, recurrent, or mixed with periodontal elements. A basic clinical feature of pulpal pain is that it does not remain the same indefinitely. Generally it resolves, becomes

Fig 11-2 Radiograph showing rampant caries and extensive periodontal disease. Such a situation presents several possible causes of odontogenous pain, pulpal and periodontal.

chronic, or proceeds to involve the periodontal structures by direct extension through the apex of the tooth root. Rarely does it remain unchanged for long periods.

Acute Pulpal Pain. Perhaps the most typical of all visceral pains is *acute pulpal pain.* It is so completely nonlocalizable by the patient that its source often cannot be determined subjectively. Objective evidence such as deep caries, erosion into the pulp chamber or root canal, or fracture or splitting may immediately identify the offending tooth. If such evidence is lacking and, especially, if more than a single tooth could be involved (Fig 11-2), clinical identification of the offending tooth may be difficult if not impossible.

The cause of acute pulpal pain is noxious stimulation of the pulpal receptors. Normally, tooth structure protects these nerve endings from superficial stimulation so that only extreme surface irritation such as electric stimulation or extremes of thermal change is sensed as pain. If the tooth structure is breached by splitting, a normal pulp

239

may immediately become painful on contact with saliva or air. This occurs especially when masticatory stress tends to open the split. If the tooth structure is breached by fracture from a submerged metallic filling, pain results from pressure exerted against the pulp and is increased when additional pressure is brought to bear on the filling by biting against it. Until the pulp becomes inflamed, pain from such cause is intermittent.

The pulp tissue responds to injury whether it be from repeated threshold stimulation of the intact surface, cervical exposure due to gingival recession, repeated irritation of occlusal trauma, breaching of the overlying protective tooth structure due to splitting or fracture, repeated thermal shocks transmitted by metallic fillings, thinning of the overlying tooth structure by erosion or abrasion, traumatic shock, or dental caries. The changes that take place are usually inflammatory. These conditions may be reversible unless congestion occurs and causes pulpal necrosis or gangrene. Once tissue death occurs, extension to the periodontal tissue through the apical foramen of the root almost invariably takes place. This is especially true if the pulpal inflammation is caused by bacteria. In multirooted teeth, irreversible pulpal changes may occur in one root, with reasonably normal pulp tissue surviving in another. Situations of this type may not occur frequently, but when they do, a confusing symptom picture may result.

The pulpal pains that result from such tissue changes should be understood. As a rule, the pain threshold of all deep receptors and nerve fibers that mediate pain is lowered by inflammation. Thus, the inflamed dental pulp is hypersensitive to all stimuli, including electric stimulation, thermal shock, probing, and percussion. Pain may be elicited by the application of some or all such stimuli to the tooth. If the tissue change is not too great, application of such stimuli causes pain only for the duration of the noxious stimulation. But if the change is greater, such stimulation may induce a prolonged toothache. As the inflammatory process progresses, spontaneous toothache may occur with no outside provocation.

Acute pulpal pain may range from occasional hypersensitivity caused by sweets and other minor stimulants to spontaneous, violent, throbbing toothache of intolerable intensity that cannot be controlled even with narcotic analgesics. It may be induced by many types of irritants or be wholly spontaneous. It may be increased by both heat and cold or increased by heat and relieved by cold. It may be intermittent or continuous. It may relate to the contact of teeth or to the presence or temperature of foods and beverages. It may be mistaken for sinus headache, sinusitis, earache, neuritis, trigeminal neuralgia, or atypical facial pain. It may induce referred pains, areas of secondary hyperalgesia almost anywhere in the face and head, localized autonomic symptoms, and secondary painful masticatory muscle co-contraction. It may induce a masticatory muscle disorder or be mistaken for temporomandibular arthritis. If the pulpal inflammation is great enough to cause severe, continuing toothache, the chance of resolution is extremely low. Under favorable circumstances, resolution does occur. Usually the condition progresses to pulpal necrosis. When this occurs, pain from the pulpal tissue ceases. Such recovery from severe toothache should be interpreted as the transition period from pulpal to periodontal involvement. This transition is extremely variable. If the pulpal inflammation is due to infection, the transition is usually rapid and consists of mixed pulpal and periodontal pains at first and terminates as an acute periodontal abscess (Fig 11-3). If the pulpal inflammation is sterile, all pain may cease, and a painless periapical granuloma or radicular cyst may develop (Fig 11-4). All gradations between these extremes may occur. If a multirooted tooth is involved, one root may exhibit symptoms of acute pulpitis, whereas another may show evidence of pulpal necrosis and periapical abscess (Fig 11-5). When this occurs, the symptom picture can become confusing.

Chronic Pulpal Pain. Under certain conditions, injured pulpal tissue may progress from an acute to a chronic inflammatory phase and thus undergo changes that proceed neither to resolution nor to necrosis but remain indefinitely as what is usually described as *chronic pulpitis*. The condition that favors this transition is traumatic injury to a young tooth, especially one with an open expansive root end that is less likely to facilitate congestion and necrosis of the pulp. Such teeth continue to respond to the pulp tester even though considerably less responsive than those with normal pulps. Frequently, internal resorption of the tooth occurs (Fig 11-6).

When chronic pulpitis develops, the pain responses change from the extremely variable character of acute pulpal pain to a milder and less variable discomfort that may not be described as pain at all (Fig 11-7). In fact, the tooth may become symptomless unless further injury to it takes place.

Recurrent Pulpal Pain. Severe acute pulpal pain is rarely recurrent in the true sense

Fig 11-3 Radiograph showing early periapical radiolucent change (mandibular second molar) indicative of periapical abscess. This tooth was split mesiodistally and had elicited recurrent acute pulpal pains on several occasions. As periapical tissues became involved, both pulpal and periodontal pain could be identified. Early in its clinical course, the first molar was suspected due to the large amalgam restoration.

Fig 11-4 Radiograph showing an extensive apical radiolucency involving the mandibular anterior teeth. The four incisors were slightly discolored and nonresponsive to thermal and electric stimulation. The condition was painless. The history was that of former trauma and acute pulpal pain that soon subsided.

241

Fig 11-5 Radiograph showing periapical radiolucent change involving the mesial root of the mandibular first molar tooth. Clinical symptoms were those of typical pulpal pain and acute periodontal pain occurring simultaneously in the tooth.

Fig 11-6 Radiograph showing central radiolucency in the maxillary central incisor tooth, indicative of internal resorption. The tooth had a normal color and responded positively to electric pulp testing but considerably less than the adjacent teeth. The patient was a 32-year-old man. There was history of trauma to his tooth 16 years previously, followed by a toothache that promptly subsided. Presently the tooth is nonsymptomatic.

Fig 11-7 Radiograph showing apical and periapical radiolucency of the maxillary central incisors. Both had a normal color and responded positively to electric pulp testing but considerably less so than the adjacent teeth. Both teeth, especially the right incisor, were described as vaguely uncomfortable, but not painful.

because the inflammation usually goes either to resolution, chronicity, or necrosis. When acute pulpal pain appears to be recurrent, it usually consists of recurring periods of inflammation in a sequential pattern.

This may occur when a partially split tooth is opened only by some unusual occlusal stress. Real *recurrent pulpal pain* ordinarily does not cause a toothache but is sensed as recurrent hypersensitivity. Such conditions

242

Fig 11-8 Radiograph showing periodontal radiolucency involving the distal root of the mandibular second molar tooth. There is extensive interradicular involvement and deep surface resorption into the mesial aspect of the distal root. Clinically, the tooth had symptoms indicative of a chronic periodontal abscess with more recent symptoms of acute pulpitis. The tooth was responsive to electric pulp testing.

are frequently associated with changes in vascular pressure or fluid balance. So-called menstrual toothache and high-altitude toothache fall into this category. The offending tooth is usually slightly inflamed, and the lowered pain threshold becomes symptomatic when the proper environmental conditions prevail. Other instances of recurrent pulpal pain include hypersensitive teeth that are stimulated to the point of pain by such factors as sweets, thermal changes, and occlusal abuse.

When the transition from pulpal inflammation through necrosis to periapical involvement is rapid, symptoms of both pulpal and periodontal pain may occur. Conversely, when the dental pulp becomes secondarily involved by direct extension from the periodontal structures, mixed symptoms may be evident (Fig 11-8). Also, especially as a result of trauma, both pulpal and periodontal symptoms may occur simultaneously. In all such instances, the cause usually is obvious and the symptoms readily explained. However, a tooth can present with pulpal and periodontal symptoms due to separate and independent causes, and if so, the symptom picture may be confusing. This can occur especially in multirooted teeth. Also, nearby teeth may be simultaneously involved and have symptoms that are misleading to examiner and patient alike (Fig 11-9).

Obscure Causes of Pulpal Pain. There are several fairly common causes of pulpal pain that are clinically difficult to recognize. Perhaps the most common of these is the mesiodistally split tooth, the margins of which are obscured by adjacent teeth and the presence of which is not radiographically visible. Another common cause is an occlusal filling that is slightly dislodged in a pulpal direction. Recurrent caries obscured both clinically and radiographically by an overlying dental restoration may be the cause. Still another cause is mechanical abrasion of the root of a tooth due to the presence of an adjacent impacted tooth (Fig 11-10). Abrasions can penetrate the substance of the root until the contents of the root canal are exposed. Another very obscure cause of pulpal involvement is direct extension from a periodontal pocket via an aberrant lateral root canal. Hematogenous infection of the dental pulp has been reported.

All such possibilities should be considered and explored when pain appears to be truly odontogenous but the cause is oba b

Fig 11-9 Radiographs showing reasonable cause for pulpal and periodontal pain in adjacent teeth. *(a)* The maxillary second premolar shows periapical radiolucency; the first molar has extensive dental caries. *(b)* There is evidence of recurrent caries beneath the mesial filling in the mandibular second molar; the distal root of the first molar shows slight but definite periapical involvement.

Fig 11-10 Radiograph of an impacted maxillary third molar that had abraded into the root of the second molar. The patient presented with symptoms of acute pulpal pain emanating from the second molar. The tooth was sacrificed. The abraded area involved the nerve canal of the distobuccal root.

more radical approach, which may be extracting such a tooth on a presumptive diagnosis. Endodontic measures can be used to salvage the tooth if a mistake is made.

Identifying Pulpal Pain. The examiner should suspect pain as being of pulpal origin when it is difficult for the patient to precisely localize it to a certain tooth. A thorough dental examination becomes mandatory. Obvious possible sources of the pulpal pain should be investigated first. This would include such conditions as primary caries, recurrent caries, defective fillings, cervical exposure, erosion, abrasion, split or fractured teeth, and deep or massive dental restorations, as indicated by clinical and radiographic findings. When a suspicious tooth is located, an attempt to induce or increase the pain by noxious stimulation of that tooth by chemical, thermal, mechanical, or electric irritants should be made. If pain is induced by applying heat to the tooth, cold should be applied to see whether the pain is relieved. The examiner

scure. Occasionally, direct exploration of the tooth is justified if the pain is severe and the patient unwilling to wait for natural localization. The risk of opening an innocent dental pulp may be justified to establish a positive diagnosis. This is better than the should carefully isolate the tooth with celluloid strips when applying thermal or electric irritants to prevent conduction to an adjacent tooth, especially if contacting metallic fillings are present. If the pain can be influenced by local irritation, the tooth should be anesthetized locally to see whether anesthesia promptly and completely arrests the pain and prevents stimulation by applied irritants. If such is the case, the offending tooth has been satisfactorily identified.

With no lead as to which tooth is the source of pain (if indeed it is a tooth at all), the examiner is obliged to be suspicious of every tooth on the side on which there is pain, maxillary and mandibular. Each tooth should be tested by inspection, probing, palpation, percussion, thermal shocking, and electric stimulation to determine whether one tooth is considerably more responsive than others. Systematic analgesic blocking should be done, first to determine whether the pain site is maxillary or mandibular, and second to more accurately identify the offending teeth.

Broad conclusions can be drawn as to whether the pain arises from maxillary or mandibular structures. If analgesic blocking fails to arrest the pain promptly and completely for the duration of anesthesia, a conclusion that the pain does not arise from dental structures is justified. If such blocking is accurately effective, the conclusion that the pain is initiated in structures thus anesthetized is usually correct, but it does not necessarily follow that the pain is in fact odontogenous.

If the pain is shown to arise from the dental area but a particular tooth cannot be identified as the offending source, it is wise to wait for pain localization to occur through the process of transition from pul-

Fig 11-11 Radiograph of extensive dental caries involving the maxillary second molar distally. The patient presented with symptoms of acute pulpal pain without evident clinical cause. Although extensive, the carious lesion was obscured clinically by the third molar.

pal to periodontal pain, as previously discussed. Eventually, localized tenderness should identify the proper tooth, probably within a few days or weeks.

Radiographic examination does not identify the source of pulpal pain other than to give clues as to its cause (Fig 11-11). Electric pulp testing has value when performed with other forms of pulpal stimulation but has very limited value by itself. The history, descriptive characteristics, and clinical behavior are extremely important in the diagnosis of pulpal pain. Recognition of secondary excitatory effects is essential, and the importance of an understanding of how such effects relate to the primary pain source cannot be overemphasized. This is especially true regarding secondary painful muscle spasms.

Dental Pains of Periodontal Origin

Periodontal pain is deep somatic pain of the musculoskeletal type. As such, it is more lo-

Fig 11-12 Radiograph of the mandibular first molar showing extensive radiolucency around tooth roots. The tooth was in "traumatic" occlusion.

calized than is pulpal (visceral) pain. It is intimately related to biomechanical (masticatory) function. It responds to provocation proportionately and in graduated increments rather than as a threshold response like pulpal pain.

The receptors of the periodontal ligament are capable of rather precise localization of the stimulus. Therefore, periodontal pain of all types presents no real diagnostic problem because the proper offending tooth is readily identified. This is true whether the pain is in the apical area of the periodontal ligament (usually designated as periapical pain) or in the lateral region of the tooth. This ability of the periodontal receptors to accurately localize the pain source characterizes all periodontal pains and prevents the uncertainty and mystery attendant with acute pulpal pains, as previously discussed.

Such localization is identified by applying pressure to the tooth laterally or axially. Under the load of occlusal pressure during chewing, the tooth feels sore or elongated. The discomfort may sometimes be felt when the biting pressure is released rather than while it is sustained. Lateral or axial pressure may be applied to the tooth by the examiner as part of his or her clinical examination.

The causes of periodontal pain are many and varied. It may occur as a primary periodontal inflammatory condition due to a local cause such as trauma, occlusal overstressing (Fig 11-12), or contact with an adjacent embedded tooth. It may occur as a result of dental prophylaxis, endodontic treatment, orthodontic therapy, preparation and manipulation of teeth for restoration, inadequate opposing occlusal contact, occlusal interference, overcontoured or undercontoured proximal contact areas, stresses applied to abutment teeth, and surgical interference of all types. It may result from a spreading inflammatory reaction incidental to nearby trauma or the healing of surgical wounds. It may occur as an acute inflammation of a preexistent chronic periodontal lesion as a result of infection, injury, food impaction, or lowered resistance (Fig 11-13). It may spread from pulpal inflammation either directly through the apical root canal and cause a typical periapical abscess (Fig 11-14) or through an aberrant lateral root canal and cause a lateral periodontal abscess. It may occur by direct extension from a nearby inflammatory condition involving an adjacent tooth (Fig 11-15), the maxillary antrum, or a spreading osseous infection (Fig 11-16).

When the periodontal pain involves several teeth, especially opposing teeth, the matter of occlusal overstressing should be considered. This may occur with little or no evidence of gross disease. Overstressing not only from occlusal interference but from clenching and bruxism may occur.

Fig 11-13 Radiographs showing periodontal lesions of various types. (a) Deep periodontal pocket associated with elongation of the maxillary second premolar. (b) Buccally located periodontal lesion involving the mandibular first molar. (c) Interradicular lesion involving the mandibular first molar. (d) Extensive generalized periodontal disease.

11-13a

11-13b

11-13c

11-13d

With multirooted teeth, one root may be periapically or periodontally involved while another shows symptoms of pulpal pain. These circumstances can certainly confuse the clinician. Sometimes the location of the electrode of the pulp tester on the tooth may give some indication of the conditions present.[23] Radiographic evidence may help in diagnosis.

Tooth Pain from Deficient Central Inhibition

All conditions that alter the effectiveness of the endogenous antinociceptive system may permit ordinarily nonnociceptive impulses to be transmitted and felt as pain. As a result, teeth may become unduly sensitive or actually painful. They may hurt when

Fig 11-14 Radiograph showing periapical radiolucency involving the maxillary central incisor. This condition followed pulpal inflammation.

Fig 11-15 Radiograph of the maxillary incisor area showing diffuse radiolucency centered from the incisors. The central and lateral incisors had been injured several years earlier.

Fig 11-16 Radiograph of the mandibular incisor area showing diffuse radiolucency due to spreading osseous infection.

touched, moved, pressed, stressed through occlusal use, or subjected to stimulants such as tooth brushing, flossing, thermal changes, or ingestion of sweets. In such situations, many or all of the teeth may become painful. Multiple toothaches without adequate local dental cause should be a warning sign.

Secondary Effects of Dental Pain

Being of the deep somatic category, odontogenous pain has the propensity to induce a variety of secondary central excitatory effects. Most acute dental pains have a component of pain that is felt in one or more adjacent teeth of the same arch, in teeth of the opposing arch, or in both. Ordinarily, such heterotopic pain does not cross the midline except when the site of primary pain is located at or close to the midline. Reference to

another major division of the trigeminal nerve usually follows a vertical laminated pattern as discussed in Chapter 4. Referred dental pain is frequently felt as a headache. It may be felt in the orbital and frontal area, in the maxillary sinus region, in the auricular and preauricular parts, or throughout the face. Sometimes, an acute pulpitis will cause pain that radiates throughout the entire face and head with no subjective localization of the primary site at all. The variable, spontaneous, nonlocalizable, and pulsatile qualities of acute pulpal pain together with its secondary effects can imitate almost every known pain disorder of the face and head.

Secondary hyperalgesia is also a common manifestation of dental pain. It may be expressed superficially as an area of touchy gingiva, skin, or scalp. It may be felt as other tender teeth. Deep secondary hyperalgesia sensed as palpable tenderness may be misdiagnosed as an area of inflammation or muscle tenderness. This is likely to involve the temporal and masseter areas especially.

It is not unusual for dental pain to induce secondary autonomic effects expressed as nasal congestion, lacrimation, and puffy swelling of the eyelids or other areas of loose facial skin. Such symptoms may be misdiagnosed as sinusitis or cellulitis.

A myalgia originating in muscles innervated by the trigeminal nerve may be induced by dental pain. Involvement of digastric or mylohyoid muscles may cause symptoms in the floor of the mouth and upper cervical region. If the tensor palatini muscle is involved, palatal soreness, difficulty with swallowing, and eustachian tube symptoms may occur. If the masticatory muscles are involved, a masticatory muscle disorder may result (see Chapter 12). If such a secondarily induced muscle condition develops into a cycling muscle pain, it becomes wholly independent of initiating cause and can remain as a separate clinical entity long after the etiologic factor has disappeared. This will be discussed in detail in Chapter 12.

Perhaps the most confusing complication of dental pain is the induction of myofascial trigger points in muscles innervated by the trigeminal nerve. Such trigger points tend to remain after the initiating pain has disappeared. As such, they can cause an orofacial complaint for long periods, sometimes in a recurrent, episodic pattern. The zone of reference from such a trigger point frequently is at or near the location of the primary pain that initiated it. Thus, continuing pain at the toothache site may be experienced despite adequate dental therapy for the original cause of pain. Clear diagnostic thinking and skillful use of examining techniques may be required to resolve such issues.

Tender Teeth from Nondental Cause

Stimulation-evoked tooth pain that simulates pain of periodontal origin may occur as the result of deep somatic pain input located elsewhere in the trigeminal area. This manifestation of secondary hyperalgesia is a central excitatory effect. It differs from spontaneous toothache due to referred pain in that it is provoked by manipulation or functional activities. As such, it is localized and can be confused with true odontogenous pain of periodontal origin, from which it should be differentiated.

Secondary hyperalgesia expressed as tender teeth is common. It occurs with pharyngeal and nasal mucosal pains in particular. Similar phenomena, however, occur with other dental pains, especially with pulpitis.

The differential diagnosis depends chiefly on a failure to find an adequate local dental cause. Confirmation may be done by analgesic blocking of the site of pain. Primary periodontal pain is arrested while secondary hyperalgesic pain is not.

Toothaches of Nondental Origin

Since dental pain is such a common cause of orofacial pain, the clinician can be easily drawn to this diagnosis. This is especially true when the patient convincingly reports that the pain is felt in a particular tooth. It is a frustrating experience for both the patient and the clinician when toothache continues long after sound dental therapy has been completed. It is not uncommon to hear patients report a history of multiple endodontic procedures followed by an extraction, with no reduction of pain. This type of experience is quite humbling to the dental clinician who is expected to be successful in managing dental pains. The clinician needs to be aware that some pains felt in the teeth do not originate from the dental structures.

There are many structures of the head and neck that can produce heterotopic pains felt in the teeth. These heterotopic pains occur as secondary effects from central sensitization or excitation of the second-order neurons produced by a constant barrage of nociceptive input from deep structures (see Chapter 4). As with any heterotopic pain, this poses a diagnostic problem for the clinician. The patient's chief complaint is toothache but the origin of the pain lies elsewhere. The clinician must have the diagnostic skills to be able to differentiate the site of pain from the source of pain. As discussed in earlier chapters, heterotopic pains are differentiated by local provocation and by the selective use of local anesthetic. When the pain complaint is heterotopic, local provocation of the site of pain fails to increase the pain. Also, local anesthetic placed at the site of pain fails to reduce the pain. These two findings are extremely important in differentiating true dental pain from heterotopic pain felt in a tooth. The clinician should use these diagnostic tests routinely for differentiating dental pain. When toothache is not accentuated by local provocation (ie, cold, hot, percussion, etc), heterotopic pain should be suspected. When there is any question regarding the diagnosis, the offending tooth should be locally anesthetized. If pain is not markedly reduced or eliminated, heterotopic pain should be suspected.

Once heterotopic toothache is suspected, the true source of the pain must be located. It is only with location of the source of pain

that effective therapy can begin. Although pain from many structures of the face can refer to the teeth, there are certain structures that refer pain more commonly; they should be immediately investigated. Common heterotopic toothaches that will be reviewed in this section are: muscular toothache, neurovascular toothache, cardiac toothache, neuropathic toothache, sinus toothache, and psychogenic toothache. Knowing the pain characteristics for each of these disorders is an essential key to diagnosis. Each of these pain disorders will be discussed in detail in later chapters. They are mentioned here to remind the clinician that they may be a source of toothache.

Muscular Toothache. Although all deep pains in the head and neck have the propensity to induce secondary referred pain felt as toothache, those of muscle origin are the most common. The masseter and temporalis muscles are the chief offenders and not uncommonly refer pain to the teeth. The clinical characteristics of a muscular toothache are:

1. Non-pulsatile, more constant aching
2. Not responsive to local provocation of the tooth
3. Pain increasing with function of involved muscle (trigger points)
4. Local anesthesia of the tooth not affecting the toothache
5. Local anesthesia of the involved muscle (trigger points) reducing the toothache

A good understanding of the muscular genesis of pain and of the overall behavior of musculoskeletal pain disorders is prerequisite to good management of such tooth-

Case 1	Heterotopic pain, felt as toothache, referred from the masseter muscle

Chief Complaint	Dull aching pain felt in the left mandibular teeth, jaw, and ear.

History	A 43-year-old woman with mild-to-severe, variable but continuous, dull aching pain diffusely located in the left mandibular teeth, jaw, and ear. The pain is usually worse in the early morning and seems to be aggravated by mandibular movement and use. The complaint began about 2 months ago and has been present ever since. During the 2 months that preceded this complaint, endodontic treatment was completed on the lower left first premolar and a fixed partial denture replacing the lower left second premolar and first molar was fabricated. This prosthesis was occlusally adjusted several times and then remade. The new bridge became loose from the lower second molar abutment and it was at that time the present complaint began. It has continued in spite of recementing the bridge, removing the bridge, temporarily crowning the abutments, treating the second molar endodontically, and using antibiotics.
	There is no history of illness, infection, or trauma. She is medically negative for cause. No medications other than analgesics are presently used.

Examination	**Intraoral:** Clinically and radiographically negative for cause of pain. The lower left first premolar and second molar have temporary crowns. All left mandibular and maxillary teeth not endodontically treated respond normally to electric pulp testing. There is no hyperalgesia of the teeth or gingiva. There is a slight decrease in the comfortable range of mandibular movement.
	TM Joints: Well within normal limits clinically and radiographically.
	Muscles: Acute palpable tenderness in the left masseter muscle.
	Cervical: Within normal limits.
	Cranial Nerves: Within normal limits.
	Diagnostic Tests: Local anesthetic blocking of the left mandibular nerve failed to stop the pain. Analgesic blocking of the left masseter muscle arrested the dental, mandibular, and auricular pain completely.

Impression	Deep somatic myofascial pain emanating from the left masseter muscle is producing a central excitatory effect that is being sensed as referred pain in the left mandible and ear. The initiating cause of the myofascial pain appears to relate to the prior dental experience and likely began as protective co-contraction. There is no evidence that the pain arises from dental or oral causes, nor is it a significant masticatory dysfunction.

Diagnosis	Myofascial pain in the left masseter muscle that is producing a left mandibular "muscular toothache."

ache complaints (Case 1). Muscle pain disorders will be discussed in detail in Chapter 12.

Neurovascular Toothache. Migraine with and without aura may cause pain that is felt as a toothache. Usually no management problem arises because such headaches are readily diagnosed, and additional pains around the face and mouth cause little concern on the part of patient or doctor.

There are, however, some migraine variants (see Chapter 16) that are not well understood and can pose some difficult diagnostic problems. Neurovascular variants, sometimes called migrainous neuralgias, can produce relatively localized pains that present with the clinical characteristic of toothache. Most accompanying toothaches are mistaken for true odontogenous pains and treated as separate entities. Unfortunately, there are several clinical characteristics that can mislead both patient and doctor. The following characteristics are common to neurovascular toothache:

1. The pain is spontaneous, variable, and pulsatile; characteristics that simulate pulpal pain. The toothache is characterized by periods of remission. Episodes of pain may pose a temporal behavior appearing at similar times during the day, week, or month.
2. The pain may follow illness, sinusitis, dental treatment, surgery, or trauma, appearing to be a complication of a former experience.
3. The pain very frequently is felt initially in teeth (the maxillary canine and premolar usually) as a toothache so convincingly that dental treatment may be undertaken without hesitation, even

when only minor dental cause can be located.

4. The pain may undergo remission following dental treatment, although recurrence is characteristic with neurovascular pains. It may spread to adjacent teeth, opposing teeth, or the entire face.
5. If the pain experience is protracted, it may induce autonomic effects manifested as nasal congestion, lacrimation, and edema of the eyelids and face, which may be mistaken for sinusitis or dental abscess.

This rather typical behavior of neurovascular variants should be well appreciated to prevent unnecessary therapy and the accompanying frustration felt by patient and dentist alike. To be suspicious of the presence of neurovascular pain is the key to diagnosis. Dental treatment, even palliative and quite innocuous, may offer the patient reason to blame the dentist for aggravating the problem if not actually initiating it (see Case 16, page 358).

Although the term neurovascular toothache is nondescriptive, it has served to alert the dental profession to an important clinical entity that has been misdiagnosed and mistreated in the past. The absence of other better known clinical characteristics of neurovascular pain has made the diagnosis difficult. The chief indications of this syndrome that mimic real odontogenous toothache are the absence of adequate local dental cause, the tendency for it to be periodic and recurrent, and the patient's ability to precisely locate the painful tooth. Confirming evidence consists of identifying the presence of a neurovascular pain disorder with the use of carotid pressure, ergotamine tartrate testing, or trial therapy. Diagnostic analgesic blocking may yield confusing data because sometimes it reduces the pain, sometimes it does nothing, and sometimes it increases the pain.

Unfortunately, dental therapy often induces a remission of the pain, thereby deluding the dentist into thinking that the condition is in fact a dental one and that a proper treatment has been applied. With recurrence, additional dental therapy may be performed without realizing that it is futile and may be harmful.

Cardiac Toothache. Dentists should be particularly aware of the incidence of jaw and tooth pain that occurs as a secondary manifestation of cardiac pain input.[24] Although other clinical evidence of cardiac distress (such as substernal chest discomfort and left arm and neck pain) is usually present, sometimes the dental symptoms may be the only ones of which the patient complains when he comes to the dentist with what he thinks is a dental problem.[25] Great care should be exercised in such situations. A lack of adequate dental cause for the pain complaint should always be an alerting sign. Failure of analgesic blocking to arrest the pain promptly and completely is confirming evidence that the primary source of pain is not the tooth. It should be noted that anesthesia is usually quite adequate for dental therapy; therefore, unless the question "Does the tooth still hurt?" is asked, the dentist may not be aware that it did not arrest the toothache. In all cases where pain is an issue and analgesic blocking is used, the patient should be carefully questioned about the effectiveness of the maneuver in arresting the pain (Case 2). A complete health history is essential when cardiac toothache

is suspected since immediate referral to proper medical personnel is mandatory. The clinical characteristics of cardiac toothache are:

1. Aching pain is cyclic.
2. Pain is increased with physical exertion or exercise.
3. The toothache is associated with chest pains.
4. The toothache is decreased with nitroglycerin tablets.

Neuropathic Toothache. Pain felt in a tooth may be the result of a projected or referred pain originating in neural structures. These pains may be either episodic or continuous and are classified in that manner.

Episodic neuropathic toothache is characterized by a sudden, sharp, spontaneous pain felt either in a tooth or radiating to a tooth. It is similar to the pain felt in paroxysmal neuralgia and in fact is likely to be related to such a neuropathic pain disorder. Trigeminal neuralgia or tic douloureux may be triggered from the teeth and felt as pain in the teeth. Unfortunately, analgesic blocking arrests the paroxysms of pain and may lead to a mistaken diagnosis of odontogenous pain. Also, dental therapy, especially if a local anesthetic block is used, may induce a remission, thereby leading both patient and dentist to assume that the diagnosis is correct and that proper treatment has been done. When the condition recurs, additional forms of dental therapy may be employed, thus compounding the mistake (see Case 24, page 410). The clinical characteristics of the episodic neuropathic toothache are:

1. Pain is unilateral, severe, lacerating, shock-like (paroxsymal) pain.
2. Pain is provoked by a trigger.

| Case 2 | Heterotopic pain, felt as toothache, referred from the cardiac muscle |

Chief Complaint

Lower left mandibular pain and toothache.

History

A 61-year-old man with mild, continuous but variable, dull aching pain diffusely located in the left mandible and teeth. Mandibular movement did not increase the pain. The pain was preceded by left shoulder discomfort. The shoulder pain began 3 days ago as a variable vague but more or less continuous pain. He went to his physician who diagnosed the complaint as bursitis and initiated some therapy. Two days later, the left "toothache" pain began even though patient had been edentulous for about 20 years. Thinking the mandibular pain stemmed from the dentures, the physician advised a dental examination. His dentist made a dental radiograph of the lower left mandibular area and saw part of a deeply impacted third molar. He was then immediately referred to an oral surgeon for removal of the tooth.

No medications are presently being taken except aspirin for pain.

Examination

Intraoral: A normal appearing edentulous mouth with satisfactory artificial dentures. There is no local hyperemia in the denture-bearing areas. There is no palpable discomfort in the area of the impacted lower third molar nor in the left submandibular triangle. A panoramic radiograph revealed a deeply impacted lower left third molar. This tooth appear to be completely covered with bone, having no coronal radiolucency indicative of dental caries, and exhibiting no osseous changes around the tooth. Mandibular functioning is clinically normal in all respects. There is no dental, oral, or masticatory cause for the complaint.

TM Joints: Clinically normal.

Muscles: Clinically negative for cause of pain.

Cervical: Within normal limits.

Cranial Nerves: Within normal limits.

Diagnostic Tests: Analgesic blocking of the left mandibular nerve did not arrest the pain. Medical consultation advised. Telephone report that electrocardiogram indicated cardiac muscle damage. Medical diagnosis of cardiac pain made.

Impression

The shoulder pain mistaken for bursitis and the mandibular pain mistaken for "toothache" were not associated with appreciable chest discomfort. It is presumed, therefore, that the primary cardiac muscle pain was wholly inhibited and only the secondary central excitatory effects were felt by the patient.

Diagnosis

Cardiac muscle pain referred as mandibular toothache.

3. Local anesthetic at the tooth will not reduce the pain unless it is also the trigger (which is very rare).
4. Local anesthetic at the trigger will reduce the attacks.

Some neuropathic toothaches produce a persistent, ongoing, unremitting pain. These pains may be increased by local provocation such as touching the tooth and surrounding gingiva, which adds confusion to the diagnosis. A key to the diagnosis of *continuous neuropathic toothache* is the presence of other neurologic complaints such as hyperesthesia, hypoesthesia, anesthesia, paresthesia, muscular tics, weakness, and paralysis as well as autonomic and special sense aberrations, depending on the fiber content at the site of neuropathy. The types of neuropathic conditions that can produce continuous pain felt in a tooth are neuritic pains, deafferentation pains, or sympathetically maintained pains.

Neuritic pain (neuritis) arising in the maxillary and mandibular divisions of the trigeminal nerve can cause dental pains along with other neurologic symptoms. Neuritis of the superior dental plexus due to extension from maxillary sinusitis may cause a toothache in and around one or more maxillary teeth. Such pain is persistent, nonpulsatile, and burning. If the accompanying maxillary sinusitis is nonsymptomatic, diagnosis may be difficult. The key usually is to recognize accompanying neurologic signs that involve other teeth or nearby structures served by the same nerve (see Case 25, page 411). A similar toothache in the mandibular teeth may occur as an expression of neuritis of the inferior alveolar nerve from direct trauma, dental sepsis, or surgery (see Case 33, page 450).

Neuropathic pain may arise following an injury such as external trauma, tooth pulp extirpation, simple extraction, or major oral surgery. Such pains are called deafferentation pains and are often mistaken for a posttraumatic or postoperative complication (see Case 32, page 442). Some of these pains may be the result of a neuroma secondary to the nerve trauma. These conditions may present as a phantom toothache and in recent years have been described under the name of atypical odontalgia.[26-29]

Atypical odontalgia is a difficult pain condition that most dentists will sooner or later face. The patient will complain of specific tooth pain and yet there will be no local signs of dental pathosis. Repeated attempts at dental therapy will fail to resolve the pain. The patient and the dentist will often both become quite frustrated and sometimes desperate. Graff-Radford et al[29] have suggested the following identifying criteria for atypical odontalgia:

1. Pain in a tooth or tooth site
2. Continuous or almost continuous pain
3. Pain persisting more than 4 months
4. No sign of local or referred pain
5. Equivocal results of a somatic block

Although much is still unknown regarding the pathophysiology of atypical odontalgia, it appears that the clinical characteristics fit best in the category of deafferentation pain and may or may not be maintained by the sympathetic activity. As with other deafferentation pain, tricyclic antidepressants can be helpful.[27-30] Treatment of deafferentation pains will be presented in Chapter 17.

Sinus or Nasal Mucosal Toothache.

Pain arising from the nasal mucosa as the result of viral or allergic rhinitis is prone to

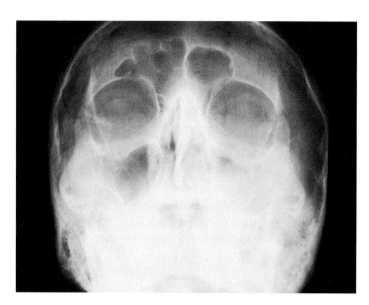

Fig 11-17 Water's view of the maxillary sinus. Note the air/fluid level in the patient's right maxillary sinus. This patient reported right maxillary first molar toothache. (Courtesy of Dr Donald Falace, Lexington, Kentucky.)

be expressed as referred pain throughout the maxilla and maxillary teeth in the form of a toothache. It may also display autonomic signs that are mistaken for symptoms of maxillary sinusitis. The so-called sinus headache may cause management problems because of the tooth pains.

Diagnostically, analgesic blocking by infiltration at the apex of the tooth in question does not arrest the toothache if it is referred from the nasal mucosa. In contrast, topical anesthesia of the nasal mucosa effectively arrests the toothache. Again, suspicion that the dental pain is referred is the key to diagnosis (see Case 19, page 386).

The clinical characteristics of sinus or nasal mucosal toothache are:

1. Pressure below the eyes
2. Increased pain with lowering of the head
3. Increased pain with applied pressure over the involved sinus

4. Local anesthesia of the tooth not eliminating the pain
5. Diagnosis able to be confirmed by air/fluid level seen with appropriate imaging studies (Fig 11-17)

Psychogenic Toothache. On occasion, a patient may report symptoms of toothache that do not appear to fit in any clinical category of orofacial pain. The clinician should always be mindful of somatoform pain disorders. This is a category of mental disorders in which a patient may complain of a physical condition with absolutely no physical signs. This condition may be thought of as a psychogenic toothache. Perhaps this condition is related to an efficiency in the descending inhibitory mechanism or the endogenous antinociceptive system. Somatoform pain disorders felt in the teeth are characterized by:

1. Multiple teeth often reported as painful with frequent changes in character and location of the pain
2. Normal or physiologic patterns of pain not applicable
3. Chronic pattern of pain
4. Lack of response to reasonable dental treatment
5. Not identifiable as any other pain condition

Somatoform pain disorders are mental disorders and are best treated by a qualified psychologist or psychiatrist. The clinician must identify these disorders to avoid unnecessary dental therapies.

Cardinal Warning Symptoms of Nondental Toothache. Toothaches of nondental origin require accurate diagnostic identification of the true source of the patient's pain. The most important step toward proper management is suspicion that the pain is not of dental origin. The cardinal warning symptoms of toothache of nondental origin are[31]:

1. Spontaneous multiple toothaches
2. Inadequate local dental cause for the pain
3. Stimulating, burning, nonpulsatile toothaches
4. Constant, unremitting, nonvariable toothaches
5. Persistent, recurrent toothaches
6. Failure of the toothache to respond to reasonable dental therapy.

Differential Diagnosis

Primary deep somatic pain of dental origin should be distinguished diagnostically from nonodontogenous pains that are felt in the teeth and presented as dental complaints. The following nondental sources of toothache should be considered:

1. Heterotopic referred pains and secondary hyperalgesias as secondary effects of deep pain originating in the following somatic structures: musculoskeletal, vascular, cardiac, or sinus mucosa
2. Neuropathic pains, either continuous or episodic
3. Somatoform pain disorders
4. Heterotopic pains of central origin

Therapeutic Options

For the management of primary deep somatic pains of dental origin, the following therapeutic options are available (see Chapter 9): analgesics for palliative relief and counseling, and cause-related therapy consisting of accurate location of the true source of pain and proper treatment.

References

1. Lipton JA, Ship JA, Larach-Robinson D. Estimated prevalence and distribution of reported orofacial pain in the United States. J Am Dent Assoc 1993; 124:115–121.

2. Willis RD, DiCosimo CJ. The absence of proprioceptive nerve endings in the human periodontal ligament: The role of periodontal mechanoreceptors in the reflex control of mastication. Oral Surg 1979; 48:108–115.

3. Hannam AG. The response of periodontal mechanoreceptors in the dog to controlled loading of the teeth. Arch Oral Biol 1969; 14:781–791.

4. Anderson DJ, Hannam AG, Matthews B. Sensory mechanisms in mammalian teeth and their supporting structures. Physiol Rev 1970; 50:171–195.

5. Cody FW, Lee RW, Taylor A. A functional analysis of the components of the mesencephalic nucleus of the fifth nerve in the cat. J Physiol (Lond) 1972; 226:249–261.

6. Azerad J, Woda A, Albe-Fessard D. Physiological properties of neurons in different parts of the cat trigeminal sensory complex. Brain Res 1982; 246:7–21.

7. de Last A. Reflexes excitable in jaw muscles and their role during jaw function and dysfunction: A review of the literature: Part 11. Central connections of orofacial afferent fibers. J Craniomand Pract 1987; 5:247–253.

8. Krauser JT. Hypersensitive teeth: Part 1. Etiology. J Prosthet Dent 1986; 56:153–156.

9. Gross D. Pain and autonomic nervous system, in Bonica JJ (ed): Advances in Neurology, vol 4. New York: Raven Press; 1974: 93–103.

10. Young RF. Effect of trigeminal tractotomy on dental sensations in humans. J Neurosurg 1982; 56:812–818.

11. Sessle BJ. Is the tooth pulp a "pure" source of noxious input? In Bonica JJ, Liebeskind JC, Albe-Fessard DG (eds): Advances in Pain Research and Therapy, vol 3. New York: Raven Press; 1979: 245–260.

12. Mumford JM, Bowsher D. Pain and protopathic sensibility: A review with particular reference to the teeth. Pain 1976; 2:223–243.

13. Chatrian GE, Fernandes de Lima JM, Lettich E, et al. Electrical stimulation of tooth pulps in humans: II. Qualities of sensation. Pain 1982; 14:233–246.

14. McGrath PA, Gracely RH, Dubner R, et al. Nonpain and nonpain sensations evoked by tooth pulp stimulation. Pain 1983; 15:377–388.

15. Narhi M, Jyvasjarvi E, Hirvonen T, et al. Activities of heat-sensitive nerve fibers in the dental pulp of the cat. Pain 1982; 14:317–326.

16. Narhi M, Virtanen A, Huopaniemi T, et al. Conduction velocities of single pulp nerve fiber units in the cat. Acta Physiol Scand 1982; 116:209–213.

17. Rozza AJ, Beuerman RW. Density and organization of free nerve endings in the corneal epithelium of the rabbit. Pain 1982; 14:105–120.

18. Nord SG. Responses of neurons in rostral and caudal trigeminal nuclei to tooth pulp stimulation. Brain Res Bull 1976; 1:489.

19. Vyklicky L, Keller O, Jastreboff P, et al. Spinal trigeminal tractotomy and nociceptive reactions evoked by tooth pulp stimulation in the cat. J Physiol (Paris) 1977; 73:379–386.

20. Hannam AG, Matthews B, Yemm R. Receptors involved in the response of the masseter muscle in tooth contact in man. Arch Oral Biol 1970; 15:17–24.

21. Sessle BJ, Schmitt A. Effects of controlled tooth stimulation on jaw muscle activity in man. Arch Oral Biol 1972; 17:1597–1607.

22. Wilson S, Fuller PM, Winfrey J. Histochemical evidence for strictly ipsilateral innervation of maxillary canine teeth in cats. Exp Neurol 1980; 70:138–145.

23. Mumford JM. Toothache and Related Pain, ed 2. Edinburgh: Churchill Livingstone; 1976: 174–187.

24. Graham LL, Schinbeckler GA. Orofacial pain of cardiac origin. J Am Dent Assoc 1982; 104:47–48.

25. Batchelder BJ, Krutchkoff DJ, Amara J. Mandibular pain as the initial and sole clinical manifestation of coronary insufficiency: Report of case. J Am Dent Assoc 1987; 115:710–712.

26. Rees RT, Harris M. Atypical odontalgia. Br J Oral Surg 1979; 16:212–218.

27. Brooke RI. Atypical odontalgia. J Oral Surg 1980; 49:196–199.

28. Kreisberg MK. Atypical odontalgia: Differential diagnosis and treatment. J Am Dent Assoc 1982; 104:852–854.

29. Graff-Radford SB, Solberg WK. Atypical odontalgia. J Craniomandib Disord Oral Facial Pain 1992; 6:260–266.

30. Rees RT, Harris M. Atypical odontalgia: Differential diagnosis and treatment. Br J Oral Surg 1988; 16:212–218.

31. Bell WE. Toothaches of nonodontogenic origin. J Calif Dent Assoc 1976; 4:50–58.

12

Pains of
Muscular Origin

Pains of muscular origin are the most frequent cause of discomfort around the head and neck. Since dental pain is the most frequent oral pain, a good rule to follow in the diagnosing of pains around the face and mouth is initially to assume that it is dental until proved otherwise, then muscular until proved otherwise. The possibility of orofacial pain being of muscle origin should be taken into account with every complaint. Even when the primary cause is not muscular, central excitatory effects tend to be expressed in the muscles, which makes this a frequent complication accompanying other sources of pain.

Muscle pain emanates from the skeletal muscles, tendons, and fascia. It is said to result from stretching, forceful or sustained contraction, ischemia, and hyperemia[1] as well as from trauma and inflammatory factors. Some muscle pain arises from the blood vessels within the muscles and fascial sheaths.[2] Myofascial genesis of pain accounts for other discomforts of muscle origin.[3]

Muscle pain usually is felt as a nonpulsatile, variable, aching sensation, sometimes with a boring quality. This more constant background discomfort may escalate to or be punctuated by sharper, more severe lancinating pains occurring both spontaneously and in response to stretching, contraction, manipulation, or manual palpation. Sometimes the pain is no more than a feeling of pressure. At other times it may increase to excruciating intensity. It may be transitory or persistent, constant, intermittent, or recurrent. Its behavior is labile, characterized by suddenness of onset and rapidity of change. It follows no time frame unless it has an inflammatory origin. Accompanying dysfunction may be expressed as tightness and weakness, or it may relate to impairment of muscle function such as stiffness, rigidity, swelling, or shortening. Pain decreases the biting strength of masticatory muscles by 33% to 50%[4] and induces a feeling of muscular weakness. Muscle pain also impairs the proprioceptive feedback mechanism, thus leading to less precise muscle action.[5] Palpable muscle tenderness and the fact that movement and functioning modify the pain and stiffness are clinical indications of the presence of muscle pain.[6]

Myogenous pains of different types may involve muscles of the mouth, face, and neck, the symptom complex depending on the kind, number, and location of muscles

Classification of Orofacial Pains

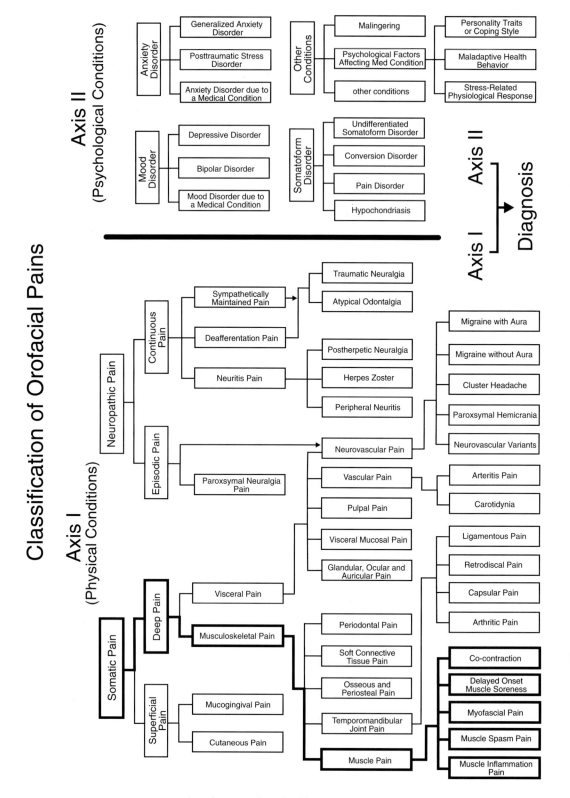

Fig 12-1 Pain classification chart highlighted to show the relationship of muscle pains to other orofacial pain disorders.

involved and the degree to which they are affected. The likelihood of secondary central excitatory effects should be considered. When the primary pain remains relatively silent, the secondary referred pain may constitute most of the complaint. Referred pain from muscles can be the source of considerable diagnostic confusion. For example, more or less silent pain arising in the sternocleidomastoid muscle may be felt in and around the ear as earache or as temporomandibular joint pain. Cardiac muscle pain may be referred to the mandible.

Behavior of Muscular Pain

Myogenous pains that emanate from the orofacial structures are classified as musculoskeletal pains of the deep somatic category (Fig 12-1). The general features exhibited by muscle pain include those of deep somatic pain: the pain has a dull, depressing quality; subjective localization is variable and somewhat diffuse; the site of pain may or may not identify the correct location of the source of pain; response to provocation at the site of pain is fairly faithful in incidence and intensity, but not in location; and central excitatory effects often accompany the pain. To these features are added characteristics peculiar to musculoskeletal pain: the pain relates reasonably to the demands of biomechanical function, and manual palpation at the site of pain, or functional manipulation, effects a graduated response.

The stimulation of skeletal muscle tissue induces a dull, aching pain felt deeply and diffusely in a broad region of the muscle. It is mediated by group III (A-delta fibers) and group IV (C fibers) afferent neurons. A crescendo of intensity indicates some temporal summation.[7] Regardless of the true source of muscle pain, movements that actively stretch the muscle, or increase its isometric tension, increase the patient's awareness of pain. If passive movement is painful, one or more antagonists should be suspected of containing an abnormally tender muscle region.[8]

Muscle pain can originate from any muscle of the head or neck. When muscle pain originates from a muscle that moves the mandible, the pain is considered a masticatory muscle pain. Generally, *masticatory pain* is defined as discomfort around the face and mouth that is induced by chewing and other jaw use but is independent of local disease involving the teeth and oral cavity proper. It describes pain that emanates from the temporomandibular joints and/or masticatory musculature[9] and is therefore a chief complaint of many temporomandibular disorders. Myalgic masticatory pain can be differentiated from arthralgic masticatory pain by manual palpation or functional manipulation and by the use of diagnostic analgesic blocking. As a rule, myalgia displays both dynamic and static pain, while arthralgia displays dynamic pain only.[10]

Types of Masticatory Muscle Pain

All masticatory muscle disorders are not the same clinically. There are at least five different types and being able to distinguish among them is important, because the treatment of each is quite different. The five types are protective co-contraction (muscle splinting), delayed onset muscle soreness (local muscle soreness), myofascial (trigger point) pain, myospasm, and myositis. A sixth condition known as fibromyalgia also needs to be discussed. The first three conditions (protective co-contraction, delayed onset muscle soreness, and myofascial pain) are commonly seen in the dental office. Myospasm and myositis are less frequently seen. Since most of these five masticatory muscle disorders occur and recover in a relatively short period they are generally considered *acute myalgic disorders*. When these conditions are not resolved, more chronic pain disorders may result. Chronic masticatory muscle disorders become more complicated and are generally called *chronic myalgic disorders*. Fibromyalgia is a chronic myalgic disorder that presents as a systemic musculoskeletal pain problem that needs to be recognized by the dentist and is best managed by referral to appropriate medical personnel.

Masticatory Muscle Pain Model

To understand the relationship between different muscle pain disorders, a masticatory muscle pain model[11] will be presented (Fig 12-2). The model begins with the assumption that the muscles of mastication are healthy and functioning normally. Normal muscle function can be interrupted by certain types of events. If an event is significant, a muscle response occurs known as *protective co-contraction (muscle splinting)*. In many instances the consequence of the event is minor and co-contraction quickly resolves allowing muscle function to return to normal. If, however, protective co-contraction is prolonged, local biochemical and later structural changes can occur, creating a condition know as *delayed onset muscle soreness*. Another disorder, myofascial pain,

is related but presents with different clinical characteristics. Both of these disorders may resolve spontaneously or with treatment. If, however, either of these disorders is allowed to continue, dystrophic changes in the muscle tissues may develop. As chronicity is approached, the clinical appearance of the disorders begin to resemble an inflammatory condition known as *myositis*.

In some instances, the central nervous system responds to certain events or local conditions by inducing an involuntary contraction of the muscle called a *myospasm*. Myospasms are not chronic but instead represent a condition of relatively short duration. At one time myospasm was thought to be the primary condition responsible for myalgia. Recent studies[12-15] suggest that true myospasms are not common in patients suffering with masticatory muscle pain.

These masticatory muscle disorders usually present as relatively acute problems and once identified and treated, the muscle returns to normal function. If, however, these acute myalgic disorders are not recognized or appropriately managed, certain perpetuating conditions can advance the problem into a chronic myalgic disorder. One such chronic musculoskeletal pain disorder is *fibromyalgia*. Although this is not primarily a masticatory pain disorder, the dentist needs to recognize this condition to avoid unnecessary dental therapy. The dentist also needs to be aware that chronic pain disorders are managed quite differently than the relatively acute, regional disorders previously mentioned.

To better understand the masticatory muscle pain model, each component of the model will be discussed in detail.

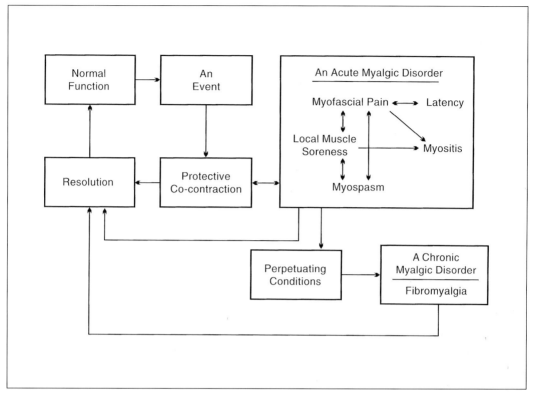

Fig 12-2 A masticatory muscle pain model. This model depicts the relationship between various clinically identifiable muscle pain disorders along with some etiologic considerations. (From Okeson JP. Management of Temporomandibular Disorders and Occlusion, ed 3. St Louis: Mosby Year Book; 1993: 181. Used with permission.)

An Event

Normal muscle function can be interrupted by various types of events. These events can arise from either local or systemic factors. Local factors represent any event that acutely alters sensory proprioceptive input in the masticatory structures; eg, the fracture of a tooth or the placement of a restoration in superocclusion. Trauma to local structures such as tissue damage caused by a dental injection represents another type of local event. Trauma might also arise from excessive or unaccustomed use of masticatory structures, such as chewing unusually hard food or chewing for a long time (ie, gum chewing). Opening too wide may produce a strain to ligaments supporting the joint and/or muscles. This may occur as a result of a long dental procedure or even by simply opening too wide (ie, yawning). Any source of constant deep pain input may also represent a local factor that alters muscle function. This pain input may have its source in local structures such as the teeth, joints, or even the muscles themselves. The source of the pain, however, is not significant since any constant deep pain, even idiopathic pain, may create a muscle response.

Systemic factors may also represent events that can interrupt normal muscle function. One of the most commonly recognized systemic factors is emotional stress.[16,17] Stress seems to alter muscle function through either the gamma efferent system to the muscle spindle or by means of sympathetic activity to the muscle tissues and related structures.[18,19] Of course, responses to emotional stress are quite individualized. Therefore the patient's emotional reaction and psychophysiologic response to stressors may vary greatly.

There are other systemic factors that can influence muscle function that are less understood, such as acute illness or viral infections. Likewise, there is a broad category of poorly understood constitutional factors that are unique to each patient. Such factors include immunologic resistance and autonomic balance of the patient. These factors can influence the response of the patient to various events. Constitutional factors are likely influenced by age, gender, diet, and perhaps even genetic predisposition. Clinicians realize that patients often respond quite differently to similar events. It is assumed therefore that certain constitutional factors do exist and can influence the individual's response. At this time, these factors are poorly understood and not well defined as they relate to muscle pain disorders.

As with local factors, constant deep pain input can represent a systemic factor that may influence muscle function. Although pain is often felt in local structures it may not necessarily have its source in these same structures. As mentioned in previous chapters, pain can be felt not only as a result of peripheral cause, but as a result of a central nervous system (CNS) effect.[20] The central nervous system has the ability to alter pain sensations, both moving toward and away from the cortex.[21,22] If the CNS enhances sensory input, pain may be felt even without organic cause. This pain modulation phenomenon can create a site of pain felt in muscle tissues. One must appreciate, therefore, that this pain modulation phenomenon can represent a systemic event that produces muscle pain and ultimately affects function.

Protective Co-contraction (Muscle Splinting)

The first response of the masticatory muscles to one of the previously described events is protective co-contraction. Protective co-contraction is a CNS response to injury or threat of injury. This response has also been called protective muscle splinting.[23] It has been described for many years, but only recently documented.[24-27] In the presence of an injury or threat of injury, normal sequencing of muscle activity seems to be altered to protect the threatened part from further injury. Protective co-contraction can be compared to the co-contraction[28] observed during many normal functional activities such as bracing the arm when attempting a task with the fingers. In the presence of altered sensory input or pain, antagonistic muscle groups seem to fire during movement in an attempt to protect the injured part. In the masticatory system for example, a patient experiencing co-contraction will demonstrate an increase in muscle activity of the elevator muscles during mouth opening.[25,27] During closing of the mouth, an increased activity is noted in the depressing muscles. This co-activation of antagonistic muscles is thought to be a normal protective or guarding mechanism and needs to be recognized by the clinician. Protective co-contraction is not a pathologic condition, although when prolonged, may lead to myalgic symptoms.

The etiology of protective co-contraction can be any change in sensory or proprioceptive input from associated structures. An example of such an event in the masticatory system is the placement of a high crown. Protective co-contraction can also be caused by any source of deep pain input or an increase in emotional stress.[29–33]

Co-contraction is reported clinically as a feeling of muscle weakness following some event. There is no pain reported when the muscle is at rest but use of the muscle usually increases the pain. The patient often presents with limited mouth opening but, when asked to open slowly, can achieve full opening. The key to identifying co-contraction is that it immediately follows an event and therefore the history is very important. Protective co-contraction only lasts a few days. If it is not resolved, an acute myalgic disorder is likely to follow.

Delayed Onset Muscle Soreness (Local Muscle Soreness)

Delayed onset muscle soreness is a primary, noninflammatory, myogenous pain disorder. It is often the first response of the muscle tissue to prolonged co-contraction. While co-contraction represents a CNS-induced muscle response, delayed onset muscle soreness represents a condition that is charac-terized by changes in the local environment of the muscle tissues. These changes are characterized by the release of certain algogenic substances (ie, bradykinin, substance P) that produce pain. These initial changes may represent nothing more than fatigue. Along with protracted co-contraction, other causes of delayed onset muscle soreness are local trauma or excessive use of the muscle. When excessive use is the cause, a delay in the onset of the muscle soreness can occur. It is common to experience muscular discomfort for several days following unaccustomed use or exercise. The symptoms are muscle stiffness, palpable tenderness, and pain with active muscular contractions. This common muscle pain problem has been a clinical enigma because of the absence of local cellular change indicative of an inflammatory process. The pathophysiology of this condition is not known. Friden et al[34] investigated experimentally induced delayed muscle soreness with histochemical analysis and electron microscopy of the muscle fibers. They found no signs at the cellular level either of ischemic fiber necrosis or fiber rupture. At the subcellular level, however, abnormalities were observed in biopsy specimens obtained 2 days after exercise. At the ultrastructural level, mechanical disruption of the Z-bands that connect adjacent sarcomeres to each other was observed. Type 2 fast-twitch fibers were predominantly affected.[35] These studies support the concept that unaccustomed exercise may overload muscle fibers, which partially distorts their contractile machinery. Later studies indicated that training caused the skeletal musculature to adapt itself in a functional manner to the extensive tension demands put upon it.[36]

When muscle soreness develops in the absence of excessive muscle use, the term *local muscle soreness* has been suggested.[11] Since delayed onset muscle soreness and local muscle soreness are both sources of deep pain, an important clinical event can occur. Deep pain produced by muscle soreness can in fact produce protective co-contraction. This additional co-contraction can, of course, produce more muscle soreness. Therefore, a clinical cycle can be created whereby muscle soreness produces more co-contraction and so on. This condition is called *cyclic muscle pain* and is an important clinical aspect of many muscle disorders.[37]

The clinician needs to be aware of the complications this might create in a diagnosis. For example, trauma occurs to a muscle, producing muscle soreness; the pain associated with the soreness produces protective co-contraction. Since protective co-contraction can lead to muscle soreness, a cycle begins. During this cycling, the original tissue damage produced by the trauma resolves. When tissue repair is complete, the original source of pain is eliminated, however, the patient may continue to suffer with a cyclic muscle pain disorder. Since the original cause of the pain is no longer part of the clinical picture, the clinician can easily be confused during the examination. The clinician needs to recognize that even though the original cause has resolved, a cyclic muscle pain condition exists and needs to be treated. This condition is an extremely common clinical finding and if not recognized often leads to incorrect treatment of the patient.

Delayed onset muscle soreness presents clinically with muscles that are tender to palpation and reveal increased pain with function. Structural dysfunction is common and when the elevator muscles are involved, there is limited mouth opening. Unlike protective co-contraction, the patient has great difficulty opening wider. With delay onset muscle soreness, there is an actual muscle weakness.[38] Muscle strength is returned to normal when the muscle soreness is resolved.[39]

Note: There is still much to be learned about muscle pain disorders. Delayed onset muscle soreness is used as the title of this category because it has been precisely described in the literature. However, other sources of muscle pain (fatigue, ischemia, etc) also present clinically in this category. Perhaps a broader term such as "local muscle soreness—unclassified" would be more appropriate until clinical criteria are developed that will differentiate the various types of muscle conditions.

Myofascial Pain (Trigger Point Myalgia)

Myofascial pain is a regional myogenous pain condition characterized by local areas of firm, hypersensitive bands of muscle tissue known as *trigger points*. This condition is sometimes referred to as myofascial trigger point pain. It is a type of muscle disorder that is not widely appreciated or completely understood, yet it commonly occurs in patients with myalgic complaints. In one study,[40] more than 50% of the cases in a university pain center were diagnosed as this type of pain.

Myofascial pain was first described by Travell and Rinzler[41] in 1952, yet the dental and medical communities have been slow to appreciate its significance. In 1969, Laskin[42] described the myofascial pain dysfunction

(MPD) syndrome as having certain clinical characteristics. Although he borrowed the term myofascial, he was not describing myofascial trigger point pain. Instead MPD syndrome has been used in dentistry as a general term to denote any muscle disorder (not an intracapsular disorder). Since the term is so broad and general, it is not useful in the specific diagnosis and management of masticatory muscle disorders. MPD syndrome should not be confused with Travell and Rinzler's description, which will be used in this textbook.

As stated, myofascial pain arises from hypersensitive areas in muscles called trigger points. These very localized areas in muscle tissues or their tendinous attachments are often felt as taut bands when palpated, which elicits pain. Tissue studies of trigger point sites have yielded very little useful information. Mild dystrophic changes similar to those seen with ischemia have been identified. Some changes have been identified in long-standing trigger point sites.[43,44] But on the whole, the local tissue changes thus far identified are hardly sufficient to account for trigger point phenomena.

The exact nature of a trigger point is not known. It has been suggested[45,46] that certain nerve endings in the muscle tissues may become sensitized by algogenic substances that create a localized zone of hypersensitivity. It is known that bradykinin is released in muscle tissue during ischemic episodes.[47] There may be a local temperature rise at the site of the trigger point, suggesting an increase in metabolic demand and/or reduction of blood flow to these tissues.[48,49] Fricton et al[50] reported a significant electromyographic (EMG) change associated with local twitch response in patients with active trigger points in the upper

trapezius muscle as compared with the contralateral normal muscle in the same individual. There is also considerable evidence that suggests an endogenous opioid system as a mediator for the beneficial effect of trigger point injections.[51]

A trigger point is a very circumscribed region in which just a relatively few motor units seem to be contracting. If all the motor units of a muscle contract, the muscle will of course shorten in length. This condition is called myospasm and will be discussed later in this chapter. Since a trigger point has only a select group of motor units contracting, there is no overall shortening of the muscle as with myospasm. The unique characteristic of trigger points is that they are a source of constant deep pain and therefore can produce central excitatory effects (see Chapter 4). If a trigger point centrally excites a group of converging afferent interneurons, referred pain will often result, generally in a predictable pattern according to the location of the involved trigger point[40] (see Figs 12-3 to 12-11). The pain is often reported by the patient as a tension-type headache.

The etiology of myofascial pain is complex. Unfortunately we are lacking in a complete understanding of this myogenous pain condition. It is therefore difficult to be specific concerning all etiologic factors. Travell and Simons have described certain local and systemic factors that seem to be associated, such as trauma, hypovitamintosis, poor physical conditioning, fatigue and viral infections.[52] Other important factors are likely to be emotional stress and deep pain input.

The most common clinical feature of myofascial pain is the trigger points, which present as local areas of firm, hypersensitive

267

bands of muscle tissue. Although palpation of trigger points produces pain, local muscle sensitivity is not the most common complaint of patients suffering from myofascial trigger point pain. The most common complaints center on the central excitatory effects created by the trigger points. In many instances, patients may be aware only of the referred pain and not even acknowledge the trigger points. A perfect example is the patient suffering from myofascial trigger point pain in the trapezius muscle that creates referred pain to the temple region[53] (see Fig 12-9). The chief complaint is temporal headache, with very little acknowledgment of the trigger point in the shoulder. This clinical presentation can easily distract the clinician from the source of the problem. The patient will draw the clinician's attention to the site of pain (the temporal headache) and not the source. The clinician must always remember that for treatment to be effective it must be directed toward the source of the pain, not the site.

Since trigger points can create central excitatory effects, it is important likewise to be aware of all the possible clinical manifestations. As stated in Chapter 4, central excitatory effects can appear as referred pain, secondary hyperalgesia, protective co-contraction, or even autonomic responses. These conditions must be considered when evaluating the patient.

An interesting clinical feature of a trigger point is that it may present in either an active or a latent state. In the active state, it produces central excitatory effects. Therefore, when a trigger point is active, a headache is commonly felt. Since referred pain is wholly dependent on its original source, palpation of an active trigger point (local provocation) often increases such pain.

Although not always present, when this characteristic appears it is an extremely helpful diagnostic aid. In the latent state, a trigger point is no longer sensitive to palpation and therefore does not produce referred pain. When trigger points are latent they cannot be found by palpation and the patient does not complain of headache pain.

It is thought that trigger points do not resolve without treatment. They may in fact become latent or dormant, creating a temporary relief of the referred pain. Trigger points may be activated by various factors,[54] such as increased use of a muscle, strain on the muscle, emotional stress, or even an upper respiratory infection. When trigger points are activated, the headache returns. This is a common finding with patients who complain of regular late afternoon headaches following a very stressful day.

Along with referred pain, other central excitatory effects may be felt. When secondary hyperalgesia is present, it is commonly felt as sensitivity to touch the scalp. Some patients will even report that their "hair hurts" or that it is painful to brush their hair. Co-contraction is another common condition associated with myofascial pain. Trigger points in the shoulder or cervical muscles can produce co-contraction in the muscles of mastication.[55] If this continues, local muscle soreness in the masticatory muscle can develop. Treatment of the masticatory muscles will not resolve the condition since its source is the trigger points of the cervicospinal and shoulder muscles. However, treatment of the trigger points in the shoulder muscle will resolve the masticatory muscle disorder. Management may become difficult when muscle soreness has been present for a long time, because it can initiate cyclic muscle pain. In these cases treatment extended to both the muscles of mastication and the trigger points in the cervicospinal and shoulder muscles will usually resolve the problem.

On occasion, autonomic effects are produced by deep pain input from trigger points. These may result in such clinical findings as a tearing or drying of the eye. There may be vascular changes (eg, blanching and/or reddening of tissue). Sometimes the conjunctiva will become red. There may even be mucosal changes that produce nasal discharge similar to an allergic response. The key to determining whether the autonomic effects are related to central excitatory effects or to a local reaction such as allergies is the unilateral appearance. Central excitatory effects in the trigeminal area rarely cross the midline. Therefore, if the deep pain is unilateral, the autonomic effects will be on the same side as the pain. In other words, one eye will be red and the other normal, one nostril draining mucus and the other not. With allergic responses both eyes or both nostrils will be involved.

Referral Patterns of Myofascial Pain in the Orofacial Region. The clinician treating orofacial pain disorders needs to have a sound understanding of myofascial pain since it is so common in pain populations. The following section will review the most common muscles of the head and neck and the typical referral pattern for each. Becoming familiar with these patterns can be extremely helpful during history taking, examination, and diagnosis.

Masseter Muscle. Trigger points located at sites in the superficial layer of the masseter muscle refer to the posterior mandibular and maxillary teeth, the jaw, and the face (Fig 12-3). Toothache is a common complaint from this source. The deep portion refers to the ear and temporomandibular joint area. Earache and preauricular pain thought to be emanating from the joint are common complaints. Moderate restriction of opening associated with ipsilateral deflection of the midline incisal path may be observed. Tinnitus described as a "low roaring noise" may occur from deep masseter trigger points. The muscle is accessible for manual palpation to identify trigger sites.

Temporalis Muscle. The reference zone of the temporalis muscle includes all the maxillary teeth and upper portion of the face (Fig 12-4). Headache and toothache are the common complaints. A restricted opening is rarely displayed. The muscle is accessible for manual palpation to identify trigger sites.

Medial Pterygoid Muscle. The reference zone for the medial pterygoid muscle includes the posterior part of the mouth and throat as well as the temporomandibular and infra-auricular areas (Fig 12-5). Throat and postmandibular (infra-auricular) pain is the common complaint. Eustachian tube symptoms may be displayed. Moderate restriction of mouth opening associated with contralateral deflection of the midline incisal path may be observed. The muscle is only partially accessible for intraoral manual palpation to identify trigger sites. Functional manipulation therefore may be needed for this purpose: a pain source within the muscle will be accentuated by opening widely (stretching the muscle) and by biting firmly (contracting the muscle).

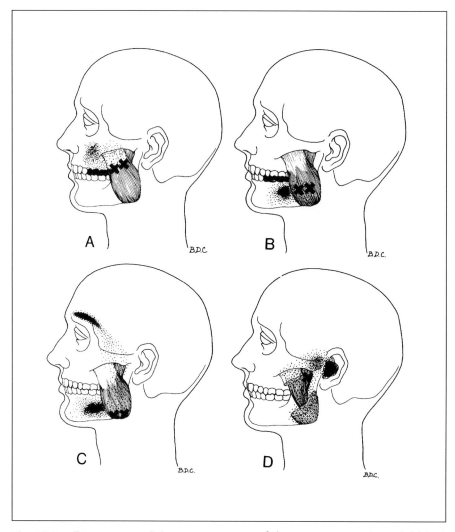

Fig 12-3 Trigger points (**x**) in various parts of the masseter muscle. Solid black shows essential reference pain zones; stippled areas are spillover pain zones. *A,* superficial layer, upper portion; *B,* superficial layer, midbelly; *C,* superficial layer, lower portion; *D,* deep layer, upper part. (From Travell JG, Simons DG. Myofascial Pain and Dysfunction. Baltimore: Williams & Wilkins; 1983: 220. Used with permission.)

Inferior Lateral Pterygoid Muscle. The lateral pterygoid muscle has been incriminated as the cause of numerous temporomandibular complaints. This probably stems from a lack of understanding of how the muscle is constructed and what its normal functions are. No doubt, the difficulty of adequately

examining the muscle clinically has provided good cover for these incriminations. Several hard facts need to be considered in evaluating the effects of this muscle on masticatory symptoms. It should be understood first that there are two lateral pterygoid muscles: the inferior lateral pterygoid and

Fig 12-4 Referred pain patterns from trigger points (**x**) in the temporalis muscle. A, anterior fibers; B and C, middle fibers; D, posterior fibers. (From Travell JG, Simons DG. Myofascial Pain and Dysfunction. Baltimore: Williams & Wilkins; 1983: 237. Used with permission.)

the superior lateral pterygoid. Only the inferior lateral pterygoid muscle protracts the mandible and therefore can act to create acute occlusal disharmony when it is shortened. The superior muscle remains inactive at all times except during power strokes in conjunction with elevator muscle action.[56]

Even when shortened, the superior lateral pterygoid muscle cannot disrupt joint functioning in the absence of structural joint disease.

The dearth of muscle spindles in the lateral pterygoid muscles reduces the chance of reflex contraction when this muscle is

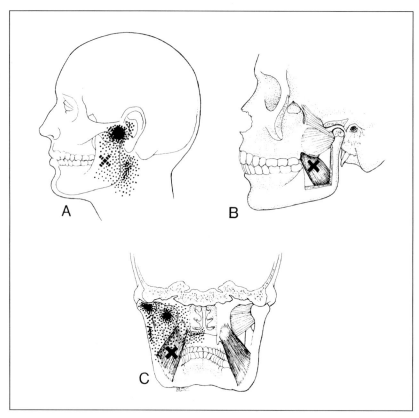

Fig 12-5 Referred pain pattern and location of responsible trigger point (**x**) in the medial pterygoid muscle. *A,* external areas of pain to which the patient can point; *B,* anatomic cutaway to show the location of the trigger point; *C,* coronal section showing internal areas of pain. (From Travell JG, Simons DG. Myofascial Pain and Dysfunction. Baltimore: Williams & Wilkins; 1983: 250. Used with permission.)

stretched. Then too, these muscles are composed chiefly of slow-twitch fibers[57] that resist fatigue and seldom undergo spastic activity. The prime reason that a diagnosis of problems with this muscle is so difficult is that it is inaccessible for manual palpation.[58] Despite voluminous testimony to the contrary, the possibility of diagnostically accurate manual or instrument palpation of the muscle is remote.

Trigger points in the inferior lateral pterygoid muscle refer to the temporomandibular joint area (Fig 12-6). Slight acute malocclu-sion may be sensed as disocclusion of the ipsilateral posterior teeth and premature occlusion of the contralateral anterior teeth (Cases 3 and 4). Since this muscle is inaccessible for palpation, functional manipulation is required to help identify the presence of myofascial pain: a pain source within the muscle will be accentuated by maximum intercuspation (stretching the muscle) and by protruding the jaw against resistance (contracting the muscle).[59]

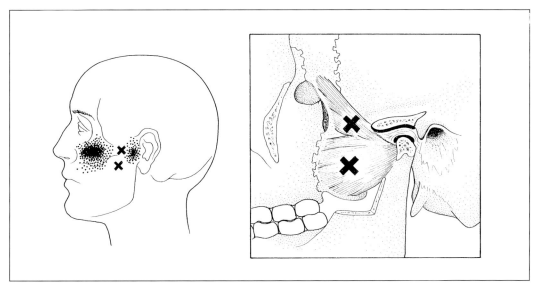

Fig 12-6   Referred pain patterns of trigger points (**x**) in the superior and inferior lateral pterygoid muscles. (From Travell JG, Simons DG: Myofascial Pain and Dysfunction. Baltimore: Williams & Wilkins; 1983: 261. Used with permission.)

Superior Lateral Pterygoid Muscle. Trigger points in the superior lateral pterygoid muscle refer to the zygomatic area (Fig 12-6). No dysfunction is observed unless there is extensive deterioration in the temporomandibular joint sufficient to permit anterior displacement of the articular disc. Diffuse pain in the malar area is the usual complaint. Since this muscle is inaccessible for manual palpation,[58] functional manipulation is required to identify the presence of myofascial pain: a pain source within the muscle will be accentuated by maximum intercuspation (stretching the muscle) and by biting on a separator (contracting the muscle). Opening widely and protruding against resistance do not involve this muscle functionally and therefore are painless.

Anterior Digastric Muscle. Trigger points in the anterior belly of the digastric muscle,

which is the trigeminal-innervated part, refer pain to the mandibular incisor area (Fig 12-7). No dysfunction is observed. This muscle is accessible for manual palpation to identify trigger points.

Sternocleidomastoid Muscle. The reference zone from the superficial sternal division of the sternocleidomastoid muscle is throughout the entire face and head (Fig 12-8). A great variety of face pain and headache complaints may arise from this source. The deeper clavicular division refers to the ear, postauricular area, and frontal region. Earache, temporomandibular pain, and frontal headache are common complaints. This muscle is a frequent source of so-called tension-type headache. Postural vertigo may be displayed. The muscle is accessible for manual palpation to identify trigger sites.

273

Chief Complaint

Diffuse left side facial pain

History

A 47-year-old woman with mild continuous protracted variable steady dull aching pain diffusely located in the right ear, preauricular area, face, and temple, aggravated by opening widely, chewing food, and clenching the teeth, and accompanied by acute malocclusion and restricted opening.

The patient has had recurring episodes of earache associated with acute upper respiratory infections for several years. About 3 weeks ago, she had such an episode with continuous severe earache on the right side. After about 7 days, she noticed her "bite was off," she could not open normally, and she had pain with opening, chewing, and occluding the teeth. This had become progressively worse even though antibiotic therapy by her ENT physician eliminated the ear infection completely. He referred her to her dentist who recognized the trismus and occlusal disharmony but declined to adjust the occlusion pending further investigation of the temporomandibular joints. She has no other physical complaints and takes no medications.

Examination

Intraoral: The teeth are clinically and radiographically normal. There is premature contact of the left anterior teeth and disocclusion of the posterior teeth on the same side of the pain. When she fully occludes the teeth, there is acute pain in the right TM area. This is decreased by biting on a tongue blade. Pain also occurs with eccentric biting, forceful lateral and protrusive movements, and opening beyond 10 mm. Opening is restricted to 31 mm with deflection to the right after 23 mm.

> **TM Joints:** Both joints appear structurally normal. The left joint functions normally but the right condyle appears to be protruded in initial occlusal contact position and fails to move properly with opening efforts.
>
> **Muscles:** There is palpable tenderness in the right masseter and temporal muscles.
>
> **Cervical:** Within normal limits.
>
> **Cranial Nerves:** Within normal limits.

Diagnostic Tests: Analgesic blocking of the right lateral pterygoid muscle arrested pain induced by fully occluding the teeth and making forceful excursions. Similar blocking of the right masseter and temporal muscles arrested all other pain.

Impression

The masticatory pain is muscular and stems from the right lateral pterygoid, masseter, and temporal muscles only. The acute malocclusion is symptomatic of spasm of the right lateral pterygoid muscle. The trismus is due to spasm of the right masseter and temporal muscles. The myospasms occurred by way of muscle co-contraction produced by central excitatory effects induced by primary otalgia. Cyclic muscle pain has occurred.

Diagnosis

Masticatory myospasm of the right lateral pterygoid, masseter, and temporal muscles, secondary to otalgia. Cycling muscle pain appears to be present.

Masticatory muscle pain expressed as spasm in the lateral pterygoid muscle.

Chief Complaint

Right ear and preauricular pain

History

A 20-year-old woman with mild variable steady dull aching pain diffusely located in the right ear and preauricular area. It is induced by clenching the teeth, chewing, and other jaw use, and lasts variable periods of time. The pains are intermittent and are significantly related to gum chewing, hard biting, and forceful jaw movements. She complains her bite is not very comfortable with premature contact of the left anterior teeth and disocclusion of the posteriors. When she brings the teeth into full occlusion, she feels the acute pain and therefore she avoids activity.

The complaint began about 2 years ago in sudden recurring episodes usually lasting only a few days and then disappearing for variable periods of time. The complaint seemed to be worse especially in the early mornings. The present episode began about 6 months ago and has remained the same ever since.

Examination

Intraoral: The teeth are clinically and radiographically negative for pulpal or periodontal pain. An acute malocclusion is evident. There is premature contact of the left anterior teeth while the posterior teeth do not occlude. When the patient is asked to bring all the teeth into firm occlusion, she experiences pain in the right TM area. This can be prevented by biting on a tongue blade to preclude full intercuspation of the teeth. She thinks her occlusion was normal 6 months ago and relates the malocclusion to her pain complaint.

> **TM Joints:** Clinical functioning of the joints is well within normal limits except for the sensation of malocclusion and the right side pain when she occludes the teeth or moves the jaw forcefully. She opens 45 mm with no deviation or deflection of the incisal path. Protrusive and lateral excursions are adequate and symmetrical. Asking the patient to push the jaw forward against resistance increases the pain. Radiographically, both joints appear to be within normal limits structurally. There is radiographically visible displacement of the right condyle as the teeth are fully occluded from the position of primary occlusal contact.
>
> **Muscles:** There is slight palpable muscle tenderness but the discomfort appears to be wholly subjective.
>
> **Cervical:** Within normal limits.
>
> **Cranial Nerves:** Within normal limits.

Diagnostic Tests: Analgesic blocking of the right lateral pterygoid muscle immediately arrests the pain complaint.

Impression

The pain is myalgic and arises from the right lateral pterygoid muscle. The malocclusion is acute and relates to muscle spasm.

Diagnosis

Myospasm of the right lateral pterygoid muscle. The cause is presumed to relate to clenching, emotional stress, bruxism, fatigue, etc.

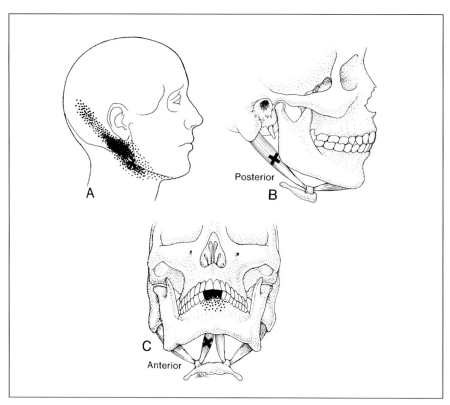

Fig 12-7 Referred pain pattern of trigger point (**x**) in the anterior belly of a digastric muscle. (From Travell JG, Simons DG. Myofascial Pain and Dysfunction. Baltimore: Williams & Wilkins; 1983: 274. Used with permission.)

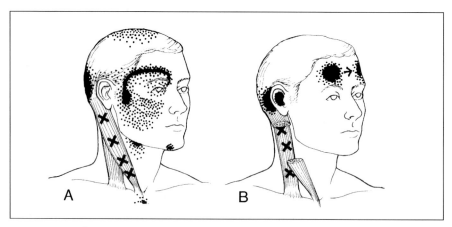

Fig 12-8 Referred pain patterns with locations of corresponding trigger points (**x**) in the sternocleidomastoid muscle. A, superficial sternal division; B, deep clavicular division. (From Travell JG, Simons DG. Myofascial Pain and Dysfunction. Baltimore: Williams & Wilkins; 1983: 203. Used with permission.)

Trapezius Muscle. The reference zone for trigger points in the upper part of the trapezius muscle is along the posterolateral part of the neck, the postauricular area, the mandibular angle, and the temple (Fig 12-9). This is a major source of so-called tension-type headache. It should be noted that tension-type headache is due neither to excessive muscular tension nor to muscle contraction because there is no statistically significant difference in the EMG activity between such muscles and those in control subjects.[60,61] This muscle is accessible for manual palpation to identify trigger sites.

Occipitofrontalis Muscle. The frontalis portion of the occipitofrontalis muscle refers as frontal headache; the occipital portion refers as lateral cranial and postocular headache (Fig 12-10). This is another major source of tension-type headache. The muscle is accessible for manual palpation to identify trigger sites. The splenius capitis, splenius cervicis, posterior cervical, and suboccipital muscles are other sources of tension-type headache.[52]

Muscles of Facial Expression. Trigger points in the orbicularis oculi muscle refer down through the nose and upper lip, those of the zygomaticus major muscle refer upward along the inner canthus of the eye to the midforehead, and those in the platysma muscle refer diffusely in the mandibular region (Fig 12-11). These muscles are all accessible for manual palpation to identify trigger sites.

Cervical Muscles. It should be noted that myofascial trigger point pain emanating from muscles innervated by cervical spinal nerves often induce heterotopic pain in the orofacial and head regions. Spontaneous referred pain is usually felt as a headache. It is possible, however, that such reference is felt as an earache, toothache, or masticatory pain. Stimulation-evoked secondary hyperalgesia is also a common form of heterotopic pain that occurs secondarily to cervical nociceptive input. Thus, areas of touchy skin or scalp may occur. Frequently, however, deeper areas of palpable tenderness that are accentuated by masticatory function may occur. Such heterotopic manifestation of cervical pain may be mistaken for true masticatory pain. Caution therefore should always be exercised when cervical and masticatory pains are felt concurrently. When this occurs, it behooves the clinician to more completely evaluate the cervical spine.

Such an examination entails observation of the neck contours for deviation or straightening of the neck, rotation or tilting of the head, or elevation of the shoulder (see Chapter 8). The mobility of the neck should be tested both actively and passively for range of motion, pain, and crepitation. Tenderness and muscle soreness can be determined by palpation. Sensory evaluation of neck pain sources as identified by dermatome distribution is important on the basis that cervical nerve pain is felt superficially in the shoulder, outer portion of the arm, and hand, whereas thoracic nerve pain is commonly felt in the axillary region and inner part of the arm. Deep tendon reflexes and motor evaluation of the shoulder and arm should be done while keeping in mind that motor innervation of the deltoid, biceps, triceps, and wrist muscles is from the cervical spinal nerves. Radial pulse changes with postural maneuvers of the arms should be tested.

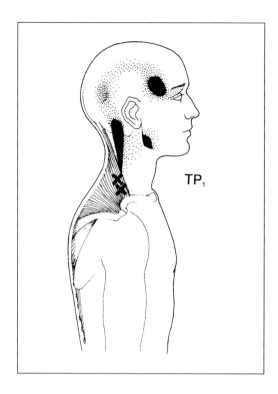

Fig 12-9 Referred pain patterns and location of trigger points (**x**) in upper part of the trapezius muscle. (From Travell JG, Simons DG. Myofascial Pain and Dysfunction. Baltimore: Williams & Wilkins; 1983: 184.)

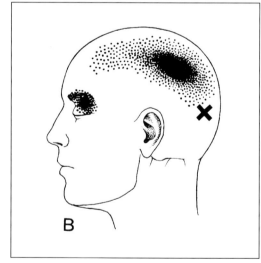

Fig 12-10 Pain patterns referred from trigger points (**x**) in the occipitofrontalis muscle. A, frontalis belly; B, occipitalis belly. (From Travell JG, Simons DG. Myofascial Pain and Dysfunction. Baltimore: Williams & Wilkins; 1983: 291.) Used with permission.

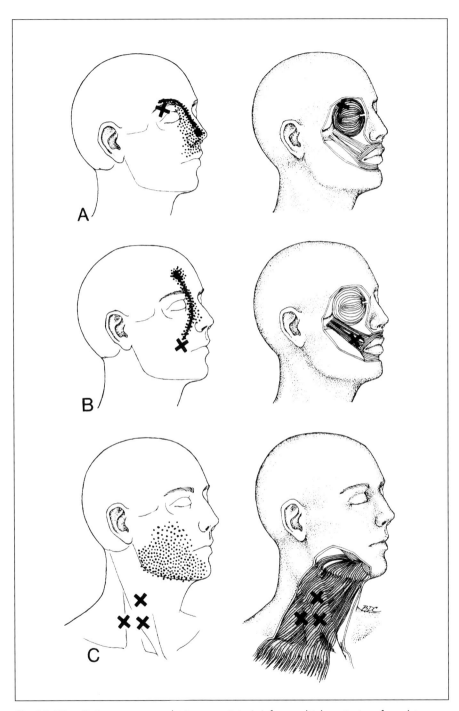

Fig 12-11 Pain patterns and trigger points (**x**) from which pain is referred in muscles of facial expression. *A*, orbital portion of orbicularis oculi muscle; *B*, zygomaticus major muscle; *C*, platysma muscle. (From Travell JG, Simons DG.: Myofascial Pain and Dysfunction. Baltimore: Williams & Wilkins; 1983: 283. Used with permission.)

Such a clinical examination may reveal not only the presence of pain sources in the neck but may help to pinpoint which cervical spinal nerves are involved. It should be noted that upper cervical spinal nerves are more likely sources of pain that refer or spread to the masticatory region than are lower ones. This examination may produce sufficient evidence to warrant an orthopedic consultation.

Among neck conditions that the dentist should be familiar with are chronic cervical myofascial pain; acute cervical strain; osteoarthritis of the cervical spine and intervertebral disc disease; and scalenus anticus syndrome[62] and other nerve entrapments in the neck.

Secondary effects of muscle pain include not only reference of pain, as previously discussed, but also the development of secondary co-contraction in other muscles, which gives the syndrome a pattern of spreading pain. A cervical strain or whiplash injury may, by central hyperexcitability, induce motor effects in the masticatory muscles. This then leads to a typical masticatory muscle disorder, the symptoms of which may become dominant. As such, the very real masticatory pain disorder may cause the patient to consider this to be the total complaint when in fact it is no more than a secondary effect of the cervical disorder. These types of disorders require astute diagnostic and therapeutic management to avoid failure and chronicity.

Persistent cervical sources of deep somatic pain, such as cervical osteoarthritis, are prone to induce central excitatory effects that include heterotopic pain and co-contraction of muscles innervated by cervical, facial, and trigeminal nerves. Thus, a masticatory muscle disorder may be initi-

ated as part of a larger, spreading muscle pain problem (Case 5). Since cyclic muscle pain can become independent of the initiating cause, such pain represents a separate therapeutic entity. Since the cause is not masticatory, treatment should not be primarily directed toward the masticatory apparatus. Therapy needs to be directed to the original source of pain, in this case, the cervical disorder. Since the masticatory muscle disorder may become independent of the original source, therapy may also need to be directed to this disorder. Treatment of only masticatory muscle pain, however, will not be successful unless proper cervical treatment is also accomplished. Pain disorders of this type can best be recognized and distinguished from those of true masticatory origin by careful history taking and by a clinical examination that includes the cervical structures.

Tension-type Headache. Tension-type headache is characterized by a constant, dull aching pain felt bilaterally in the temporal and frontal regions and is often described as wearing a tight headband. Previously this type of headache was referred to as a muscular contraction headache or muscle tension headache. More recent studies[12-13,64,65] demonstrate that there is no significant increase in EMG activity of these muscles and therefore these names are not appropriate. Certainly not all tension-type headaches are related to myofascial pain but many are likely to be secondary to myofascial trigger point pain originating in head and neck muscles. Sometimes, a vague low-grade muscular discomfort is sensed in the cervical and occipital area. As just reviewed, pain referred from the frontalis portion of the occipitofrontalis muscle is felt as

Case 5	Myofascial pain of the maticatory muscles secondary to a cervical pain condition

Chief Complaint

Generalized facial pain and headache

History

A 52-year-old female with mild continuous protracted steady dull aching pain diffusely located bilaterally in the temporal, preauricular, and occipital areas. The pain is aggravated by head movements, emotional stress, fatigue, and jaw use.

During the past 6 to 7 years, the patient has had recurring episodes of bilateral occipital, temporal, and frontal headaches lasting up to 2 to 3 months and occurring at irregular intervals. They are aggravated by head movements, emotional stress, and fatigue and have been treated as tension-type headaches by her osteopathic physician. About 8 to 9 months ago, the present episode began, first intermittently, then becoming constant. During recent months, the pains have been aggravated by chewing and opening widely and she has noticed moderate restriction of mouth opening. Her physician therefore has advised a dental examination. She also has neck, finger, arm, and leg complaints but she has been cleared medically and neurologically for cause except minor osteoarthritis of the cervical vertebrae. No medications or therapy presently in use.

Examination

Intraoral: No dental or oral cause for the pain is evident clinically or radiographically. The teeth respond normally to pulp testing. She has bilateral preauricular pain with opening, sustained clenching, and hard biting eccentrically. Her maximum mouth opening is about 34 mm with no deflection. Lateral and protrusive movements are normal. She has moderate joint noise with extended or strained movements only. There is no discernible occlusal disharmony.

TM Joints: Clinically and radiographically normal except for moderate restriction of condylar movement bilaterally with opening.

Muscles: Palpable tenderness in the masseter, temporal, medial pterygoid, sternocleidomastoid, occipital, and trapezius muscles bilaterally.

Cervical: Significant pain to palpation of the cervical spine and associated muscles. Restriction of cervical function to rotation and bending.

Cranial Nerves: Within normal limits.

Impression

The masticatory pain and dysfunction appear originating from muscular origin and are intimately related to preexistent muscle pain emanating from the cervical musculature bilaterally. By history, the cervical component preceded the more recent masticatory complaint and the entire symptom complex is highly suggestive of a cervical myofascial pain disorder that has spread to involve the masticatory muscles. It is presumed that cervical arthritis is a likely predisposing cause and this possibility deserves serious investigation on a medical level. There is no identifiable dental, oral, or masticatory cause for the patient's complaint.

Diagnosis

Masticatory myofascial pain expressed in the elevator muscles secondary to a cervical pain condition of undetermined origin.

frontal headache while that from the occipitalis portion is felt as postocular and lateral headache. While pain referred from the sternal division of the sternocleidomastoid muscle is felt diffusely throughout the face and head, that from the clavicular division is felt as postauricular and frontal headache. The upper part of the trapezius muscle refers pain that is felt as postauricular and temporal headache. The splenius capitis, splenius cervicis, and other posterior cervical and suboccipital muscles may contribute also to tension-type headache. Tension-type headache will be discussed more completely in Chapter 16.

Tension-type Headache Mistaken for Masticatory Pain. It is not unusual for the heterotopic referred pain of tension-type headache to be accompanied by secondary hyperalgesia that is felt as discomfort with jaw movements and deep tenderness due to manual palpation. The "chewing pain" thus created, which can be "manually palpated" and is accompanied by "headache," may be misdiagnosed as a masticatory disorder and treated accordingly. This fairly common complaint can be distinguished from true masticatory pain in that coincidental masticatory dysfunction is lacking and the discomfort is not arrested by analgesic blocking at the site of pain.

The clinical symptoms reported with myofascial pain are most commonly associated with the central excitatory effects created by the trigger points and not the trigger points themselves. The clinician must be aware of this and find the involved trigger points. When these are palpated, they appear as hypersensitive areas often felt as taut bands within the muscle. There is usually no local pain when the muscle is at rest but some pain when the muscle is used. Often slight structural dysfunction will be seen in the muscle harboring the trigger points. This is commonly reported as a stiff neck.

Myospasms (Tonic Contraction Myalgia)

By definition, muscle spasm is a sudden, violent, involuntary contraction of a muscle or group of muscles that is attended by pain and interference with function and produces involuntary movement and distortion.[63] For many years, the dental profession thought that myospasms were a significant source of myogenous pain. Recent studies, however, shed new light on muscle pain and myospasms. It is reasonable to expect that a muscle in spasm or tonic contraction would reveal a relatively high level of electromyographic activity. Studies, however, do not support that painful muscles have a significant increase in their EMG output.[64,65] These studies have forced us to rethink the classification of muscle pain and differentiate myospasms from other muscle pain disorders. Although myospasms of the muscles of mastication do occur, this condition is not common and, when present, is easily identified by clinical characteristics.

The cause of myospasms has not been well documented. There are likely to be several factors that combine to promote myospasms. There appears to be certainly local muscle conditions that seem to foster myospasms. These conditions involve muscle fatigue and changes in local electrolyte balance. Deep pain input may also precipitate myospasms.

Myospasms are easily recognized by the structural dysfunction that is produced. Since a muscle in spasm is contracted, major jaw positional changes result according to the muscle or muscles in spasm. These changes in the position of the jaw create what is known as an *acute malocclusion*. An acute malocclusion is a sudden change in the occlusal condition as a result of a disorder. Since the malocclusion is secondary to a disorder, the clinician should not focus treatment on correcting the malocclusion but instead on the disorder that has caused the malocclusion. Myospasms are also characterized by very firm muscles as noted by palpation.

When the inferior lateral pterygoid muscle shortens due to myospastic activity, acute malocclusion results. This is recognized as disocclusion of the ipsilateral posterior teeth and premature occlusion of the contralateral anterior teeth. The presence of pain sites within the muscle is identified by functional manipulation: pain is accentuated by maximum intercuspation (stretching the muscle) and by protrusion against resistance (contracting the muscle). It should be noted that pain with clenching of the teeth is relieved by biting ipsilaterally on a tongue blade because this prevents intercuspation of the teeth that stretches the muscle. Unless acute malocclusion can be identified and pain induced by functional manipulation, a diagnosis of spasm of this muscle is invalid.

Local analgesic blocking of the inferior lateral pterygoid muscle promptly arrests all pain emanating from this source and offers the best clinical means of accurately locating the source of pain.

Myositis (Inflammatory Myalgia)

Myositis, by definition, represents an inflammatory condition within the muscle tissue. This condition is not common in early stages of myogenous pain. Like other inflammatory conditions, myositis becomes more predominant as the acute myalgic disorder becomes protracted. In other words, the longer the patient complains of myogenous pain, the greater the likelihood of myositis. It should be noted that myositis is more closely associated with continuity of muscle pain rather than actual duration. Many muscle pain disorders are episodic, intermittent periods of no muscle pain. Periodic episodes of muscle pain do not produce myositis. A prolonged and constant period of muscle pain, however, is likely to lead to myositis.

On occasion, a bacterial or viral infection can spread to a muscle, producing an infectious myositis. This condition is not common but when present needs to be identified and properly treated.

The more common type of myositis is produced by protracted muscle soreness or myofascial pain. Since this condition has no invading organism, it is thought of as noninfectious or sterile myositis. The clinical characteristics of this muscle disorder closely resemble the clinical characteristics of many other inflammatory disorders. It should be noted, however, that results of tissue biopsies often fail to depict a true inflammatory response in the muscle tissues. Therefore, some question exists as to whether this is a genuine inflammatory disorder. Since this condition clinically presents as an inflammatory condition and it responds to management as an inflammatory condition, it will be described in this text as myositis.

A clinical characteristic of myositis is the presence of constant, aching myogenous pain. The pain is present during rest and increases with function. The muscles are very tender to palpation and structural dysfunction is common. The most common clinical feature is the extended duration of the symptoms (Case 6).

Other inflammatory myogenous pains are fasciitis, tendinitis, and bursitis. Fasciitis is an inflammatory condition of the muscle sheath that occurs in conjunction with and is diagnostically inseparable from inflammation of the body of the muscle. Although myofascial pain is not inflammatory, it may be designated myofasciitis for administrative or insurance purposes.[52] Tendinitis is an inflammatory condition of a tendon or tendon-muscle attachment. Abusive use and trauma are the most frequent causes. Bursae are synovial membrane–lined antifriction structures that facilitate muscle movements, especially when bidirectional. A bursa is found at the hamular process of the sphenoid bone to facilitate tensor palatini muscle action. One lies beneath the tongue. Several facilitate muscle action involving the hyoid bone. Bursitis is an inflammatory condition of a bursa and usually results from trauma. It may be a manifestation of rheumatoid arthritis.

Acute vs Chronic Muscle Disorders

The myalgic disorders that have been described are commonly seen in the general practice of dentistry and usually represent problems of short duration. With proper therapy, these disorders can be completely resolved. However, when myogenous pain persists, more chronic and often complex muscle pain disorders can develop. With chronicity, myogenous pain disorder symptoms become less local and more regional or even occasionally global. Often cyclic muscle pain becomes an important feature that perpetuates the condition.

As a general rule, chronic pain is considered pain that has been present for 6 months or longer. As mentioned with myositis, however, the duration of pain may not be the most important factor that determines chronicity. There are some pains that are experienced for years that never become chronic pain conditions. Likewise, there are some pain conditions that become clinically chronic in a matter of months. The additional factor that must be considered is the continuity of the pain. When a pain experience is constant, with no periods of relief, the clinical manifestations of chronicity develop quickly. On the other hand, if the pain is interrupted with periods of remission (no pain), the condition may never become a chronic pain disorder. For example, trigeminal neuralgia is an extremely painful neuropathic condition that may last for years and never become a chronic pain disorder. The reason for this is the significant periods of relief between episodes of the pain. Conversely, the constant pain associated with myositis, when left untreated, can develop the clinical manifestations of chronicity within several months.

It is important for the clinician to recognize that when myalgic complaints progress from an acute myalgic disorder to a chronic myalgic disorder the effectiveness of local treatment is greatly reduced. Chronic pain disorders often need to be managed with a multidisciplinary approach. In many instances, the dentist alone is not equipped to manage these disorders. It is important,

| Case 6 | Masticatory muscle pain expressed as significant co-contraction and myositis |

Chief Complaint

Limited mouth opening associated with left face pain.

History

A 67-year-old man with mild continuous protracted steady dull aching pain diffusely located in the left face, temple, and jaw. The pain is accompanied by marked reduction in mouth opening and aggravated by any attempt to open the mouth or chewing.

The complaint occurred as a postoperative complication following the removal of the lower left third molar about 30 days ago. Prior to the extraction, there was moderate soreness in the lower left molar area but no acute pain or trismus. The removal of the tooth was described as a difficult and painful experience. Swelling and pain of the surgical site followed the surgery and after about 3 to 4 days the mouth was restricted to only 10 mm of opening. Generalized pain, localized swelling, and inability to open the mouth have persisted. No therapy other than the application of heat and suggestion to encourage jaw use have been prescribed. Presently, no medications are in use.

Examination

Intraoral: Due to the mouth restriction the teeth cannot be adequately examined. Panoramic radiograph of the mandible shows no osseous change and the lower left alveolus appears normal. There is localized swelling and tenderness in the lower left area intraorally, moderate tenderness in the left submandibular triangle, and slight swelling and tenderness above the left zygomatic arch. Opening is restricted to about 10 mm with little or no deflection and accompanied by pain in the left temporal and postmandibular areas. Lateral and protrusive movements are only moderately restricted and painful.

TM Joints: Both joints appear structurally normal. The restricted condylar movement appears to be the result of an extracapsular restriction associated with pain in the left temporal and medial pterygoid muscles.

Muscles: Palpable tenderness in the left temporal muscle area. The left medial pterygoid muscle is not accessible for palpation. The left masseter muscle appears to be clinically normal.

Cervical: Within normal limits.

Cranial Nerves: Within normal limits.

Impression

The history, clinical course, and present clinical and radiographic evidence indicate that inflammation in the left pterygomandibular space followed the surgical removal of the lower left third molar. As this progressed superiorly, the left infratemporal space also became involved, hence the swelling above the left zygomatic arch. Some inflammation still persists as evidenced by intraoral and suprazygomatic symptoms. The left medial pterygoid and temporal muscles were likely affected by the pain first with protected co-contraction and later by inflammation.

Diagnosis

Significant co-contraction or trismus due to myositis of the left temporal and medial pterygoid muscles.

therefore, for the clinician to recognize chronic pain disorders and consider referring the patient to a team of appropriate therapists who are better able to manage the pain condition.

Perpetuating Factors

When an acute myalgic disorder is not resolved it may progress into a chronic pain disorder. Certain perpetuating factors may contribute to this progression. These perpetuating factors can be divided into those of local source and those of systemic source.

Local Perpetuating Factors. The following conditions represent local factors that can be responsible for the progression of an acute muscle disorder into a chronic pain condition.

Protracted Cause. If the clinician fails to eliminate the cause of an acute myalgic disorder, a more chronic condition will likely develop.

Recurrent Cause. If the patient experiences recurrent episodes of the same etiology that produced an acute myalgic disorder it is likely that the disorder will progress to a more chronic condition (ie, bruxism, repeated trauma, etc).

Therapeutic Mismanagement. When a patient is improperly treated for an acute myalgic disorder, symptoms will not resolve. This can lead to a chronic condition. This type of perpetuating factor emphasizes the importance of establishing the proper diagnosis and initiating effective therapy.

Systemic Perpetuating Factors. The following conditions represent systemic factors that can be responsible for the progression of an acute muscle disorder into a chronic pain condition.

Continued Emotional Stress. Since increased emotional stress can be an etiologic factor in the development of an acute muscle disorder, continued experience of significant levels of emotional stress can represent a perpetuating factor that may advance the condition to a more chronic pain disorder.

Constitutional Factors. Each individual has certain constitutional factors that influence his or her response to events. Constitutional factors may be influenced by such variables as nutritional deficiency, metabolism, and physical fitness. Although the idea of individual variation of constitutional factors is well appreciated by the clinician, these factors have yet to be adequately documented.

Sleep Disturbances. It appears that sleep disturbances are commonly associated with many chronic myalgic pain disorders.[66–69] It is presently unknown whether the chronic pain condition produces a sleep disturbance or whether a sleep disturbance is a significant factor in the initiation of the chronic pain condition. Regardless of this cause-and-effect question, the relationship between sleep disturbances and chronic pain disorders must be recognized since it may need to be addressed during therapy.

Learned Behavior. Patients who experience prolonged suffering can develop an illness behavior that seems to perpetuate the pain disorder. In other words, people learn to be sick instead of well. Patients who present with illness behavior need to receive therapy to promote wellness behavior before complete recovery can be accomplished.

Secondary Gain. Chronic pain disorders can produce certain secondary gains for the suffering patient.[70] When a patient learns that chronic pain can be used to alter normal life events, the patient may have difficulty giving up the pain and going back to normal responsibilities. For example, if chronic pain becomes an excuse to avoid work, it will be difficult for the clinician to resolve the pain problem unless the patient wishes to return to work. It is important that the therapist recognize the presence of secondary gains so they can be properly addressed. Failure to eliminate secondary gains will lead to failure in resolving the chronic pain disorder.

Depression. Psychologic depression is a common finding in patients with chronic pain.[71,72] It is well-documented that patients who suffer for long periods will frequently become depressed.[73,74] Since depression can result in an independent psychologic problem, it must be properly addressed to treat the patient completely.[75] Elimination of the pain problem alone will not necessarily eliminate depression. This is reflected in the Axis II diagnosis of mood disorders.

Psychogenic Intensification. The longer an individual suffers, the greater the intensity of the pain. This phenomenon can occur even when nociceptive input remains unchanged. This may be explained by a decrease in the patient's ability to modulate pain. Psychogenic intensification is a common perpetrating factor in chronic pain disorders.

Chronic Myalgic Pain Disorders

Chronic pain disorders need to be recognized as such because therapy demands it. There are many types of chronic pain disorders. One method of classifying these conditions is by the structures that are most involved. A broad term that might be used for muscle problems is chronic myalgic disorders. Some of the same disorders discussed as acute myalgic disorders can become chronic when significant perpetuating factors are present. Myositis and myofascial pain may commonly present as a part of a chronic myalgic disorder. The treatment becomes more complicated, however, because perpetuating factors and cyclic muscle pain also need to be addressed. Another complicating factor in chronic myalgic disorders is that the area involved in the condition often seems to broaden. In other words, pain that begins in the masseter muscle spreads to involve the temporalis and medial pterygoid muscles and perhaps even later the cervical muscles. Often as pain becomes chronic, it becomes more regional or even global. This, of course, complicates treatment.

A chronic myalgic disorder that the dentist needs to aware of is *fibromyalgia*. This condition represents a global musculoskeletal pain disorder that can often be confused with an acute masticatory muscle disorder. In the past, fibromyalgia has been referred to in the medical literature as fibrositis. According to a recent consensus report,[76] fibromyalgia is a widespread musculoskeletal pain disorder in which tenderness that has been present for more than 3 months is found in 11 or more of 18 specific tender point sites in at least three of the four body quadrants. Fibromyalgia is not an orofacial pain disorder and therefore needs to be recognized and the patient referred to appropriate medical personnel.

Sequelae to Immobilization of a Muscle. When muscle pain is present, the patient will often decrease function of the involved muscle(s). Immobilization of a muscle may cause changes that require special therapy when the pain condition resolves. Disuse atrophy in a muscle begins almost immediately when it is immobilized, and if such immobilization lasts more than a few days, the degree of atrophic change may become significant. Reversal can usually be accomplished by isometric exercises. It is estimated, however, that it requires at least twice as long to resolve disuse atrophy as it takes to induce it.

If immobilization prevents periodic stretching of a muscle, its resting length decreases due to inactivity of the inverse stretch reflex. This is termed *myostatic contracture*. It is usually reversible, however, by momentarily stretching the muscle many times a day. Resolution is slow and time-consuming (Case 6).

Therapeutic consideration, therefore, should be given to treating weakened and shortened muscles that have been involved in a muscle pain problem.

Muscular Toothache

Heterotopic pain manifested as a spontaneous toothache (referred pain) or palpable tenderness of the teeth (secondary hyperalgesia) may occur as a result of myofascial trigger points in the orofacial musculature (see Chapter 11 and Case 1). Trigger points in the temporalis muscle may induce pain felt as maxillary toothache. Superficial masseter muscle trigger points cause pain felt in the maxillary and mandibular posterior teeth. Trigger points in the anterior digastric muscle refer to the mandibular anterior teeth. Muscle-induced heterotopic tooth pain can be distinguished from odontogenous pain in that there is inadequate local dental cause, and the pain is not arrested by analgesic blocking of the tooth.

Referred Pain Mistaken for Masticatory Pain

Heterotopic pain referred to the auricular and preauricular area or from nonmasticatory muscles may be mistaken for pains that emanate from the masticatory apparatus (see Case 18, page 363). The source of such pain is myofascial trigger points located in the inferior lateral pterygoid, the medial pterygoid, the deep masseter, or the clavicular division of the sternocleidomastoid muscle. Such pain can be distinguished from true masticatory pain in that it is not accompanied by coincidental symptoms of masticatory dysfunction, and it is not arrested by analgesic blocking of the joint proper.

Differentiating Various Masticatory Muscle Pains

Masticatory muscle pain is experienced by the patient as a diffuse, commonly bilateral, complaint. The location of the discomfort felt by the patient may be wholly inaccurate as a means of identifying its source. The overriding painful sensation is usually described as having a dull, aching quality. Spontaneous lancinating pains may occur, shooting to the ear, temple, or face. Such pains may also relate to chewing and opening. Palpable tenderness over the joint is frequently masseteric in origin. Infra-auricular, postmandibular, and pharyngeal discomfort is usually due to the medial pterygoid muscle. Earache is usually masseteric in origin. Although secondary referred pains may be felt widely over the auricular, preauricular, infra-auricular, temporal, and facial areas, such pain is rarely described as located in the postauricular, occipital, or cervical areas unless cervical muscles are simultaneously involved. Headache occurs frequently.

Elevator Muscle Pain

Pain of an elevator muscle will often restrict opening movement to the extent of the shortened muscle but does not appreciably restrict protrusive or contralateral excursion except that due to the inhibitory effect of pain. The mandibular incisal path is deflected to the affected side when the masseter or temporalis is shortened unilaterally. It is deflected to the opposite side when the medial pterygoid is shortened unilaterally. Deflection does not occur when both the masseter and medial pterygoid are shortened unilaterally or with any combination of bilateral muscle shortening. Deflection of protrusive excursion does not occur except that due to pain inhibition.

Some poorly defined acute malocclusion may occur, more readily sensed subjectively by the patient than witnessed objectively by the examiner.

Pain originating in elevator muscles is accentuated when the patient attempts to open the mouth, chew food, or clench the teeth. The clenching pain is not decreased by biting on a tongue blade placed between the teeth on the painful side. Pain with opening is due to stretching the painful muscle. Pain with chewing food and clenching the teeth is due to contracting the painful muscle. Eccentric movement of the mandible will not usually increase pain since this type of movement does not significantly lengthen the elevator muscles.

The pain of an elevator muscle spasm may be felt in and around the ear, temple, and face. Pain increases with opening, chewing food, and clenching the teeth, the latter pain not being reduced by biting on a tongue blade. The masticatory pain is accompanied by a restriction of opening. Deflection of the incisal path depends on the muscles involved. There is minimal restriction of lateral and protrusive movements except when caused by the inhibitory influence of pain or secondary disc interference. The pain sources are identified by manual palpation and arrested by analgesic blocking of the muscles in a painful spasm (Case 7).

Lateral Pterygoid Muscle Pain

Pain originating in the inferior lateral pterygoid muscles may cause an acute malocclusion that is described as anterior premature contact or overstressing accompanied by bilateral disocclusion posteriorly. Bilateral local analgesic blocking promptly arrests the pain emanating from these muscles.

Case 7	Masticatory muscle pain expressed as inflammation of the elevator muscles

Chief Complaint Right preauricular pain.

History A 42-year-old woman with recurrent episodes of mild continuous protracted dull aching pain diffusely located in the right auricular and preauricular area, induced by attempts to open the mouth beyond 22 mm. There is a history of progressive restriction of opening during painless as well as painful periods.

The complaint began about 10 years ago as recurrent episodes of right earache lasting a few days and disappearing. She has been aware of some progressive restriction of opening that she reports was initiated by a painful experience of right joint dislocation about 25 years ago. Prior to that, she had "loose noisy joints." About 2 years ago, her ENT physician found the ears to be normal and suggested it was a right joint condition. Her physician has since treated her periodically for arthritis without significant change in the complaint. Recently, she had an episode of earache following minor dental treatment, so her dentist referred her for a TM joint examination. Presently, she takes no medications.

Examination **Intraoral:** There is no dental or oral cause for the pain. There is minor palpable tenderness of the right masseter muscle and increasing discomfort as she tries to open beyond 22 mm. There is no pain with other movements. Mouth opening is restricted to 22 mm with deflection to the right. Protrusive and lateral movements are within normal limits.

TM Joints: Both joints appear to be structurally normal. There is restriction of right condylar movement with maximum opening, interpreted as indicative of contracture of the right masseter muscle.

Muscles: Moderate tenderness and shortening of the right masseter muscle.

Cervical: Within normal limits.

Cranial Nerves: Within normal limits.

Impression Recurrent mild myositis due to injudicious stretching of preexistent myofibrotic contracture of the right masseter muscle presumed to be related to an experience of painful dislocation of the right temporomandibular joint some 25 years ago. The contracture appears to be progressive.

Diagnosis Painful extraarticular adhesions that restrict mouth opening. Also, muscle contracture involving the right masseter muscle.

Inferior Lateral Pterygoid Muscle

Pain originating from the inferior lateral pterygoid muscle is usually felt in the joint proper, but this may vary. It is most severe when the teeth are fully occluded. This is reduced by insertion of a tongue blade between the molar teeth to prevent intercuspation. Pain occurs with a resisted protrusive movement. Discomfort is slight with relaxed translatory movements except when extended to maximum range. The pain is promptly arrested by analgesic blocking of the offending muscle.

Differential Diagnosis

Primary deep somatic musculoskeletal pains that emanate from the musculature of the face and jaws should be distinguished from the following:

1. Odontogenous pains
2. Arthralgic pains that emanate from the temporomandibular joints
3. Neurovascular pain disorders
4. Heterotopic referred pains and secondary hyperalgesia due to other deep somatic pain input
5. Heterotopic projected neuropathic pains
6. Heterotopic pains of central origin
7. Pains of Axis II origin

Therapeutic Options

For the management of primary deep somatic musculoskeletal pains arising from orofacial muscles, the following general therapeutic options are available (see Chapter 9):

1. Restriction of functional activities within painless limits, analgesics and muscle relaxants for palliative relief, and counseling.
2. Cause-related therapy consisting of identification and treatment of etiologic factors and contributing conditions.
3. Specific therapy for masticatory pain of muscle origin:
   a. For protective co-contraction:
      1. Direct therapy toward the cause of the co-contraction.
      2. Set the muscle at rest.
      3. No therapy other than a muscle relaxant and/or mild analgesics.
   b. For delayed onset muscle soreness (local muscle soreness):
      1. Restrict use within painless limits.
      2. Maximum normal use but restrained well within painless limits.
      3. Occlusal disengagement.
      4. Analgesic blocking and functional manipulation.
      5. Exercises to reflexly relax muscle.
      6. Biofeedback training.
   c. For myofascial trigger points:
      1. Coolant spray and stretch manipulation.
      2. Deep massage and kneading.
      3. Compressive force of 20 to 30 lb sustained for 1 to 2 minutes.
      4. Ultrasound therapy.
      5. Local anesthesia injections and stretch manipulation.
   d. For muscle spasm:
      1. Immediate reduction of pain (ie, massage, cold, local anesthesia, etc).
      2. Followed by passive lengthening of the involved muscle.
   e. For muscle inflammation pain:

1. Until acute symptoms subside:
   a. Restrict use within painless limits.
   b. No exercises, massage, or injections.
   c. Anti-inflammatory therapy.
   d. Deep heat judiciously applied with increasing use as acute symptoms subside.
2. When the acute symptoms have subsided:
   a. Stop anti-inflammatory therapy.
   b. Institute active exercise therapy and increase it vigorously as resolution occurs.
3. Near the end of the resolution period:
   a. Add therapy to counteract muscle atrophy (isometric exercises), and myostatic contracture (momentary stretching exercises).
4. Medical consultation.

References

1. Layzer RB. Muscle pain, cramps and fatigue. In: Engel AG, Franzini-Armstrong C (eds). Myology. New York: McGraw-Hill; 1994: 1754–1768.

2. Jerusalem F. The microcirculation of muscle. In: Engel AG, Franzini-Armstrong C (eds). Myology. New York: McGraw-Hill; 1994: 316–374.

3. Travell J, Rinzier SH. The myofascial genesis of pain. Postgrad Med 1952; 11:425–434.

4. Molin C. Vertical isometric muscle forces of the mandible: A comparative study of subjects with and without manifest mandibular pain dysfunction syndrome. Acta Odontol Scand 1972; 30:485–499.

5. Nielsen IL, Ogro J, McNeill C, et al. Alteration in proprioceptive reflex control in subjects with craniomandibular disorders. J Cranomandib Disord Facial Oral Pain 1987; 1:170–178.

6. Wolff HG. Headache and Other Head Pain, ed 2. New York: Oxford University Press; 1963.

7. Ochoa JL, Torebjork HE. Pain from skin and muscle. Pain 1981; 11 (suppl 1):87.

8. MacDonald AJR. Abnormally tender muscle regions and associated painful movements. Pain 1980; 8:197–205.

9. Bell WE. Management of masticatory pain. In Alling CC (ed): Facial Pain. Philadelphia: Lea & Febiger; 1968: 191–212.

10. Hansson TL. Temporomandibular joint anatomical findings relevant to the clinician. In Clark GT, Solberg WK (eds): Perspectives in Temporomandibular Disorders. Chicago: Quintessence; 1987: 45–54.

11. Okeson JP. Management of Temporomandibular Disborders and Occlusion, ed 3. St Louis: Mosby Year Book; 1993:180–191.

12. Carlson CR, Okeson JP, Falace DA, et al. Comparison of psycholgical and physiological functioning between patients with masticatory muscle pain and matched controls. J Orofacial Pain 1993; 7:15–22.

13. Yemm R. A neurophysiological approach to the pathology and aetiology of temporomandibular dysfunction. J Oral Rehabil 1985; 12:343–353.

14. Schroeder H, Siegmund H, Santibanez G, Kluge A. Causes and signs of temporomandibular joint pain and dyfunction: An electromyographical investigation. J Oral Rehabil 1991; 18:301–331.

15. Flor H, Birbaumer N, Schulte W, Roos R. Stress-related electromyographic responses in patients with chronic temporomandibular pain. Pain 1991; 46:145–152.

16. Sternbach RA. Pain and hassles in the United States: Findings of the Nuprin pain report. Pain 1986; 27:69–80.

17. Selye H. Stress without distress. Philadelphia: JB Lipincott; 1974: 25–59.

18. Grassi C, Passatore M. Action of the sympathetic system on skeletal muscle. Ital J Neurol Sci 1988; 9:23–28.

19. Passatore M, Grassi C, Filippi GM. Sympathetically induced development of tension in jaw muscles: The possible contraction of intrafusal muscle fibers. Pflug Arch 1985; 405:297–304.

20. Wall PD, Devor M. Sensory afferent impluses originate from dorsal root ganglia as well as from the periphery in normal and nerve injured rats. Pain 1983; 17:321–339.

21. Melzack R, Wall PD. Pain mechanisms: A new theory. Science 1965; 150:971–979.

22. Wall PD. The gate theory of pain mechanisms: A reexamination and restatement. Brain 1978; 101:1–18.

23. Bell WE. Temporomandibular Disorders, ed 3. Chicago: Year Book; 1990: 60–61.

24. Lund JP, Olsson KA. The importance of reflexes and their control during jaw movements, Trends Neurosci1983; 6:456.

25. Stohler CS, Wang JS, Veerasarn P. Motor unit behavior in response to experimental muscle pain. J Dent Res 1990; 69:273.

26. Stohler C, Yamada Y, Ash MM. Antagonistic muscle stiffness and associated reflex behaviour in the pain-dysfunctional state. Schweiz Monatsschr Zahnmed 1985; 95:719–726.

27. Ashton-Miller JA, McGlashen KM, Herzenberg JE, Stohler CS. Cervical muscle myoelectric response to acute experimental sternocleidomastoid pain. Spine 1990; 15:1006–1012.

28. Smith AM. The coactivation of antagonist muscles. Can J Physiol Pharmacol 1981; 59:733–747.

29. Moulton RE. Psychologic considerations in treatment. In Schwartz LL (ed): Disorders of the Temporomandibular Joint. Philadelphia: WB Saunders; 1959: 307–312.

30. Moulton RE. Emotional factors in nonorganic temporomandibular joint pain. Dent Clin North Am 1966 (Nov); 609–620.

31. Lupton DE. A preliminary investigation of the personality of female temporomandibular joint dysfunction patients. Psychother Psychosom 1966; 14:199–216.

32. Moulton RE. Emotional factors in nonorganic temporomandibular joint pain. In Schwartz LL, Chayes CM (eds): Facial Pain and Mandibular Dysfunction. Philadelphia: WB Saunders; 1968: 318–334.

33. Laskin DM, Greene CS. Influence of the doctor-patient relationship on placebo therapy for patients with myofascial pain-dysfunction (MPD) syndrome. J Am Dent Assoc 1972; 85: 892–894.

34. Friden J, Sjostrom M, Ekblom B. A morphological study of delayed muscle soreness. Experimentia 1981; 37:506–507.

35. Friden J, Sjostrom M, Ekblom B. Myofibrillar damage following intense eccentric exercise in man. Int J Sports Med 1983; 4:170–176.

36. Friden J, Seger J, Sjostrom M, et al. Adaptive response in human skeletal muscle subjected to prolonged eccentric training. Int J Sports Med 1983; 4:177–183.

37. Mense S. Considerations concerning the neurobiological basis of muscle pain. Can J Physiol Pharmacol 1991; 69:610–616.

38. Sorini M, Pasero F, Rapetti A, et al. Masticatory muscle tenderness and masseteric clenching EMG activity. J Dent Res 1991; 70:330.

39. High AS, MacGregor AJ, Tomlinson GE. A gnathodynanometer as an objective means of pain assessment following wisdom tooth removal. Br J Oral Maxillofac Surg 1988; 26:284.

40. Fricton JR, Kroenig R, Haley D, Siegert R. Myofascial pain syndrome to the head and neck: a review of clinical characteristics of 164 patients. Oral Surg 1985; 60:615–623.

41. Travell JG, Rinzler SH. The myofascial genesis of pain. Postgrad Med 1952; 11:425–434.

42. Laskin DM. Etiology of the pain-dysfunction syndrome. J Am Dent Assoc 1969; 79:147–153.

43. Lange M. Die Muskelharten (Myogelosen). Munich: JF Lehman Verlag; 1931.

44. Glogowski G, Wallraff J. Ein Beitrag zur Klinik und Histologie der Muskelharten (Myogelosen). Z Orthop 1951; 80:238–245.

45. Simons DG, Travell JG. Letter to the editor. Pain 1981; 10:106–109.

46. Mense S, Meyer H: Bradykinin-induced sensitization of high-threshold muscle receptors with slowly conducting afferent fibers. Pain 1981; S204.

47. Foreman RD, Blair RW, Weber RN. Effect on T3 to T5 primate spinothalamic tract cells of injecting bradykinin into the heart. Pain 1981; 11 (suppl 1):212.

48. Travell J. Introductory comments. In Ragan C (ed): Connective Tissues. Transactions of the Fifth Conference. New York: Josiah Macy Jr Foundation; 1954: 12–22.

49. Travell JG, Simons DG. Myofasical Pain And Dysfunction: A Trigger Point Manual. Baltimore: Williams & Wilkins; 1983: 32–37.

50. Fricton JR, Auvinen MD, Dykstra D, et al. Myofascial pain syndrome: Electromyographic changes associated with local twitch response. Arch Phys Med Rehabil 1985; 66:314–317.

51. Fine PG, Milano R, Hare BD. The effects of myofascial trigger point injections are naloxone reversible. Pain 1988; 32:15–20.

52. Travell JG, Simons DG. Myofasical Pain and Dysfunction: A Trigger Point Manual, Baltimore: Williams & Wilkins; 1983: 103–164.

53. Giunta JL, Kronman JH. Orofacial involvement secondary to trapezius muscle trauma. Oral Surg 1985;60:368–369.

54. Travell JG, Simons DG. Myofasical Pain and Dysfunction: A Trigger Point Manual, Baltimore: Williams & Wilkins; 1983: 55–56.

55. Carlson CR, Okeson JP, Falace DA, Nitz AJ, Lindroth JE. Reduction of pain and EMG activity in the masseter region by trapezius trigger point injection. Pain 1993; 155:397–400.

56. McNamara JA Jr. The independent functions of the two heads of the lateral pterygoid muscle. Am J Anat 1973; 138:197–205.

57. Eriksson PO. Muscle-fiber composition of the human mandibular locomotor system. Swed Dent J 1982; 20:8–44.

58. Johnstone DR, Templeton M. The feasibility of palpating the lateral pterygoid muscle. J Prosthet Dent 1980; 44:318–323.

59. Thomas CA, Okeson JP. Evaluation of lateral pterygoid muscle symptoms using a common palpation technique and method of functional manipulation. J Craniomand Pract 1987; 5: 125–129.

60. Martin PR, Mathews AM. Tension headaches: Psychophysiological investigation and treatment. J Psychosom Res 1978; 22:389–399.

61. Sutton EP, Belar CD. Tension headache patients versus controls: A study of EMG parameters. Headache 1982; 22:133.

62. Finneson BE. Diagnosis and Management of Pain Syndromes, ed 2. Philadelphia: WB Saunders; 1969.

63. Dorland's Illustrated Medical Dictionary, ed 28. Philadelphia: WB Saunders; 1994: 1550.

64. Lund JP, Widmer CG. Evaluation of the use of surface electromyograph in the diagnosis, documentation and treatment of dental patients. J Crainomandib Disord Facial Oral Pain. 1989; 3:125–137.

65. Lund JP, Donga R, Widmer CG, Stohler CS. The pain-adaptation model: A discussion of the relationship between chronic musculoskeletal pain and motor activity. Can J Physiol Pharmacol 1991; 69:683–694.

66. Moldofsky H, Scarisbrick P. Induction of neurasthenic musculoskeletal pain syndrome by selective sleep deprivation. Psychsom Med 1976; 38:35–44.

67. Moldofsky H, Scarisbrick P, England R, Smythe H. Musculoskeletal symptoms and non-REM sleep disturbance in patients with fibrositis and healthy subjects. Psychosom Med 1975; 37: 341–351.

68. Moldofsky H, Tullis C, Lue FA. Sleep related myoclonus in rheumatic pain modulation disorder (fibrosis syndrome). J Rheumatol 1986; 13:614–617.

69. Molony RR, MacPeek DM, Schiffman PL, et al: Sleep, sleep apnea, and the fibromyalgia syndrome. J Rheumatol 1986;13:797–800.

70. Marbach JJ, Lennon MC, Dohrenwend BP. Candidate risk factors for temporomandibular pain and dysfunction syndrome: Psychosocial, health behavior, physical illiness and injury. Pain 1988; 34:139–151.

71. Tauschke E, Merskey H, Helms E. Psychological defence mechanisms in patients with pain. Pain 1990; 40:161–170.

72. Marbach JJ, Lund P. Depression, anhedonia, and anxiety in temporomandibular joint and other facial pain syndromes. Pain 1981; 11:73–84.

73. Fine E. Psychological factors associated with non-organic temporomandibular joint pain-dysfunction syndrome, Br Dent J 1971; 131: 402–404.

74. Haley WE, Turner JA, Romano JM. Depression in chronic pain patients: Relation to pain, activity and sex differences. Pain 1985; 23:337–343.

75. Dworkin RH, Richlin DM, Handlin DS, Brand L. Predicting treatment response in depressed and non-depressed patients with pain. Pain 1986; 24:343.

76. Wolfe F, Smythe HA, Yunus MB, et al. The American College of Rheumatology 1990 Criteria of the Classification of Fibromyalgia. Arthritis Rheum 1990; 33:160–172.

13 | Temporomandibular Joint Pains

Masticatory pain that emanates from the temporomandibular joints is called masticatory arthralgia (Fig 13-1). Arthralgic pains can arise only from pain-sensitive structures of the joint and its ligaments. Normally, the pressure-bearing articular surfaces as well as the articular disc are noninnervated and therefore are incapable of initiating sensory response of any kind, including nociception. Proprioceptive input needed for functional guidance does not come from the articular surfaces but from proprioceptors located in the ligaments and muscles. Pain from the temporomandibular joints can therefore emanate from the associated soft tissue structures of the joint or the osseous tissues themselves. Pain emanating from the osseous structures usually only occurs after loss of the fibrous articular surface of the joint. When this occurs, it is commonly referred to as *arthritis*. Not all joint pains, however are arthritis. When the soft tissues of the joint produce pain, the condition is classified according to the tissues involved (ie, retrodiscitis, capsulitis, etc).

Behavior of Temporomandibular Joint Pains

Pains that emanate from the structures of the temporomandibular joint are of the deep somatic category. As such, they display the clinical characteristics of deep somatic pain. Additionally, they are of the musculoskeletal type and therefore display the features that identify such pains: there is a strong relationship to the demands of masticatory function, and the pain is accentuated in a graduated manner by manual palpation or functional manipulation.

It should be noted that most arthralgia is related to functional abuse and trauma, which may be accompanied by inflammation. Thus, arthralgia frequently displays clinical characteristics of inflammatory pain that are influenced by the location, degree, and phase of inflammation present. Such pains exhibit features that depend on local provocation and functional manipulation as well as on the extent and confinement of inflammatory exudate. As long as joint pain occurs intermittently, it remains diffusely localized to the joint region and does not initiate secondary central excitatory effects. If arthralgia becomes continuous, however, a variety of secondary effects may become ev-

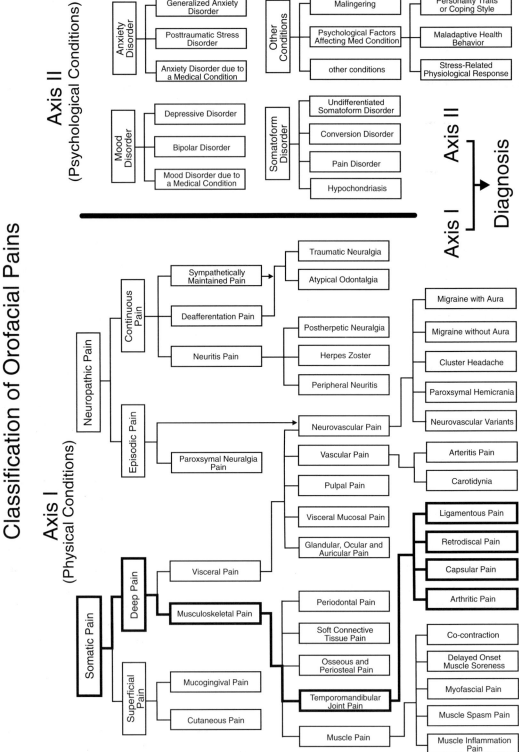

Fig 13-1 Pain classification chart highlighted to show the relationship of temporomandibular joint pains to other orofacial pain disorders.

ident such as referred pain that may be felt as headache, secondary hyperalgesia expressed as areas of deep palpable tenderness, and co-contraction activity in the masticatory musculature.

Normal Anatomy and Function of the Temporomandibular Joint

The temporomandibular joint represents the articulation of the mandible to the temporal bone of the cranium (Fig 13-2). The bony components of the joint are separated by a structure composed of dense fibrous connective tissue called the *articular disc.* Like any mobile joint, the integrity and limitations of the joint are maintained by ligaments. Ligaments are composed of collagenous fibers that have specific lengths. As in all mobile joints, ligaments do not actively participate in function of the joint. Ligaments act as guide wires to restrict certain movements (border movements) while allowing other movements (functional movements). If joint movements consistently function against ligaments, the length of the ligaments can become altered. Ligaments have a poor ability to stretch and therefore, when this occurs, they often permanently elongate. This elongation creates a change in joint biomechanics and can lead to certain clinical changes that will be discussed later.

The temporomandibular joint is capable of both hinging and gliding movements and therefore is known as a ginglymoarthrodial joint. To simplify the mechanics of this extremely complex joint, it can be separated into two distinct joints. The lower joint is made up of the condyle and disc, which are attached to each other by ligaments. This combined structure is referred to as the condyle-disc complex. The condyle-disc complex allows rotational movement between the disc and the condyle. The upper joint is formed by the condyle-disc complex articulating with the glenoid fossa. It is between these structures that translation occurs as the condyle-disc complex moves out of the fossa during opening.

Careful examination of the condyle and disc reveals that the disc is attached to the condyle both medially and laterally by the discal collateral ligaments (Fig 13-3). These ligaments allow rotation of the disc across the articular surface of the condyle in an anterior and posterior direction while restricting medial and lateral movements. The range of anterior and posterior rotation of the disc is also restricted by ligaments. The inferior retrodiscal lamina limits anterior rotation of the disc on the condyle whereas the anterior capsular ligament limits posterior rotation of the disc (see Fig 13-2).

The morphologic characteristics of the disc are extremely important. It is thinnest in the intermediate zone, thicker in the anterior border, and thickest in the posterior border. The condyle articulates on the intermediate zone of the disc and is maintained in this position by constant interarticular pressure provided by the elevator muscles (masseter, temporalis, and medial pterygoid). Although the pressure between the condyle, disc, and fossa can vary according to the activity of the elevator muscles, some pressure is always maintained to prevent separation of the articular surfaces. If contact between the articular surfaces is lost, a condition of dislocation exists (dislocation means separation of the articular surfaces).

Posterior to the disc are the retrodiscal tissues. These tissues are highly vascularized

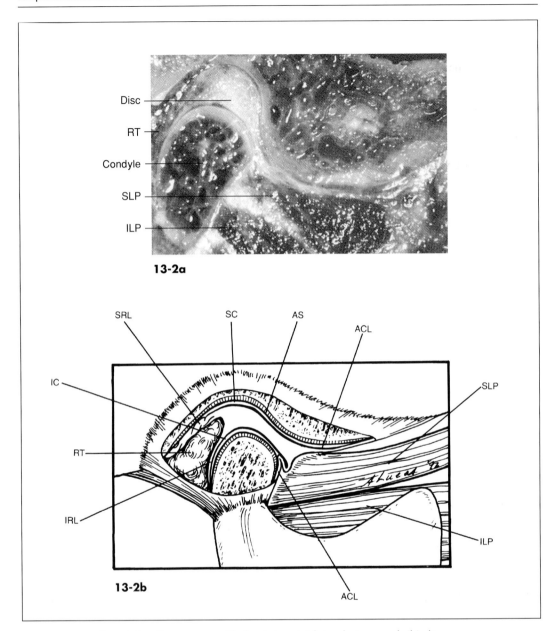

Fig 13-2 Temporomandibular joint. *(a)* lateral view and *(b)* diagram showing the anatomic components: *RT* = retrodiscal tissues; *SRL* = superior retrodiscal lamina (elastic); *IRL* = inferior retrodiscal lamina (collagenous); *ACL* = anterior capsular ligament (collagenous); *SLP* and *ILP* = superior and inferior lateral pterygoid muscles; *AS* = articular surface; *SC* and *IC* = superior and inferior joint cavity; the discal (collateral) ligament has not been drawn. (From, Okeson JP. Management of Temporomandibular Disorders and Occlusion, ed 3. St Louis: Mosby Year Book; 1993: 11. Used with permission.)

Fig 13-3 Temporomandibular joint (anterior view). The following are identified: *AD* = articular disc; *CL* = capsular ligament; *LDL* = lateral discal ligament; *MDL* = medial discal ligament; *SC* = superior joint cavity; *IC* = inferior joint cavity. (From Okeson JP. Management of Temporomandibular Disorders and Occlusion, ed 3. St Louis: Mosby Year Book; 1993:12. Used with permission.)

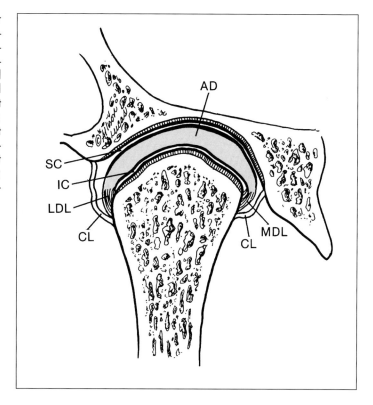

and well innervated. Anterior to the condyle-disc complex are the superior and inferior lateral pterygoid muscles. The inferior pterygoid muscle inserts on the neck of the condyle whereas the superior lateral pterygoid muscle inserts on both the neck of the condyle and the articular disc. Although the inferior lateral pterygoid is active with the depressing muscles (mouth opening), the superior lateral pterygoid muscle has been shown to be active in conjunction with the elevator muscles (mouth closing).[1,2] The superior lateral pterygoid muscle appears to be a stabilizing muscle for the condyle-disc complex, especially during unilateral chewing.[3]

When the condyle-disc complex translates down the articular eminence (mouth opening), the disc rotates posteriorly on the condyle as seen in Figure 13-4. The superior surface of the retrodiscal tissues is unlike any other structure in the joint. The superior retrodiscal lamina is composed of loose connective tissue and elastin fibers that allow the condyle-disc complex to translate forward without damage to the retrodiscal tissues. In the closed mouth position, the superior retrodiscal tissues are passive and have very little influence on disc position. During full mouth opening however, the superior retrodiscal lamina is fully stretched and produces a mild posterior retractive force on the disc. It is important to remember that this is the only structure in the temporomandibular joint capable of providing a retractive force on the articular disc.

299

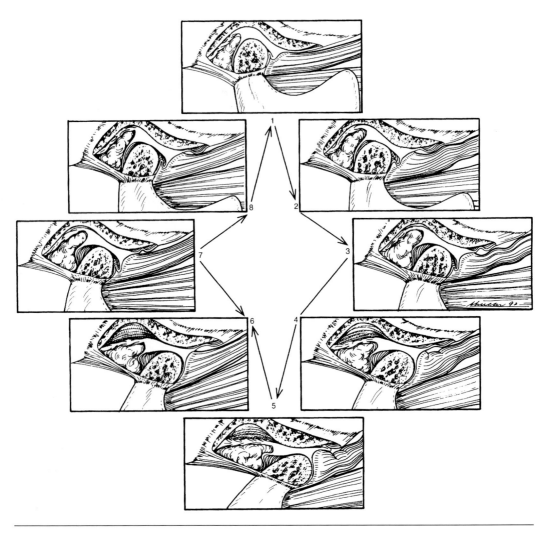

Fig 13-4 Normal functional movement of the condyle and disc during the full range of opening and closing. Note that the disc is rotated posteriorly on the condyle as the condyle is translated out of the fossa. The closing movement is the exact opposite of opening. (From Okeson JP. Management of Temporomandibular Disorders and Occlusion, ed 3. St Louis: Mosby Year Book; 1993: 24–25. Used with permission.)

During opening and closing, the disc and condyle move together, not because of ligamentous attachments, but because of two fundamental features: the morphologic characteristics of the disc and interarticular pressure (pressure between the articular surfaces). Because some degree of interar-ticular pressure is always present, the condyle maintains itself on the thinnest intermediate zone of the disc. The thicker anterior and posterior borders of the disc force it to translate with the condyle during mouth opening and closing. The morphologic characteristics of the disc, therefore, require it to move with the condyle. If there is an alteration in interarticular pressure or a change in the characteristics of the disc, condyle-disc movement can be altered. This, in fact, begins the biomechanical changes associated with many intracapsular symptoms.

Normally the thinnest portion of the disc is centered on the condyle when the interarticular space is minimal, as during maximum intercuspation. Biting on one side against a bolus of food depresses the condyle on the ipsilateral side and widens the articular space. When this occurs, the disc is rotated anteriorly by the superior lateral pterygoid muscle, which contracts in conjunction with elevator muscle action. Thus, the thicker posterior part of the disc firmly fills the articular disc space, and adequate stability of the joint is maintained. Then, as the teeth bite through the bolus and the space narrows accordingly, disc contour causes it to rotate posteriorly, thereby bringing the thinner portion of disc back into position. It becomes fully centered when maximum intercuspation is accomplished. As the resting position is assumed, the space increases, with compensating rotation of the disc anteriorly as the result of muscle tonus in the resting superior lateral pterygoid muscle. This permits synovial fluid to bathe the surfaces from which it was expelled by pressure during the biting effort.

Subtle but essential disc rotary movement is constantly going on. This is in addition to that necessary for keeping the upper surface of the disc in proper contact with the eminence during translatory movement as well as for gross separation of the jaws for opening. The more steeply inclined the articular eminence, the greater the disc movement required for condylar translation.[4]

Types of Temporomandibular Joint Pains

Arthralgic pain that emanates from non-arthritic temporomandibular joint structures must arise from structures that are innervated: the collateral discal ligaments; the retrodiscal tissue; and the joint capsule itself, which includes the strong temporomandibular (lateral) ligament that reinforces its lateral wall.[4] Therefore, depending on the structure from which the pain emanates, nonarthritic temporomandibular arthralgia may be identified as ligamentous pain, retrodiscal pain, or capsular pain, or some combination of the three. Arthritis comprises a fourth source of arthralgia that may be identified as arthritic pain.

The ligamentous structures of the joint are innervated for proprioceptive function. They therefore are particularly responsive to such biomechanical factors as pressure, traction, stress, strain, torque, and movement. If such mechanical influence becomes noxious, pain results.[5] Both proprioceptive and nociceptive responses are dependent on the presence of normal neural structures.[6] As ligamentous deterioration takes place, the proprioceptive response as well as pain diminishes. It is a paradox that decreasing pain emanating from such structures may be indicative of a worsening condition of the ligaments from which it arises. It is important that this be kept in mind when evaluating the seriousness of joint pains. It should also be noted that proprioceptive responses are answered by skeletal muscle activity. Muscle co-contraction is a normal protective reaction of muscles in response to altered proprioceptive input. Therefore, muscle pain of the protective co-contraction type may accompany noxious biomechanical forces that affect the joint. Again, such response depends on normal innervation of the ligamentous structures of the joint. Acute muscle effects are indicative of normally functioning proprioceptors and therefore identify a lesser degree of deterioration in the ligaments. As deterioration takes place due to continued functional abuse and trauma, such muscle effects are less likely to occur.

It should be recognized that masticatory pain emanates from masticatory muscles, from pain-sensitive structures of the temporomandibular joints, or from both. Effective therapy depends on accurate identification of pain source. It is therefore of considerable importance that, not only should myalgia be distinguished from arthralgia, but the type of myalgia or arthralgia be correctly identified. Arthralgia emanating from the temporomandibular joints may be classified as: ligamentous pain, retrodiscal pain, capsular pain, and arthritic pain.

Ligamentous Pain

Pain originating from the ligamentous attachments of the condyle-disc complex may present as a range of conditions, some of which can be viewed as a continuum of progressive events. They occur secondary to changes in the relationship between the articular disc and the condyle. These conditions are often referred to as *disc-interference or internal derangement disorders.*

If the apprearance of the disc is altered and the discal ligaments become elongated, the disc is then permitted to slide (translate) across the articular surface of the condyle. This type of movement is not present in the healthy joint. Its degree is determined by

changes that have occurred in the appearance of the disc and the degree of elongation of the discal ligaments.

Assume for purposes of discussion that the discal ligaments become elongated. (Ligaments can be only elongated. They cannot be stretched. Stretch implies extension followed by a return to the original length. Ligaments do not have elasticity and therefore, once elongated, generally remain at that length.) In the normal closed joint position and during function, interarticular pressure still allows the disc to position itself on the condyle and no unusual symptoms are noted. Alteration in the morphologic characteristics of the disc accompanied by elongation of the discal ligaments can change this normal functioning relationship. In the resting closed-joint position, the interarticular pressure is very low. If the discal ligaments become elongated, the disc is free to move on the articular surface of the condyle. Since in the closed joint position the superior retrodiscal lamina does not provide much influence on disc position, tonicity of the superior lateral pterygoid will encourage the disc to assume a more forward position on the condyle. The forward movement of the disc will be limited by the length of the discal ligaments, inferior retrodiscal lamina, and the thickness of the posterior border of the disc. As this area is thinned, the disc may be displaced more in the anteromedial direction. Since the superior retrodiscal lamina provides little resistance in the closed joint position, the medial and anterior position of the disc is maintained. As the posterior border of the disc becomes thinned, it can be displaced further into the discal space so that the condyle becomes positioned on the posterior border of the disc. This condition is

Fig 13-5 *(a)* Normal position of the disc on the condyle in the closed joint position. *(b)* Functional displacement of the disc. Its posterior border has been thinned and the discal and inferior retrodiscal ligaments are elongated, allowing activity of the superior lateral pterygoid to displace the disc anteriorly (and medially). *(c)* In this specimen the condyle is articulating on the posterior band of the disc *(PB)* and not on the intermediate zone *(IZ)*. This depicts an anterior displacement of the disc. (From Okeson JP. Management of Temporomandibular Disorders and Occlusion, ed 3. St Louis: Mosby Year Book; 1993: 195. Used with permission.)

known as *functional disc displacement* (Fig 13-5). Most persons report functional displacements of the disc initially as a momentary altered sensation during movement but not usually pain. Pain may occasionally be experienced when the person bites (a power stroke) and activates the superior lateral pterygoid. As this muscle pulls, the disc is displaced further and tightness in the already elongated discal ligament can produce joint pain.

With the disc in this more forward and medial position, function of the joint can be somewhat compromised. As the mouth opens and the condyle moves forward, a short distance of translatory movement can occur between the condyle and the disc until the condyle once again assumes its normal position on the thinnest area of the disc (intermediate zone). Once it has translated over the posterior surface of the disc to the intermediate zone, interarticular pressure maintains this relationship and the disc is again carried forward with the condyle through the remaining portion of the translatory movement. After the full forward movement is completed, the condyle begins to return and the stretched fibers of the superior retrodiscal lamina actively assist in returning the disc with the condyle to the closed joint position. Again, the interarticular pressure maintains the articular surface of the condyle on the intermediate zone of the disc by not allowing the thicker anterior border to pass between the condyle and the articular eminence. Once in the closed joint position, again the disc is free to move according to the demands of its functional attachments. The presence of muscle tonicity will again encourage the disc to assume its most anteromedial position allowed by the discal attachments and its own morphologic characteristics. One can imagine that if muscle hyperactivity were present (as with bruxism), the superior lateral pterygoid muscle would have even a greater influence of the disc position.

The important feature of this functional relationship is that the condyle translates across the disc to some degree when movement begins. This type of movement does not occur in the normal joint. During such movement, the increased interarticular pressure may prevent the articular surfaces from sliding across each other smoothly. The disc can stick or be bunched slightly, causing an abrupt movement of the condyle over it into the normal condyle-disc relationship. Accompanying this abrupt movement is often a clicking sound. Once the joint has clicked, the normal relationship of the disc and condyle is reestablished and this relationship is maintained during the rest of the opening movement. During closing of the mouth, the normal relationship of the disc and condyle is maintained because of interarticular pressure. However, once the mouth is closed and the interarticular pressure is lower, the disc can once again be displaced forward by tonicity of the superior lateral pterygoid muscle. In many instances if the displacement is slight and the interarticular pressure is low, no click is noted during this redisplacement. This single click observed during opening movement represents the very early stages of disc derangement disorder or what is also called internal derangement.

If this condition persists, a second stage of derangement is noted. As the disc is more chronically repositioned forward and medially by muscle action of the superior lateral pterygoid, the discal ligaments are further elongated. Continued forward positioning of the disc also causes elongation of the inferior retrodiscal lamina. Accompanying this breakdown is a continued thinning of the posterior border of the disc, which permits the disc to be repositioned more anteriorly, resulting in the condyle being positioned more posteriorly on the posterior border.[7] The morphologic changes of the disc at the area where the condyle rests can create a second click during the later stages of condylar return just prior to the closed joint position. This stage of derangement is called the reciprocal click[8] (Fig 13-6).

The opening click can occur at any time during that movement depending on disc-

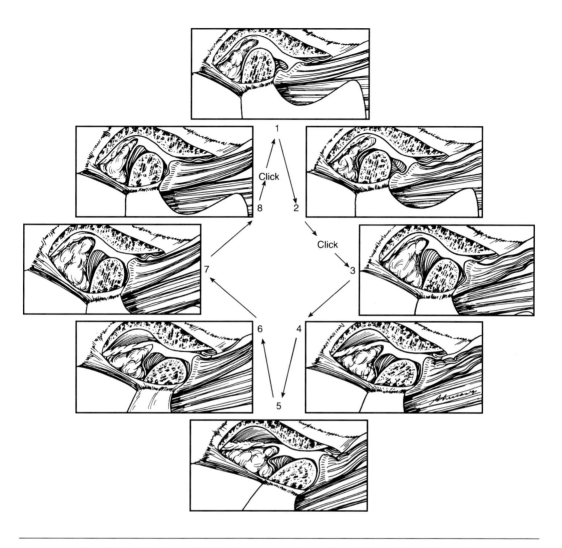

Fig 13-6 Reciprocal click. Between positions *2* and *3,* a click is felt as the condyle moves across the posterior border of the disc. Normal condyle-disc function occurs during the remaining opening and closing movement until the closed joint position is approached. Then a second click is heard as the condyle once again moves from the intermediate zone to the posterior border of the disc (between *8* and *1*). (From Okeson JP. Management of Temporomandibular Disorders and Occlusion, ed 3. St Louis: Mosby Year Book; 1993: 198. Used with permission.)

condyle morphologic characteristics, muscle pull, and the pull of the superior retrodiscal lamina. The closing click almost always occurs very near the closed or intercuspal position.

The longer the disc is anteriorly displaced, the longer the superior retrodiscal lamina is being elongated. If this condition is maintained for a prolonged period, the elasticity of the superior retrodiscal lamina can break down and be lost. It is important to remember that this area is the only structure that can apply retractive force on the disc. Once this force is lost, there is no mechanism to retract the disc posteriorly.

Some authors[9] debate that the superior lateral pterygoid muscle is not the major influencing factor on the anterior medial displacement of the disc. Although this would appear to be the obvious influencing factor, certainly other features need to be considered. Tanaka[10,11] has identified a ligamentous attachment of the medial portion of the condyle-disc complex to the medial wall of the fossa. If this ligament were tightly bound, forward movement of the condyle could create a tethering of the disc to the medial. Tanaka[12] has also identified that the retrodiscal tissues are tightly attached in the medial aspect of the posterior fossa but not in the lateral aspect. This might suggest that the lateral aspect of the disc can be more easily displaced then the medial, allowing the direction of the disc displacement to be more anteromedially. There are likely to be still other factors that have not yet been described. Further investigation in this area is needed.

With this in mind, we can now begin a discussion of the next stage of disc derangement. The longer the disc is displaced anteriorly and medially, the greater will be the thinning of its posterior border and the more the lateral discal ligament and inferior retrodiscal lamina will be elongated. Also, protracted anterior displacement of the disc leads to a greater loss of elasticity in the superior retrodiscal lamina. The more the shape of the disc changes to accommodate the pull of the muscle and position of the condyle, the greater is the likelihood that the disc will be forced through the discal space, collapsing the joint space behind. In other words, if the posterior border of the disc becomes thin, the disc can slip completely through the discal space. When this occurs, interarticular pressure will collapse the discal space, trapping the disc in the forward position. Then the next full translation of the condyle is inhibited by the anterior and medial position of the disc. The person feels the joint being locked in a limited closed position. Since the articular surfaces have actually been separated, this condition is referred to as a functional dislocation of the disc (Fig 13-7).

As already described, a functionally displaced disc can create joint sounds as the condyle skids across the disc during normal translation of the mandible. If the disc becomes functionally dislocated, the joint sounds are eliminated since no skidding can occur. This can be helpful information in distinguishing a functional displacement from a functional dislocation.

Some persons with a functional dislocation of the disc are able to move the mandible in various lateral directions to accommodate the movement of the condyle over the posterior border of the disc and the locked condition is resolved. If the lock occurs only occasionally and the person can resolve it with no assistance, it is referred to as a *functional dislocation with reduction* (Fig 13-8). The patient will often report that the jaw catches when opening wide. This condition may or may not be painful depending on the severity and duration of the lock and the integrity of the structures in the joint. If it is acute, with a short history and duration, joint pain may only be associated with elongation of the joint ligaments (such as trying to force the jaw open). As episodes of catching or locking become

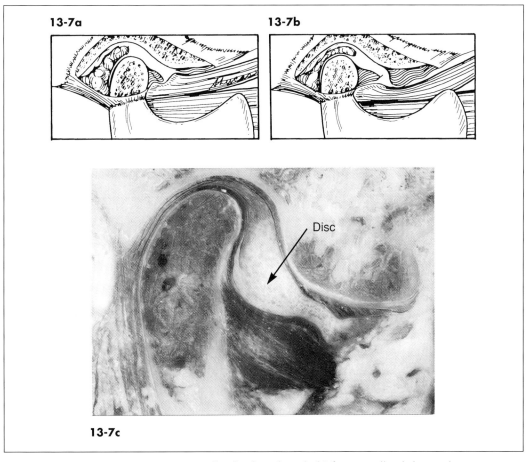

Fig 13-7 *(a)* Functionally displaced and *(b)* functionally dislocated discs. In the functionally dislocated disc, the joint space has narrowed and the disc is trapped anteriorly (and medially). *(c)* In this specimen the disc is functionally dislocated anterior to the condyle. (From Okeson JP. Management of Temporomandibular Disorders and Occlusion, ed 3. St Louis: Mosby Year Book; 1993: 200. Used with permission.)

more frequent and chronic, ligaments break down and innervation is lost. Pain becomes less associated with ligaments and more related to forces placed on the retrodiscal tissues.

The next stage of disc derangement is known as *functional disc dislocation without reduction*. This condition occurs when the person is unable to return the dislocated disc to its normal position on the condyle.

The mouth cannot be opened maximally because the position of the disc does not allow full translation of the condyle (Fig 13-9). Typically the initial opening will be only 25 to 30 mm interincisally, which represents the maximum rotation of the joint. The person usually is aware of which joint is involved and can remember the occasion that led to the locked feeling. Since usually only one joint becomes locked, a distinct pattern

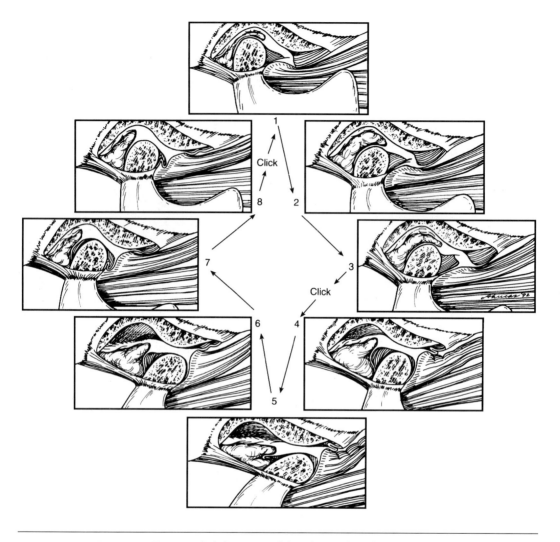

Fig 13-8 Functional dislocation of the disc with reduction. Note that during opening the condyle passes over the posterior border of the disc onto the intermediate area of the disc, thus reducing the dislocated disc. This may be felt as a catching sensation and is often associated with reciprocal clicking. (From Okeson JP. Management of Temporomandibular Disorders and Occlusion, ed 3. St Louis: Mosby Year Book; 1993: 198. Used with permission.)

of mandibular movement is observed clinically. The joint with the functionally dislocated disc without reduction does not allow complete translation of its condyle whereas the other joint functions normally. Therefore, when the patient opens wide, the midline of the mandible is deflected to the affected side. Also the patient is able to perform a normal lateral movement to the affected side (the condyle on the affected side only rotates). However, when movement is attempted to the unaffected side, a restric-

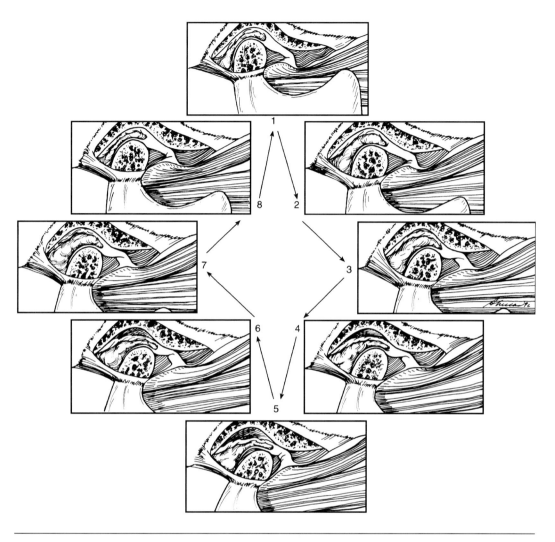

Fig 13-9 Closed lock. Note that the condyle never assumes a normal relationship on the disc but instead causes the disc to move forward ahead of it. This condition limits the distance it can translate forward. (From Okeson JP. Management of Temporomandibular Disorders and Occlusion, ed 3. St Louis: Mosby Year Book; 1993: 203. Used with permission.)

tion develops (the condyle on the affected side cannot translate past the anterior functionally dislocated disc): The dislocation without reduction is known as a *closed lock*. Patients may report pain when the mandible is moved to the point of limita-

tion, but pain is not necessarily an accompaniment of this condition.[13]

If the closed lock continues, the condyle will be chronically positioned on the retrodiscal tissues. These tissues are not anatomically structured to accept force. Therefore, as force is applied, there is a great likelihood that the tissues will break down.[14] With this breakdown comes tissue inflammation. This disorder will be discussed in the next category of temporomandibular joint pains.

Any condition or event that leads to elongation of the discal ligaments or thinning of the disc can cause these derangements of the condyle-disc complex disorders. Certainly one of the most common factors is trauma. Two general types of trauma need to be considered: macrotrauma or microtrauma.

Macrotrauma. Macrotrauma is any sudden force to the joint that causes structural alterations. The major type of injury that can elongate the discal ligaments is a blow to the mandible when the teeth are separated. This open-mouth trauma can produce a sudden displacement of the condyle within the fossa. This sudden movement of the condyle is resisted by the ligaments. If the force is great, the ligaments can become elongated, which may compromise normal condyle-disc mechanics. The resulting increased looseness can lead to discal displacement and to the symptoms of clicking and catching. Unexpected macrotrauma to the jaw (as might be sustained during a fall or in a motor vehicle accident) may lead to discal displacement and/or dislocation.[15-22]

Macrotrauma can also occur when the teeth are together (closed mouth trauma). If trauma occurs to the mandible when the teeth are together, the intercuspation of the teeth maintains the jaw position resisting joint displacement. Closed mouth trauma is therefore less injurious to the condyle-disc complex. This reduction of potential injury becomes obvious when one examines the incidence of injury associated with athletic activity. Athletes who wear soft protective mouth appliances have significantly fewer jaw-related injuries then those that do not.[23,24] It would be wise, therefore, that if facial trauma was expected, a soft appliance should be in place or at least the teeth held tightly in the intercuspal position. Unfortunately most macrotrauma is unexpected (ie, motor vehicle accident) and therefore the teeth are separated, commonly resulting in injury to the joint structures.

Closed mouth trauma is not likely to be without some consequence. Although ligaments may not be elongated, articular surfaces can certainly receive sudden traumatic loading. This type of impact loading may disrupt the articular surface of the condyle, fossa, or disc. This may lead to alterations in the smooth sliding surfaces of the joint causing roughness and even sticking during movement. This type of trauma therefore, may result in adhesions, which can further compromise condyle-disc function.

On occasion, trauma can result in an alteration of the articular surfaces of the condyle and/or fossa. If such changes occur, they can also interrupt the normal smooth sliding movements of the joint. Structural incompatibility, whether secondary to trauma or developmentally related, represents another type of intracapsular disorder that can lead to disc attachment pain.

Macrotrauma may also be iatrogenic. Anytime the jaw is overextended, elongation of the ligaments can occur. Patients are more at risk for this type of injury if they have been sedated, reducing normal joint stabilization by the muscles. A few common examples of iatrogenic trauma are intubation procedures,[25] third molar extraction procedures, and a long dental appointment.

In fact, any extended wide opening of the mouth (eg, a yawn) has the potential of elongating the discal ligaments. The medical and dental professions need to be acutely aware of these conditions so a disc derangement problem that might last the patient's lifetime is avoided.

Microtrauma. Microtrauma is any small force to joint structures that occurs repeatedly over a long period. A good example would be muscle hyperactivity. A patient who clenches or bruxes consistently activates the superior lateral pterygoid muscle. As already described, this activity may encourage the disc to assume a more antero-medial position on the condyle. This positioning in turn may lead to thinning of the posterior border of the disc and subsequent elongation of the inferior retrodiscal lamina. The end result is disc displacement.

Another type of microtrauma may result when there is a lack of orthopedic stability within the masticatory system. Orthopedic stability exists when the stable intercuspal position of the teeth is in harmony with the musculoskeletally stable position of the condyles.[26] When this condition does not exist, microtrauma may result. This trauma occurs not when the teeth are initially brought into contact but only during loading of the masticatory structures by the elevator muscles. Once the teeth are in the intercuspal position, elevator muscle activity loads the teeth and the joints. Since the intercuspal position represents the most stable position for the teeth, loading is accepted by the teeth without consequence. If the condyles are also in a stable relationship in the fossae, loading occurs with no adverse effect to the joint structures. If, however, loading occurs when a joint is not in a sta-ble relationship with the disc and fossa, unusual movement can occur in an attempt to gain stability. This movement is often a translatory shift between disc and condyle. This movement can lead to elongation of the discal ligaments and thinning of the disc.[27] It should be remembered that the amount and intensity of the loading greatly influence whether the orthopedic instability will lead to a disc derangement disorder. Patients with bruxism and orthopedic instability, therefore, are more likely to create problems than those without bruxism and the same occlusion.

Occlusion and Disc Derangement Disorders. An important question that arises in dentistry is "What occlusal conditions are commonly associated with disc derangements?" It has been demonstrated that when an occlusal condition causes a condyle to be positioned posterior to the musculoskeletally stable position, the posterior border of the disc can be thinned.[28] A common occlusal condition that appears to provide this environment is the skeletal class II deep bite, which seems to be further aggravated when a division 2 anterior relationship also exists.[29-34] One needs to be aware however, that not all patients with class II malocclusions present with disc derangement disorders. Some studies show no relationship between class II malocclusion and these disorders.[35-43] Other studies show no association between the horizontal and vertical relationship of the anterior teeth and disc derangement disorders.[44,45] The important feature of an occlusal condition that leads to disc derangement disorders is the lack of joint stability when the teeth are tightly occluded. It is likely that some class II malocclusions provide joint stability while others do not. Another factor that must be considered is the amount of joint loading. Perhaps joint loading is more damaging with certain class II malocclusions. It becomes obvious that no simple relationship exists. It is vitally important however, that when orthopedic instability exists it be identified as a potential etiologic factor; successful management may depend on prompt alteration of the damaging relationship (see Case 11).

The following are clinical symptoms by which ligamentous pain can be recognized:

1. The pain occurs intermittently in conjunction with clinically evident disc interference of some type.
2. Pain that occurs in conjunction with condylar translatory movements relates specifically to one of the following etiologic groups of disc-interference disorders[4]:
   a. Excessive passive interarticular pressure.
   b. Structural incompatibility between the sliding parts.
   c. Degeneration of the articular surfaces.
   d. Impaired disc-condyle complex.
3. Protective muscle co-contraction may be displayed.
4. Dysfunction in the form of interference during mandibular movements is characteristic. If such interference is sufficient to arrest condylar movement, dysfunction in the form of restricted range of motion is displayed.
5. Ordinarily, central excitatory effects are not seen. (If the ligaments become inflamed, the clinical characteristics of capsular pain will be displayed. Then, secondary effects may become evident.)

Retrodiscal Pain

The retrodiscal tissues are located posterior to the articular disc and extend back to the posterior wall of the joint capsule. As previously mentioned, these tissues are composed of highly vascularized, loose connective tissue. The inferior retrodiscal lamina is composed of collagenous tissue and serves as a ligament that restricts anterior rotation of the disc on the condyle and delineates the inferior synovial sac between the articular disc and the mandibular condyle posteriorly. The superior retrodiscal lamina is composed of elastic tissue and serves, not as a ligament, but as a tractive force on the articular disc when the condyle is translated forward. In the closed mouth occluded position, however, both laminae are relaxed and exert no traction on the disc. The superior retrodiscal lamina delineates the superior synovial sac between the articular disc and the tympanic plate posteriorly. The retrodiscal tissue is sometimes referred to as the posterior attachment of the disc.

Both retrodiscal laminae are surfaced with synovial membrane. The vascularity of the retrodiscal tissue is a major source of synovial fluid to both compartments of the joint. This tissue is structured so that full and extensive translatory movements of the condyle do not interfere with the continuous flow of nutrients and metabolic exchange supplying the nonvascularized articular surfaces and articular disc. The retrodiscal tissue is innervated as other loose connective tissue with somatic and visceral afferents including nociceptors and with visceral efferents to the blood vessels.[6] It has little or no proprioceptive capability; its chief function is nutritional.

The vital retrodiscal tissue is not subject

to injury under normal conditions of mandibular function. If condylar encroachment does occur, inflammation may take place. This is marked by extensive swelling, extravasation of inflammatory fluid into the synovial sacs, and pain, especially when the condyle presses against the swollen tissue during maximum intercuspation. Trauma to the mandible can therefore induce an acute retrodiscitis. Such a condition causes acute malocclusion in the resting occluded position due to swelling of the retrodiscal tissue and excessive intracapsular fluid. The pain that occurs when the teeth are firmly occluded may be reduced considerably by biting against a separator that prevents intercuspation of the teeth. There may be some accentuation of pain when forceful ipsilateral excursions are made (Case 8).

Retrodiscitis displays symptoms that may be misdiagnosed as an inferior lateral pterygoid muscle spasm or as disc-attachment (ligamentous) pain due to orthopedic instability that occurs when the teeth are clenched in maximum intercuspation. It is important that these conditions be differentiated because treatment is not the same. Spastic shortening of the muscle is identified by pain induced by a resisted protrusive effort. Disc-attachment pain due to orthopedic instability displays no acute malocclusion in the resting occluded position. Radiographically, these three conditions may appear the same. Radiographic evidence therefore should not be accepted as conclusive unless it is confirmed by clinical symptoms.

The possibility of acute retrodiscitis should be considered in traumatic incidents that involve the mandible, both with and without osseous fracture (Case 9). The symptoms may be misdiagnosed as a man-dibular fracture when none exists. Therapy should also take into consideration the possibility of hemarthrosis, which presents the chance of adhesions between the disc and temporal fossa (ankylosis) or between the disc and condyle.

An insidious chronic form of retrodiscitis may occur as the result of functional encroachment of the condyle on the retrodiscal tissue due to orthopedic instability that displaces the condyle posteriorly when the teeth are firmly clenched in maximum intercuspation. The resultant deterioration in the discal ligaments, the disc proper, and the temporomandibular ligament permits condylar encroachment on the retrodiscal tissue. Such a condition is insidious, so that inflammatory changes sufficient to elicit symptoms usually do not occur. Such condylar encroachment involves the inferior retrodiscal lamina first, then the body of retrodiscal tissue. This usually leaves the vital superior retrodiscal lamina to function within normal limits. As metaplasia converts the retrodiscal loose connective tissue into a denser fibrotic tissue, the decreased vascularity may affect the synovial fluid metabolism. This may further complicate the already difficult problem of functional displacement of the articular disc upon which the retrodiscal condition is superimposed. If the matter of functional displacement proceeds to the point of anterior dislocation of the articular disc, biting pressure of the condyle against the remaining unprotected retrodiscal tissue may induce retrodiscal pain. This would disappear as further metaplasia of the tissue takes place.

Case 8 Temporomandibular arthralgia originating in the retrodiscal tissues

Chief Complaint

Right TMJ pain.

History

A 45-year-old woman with mild-to-severe intermittent steady dull aching pain diffusely located in the right preauricular area. The pain is induced by clenching the teeth, and lasts from a few minutes to an hour or longer. The pain is accompanied by sensations of interference and disc noise especially associated with occluding the teeth firmly.

The complaint began about 6 months ago. One day while chewing, she bit down firmly and sensed a locking of the right joint. As she opened, it popped very loudly and she felt severe sharp pain in the TMJ area. The noise and pain have occurred with firmly occluding the teeth ever since. She reports that for several years prior to this, she had noisy TM joints with chewing. She presently has no complaint of restriction of mandibular movements or any recent alteration in her "bite." She is taking no medications of any kind.

Examination

Intraoral: Clinical examination fails to identify any dental or oral cause for the pain except for the orthopedic instability provided by the occlusal condition as indicated by sensing premature contact of the right premolars, a feeling of increased pressure on those teeth in the fully occluded position, and some movement from primary contact to the full occlusal position. She feels right preauricular pain when she clenches the teeth and this is accompanied by a "binding sensation." As she releases the teeth, moderate right disc noise is heard. All this is readily prevented by biting on a tongue blade. Otherwise, masticatory functioning is clinically normal.

TM Joints: Both joints present clinical evidence of changes in the articular discs positions. When the condyles are positioned by bilateral manual manipulation into the musculoskeletal stable position, the teeth do not occlude soundly. When the patient is asked to fully close the teeth together, a 3-mm shift forward and to the left is noted.

Muscles: No palpable tenderness in the masticatory muscles. All functioning appears to be well within normal limits.

Cervical: Within normal limits.

Cranial Nerves: Within normal limits.

Impression

The patient presents with an orthopedically unstable relationship between the stable occlusal position and the orthopedically stable position for the joints. Over the years, this instability coupled with chewing and other loading factors has resulted in alteration in normal condyle/disc function leading to the joint sounds. A few months ago, she accidentally impinged the right disc with sufficient force to injure its attachments to the condyle, thus causing the symptoms of acute retrodiscitis.

Diagnosis

Acute retrodiscitis of the right TM joint, due to intrinsic injury.

| Case 9 | Acute retrodiscitis secondary to trauma |

Chief Complaint Left TMJ area pain.

History A 46-year-old woman with mild intermittent steady dull aching pain diffusely located in the left preauricular area induced by clenching the teeth and accompanied by acute malocclusion described as premature contact of the right anterior teeth with disocclusion of the posterior teeth unless forced into full occlusion.

The complaint began a week ago following an automobile accident in which she sustained a heavy blow to the right chin. Radiographs failed to identify a mandibular fracture. Because of the acute malocclusion the oral surgeon was suspicious of an unidentified fracture and placed arch bars and inter-arch elastics to bring the teeth into normal occlusion. In doing so, however, pain increased until it became intolerable, and he was forced to remove the intermaxillary elastics and refer the patient for a TM joint examination. Only ibuprofen was being taken for the pain.

Examination **Intraoral:** There is no dental or oral cause for the complaint other than the obvious malocclusion. Deep tenderness in the left joint is sensed with heavy manual palpation and this increases considerably with forced occlusion of the teeth. There is slight discomfort with maximum opening and extended lateral and protrusive movements and the patient senses a feeling of muscular weakness with these movements as well as with attempting to fully occlude the teeth. The pain produced by forcing the teeth into occlusion is prevented by biting on a tongue blade on the same side as the pain. There is no discomfort with eccentric biting or with manually straining the mandible as long as the teeth are slightly separated.

TM Joints: Both joints appear to be structurally normal on radiograph. The left condyle is displaced anteriorly in primary occlusal contact position, interpreted as possibly due to inflammatory swelling of the left retrodiscal tissues.

Muscles: There is no marked palpable tenderness in any masticatory muscle and no muscular dysfunction of any kind.

Cervical: Within normal limits.

Cranial Nerves: Within normal limits.

Diagnostic Tests: Analgesic blocking of the left lateral pterygoid muscle did not arrest the pain or acute malocclusion, confirming that it is not of muscle origin.

Impression It is presumed that the blow on the chin forced the left condyle posteriorly and traumatized the retrodiscal tissues. The ensuing retrodiscitis produced swelling that displaced the condyle forward causing the acute malocclusion.

Diagnosis Acute retrodiscitis of the left TM joint, traumatically induced.

Since the retrodiscal tissue is not responsive proprioceptively, protective muscle co-contraction does not occur. Also, the pain is frequently intermittent and may not induce secondary central excitatory effects. Acute retrodiscitis from trauma, however, may induce referred pain and secondary co-contraction of the masticatory muscles.

The following are clinical symptoms by which acute retrodiscal pain can be recognized:

1. The pain is accentuated by clenching the teeth in maximum intercuspation.
2. Such pain is decreased by biting against a separator that prevents intercuspation of the teeth.
3. The pain is accentuated by forced ipsilateral excursive movement of the mandible.
4. Pain is not induced by resisted protrusion of the mandible.
5. Dysfunction may be displayed as acute malocclusion in the resting occluded position.
6. Secondary central excitatory effects may be displayed.

Capsular Pain

Capsular pain results from inflammation of the synovial and fibrous capsules, which is referred to as synovitis and capsulitis, respectively. To distinguish between the two is difficult if not impossible clinically. Pain occurs when the inflamed capsule is stretched by translatory movement of the condyle. It is accentuated therefore by protrusion, contralateral excursion, and opening widely. There is palpable tenderness directly over the condyle and on occasion fluctuant swelling as well. Although acute capsulitis may cause restriction in the outer ranges of condylar movement due to swelling, most masticatory dysfunction results only from the inhibitory influence of pain.

Synovitis causes swelling due to effusion within the joint cavity, discomfort with joint movements, and alteration of the synovial fluid. The increased intracapsular fluid may induce a measure of acute malocclusion. In more chronic form, gelation of the synovial fluid may alter joint movements and cause some stiffness, especially after periods of inactivity. This may be accompanied by peculiar joint sounds. Such symptoms usually decrease as normal activity is resumed. Synovitis may result from localized trauma, abusive use, toxemias, specific infection, or as an allergic response. It frequently occurs as a manifestation of arthritis.

Capsulitis may result from acute trauma or from intrinsic strains that injure the capsular ligament (Case 10). A frequent cause has to do with inflammatory conditions of the discal ligaments and the temporomandibular ligament as a result of orthopedic instabilities between the stable intercuspal position and the stable joint position. This disharmony can result in the condyle being positioned away from its most stable loaded position and into the capsular ligament(s). Bruxism combined with such orthopedic instability is an important activating factor. Capsulitis may result from habits that entail excessive mandibular movements and from abusive joint hypermobility.

Inflammatory conditions of the capsule may cause varying degrees of capsular fibrosis that may restrict the outer ranges of condylar movement. Ordinarily, capsular fibrosis is entirely painless. If abused by excessive condylar movement, however, acute capsulitis may result (Case 11).

Chief Complaint

Left TMJ area pain.

History

A 20-year-old woman with mild continuous protracted steady dull aching pain diffusely located in the left preauricular area described as deep tenderness to pressure over the left condyle that increases considerably with opening beyond 30 mm as well as with extended protrusive and contralateral excursions. There is no complaint of restricted mandibular movements, interference with movements, or acute malocclusion.

The complaint began about 3 weeks ago following a volleyball accident in which she received a sharp blow on the left mandible. She thinks her mouth was partly open at the time. The blow was painful and after 24 hours the left TM joint became acutely sore and slightly swollen. All jaw use was painful and difficult for several days. Then it subsided to the present level. When the complaint persisted, she consulted her dentist who promptly referred her for a TM joint examination. No medications are presently being taken.

Examination

Intraoral: There is no dental or oral cause for the pain nor any evidence of injury to the dentition. She has deep tenderness to pressure over the left condyle. The discomfort increases with all condyle movements that tend to stretch the capsule. She has a feeling of muscular weakness with these movements and they may be slightly inhibited by pain but there is no identifiable orthopedic instability or masticatory dysfunction.

> **TM Joints:** Both joints are radiographically normal structurally and functionally except for slight decrease in distance of translatory movement in the left joint, interpreted as the effect of pain inhibition.

> **Muscles:** There is no palpable tenderness in any masticatory muscle and no muscular dysfunction.

> **Cervical:** Within normal limits.

> **Cranial Nerves:** Within normal limits.

Diagnostic Tests: Analgesic blocking of the left lateral pterygoid muscle did not arrest the pain, confirming that the discomfort was not muscular.

Impression

By history, clinical course, and the present behavioral characteristics of the complaint, it is presumed that the left capsular ligament was traumatized by the blow causing acute immobilizing capsulitis which has not subsided to a subacute non-immobilizing stage.

Diagnosis

Subacute capsulitis of the left TM joint, traumatically induced.

Capsular pain due to inflamed capsular fibrosis

Chief Complaint   Left TMJ area pain.

History

A 46-year-old woman with mild-to-severe recurring episodes of continuous pro-tracted steady dull aching pain diffusely located in the left preauricular area, in-duced by forceful or prolonged opening of the mouth, and aggravated by jaw use.

The complaint appears to relate to moderate restriction of opening (about 32 mm interincisal distance) which dates from a childhood injury. The present pain com-plaint began about 6 months ago following extensive dental treatment that re-quired extended and prolonged opening of the mouth. This was immediately fol-lowed by soreness in the left joint area and acute pain when opening fully. The episodes of discomfort depend on the amount and type of force used to open the mouth beyond her "normal" range. Her physician has treated her with systemic as well as local injections of corticosteroid medications with only transitory bene-fit. He then advised "correction of her bite" by her dentist. The dentist saw no reason for occlusal alteration and referred her for a temporomandibular joint ex-amination.

Examination

Intraoral: Three first molar teeth are missing and the spaces moderately closed leaving considerable loss of vertical support, but there is no significant orthope-dic instability. She feels sharp pain in the left TM area with opening beyond 28 mm and dull tenderness with protrusive and contralateral movements. Opening is restricted to 32 mm with slight deflection to the left. Protrusive and contralateral movements appear to be adequate.

TM Joints: Both joints appear to be structurally normal. There is restriction of left condylar movement that is interpreted as capsular, presumed to be due to preexistent capsular fibrosis or contracture, probably of traumatic origin.

Muscles: Essentially negative for cause of pain.

Cervical: Within normal limits.

Cranial Nerve: Within normal limits.

Impression

Capsular fibrosis appears to be responsible for the left condylar movements. When strained by excessive and prolonged opening, often associated with den-tal treatment, the capsule became inflamed and episodes of capsulitis have con-tinued ever since.

Diagnosis   Painful adhesions that restrict condyle movements (capsular fibrosis).

Since capsular pain is more or less continuous, some secondary central excitatory effects may be induced. This may be manifest as referred pain including headache, areas of heterotopic deep palpable tenderness, and secondary co-contraction of the masticatory muscles.

The following are clinical symptoms by which capsular pain can be recognized:

1. Palpable tenderness directly over the condyle.
2. Occasional palpable fluctuant swelling over the joint proper.
3. The pain is accentuated by translatory movements that stretch the capsule.
4. There is no increase in pain by clenching the teeth, nor is there any alteration in pain by biting against a separator.
5. Dysfunction occurs in the form of restricted mandibular movement, especially in extended ranges. Most restriction is due to the inhibitory influence of pain. Joint stiffness and strange joint sounds may occur during the first few movements following periods of inactivity. Acute malocclusion may occur as the result of increased intracapsular fluid.
6. Secondary central excitatory effects may be displayed.

Arthritic Pain

Inflammation of the articular surfaces of the joint is termed inflammatory arthritis. Normally these surfaces are nonvascularized so that an inflammatory reaction cannot occur. They are also noninnervated so that painful sensation cannot be felt. For the joint surfaces to become inflamed, fundamental arthropathic change must occur.

Such change may be due to trauma (traumatic arthritis). It can occur as a result of proliferation of inflamed synovial membrane onto the articular surfaces (rheumatoid arthritis). It can occur as a result of degeneration of the avascular fibrous tissue that normally constitutes the articular surfaces. When degenerative changes proceed until this tissue no longer is protective, the underlying innervated and vascularized osseous tissue may become exposed to the effects of movement, attrition, and articular pressures, thus becoming inflamed. This is termed *degenerative joint disease* or *osteoarthritis*.

Inflamed articular surfaces are the source of persistent though variable arthralgia. Although usually felt as a dull aching sensation, sometimes it is described as persistent burning pain. The irritation of occlusal pressure usually increases the discomfort, but sometimes the pressure of clenching the teeth temporarily relieves the pain. Usually pain is increased by chewing food and by all movements that press upon, rub, or irritate the inflamed articular surfaces.

If the inflammation is acute and widespread, the capsule may become involved so that symptoms of capsulitis are added, mainly, pain with movements, swelling of the joint, and palpable tenderness over the joint proper. Lesser degrees of inflammation may be accompanied by little or no gross dysfunction other than interference with mandibular movements that are expressed as discal noise and sensations of altered movements. As acute inflammation occurs and functioning of the joint is decreased due to pain inhibition, inflammatory exudate, or secondary muscle effects, the former noninflammatory dysfunction symptoms may decrease or subside. This effect is

Fig 13-10 Progressive anterior open bite due to an osseous change in the temporomandibular joints as a result of advanced rheumatoid arthritis in a woman aged 49. (From Bell WE. Management of temporomandibular joint problems. In Goldman HM, Gilmore HW, Royer RQ, et al (eds): Current Therapy in Dentistry, vol 4. St Louis: CV Mosby; 1970. Used with permission.)

Fig 13-11 Radiograph of the temporomandibular joint of a patient with rheumatoid arthritis. Note the gross flattening of the condyle.

Fig 13-12 Radiograph of a temporomandibular joint with advanced rheumatoid arthritis. (Courtesy of Dr Jay Mackman, Radiology and Dental Imaging Center of Wisconsin, Milwaukee, Wisconsin.)

presumably due to restraint of condylar movements. If intracapsular edema occurs, some sensation of acute malocclusion may be sensed. This is described as premature occlusion of the teeth on the opposite side. If osseous resorption decreases the vertical height of the mandibular ramus, some occlusal disharmony may be sensed; this is described as overstressing of the ipsilateral posterior teeth during maximum intercuspa-

tion. When such occlusal disharmony is advanced, clinical evidence of a progressive anterior open bite may result (Fig 13-10).

Radiographic evidence of osteoarthritis may be variable. Prior to gross structural change, rheumatoid arthritis may present some loss of definition of the osseous articular surfaces that is suggestive of diffuse surface resorption bilaterally (Fig 13-11). Although not diagnostic, this appearance is

Fig 13-13 Radiograph of a temporomandibular joint undergoing degenerative change expressed as flattening and paralleling of the osseous surfaces.

Fig 13-14 Radiograph of a temporomandibular joint with advanced degenerative joint disease. Note the flattened articular surfaces and anterior lipping of the condylar surface.

Fig 13-15 Radiographic appearance of osseous change in the left temporomandibular joint due to advanced osteoarthritis in a woman aged 45. The right joint is not affected.

sufficient to warrant medical investigation of the possibility of rheumatoid arthritis. Advanced rheumatoid arthritis may present with gross bizarre resorption of bone (Fig 13-12). Such changes do not necessarily relate functionally to the clinical symptoms. Fibrous ankylosis may be identified. The inhibitory effect of pain also may be recorded as restricted range of motion.

Osteoarthritis may show little or no radi-

ographic evidence in the early phase. As degenerative changes in the osseous surfaces occur, alterations in contour may become evident radiographically. These changes may be identified as flattened, parallel surfaces (Fig 13-13), anterior lipping (Fig 13-14), loss of definition indicative of active osseous resorption (Fig 13-15), or gross change in condylar form (Fig 13-16). Radiographic changes in the contour of the

Fig 13-16 Radiograph of a temporomandibular joint exhibiting marked lipping of the condyle.

condyle and/or fossa do not necessarily correlate with pain. It appears that for many patients osteoarthritic changes do not progress throughout their lifetime. Therefore the bony changes can persist long after adaptation of the osseous structures. Once adaptive changes have occurred, and the joint structures have stabilized, the condition is called *osteoarthrosis*. This will be discussed in more detail later in this chapter.

Traumatic arthritis may present similar radiographic changes. In addition, some evidence of former trauma such as malposition due to fracture may be seen. Other changes are condylar hyperplasia and malformation (Figs 13-17, 13-18).

In acute inflammatory arthritis, intracapsular edema is sufficient to cause an acute malocclusion. This condition appears clinically as a loss of posterior occlusal contact on the ipsilateral side. If inflammatory swelling immobilizes the joint, restriction of condylar movements will be observed both clinically and radiographically. Restriction of condylar movement due to disc jamming and the inhibitory influence of pain may also be observed (Case 12).

The following are clinical symptoms by which arthritic pain can be recognized:

1. There is usually some degree of capsular pain as well as other symptoms of synovitis/capsulitis.
2. The pain is accentuated by biting pressure, fast movements, and forced movements.
3. The pain is decreased by biting against a separator on the ipsilateral side
4. The pain is increased by biting against a separator on the contralateral side.
5. Dysfunction is expressed as restricted movement, interference during movements, and acute malocclusion. Restricted movement may be due to inflammatory swelling, capsular inflammation, altered synovial fluid function, and the inhibitory influence of pain (muscle co-contraction). Interference during movement results from damaged articular surfaces or condyle-disc complex impairment. Acute malocclusion may be due to increased intracapsular fluid or osseous change.

Fig 13-17 Panoramic radiograph revealing the effects of traumatic arthritis of the right temporomandibular joint due to a former injury. The left TMJ also reveals osteoarthritic changes.

Fig 13-18 Panoramic radiograph reveals deformed left mandibular condyle as a result of a former injury.

Periarticular Inflammation. Periarticular inflammation that envelops the joint may cause swelling, pain, and immobilization of the joint, the severity of symptoms depending on the degree, extent, location, and phase of the inflammatory reaction. Both rheumatoid arthritis and hyperuricemia may so involve the temporomandibular joints. When periarticular inflammation occurs without other obvious local cause, the examiner should consider the possibility of these causes (Case 13).

Periarticular inflammation may occur as a result of trauma or by direct extension from

323

Case 12 — Temporomandibular arthralgia expressed as degenerative joint disease or osteoarthritis

Chief Complaint

Right TMJ area pain.

History

A 61-year-old man with mild-to-severe continuous protracted steady dull aching and throbbing pain diffusely located in the right preauricular area. The pain is accompanied by tenderness and slight swelling over the TM joint and marked restriction of all jaw movements. The pain is aggravated by clenching the teeth, opening, chewing, and talking. Recently the patient reports a change in his occlusion.

The complaint began after an episode of extraordinary chewing about 2 weeks ago. Prior to that, the right joint was asymptomatic. For a few days, he noticed mild stiffness and vague discomfort in the right TM joint, gradually increasing in severity. After a week, the swelling, localized pain, fixation of the joint, and the sensation of acute malocclusion occurred. These symptoms have remained much the same ever since. Antibiotics prescribed by his physician have not controlled the complaint. No medications are presently in use other than simple analgesics.

Examination

Intraoral: The teeth and mouth are clinically and radiographically negative for cause of pain except that there is subjective acute malocclusion described as a sensation of premature contact of the left canine with slight disocclusion of the right posterior teeth. The pain increases when he attempts to fully occlude the teeth. This is reduced by insertion of a tongue blade on either side to prevent intercuspation. There is slight swelling over the right condyle and acute palpable tenderness both directly over the condyle and intra-aurally. Pain increases with all joint movements and there is described a feeling of muscular weakness when he moves the mandible. Mouth opening is restricted to about 26 mm and deflects to the right. Protrusion is restricted and deflects to the right. Left lateral excursion is only 2 mm.

TM Joints: The left joint appears to be normal. The right joint presents radiographic evidence of degenerative changes

Muscles: Essentially negative except for minor tenderness and weakness presumed to represent the inhibitory influence of pain.

Cervical: Some restriction to head flexion and extension but not related to present complaint. He reports a history of cervical arthritis that is being managed by his physician.

Cranial Nerves: Within normal limits.

Impression

Radiographic evidence of preexistent degenerative changes of both the right and left condyles. The acute activating cause was no doubt the extraordinary chewing episode. As a result, acute inflammatory changes of the joint have occurred resulting in the acute malocclusion.

Diagnosis

Degenerative joint disease with acute inflammatory arthritis of the right joint.

Case 13 Temporomandibular arthralgia expressed as arthritic pain secondary to hyperuricemia

Chief Complaint

Right TMJ pain.

History

A 70-year-old man with mild continuous variable steady dull aching pain diffusely located in the right TM joint area and aggravated by all joint use. There is localized tenderness to touch and pressure directly over the lateral pole of the joint.

The complaint began about 8 weeks ago as very mild tenderness over the right joint and minor discomfort with jaw movements. Some stiffness of the joint was noticed especially in the early mornings. The discomfort has gradually increased until the last 2 weeks the pain has become great enough to interfere with normal chewing and talking. Increasing restriction of mouth opening and pain with opening has been noticed. During the last 2 weeks he has also noticed some soreness in little finger and big toe. He sought aid from his physician who in turn referred him for a temporomandibular joint examination. He presently is receiving an NSAID but no other form of therapy.

Examination

Intraoral: Several missing mandibular posterior teeth were replaced satisfactorily with a partial denture. The remaining teeth are clinically and radiographically negative for cause of pain. No occlusal instability is identified. There is pain with lateral and protrusive movements as well as opening beyond 23 mm. Left lateral movement is restricted. Protrusive movement is restricted and deflects to the right. Opening is restricted to about 30 mm and deflects to the right.

TM Joints: Both joints appear to be structurally within normal limits and the left joint appears to function normally. The right joint presents restricted condylar movement interpreted as being due to periarticular and capsular inflammation plus the effect of pain inhibition.

Muscles: There is moderate palpable tenderness in the right masseter muscle. All other muscles are normal to palpation.

Cervical: Within normal limits.

Cranial Nerves: Within normal limits.

Diagnostic Tests: Serum uric acid: 8.9 mg%.

Impression

The right TMJ appears to be acutely inflamed due presumably to hyperuricemia involving the periarticular and capsular structures of the joint. There is moderate secondary muscle pain emanating from the right masseter muscle.

Diagnosis

Periarticular and capsular inflammation of the right TM joint, due presumably to hyperuricemia.

another contiguous inflammatory process such as otitis media. Under such circumstances, the cause should be so obvious as to present no diagnostic problem. If the injury or infection penetrates the capsule, acute inflammatory or infectious arthritis may follow, and the condition may terminate as a chronic mandibular hypomobility.

In periarticular inflammation, the joint appears normal radiographically except for possible restriction of translatory movement due either to the inflammatory exudate or to the inhibitory influence of inflammatory pain.

Painful Chronic Mandibular Hypomobilities. As the result of periarticular and articular inflammation, scar tissue may form around the joint, in the fibrous capsule, or between the joint surfaces, depending on the location of the inflammatory process. Such fibrosis, contracture, or adhesions restrict condylar movements, depending on the location and extent of cicatrization. As long as the mandibular movements do not exceed the limitations thus imposed, these conditions usually remain painless. As such, they are classified as chronic mandibular hypomobilities. If the adhesions are injured by straining or applying force to move the mandible beyond such limitation, the adhesions may become inflamed and painful.

Painful fibrous ankylosis presents with clinical symptoms of acute inflammatory arthritis. When the acutely painful condition resolves, clinical and radiographic evidence of preexistent fibrous ankylosis remains (Case 14).

Painful Growth Disorders. Most growth problems involving the temporomandibular joints are painless and do not come within the scope of this text. However, if the lack of structural harmony between the condyle and fossa, between the two joints bilaterally, or between the joints and the dentition becomes sufficient to interfere seriously with normal functioning, painful conditions may arise. Pain in such instances would probably relate to intrinsic trauma, with symptoms of capsulitis, retrodiscitis, or inflammatory arthritis, depending on what structures are inflamed. Radiographic evidence of malformation may confirm the diagnosis.

Rarely do malignant tumors involve the temporomandibular joints. The characteristic feature is slow progressive immobilization of the joint without apparent cause and usually is painless at first. The early clinical and radiographic features suggest fibrous ankylosis. It is usually the progressiveness of the condition and finally pain with all joint use that lead the examiner to believe that the condition is not a simple chronic mandibular hypomobility (Case 15).

Diagnostic Considerations

To plan effective therapy, accurate identification of the pain source is needed. Masticatory pains constitute a major segment of orofacial pain complaints. Frequently, the complaint consists of both myalgic and arthralgic components, which should be differentiated. Primary and secondary pains also must be distinguished. This may require considerable diagnostic effort. However, the more accurately it is done, the less complex the management problem and the more predictive the treatment.

Case 14 Temporomandibular arthralgia expressed as arthritic pain secondary to inflamed fibrous ankylosis

Chief Complaint

Left TMJ pain and mouth opening restriction.

History

A 34-year-old woman with mild continuous intermittently severe variable dull aching pain diffusely located in the left preauricular area. The pain is induced by forceful opening and excursive movements, and accompanied by restricted movement of the left mandibular condyle.

The complaint followed an motor vehicle accident about 18 months ago in which the patient sustained multiple fractures of the mandible, one through the left condylar process. Soreness and restricted movement of the left joint persisted after treatment of the fractures and have been present ever since. The pain is related chiefly to efforts to open the mouth. Physiotherapy, muscle relaxants, and corticosteroid injection therapy have failed to give much benefit. Patient was therefore referred for evaluation of the temporomandibular joints. No medications are presently being used.

Examination

Intraoral: No dental or oral cause for the complaint is evident clinically or radiographically. There is palpable tenderness over the left condyle but no pain described in resting or in any occlusal positions. There is a stable occlusal condition. All pain appears to occur with movements that tend to induce translation of the left condyle beyond about 22 mm. The severity of pain relates directly to the degree of attempted movement. Protrusion movement deflects the mandible to the left. Right lateral excursion is 2 mm. Maximum opening is 24 mm and deflects the mandible to the left.

> **TM Joints:** Both joints appear to be structurally normal. Radiographs reveal a restriction of left condylar movement that is interpreted as representing fibrous ankylosis.
>
> **Muscles:** Essentially negative.
>
> **Cervical:** Within normal limits.
>
> **Cranial Nerves:** Within normal limits.

Impression

Fibrous ankylosis of the left TM joint appears to have developed as a posttraumatic sequela. As the adhesions matured, continued efforts to execute normal left condylar movements induced inflammation, making them painful.

Diagnosis

Painful adhesions that immobilize the left mandibular condyle (ankylosis.).

| Case 15 | Temporomandibular arthralgia expressed as arthritic pain secondary to an invasive malignant tumor |

Chief Complaint

Left ear, TMJ, and temple pain.

History

A 54-year-old woman with mild-to-severe continuous variable protracted steady dull aching pain diffusely located in the left ear and preauricular area spreading to the temple, face, and submandibular triangle, aggravated by opening 13 mm and accompanied by restricted mandibular movements.

The complaint began about 4 years ago with no history of injury. It began insidiously as left eustachian blockage, followed soon by restriction of opening to about 25 mm. ENT therapy was ineffective. Three years ago her dentist made an occlusal splint to "correct the bite." After 2 to 3 months, mild pain began and has gradually increased ever since. After a year, the splint was discarded. About a year ago, surgery on the opposite ear was followed by an increase in the pain and trismus. Six months ago, she was given a general anesthetic and the muscles stretched, without any benefit. Recent muscle relaxant therapy and a corticosteroid injection into the left joint have not been beneficial.

Examination

Intraoral: There is no dental or oral cause for her complaint. The left face and ear pain increases with opening beyond 13 mm. There is no palpable tenderness over the left condyle. Opening is restricted to 18 mm with deflection to the right (suggestive of medial pterygoid myospasm). Protrusion deflects to the left. There is almost no right lateral excursion movement.

TM Joints: Both joints appear structurally normal. There is marked restriction of the left condylar movement interpreted as being indicative of fibrous ankylosis.

Muscles: There is only very slight palpable tenderness in the left temporal and masseter muscles. The medial pterygoid cannot be palpated due to the restricted opening.

Cervical: Within normal limits.

Cranial Nerves: The left side of the face exhibited marked anesthesia and paresthesia. Normal motor function for both CN V and CN VII.

Diagnostic Tests: Analgesic blocking of the left medial pterygoid muscle via the sigmoid notch arrested about 75% of the pain but did not alter the dysfunction.

A 1-week trial therapy for normalization of the medial pterygoid muscle was not effective. The patient was referred for comprehensive evaluation by a neurologist. Magnetic resonance imaging confirmed a diagnosis of carcinoma in the left nasopharynx invading the periarticular structures of the left TM joint.

Impression

In retrospect, no doubt the invasive neoplasm caused the symptoms clinically and radiographically interpreted as fibrous ankylosis complicated by spasm of the left medial pterygoid muscle.

Diagnosis

Immobilization of the left TM joint due to an invasive malignant tumor.

Intermittent Arthralgia

Intermittent arthralgic pains relate primarily to the effect of biomechanical abuse. As such, little or no secondary referred pain, secondary hyperalgesia, or muscle co-contraction results. The pain remains relatively "clean-cut." It is diffusely localizable to the joint region and responds rather faithfully to manual palpation and functional manipulation. Acute intermittent arthralgic pain may induce protective muscle co-contraction of the masticatory muscles. This may occur bilaterally. However, protracted muscle co-contraction may develop into local muscle soreness that, if persistent, may become inflammatory. Thus, it is important to eliminate such pains before complications develop, or else therapy must be instituted for the muscle condition as well.

Intermittent arthralgic pains may cause a change in muscle activity patterns. It is hypothesized that latent memory traces may persist after neural stimulation; thus, repeated stimulation may induce altered habitual patterns of muscle activity. It is presumed that such muscle engrain change is responsible for deviations in the midline incisal path during opening-closing movements. (Deviation refers to an alteration in the opening pathway away from midline that returns again with further opening to the centered position.) This may account also for such anomalies as avoidance closure movements, slides in centric and convenience occlusal positions, as well as various habitual jaw movements and mannerisms. Time and repetition are required. Acute and changing conditions do not cause such effects; they induce muscle co-contraction instead.

Inflammatory Arthralgia

When the condition that induces arthralgic pain becomes inflammatory, continuity of input results and, with it, the propensity to induce secondary central excitatory effects. Thus, inflammatory arthralgia (retrodiscal pain, capsular pain, and arthritic pain) may be complicated by a variety of secondary effects such as referred pains including headache, secondary hyperalgesia displayed as superficial touchy spots or areas of deep palpable tenderness, or secondary muscle symptoms. Careful differentiation between primary sources of pain input and the secondary effects of deep somatic pain is essential to accurate diagnosis and effective management. While muscle co-contraction may be induced by deep pain input, it may soon develop local muscle soreness, which in turn becomes painful. This pain can then induce continued co-contraction and a cycling mechanism can begin. This cycling condition is known as *cycling muscle pain.* As such, it may become wholly independent of the initiating cause, thus requiring a separate therapeutic effort for resolution.

Arthralgia of Nonmasticatory Origin

From the dental standpoint, it is important to distinguish between arthralgia of masticatory origin, which can reasonably be expected to respond to proper masticatory therapy, and arthralgia of nonmasticatory origin, which may require medical therapy, surgical intervention, or both. Arthralgias from hyperuricemia and rheumatoid arthritis are essentially medical problems in which treatment of the masticatory apparatus would be secondary and supplemental.

Infections, traumatic arthritis, and temporomandibular involvement from adjacent pathosis may require considerable interdisciplinary attention. Chronic mandibular hypomobilities and growth disorders are usually surgical problems.

Painful Scar Tissue in the Joint

Neuropathic pain may emanate from traumatic neuroma formation in scar tissue residual to lacerating injuries or surgery of the joint. Such pain displays the clinical characteristics of neuropathic rather than deep somatic pain. There may be no discomfort except when a certain mandibular movement puts the affected scar tissue under stretch. Such pain can be replicated at will by repeating the same jaw movement (see Case 32, page 442).

Referred Pain Felt in the Joint Area

True arthralgia that emanates from the temporomandibular joint must be differentiated from heterotopic pain that is felt in the joint area. As discussed in Chapter 12, myogenous pain may be referred to the joint. This is especially true of myofascial trigger point pain involving the sternocleidomastoid, masseter, medial pterygoid, and lateral pterygoid muscles (see Case 18, page 363). But referred pain from any source within the vast trigeminal distribution may also be felt in the joint area. The salivary glands are known sources of such reference (see Case 17, page 361).

Eagle's Syndrome

Eagle's syndrome[46–49] may be confused with temporomandibular pain because it typically induces a sensation of persistent raw throat, pain and difficulty with swallowing, pain referred to the auricular area, and limited neck movement. The condition is due to elongation of the styloid process or calcification of the stylohyoid ligament. The elongated styloid process may encroach on the carotid artery, thus causing carotid arteritis. The resulting carotodynia may refer pain through the face to the ophthalmic area. Encroachment on the carotid artery is said to cause faintness or syncope when the head is turned from side to side.[50]

Glossopharyngeal Neuralgia

A neuropathic pain that may be confused with temporomandibular joint pain is glossopharyngeal neuralgia. This paroxysmal neuralgia is triggered by stimulation of receptors in the pharyngeal mucosa. It is associated therefore with talking as well as with jaw and throat movements incidental to chewing and swallowing. The pain usually is felt deeply in the postmandibular and infra-auricular area. It presents the clinical characteristics of neuropathic rather than deep somatic pain and is temporarily arrested by topical anesthesia of the pharyngeal mucosa (see Case 25, page 411).

Differential Diagnosis

The primary deep somatic musculoskeletal pains that emanate from the temporomandibular joints should be distinguished diagnostically from the following conditions:

1. Masticatory myalgia
2. Odontogenous pains
3. Arthralgia of nonmasticatory origin such as rheumatoid arthritis and hyperuricemia.
4. Adjacent inflammatory and neoplastic conditions such as pseudoankylosis and Eagle's syndrome
5. Heterotopic referred pains and secondary hyperalgesias felt in the temporomandibular or preauricular area as secondary effects of other deep pain input
6. Heterotopic projected neuropathic pains, especially glossopharyngeal neuralgia
7. Somatoform pain disorders
8. Heterotopic pains of central origin.

Therapeutic Options for Disc-Interference Disorders

During the past 20 years, the dental profession has proposed a variety of different approaches to the management of intracapsular pain conditions. Since these pain conditions are common, a specific discussion of these therapies is in order. Disc-interference or internal derangement disorders actually represent a continuum of the pain conditions that have already been discussed. Early in these disorders, disc-attachment pain is the predominant complaint. Later, capsulitis and synovitis are common. As the disc is further displaced, retrodiscal pain becomes the predominant feature. Finally, the articular surfaces become affected, resulting in osteoarthritis. This discussion is therefore appropriate for many of the pain conditions discussed in this chapter.

The rationale for any therapy begins with a thorough understanding of the disease and its natural course. As a general rule, diseases that are progressive and destructive need to be treated quickly and aggressively. Diseases that are nonprogressive and characterized by reparative processes can often be treated more palliatively and observed over time. The rationale for the management of intracapsular disorders begins with an understanding of the natural course of these disorders. The clinician must appreciate, however, that in the practice of dentistry the natural course of the disease can be misinterpreted. Patients most often seek care when pain and/or dysfunction becomes great. When the clinical examination reveals signs and symptoms associated with disc-interference disorders, the condition is easily interpreted as progressive and in need of aggressive treatment. Well-controlled, longitudinal studies are the only reliable method of evaluating the natural course of these disorders as well as the effects of therapy on the outcome. Although these studies are the most difficult to accomplish, we are most fortunate to have a few studies that shed light on these common disorders.

When the long-term effects of dysfunction on the temporomandibular joints are being studied, certain stages need to be identified for assessment purposes. There are three clinical stages that have been commonly used.[51] The first stage is that of disc displacement with reduction. This stage is characterized by joint clicking with movement but no radiographic signs of any abnormalities in the condyle or articular eminence. The second stage is that of disc displacement without reduction. This stage is characterized by a sudden restriction in mouth opening and a loss of joint sounds during movement. Radiographic changes may or may not be present during this stage depending on the chronicity of the disorder. The third stage is that of permanent disc displacement with osteoarthritic changes as depicted with radiographic studies.

It appears that long-term studies support the concept that many patients seem to progress through these three stages.[52-57] Initially it would therefore appear that these disorders are progressive and need to be aggressively treated. However, when one looks carefully at these studies it is found that the final stage of the disorder is not often painful or debilitating. In fact, in one longitudinal study, patients with internal derangements who were observed over 30 years were found to be no different than a control group in most evaluation parameters.[51] The greatest differences that existed between these groups were that the patients experienced a slight reduction in mouth opening compared to that in the control subjects and the patients expressed a greater concern that if they opened widely the joint would hurt.[51] There was, however, no difference in the general musculoskeletal complaints of the patients and the control subjects in this study. Another significant difference was in the radiographic evidence of bony changes that had commonly occurred in the internal derangement group. These changes, however, were not necessarily correlated with pain nor often even with dysfunction.[52-55] This would suggest an adaptive condition clinically known as osteoarthrosis.

These long-term studies leave the impression that the natural course of disc-interference disorders or internal derangements is toward disc displacement without reduction and osteoarthritic changes. This is not al-ways the case, however, as depicted by long-term studies that do not show consistent progression of clicking joints to disc dislocation without reduction.[58-63] Therefore, long-term studies suggest that internal derangements may be progressive, but even when they are, for many patients they seem to be rather self-limiting, resulting in no significant disability. Understanding the natural course of these disorders allows the clinician to assume the most appropriate role as therapist. If these disorders are self-limiting for most patients, then one might question any need for aggressive therapy. Instead, the role of the therapist should be one that assists the patient through the symptomatic phase of the disorder. Palliative therapy is often the most appropriate therapy, especially early in the disorder. There may, however, be some patients who will suffer greatly through this disorder and therefore, more assistance may be needed for these patients. The aggressiveness of the therapy should only be escalated when more palliative therapy fails to control symptoms and the patient's quality of life becomes markedly decreased.

Since tissue adaptation seems to play a major role in the natural course of these disorders, treatment should be oriented toward promoting a joint condition that is most likely to repair or adapt.[64] An important part of this therapy is directed toward reducing mechanical loading of the articular surfaces. There are four types of therapies that should be initially considered for each patient with a symptomatic internal derangement disorder: patient education, physical therapy, pharmacologic therapy, and occlusal appliance therapy.

Patient Education

It is very important that each patient understand the mechanism that is causing his or her disorder. There are several important reasons for this education. The first relates to the nature of internal derangements. Since these disorders have a significant biomechanical component, the well-informed patient can play a significant role in therapy. The patient should be instructed to decrease loading of the joint as much as possible. Softer foods, slower chewing, smaller bites should be promoted. The patient should be told, when possible, not to allow the joint to click. The mechanics of some joints allow certain movements to occur with minimal dysfunction. When possible these movements should be encouraged while painful movements discouraged.

Each clinician treating internal derangement disorders should have a model or well-drawn illustration of the temporomandibular joint (TMJ) in the office so that the patient can visualize the mechanical dysfunction. This will not only help the patient understand the condition but it subtlely informs the patient that the disorder is common and one of which the clinician is well informed. This understanding will enhance the patient's confidence in the doctor, which will likely help the patient through the adaptive phase of the disorder. The patient should also be informed of the natural course of the disorder so that reasonable expectations can be met. It is important that the patient be told that in many instances this condition is self-limiting; however, the pain and dysfunction may be present for a considerable time. The patient should be told of the therapies that will be used and if they are not satisfactory, the clinician can offer more aggressive therapy. In the event more aggressive therapies are needed, the patient should always take part in the decision-making process. It is important that the patient realize that the disorder is not an aggressive, tissue-destructive disease such as cancer. This information will likely decrease anxiety and stress, promoting a better environment for healing.

In those patients with a disc displacement without reduction, the patient should be shown with a model or illustration the reason for limitation in mouth opening . The patient should be instructed not to attempt to force the mouth open, especially when pain is present. Instead the patient should be told that with time, the mouth will return to a more normal opening. If the patient attempts to force the mouth open too soon, tissues may be damaged and repair delayed. Once the condition has become relatively asymptomatic, the patient should than be encouraged to attempt to return back to a more normal opening as discussed in the next section.

Physical Therapy

Physical therapy modalities can be helpful in managing some of the symptoms associated with disc-interference disorders. These therapies can be divided into two broad types: those that reduce pain and those that improve function.

Physical Therapy for Pain. In instances when pain is significant, moist heat or ice applied over the joint region can often be helpful. Thermotherapy utilizes heat as a prime mechanism and is based on the premise that heat increases circulation to the applied area. Surface heat is applied by laying a hot moist towel over the symptomatic area.[65] A hot water bottle over the towel will help maintain the heat. This combination should remain in place for 10 to 15 minutes, not to exceed 30 minutes. An electric heating pad may be used, but care must be taken not to leave it unattended.

Like thermotherapy, coolant therapy has proved to be a simple and often effective method of reducing pain. Ice should be applied directly to the symptomatic joint and/or muscles and moved in a circular motion without pressure to the tissues. The patient will initially experience an uncomfortable feeling that will quickly turn into a burning sensation. Continued icing will result in a mild aching and then numbness.[66] When numbness begins the ice should be removed. The ice should not be left on the tissues for longer than 5 to 7 minutes. After a period of warming a second application may be desirable. It is thought that during warming there is an increase in blood flow to the tissues, assisting in tissue repair.

A common coolant therapy utilizes a vapor spray. Two of the most common sprays used are ethyl chloride and fluoromethane. Vapocoolant spray is applied to the desired area from a distance of 1 or 2 feet for approximately 5 seconds. After the tissue has been rewarmed, the procedure can be repeated. Care must be taken not to allow the spray to contact the eyes, ears, nose, or mouth. A towel should be placed to protect these areas. Vapocoolant sprays do not penetrate tissue like ice and therefore it is likely that the reduction in pain is more associated with the stimulation of cutaneous nerve fibers that in turn shut down the smaller pain fibers (the C fibers). This type of pain reduction is likely to be of short duration.

The clinician should suggest both heat and cold modalities to the patient since the results can be very individual. The patient should determine the most effective modality for his or her pain. Both these modalities are very conservative and can be used as often as the patient finds it necessary.

Two other physical therapy modalities that have been investigated are iontophoresis and cold laser. Iontophoresis is a technique by which certain medications are introduced into the tissues without affecting any other organs. With iontophoresis, the medication is placed in a pad and the pad is placed over the involved joint. Then a low electrical current is passed through the pad driving the medication into the tissue.[67] Local anesthetics and anti-inflammatory are common medications used with iontophoresis.[68,69] If the medication is driven into the tissues with ultrasound therapy the modality is known as phonopheresis.[70]

In recent years, the cold or soft laser has been investigated for wound healing and pain relief. Presently it is not considered to be a routine physical therapy modality but is included in this section for completeness. Most studies on the cold laser report on its use in chronic musculoskeletal, rheumatic, and neurologic pain conditions.[71-74] It is thought that cold laser accelerates collagen synthesis, increases vascularity of healing tissues, decreases the number of microorganisms, and decreases pain. Several case studies have been published in which cold laser therapy has been used on persistent TMJ pain.[75-77] Although the results of the studies investigating iontophoresis and cold laser have been favorable, the studies generally lack control subjects and adequate sample sizes. More investigations will be needed to better understand their effectiveness.

Physical Therapy to Improve Function.
Early in a disc-interference disorder or osteoarthritis, pain may cause the patient to restrict joint function. Although this can be helpful at first, restricting joint function can lead to chronic hypomobility and muscle atrophy. A few passive exercises can be helpful in returning the jaw to normal function. The patient should be instructed to gently open the mouth to resistance and close. The jaw should then be moved eccentrically. Early in the process of healing these exercises should not produce any significant pain. Later, as tissue adaptation progresses, the exercises should become more active so that normal range of movement can be returned.

Passive distraction of a joint can increase mobility as well as inhibit the activity of muscles that pull across the joint (elevator muscles). Distraction of the TMJ is accomplished by placing the clinician's thumb in the patient's mouth over the mandibular second molar area on the side to be distracted. With the cranium stabilized by the other hand, the clinician places downward force on the molar with the thumb (Fig 13-19). Distraction for relaxing muscles does not require translation of the joint but merely unloading in the closed joint position. The distraction should be maintained for several seconds and then released. It can be repeated several times. When joint mobility is the problem, distraction should be combined with manual translation of the joint.

Joint distraction has been suggested as a method of reducing a disc that has become permanently displaced.[78] Although this technique may provide some immediate success, there are few studies that evaluate the long-term success. When the disorder is an acute

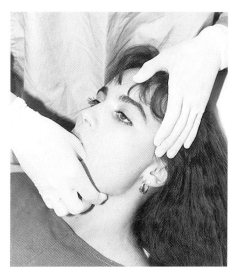

Fig 13-19 Manual distraction of the temporomandibular joint may be helpful in improving joint mobility.

disc dislocation without reduction (less than a week), the technique should be attempted. If the clinician successfully reduces the disc, an anterior repositioning appliance is indicated (discussed later). Discs that have been displaced for more than several weeks are very difficult to reduce and maintain; therefore the distraction procedure will likely fail. If the disc cannot be reduced, a muscle relaxation appliance is indicated merely to reduce loading forces in the joint associated with bruxing activity (discussed later).

Pharmaocolgic Therapy

Pharmacologic therapy can be an effective adjunct in managing symptoms associated with an intracapsular disorder. Patients should be aware that medication will not likely offer a solution or cure to the problem. However, medication in conjunction with appropriate physical therapy and definitive treatment does offer the most complete approach to many problems. The two most common types of medications used for internal derangement disorders are analgesics and anti-inflammatories.

Analgesic Medications. Analgesic medications can often be an important part of supportive therapy for many intracapsular disorders. Control of pain is not only appreciated by the patient but it also reduces the likelihood of other complicating pain disorders such as muscle co-contraction,[79] referred pain,[80] and central sensitization.[81] The nonsteroidal anti-inflammatory drugs (NSAIDs) are very helpful with most intracapsular pains. Included in this category are aspirin, acetaminophen, and ibuprofen. Ibuprofen (Motrin, Advil, Nuprin) has proven to be very effective in reducing musculoskeletal pains. A common dosage of 600 to 800 mg three times a day will often reduce pain and stop the cyclic effects of the deep pain input. There are numerous other NSAIDs and if ibuprofen does not reduce the pain, another should be tried. Individual patients may respond differently to these medications. Continued use may result in stomach irritation, so the patient should be questioned for prior stomach problems before use and monitored closely during treatment. It is suggested that these medications be taken with meals to lessen the likelihood of stomach irritation.

Anti-Inflammatory Medications. When inflammatory conditions are present, anti-inflammatories can be helpful in altering the course of the disorder. These agents suppress the body's overall response to the irritation. Anti-inflammatory agents can be administered orally or by injection.

Oral NSAIDs have already been discussed under the category of analgesics. When taken on a regular basis, these medications are quite useful in the management of inflammatory joint disorders. Aspirin or ibuprofen can serve in this capacity while providing an analgesic effect. Other oral anti-inflammatories (eg, naproxen, flurbiprofen) are appearing with increasing frequency on the market. It should be remembered, however, that these drugs do not immediately achieve good blood levels and therefore should be taken on a regular schedule for a minimum of 2 to 3 weeks. The general health and condition of the patient must always be considered before these (or any) medications are prescribed; and, as is often the case, it may be necessary to consult the patient's physician regarding the advisability of such drug therapy.

The injection of an anti-inflammatory such as hydrocortisone into the joint has been advocated[82-86] for the relief of pain and restricted movements. A single intra-articular injection seems to be somewhat helpful in older patients; however, less success has been observed in patients under age 25.[87] Although a single injection is occasionally helpful, it appears[88,89] that multiple injections may be harmful to the structures of the joint and should be avoided. Therefore, the intra-articular anti-inflammatory agents should be used only in selected cases.

Occlusal Appliance Therapy

During the past 20 years the dental profession's attitude toward management of internal derangements has changed greatly. This is especially true with regards to the use of occlusal appliances. In the early 1970s,

Farrar[90] introduced the anterior mandibular repositioning appliance. This appliance provided an occlusal relationship that required the mandible to be maintained in a forward position. This purpose of this type of appliance was an attempt to position the condyle back on the disc (recapture the disc). It was originally suggested that this appliance be worn 24 hours a day for as long as 3 to 6 months.

It was quickly discovered that the anterior mandibular repositioning appliance was useful in reducing painful joint symptoms.[91,92] When this appliance successfully reduced symptoms, a major treatment question was then asked: What next? Some clinicians believed that the mandible needed to be permanently maintained in this forward position. Dental procedures were suggested to create an occlusal condition that maintained the mandible in this therapeutic relationship. Accomplishing this task was never a simple dental procedure. Others thought that once the discal ligaments repaired, the mandible should be returned to its normal position in the fossa (the musculoskeletally stable position) and the disc would still remain in proper position (recaptured). Although one approach was more conservative than the other, neither has been supported by long-term data.

In early short-term studies,[17,63,91,93–96] the anterior repositioning appliance proved to be much more effective in reducing intracapsular symptoms then the more traditional centric relation (muscle relaxation) appliance. This, of course, lead the profession to believe that returning the disc to its proper relationship with the condyle was an essential part of treatment. The greatest insight regarding the appropriateness of a treatment modality, however, is gained from long-term studies. Forty patients with various derangements of the condyle-disc complex were evaluated 2½ years after anterior repositioning therapy and a step-back procedure.[63] No patients received any occlusal alterations. It was reported that 66% of the patients still had joint sounds, but only 25% were still experiencing pain problems. If the criteria for success in this study were the elimination of both pain and joint sounds, then success was achieved in only 28%. Other long-term studies[17,61] have reported similar findings. If the presence of asymptomatic joint sounds is not a criterion for failure, however, then the success rate for anterior repositioning appliances rises to 75%. The issue that must be addressed, therefore, is the clinical significance of asymptomatic joint sounds.

As already stated, joint sounds are very common in the general population. In many cases,[97,98] it appears that they are not related to pain or decreased joint mobility. If all clicking joints always progressed to more serious disorders, then this would be a good indication to treat each and every joint that clicked. The presence of unchanging joint sounds over time, however, indicates that the structures involved can adapt to less than optimum functional relationships.

Long-term studies reveal that anterior repositioning appliances are not as effective as once thought. They appear to be helpful in reducing pain in 75% of the patients, but joint sounds appear to be much more resistant to therapy. The fact that these sounds persist over time does not necessarily indicate a progressive disorder. These studies do, however, give insight as to how the joint responds to anterior repositioning therapy. In many patients, advancing the mandible forward for a time prevents the condyle from articulating with the highly vascular-

13-20a **13-20b** **13-20c**

Fig 13-20 *(a)* An anteriorly displaced disc with the condyle articulating on the retrodiscal tissues producing pain. *(b)* An anterior repositioning appliance is placed in the mouth to bring the condyle forward off of the retrodiscal tissues onto the disc. This relationship lessens the loading of the retrodiscal tissues, which decreases the pain. *(c)* Once the tissues have adapted, the appliance is removed, allowing the condyle to assume the original musculoskeletally stable position. The condyle now functions on adaptive fibrotic tissues resulting in a painless functioning joint but because the disc is still displaced, clicking can be present. (From Okeson JP. Management of Temporomandibular Disorders and Occlusion, ed 3. St Louis: Mosby Year Book; 1993: 410. Used with permission.)

ized, well-innervated, retrodiscal tissues. This is the likely explanation for an almost immediate reduction of intracapsular pain. During the forward repositioning the retrodiscal tissues undergo adaptive and reparative changes.[99] These tissues can become fibrotic[100–107] and avascular (Fig 13-20).

We know now that discs are not generally recaptured by anterior repositioning appliances.[108] Instead, as the condyle returns to the fossa, it moves posteriorly to articulate on the adapted retrodiscal tissues. If these tissues have adequately adapted, loading occurs without pain. The condyle now functions on the newly adapted retrodiscal tissues although the disc is still anteriorly displaced. The result is a painless joint that may continue to click with condylar movement. At one time the dental profession believed that the presence of joint sounds indicated treatment failure. Long-term follow-up studies have given the profession new insight regarding success and failure. We, like our orthopedic colleagues, have learned to accept that some dysfunction is

likely to persist once joint structures have been altered. Controlling pain, while allowing joint structures to adapt, appears to be the most important role of the therapist.

A few long-term studies[95,109] do support the concept that permanent alteration of the occlusal condition can be successful in controlling most major symptoms. This treatment, however, requires extensive dental therapy and one most questions the need when natural adaptation appears to work well for most patients. Reconstruction of the dentition or orthodontic therapy should be reserved only for those patients who present with a significant orthopedic instability.

The use of anterior repositioning appliance therapy is not without adverse consequences. A certain percentage of patients who wear these appliances develop a posterior open bite. This may be the result of a reversible, myostatic contracture of the inferior lateral pterygoid muscle. When this condition exists, a gradual relengthening of the muscle can be accomplished by slowly stepping the condyle back to the more musculoskeletally stable (anterosuperior) position in the fossa. This can be accomplished by slowly adjusting the appliance to allow the condyle to return to the musculoskeletally stable position, by slowly decreasing use of the appliance, or both. The degree of myostatic contracture that develops is likely to be proportional to the length of time the appliance has been worn. As already mentioned, when these appliances were first introduced, it was suggested that they be worn 24 hours a day for 3 to 6 months. The philosophy now is to reduce the wearing time as much as possible to limit the adverse effects on the occlusion. For many patients, full-time use is not necessary to reduce symptoms. When possible, the patient should wear the appliance only at night to protect the retrodiscal tissues from heavy loading (bruxism). If the symptoms can be controlled without wearing the appliance during the day, myostatic contracture will be avoided.

For some patients with a disc-interference disorder, a more traditional muscle relaxation (centric relation) appliance can reduce symptoms. This is the appliance of choice since the risk of altering the occlusion is minimized. Both of these appliances should provide full arch coverage so as to avoid tooth eruption.

If symptoms persist with only nighttime use of the appliance, the patient may need to wear it more often. Daytime use may be necessary for a few weeks. As soon as the patient becomes symptom-free, the use of the appliance should be gradually reduced. If reduction of use creates a return of symptoms, either there has not been adequate time for tissue repair or significant orthopedic instability is present. It is best to assume that inadequate time for tissue repair is the

reason for return of symptoms. The anterior repositioning appliance should therefore be reinstituted and more time given for tissue repair.

When repeated attempts to eliminate the appliance fail to control symptoms, orthopedic instability should be suspected. When this occurs, the appliance should be gradually reduced, allowing the condyle to return to the musculoskeletally stable (anterosuperior) position. Once the condyles are in the musculoskeletally stable position, the occlusal condition should be assessed for orthopedic stability. Orthopedic instability is not a common finding but when it is present, dental therapy may be indicated.

If the disc is permanently displaced without reduction, an anterior repositioning appliance is contraindicated. This type of appliance will likely only aggravate the anteriorly positioned disc. Patient education, physical therapy, and medications are the best methods of promoting adaptation of the permanently displaced disc. If the patient is suspected to have significant bruxing or clenching, a muscle relaxation or flat plane appliance is indicated to reduce loading of the retrodiscal tissues during sleep. A lack of adaptation is usually accompanied by pain. When nonsurgical therapies fail to adequately reduce symptoms over a reasonable time, surgical evaluation is indicated.

Other therapeutic options include:

A. Muscle therapy (see Chapter 12) for interrelated muscle symptoms.

B. Cause-related therapy consisting of the identification and treatment of causative factors and contributing conditions. This applies especially to preexistent, causative occlusal disharmonies, abusive use and habits, and bruxism.[110–114]

C. Medical management for appropriate

arthritic conditions such as rheumatoid arthritis and hyperuricemia.

D. Surgical consultation for the following painful conditions:

1. Recalcitrant degenerative arthritis

2. Chronic mandibular hypomobilities

3. Growth disorders of the joint

E. Medical consultation

References

1. McNamara, JA. The independent functions of the two heads of the lateral pterygoid muscle. Am J Anat 1973; 138:197–205.

2. Gibbs CH, Mahan PE, Wilkinson TM, et al. EMG activity of the superior belly of the lateral pterygoid muscle in relation to other jaw muscles. J Prosthet Dent 1984; 51:691–702.

3. Okeson JP. Management of Temporomandibular Disorders and Occlusion, ed 3. St Louis: Mosby Year Book; 1993: 3–27.

4. Bell WE. Temporomandibular Disorders, ed 3. Chicago: Year Book; 1990: 35–103.

5. DuBrul EL. Sicher's Oral Anatomy, ed 7. St Louis: CV Mosby; 1980: 174–209.

6. Thilander B. Innervation of the temporomandibular joint capsule in man. Trans R Sch Dent 1961; 7:1.

7. Westessen PL, Bronstein SL, Liedberg J. Internal derangement of the temporomandibular joint: morphologic description with correlation to joint function. Oral Surg 1985; 59:323–331.

8. Farrar WB, McCarty WL. The TMJ dilemma. Ala Dent Assoc 1979; 63:19.

9. Wilkinson T. The relationship between the disk and the lateral pterygoid muscle in the human temporomandibular joint. J Prosthet Dent 1988; 60:715–724.

10. Tanaka TT. Advanced dissection (videotape). San Diego: Clinical Research Foundation; 1989.

11. Tanaka TT. TMJ microanatomy, an approach to current controversies (videotape). San Diego: Clinical Research Foundation; 1992.

12. Tanaka TT. Head, Neck and TMD Management, ed 4. San Diego: Clinical Research Foundation; 1989.

13. Roberts CA, Tallents RH, Espeland MA, et al. Mandibular range of motion versus arthrographic diagnosis of the temporomandibular joint. Oral Surg 1985; 60:244–251.

14. Isberg A, Isacsson G, Johansson AS, Larson O. Hyperplastic soft-tissue formation in the temporomandibular joint associated with internal derrangement. Oral Surg 1986; 61:32–38.

15. Bakland LK, Christiansen EL, Strutz JM, Mohn R. Frequency of dental and traumatic events in TMJ symptomatology (abstract). J Dent Res, 1987; 65 :182.

16. Harkins SJ, Marteney JL. Extrinsic trauma, a significant precipitating factor in temporomandibular dysfunction. J Prosthet Dent 1985; 54:271–272.

17. Moloney F, Howard JA. Internal derangements of the temporomandibular joint. III. Anterior repositioning splint therapy. Aust Dent J 1986; 31:30–39.

18. Wienberg S, LaPointe H. Cervical extension-flexion injury (whiplash) and internal derangement of the temporomandibular joint. J Oral Maxillofac Surg 1987; 45:653–656.

19. Pullinger AG, Seligman DA. Trauma history in diagnositic groups of temporomandibular disorders. Oral Surgery 1991; 71:529–534.

20. Westling L, Carlsson GE, Helkimo M. Background factors in craniomandibular disorders with special reference to general joint hypermobility, parafunction and trauma. J Craniomandib Disord Facial Oral Pain 1990; 4:89–98.

21. Pullinger AG, Seligman DA. Association of TMJ subgroups with general trauma and MVA (abstract). J Dent Res 1988; 67:403.

22. Pullinger AG, Monteriro AA. History factors associated with symptoms of temporomandibular disorders. J Oral Rehabil 1988; 15:117–124.

23. Seals RR, Morrow RM, Kuebker WA, Farney WD. An evaluation of mouth guard programs in Texas high school football. J Am Dent Assoc 1985; 110:904–909.

24. Garon MW, Merkle A, Wright JT. Mouth protector and oral trauma: A study of adolescent football players. J Am Dent Assoc 1986; 112:663–665.

25. Knibbe MA, Carter JB, Frokjer GM. Postanesthetic temporomandibular joint dysfunction. Anesth Prog 1989; 36:21–25.

26. Okeson JP. Management of Temporomandibular Disorders and Occlusion, ed 3. St Louis: Mosby Year Book; 1993: 111–126.

27. Okeson JP. Management of Temporomandibular Disorders and Occlusion, ed 3. St Louis: Mosby Year Book; 1993: 168–171.

28. Isberg AM, Isacsson G. Tissue reactions of the temporomandibular joint following retrusive guidance of the mandible. J Craniomand Pract 1986; 4:143–148.

29. Wright JW. Temporomandibular disorders: occurrence of specific diagnosis and response to conservative management. J Craniomand Pract 1986; 4:149–155.

30. Riolo ML, Brandt D, Tenhave T. Early development of signs and symptoms of TMJ dysfunction (abstract). J Dent Res 1986; 65:307.

31. Hilty J, Burch J, Dimauro M. Incidence of temporomandibular disorders in pre-orthodontic patients (abstract). J Dent Res 1986; 65:342.

32. Solberg WK, Bibb CA, Nordstrom BB, Hansson TL. Malocclusion associated with temporomandibular joint changes in young adults at autopsy. Am J Orthod 1986; 89:326–330.

33. Seligman DA, Pullinger AG. Association of occlusal variables among refined TM patient diagnostic groups. J Craniomandib Disord Facial Oral Pain 1989; 3:227–236.

34. White CS, Dolwick MF. Prevalence and variance of TMD orthognathic surgery (abstract). J Dent Res 1991; 70:466.

35. Williamson EH, Simmons MD. Mandibular asymmetry and its relation to pain dysfunction. Am J Orthod 1979; 76:612–617.

36. DeBoever JA, Adriaens PA. Occlusal relationship in patients with pain-dysfunction symptoms in the temporomandibular joint. J Oral Rehabil 1983; 10:1–7.

37. Brandt D. Temporomandibular disorders and their association with morphologic malocclusion in children. In Carlson DS, McNamara JA, Ribbens KA (eds): Developmental Aspects of Temporomandibular Joint Disorders. Ann Arbor, Mich: University of Michigan Press; 1985:279.

38. Thilander B. Temporomandibular disorders and their association with morphologic malocclusion in children. In Carlson DS, McNamara JA, Ribbens KA (eds): Developmental Aspects of Temporomandibular Joint Disorders. Ann Arbor, Mich: University of Michigan Press; 1985:89.

39. Bernal M, Tsamtsouris A. Signs and symptoms of temporomandibular joint dysfunction in 3 to 5 year old children. J Pedodont 1986; 10:127–140.

40. Nilner M. Functional disturbances and diseases of the stomatognathic system. A cross-sectional study. J Pedodont 1986; 10:211.–238

41. Stringert HG, Worms FW. Variations in skeletal and dental patterns in patients with structural and functional alterations of the temporomandibular joint: A preliminary report. Am J Orthod 1986; 89:285–297.

42. Gunn SM, Woolfolk MW, Faja BW. Malocclusion and TMJ symptoms in migrant children. J Craniomandib Disord Facial Oral Pain 1988; 2:196–200.

43. Dworkin SF, Huggins KH, LeResche L, et al. Epidemiology of signs and symptoms in temporomandibular disorders: clinical signs in cases and controls. J Am Dent Assoc 1990; 120:273–281.

44. Ronquillo HI, Guay J, Tallents RS, et al. Comparison of internal derangements with condyle-fossa relationship, horizontal and vertical overlap, and angle class. J Craniomandib Disord Facial Oral Pain 1988; 2:137–140.

45. Pullinger AG, Seligman DA, Solberg WK. Temporomandibular disorders. Part II: Occlusal factors associated with temporomandibular joint tenderness and dysfunction. J Prosthet Dent 1988; 59:363–367.

46. Eagle WW. Elongated styloid process: Further observations and a new syndrome. Arch Otolaryngol 1948; 47:630–640.

47. Eagle WW. Symptomatic elongated styloid process. Arch Otolaryngol 1949; 49:490–503.

48. Breault MR. Eagle's syndrome: Review of the literature and implications in craniomandibular disorders. J Craniomand Pract 1986; 4:323–337.

49. Lawrence FR, Cornielson E. Eagle's syndrome. J Oral Maxillofac Surg 1962; 40:307–309.

50. Correll RW, Wescott WB. Eagle's syndrome diagnosed after history of headache, dysphagia, otalgia, and limited neck movement. J Am Dent Assoc 1982; 104:491–492.

51. de Leeuw R, Boering G, Stegenga B, de Bont LGM. Temporomandibular joint osteoarthrosis: Clinical and radiographic characteristics 30 years after nonsurgical treatment: A preliminary report. J Craniomand Pract 1993; 11:15–24.

52. Boering G. Arthrosis deformans van het kaakgewricht (thesis). Groningen, The Netherlands: University of Groningen; 1966.

53. Boering G, Stegenga B, deBont LGM. Temporomandibular joint osteoarthritis and internal derangement. Part I: Clinical course and initial treatment. Int Dent J 1990; 40:339–346.

54. Rasmussen OC. Clinical findings during the course of temporomandibular arthropathy. Scand J Dent Res 1981; 89:283–288.

55. Rasmussen OC. Temporomandibular arthropathy. Int J Oral Surg 1983; 12:365–397.

56. Stegenga B, de Bont LGM, Boering G. Osteoarthrosis as the cause of craniomandibular pain and dysfunction: A unifying concept. J Oral Maxillofac Surg 1989; 47:249–256.

57. Nickerson JW, Boering G. Natural course of osteoarthrosis as it relates to internal derangements of the temporomandibular joint. Oral Maxillofac Surg Clin North Am 1989; 1:27–45.

58. Bush FM, Carter WH. TMJ clicking and facial pain (abstract). J Dent Res 1983; 62:304.

59. Greene CS, Turner C, Laskin D. Long-term outcome of TMJ clicking in 100 MPD patients (abstract). J Dent Res 1982; 61:218.

60. Greene CS, Laskin D. Long-term status of TMJ clicking in patients with myofascial pain and dysfunction. J Am Dent Assoc 1988; 117:461–465.

61. Lundh H, Westesson PL, Kopp S. A three-year follow-up of patients with reciprocal temporomandibular joint clicking. Oral Surg 1987; 63:530–533.

62. Magnusson T. Five-year longitudinal study of signs and symptoms of mandibular dysfunction in adolescents. J Craniomand Pract 1986; 4:338–344.

63. Okeson JP. The long-term treatment of disc-interference disorders. J Prosthet Dent 1988; 60:611–616.

64. de Leeuw R, Boering G, Stegenga B, de Bont LGM. TMJ osteoarthrosis and internal derangement 30 years after nonsurgical treatment. J Orofacial Pain 1994; 8:18–24.

65. Nelson SJ, Ash MM. An evaluation of a moist heat pad for the treatment of TMJ/muscle pain dysfunction. J Craniomand Pract 1988; 6:355–359.

66. Satlerthwaite JR. Ice massage. Pain Manage 1989; 2:116.

67. Lark MR, Gangarosa LP. Iontophoresis: An effective modality for the treatment of inflammatory disorders of the temporomandibular joint and myofascial pain. J Craniomand Pract 1990; 8:108–119.

68. Gangarosa LP. Monograph: Iontophoresis in Dental Practice. Chicago: Quintessence; 1983.

69. Gangarosa LP, Ikeshima A, Morihana A, et al. Ionotophoresis (IONTO) of lidocaine (Lido) into the TMJ of rabbits (abstract). J Dent Res 1991; 70:444.

70. Kleinkort JA, Wood F. Phonophoresis with one percent versus ten percent hydrocortisone. Phys Ther 1975; 55:1320–1324.

71. Kleinkort JA, Foley R. Laser acupuncture. Its use in physical therapy. Am J Acupuncture 1984; 12:51.

72. Synder-Mackler L, Bork CE. Effect of helium-neon laser irradiation on peripheral sensory nerve latency. Phys Ther 1988; 68:223–225.

73. Walker J. Relief from chronic pain from low-power laser irradiation. Neurosci Lett 1983; 43:339–344.

74. Bliddal H, et al. Soft laser therapy of rheumatoid arthritis. Scand J Rheumatol 1987;16:225–228.

75. Hanson TL. Infrared laser in the treatment of craniomandibular arthrogenenous pain. J Prosthet Dent 1989; 61:614–617.

76. Palano D, Martelli M, et al. A clinic statistical investigation of laser effect in the treatment of pain and dysfunction of the temporomandibular joint (TMJ). Med Laser Rep 1985; (No 2) 21.

77. Bezuur NJ, Habets LLMH, Hansson TL. The effect of therapeutic laser treatment in patients with craniomandibular disorders. J Craniomandib Disord Facial Oral Pain 1988; 2:83–86.

78. Okeson JP. Management of Temporomandibular Disorders and Occlusion, ed 3. St Louis: Mosby Year Book; 1993: 413–416.

79. Okeson JP. Management of Temporomandibular Disorders and Occlusion, ed 3. St Louis: Mosby Year Book; 1993: 182–183.

80. Bell WE. Orofacial Pains, Classification, Diagnosis, and Management, ed 4. Chicago: Year Book; 1989: 67–75.

81. Woolf CJ, Thompson SWN. The induction and maintenance of central sensitization is dependent on N-methyl-D-aspartic acid receptor activation: Implications for the treatment of post-injury pain hypersensitivity. Pain 1991; 44:293–300.

82. Henny FA. Intra-articular injection of hydrocortisone into the temporomandibular joint. J Oral Surg 1954; 12:314–319.

83. Toller PA. Osteoarthritis of the mandibular condyle. Br Dent J 1973; 134:223–231.

84. Toller PA. Non-surgical treatment of dysfunctions of the temporomandibular joint. Oral Sci Rev 1976; 7:70–85.

85. Kopp S, Carlsson GE, Haraldson T, Wenneberg B. Long-term effects of intra-articular injections of sodium hyaluronate and corticosteroids on temporomandibular joint arthritis. J Oral Maxillofac Surg 1987; 45:929–935.

86. Wenneberg B, Kopp S, Grondahl, HG. Long-term effect of intra-articular ingections of a glucocorticosteroid into the TMJ: A clinical and radiographic 8-year follow-up. J Craniomandib Disord Facial Pain 1991; 5:11–18.

87. Toller PA. Non-surgical treatment of dysfunctions of the temporomandibular joint. Oral Sci Rev 1976; 7:70–85.

88. Poswillo DE. Experimental investigation of the effects of intra-articular hydrocortisone and high condylectomy on the mandibular condyle. Oral Surg 1970; 30:161–173.

89. Zarb GA, Spech JE. The treatment of mandibular dysfunction. In Zarb GA, Carlsson GE (eds): Temporomandibular Joint: Function and Dysfunction. St Louis: CV Mosby; 1979: 373–389.

90. Farrar WB. Differentiation of temporomandibular joint dysfunction to simplify treatment. J Prosthet Dent 1972; 28:629–636.

91. Anderson GC, Schulte JK, Goodkind RJ. Comparative study of two treatment methods for internal derangements of the temporomandibular joint. J Prosthet Dent 1985; 53:392–397.

92. Gazit E, Lieberman M, Eini R, et al. Prevalence of functional disturbances in 10-18 year old Israeli school children. J Oral Rehabil 1984; 11:307–317.

93. Burns R, McKinney J, Chase D, Anderson D. Occlusal splint therapy for treatment of internal derangements: retrospective study (abstract). J Dent Res 1983; 62:304.

94. Lundh H, Westesson PL, Kopp S, Tillstrom B. Anterior repositioning splint in the treatment of temporomandibular joints with reciprocal clicking: Comparison with a flat occlusal splint and an untreated control group. Oral Surg 1985; 60:131–136.

95. Lundh H, Westesson PL, Jisander S, et al. Disk-repositioning onlays in the treatment of temporomandibular joint disk displacement: Comparison with a flat occlusal splint and with no treatment. Oral Surg 1988; 66:155–162.

96. McGowan P, McKinney J, Chase D, Anderson D. Treatment of anterior disc displacement with Jankelson Myosplint: Retrospective study (abstract). J Dent Res 1983; 62:304.

97. Heikinheimo K, Salmi K, Myllarniemi S, Kirveskari P. Symptoms of craniomandibular disorders in a sample of Finnish adolescents at the ages of 12 and 15 years. Eur J Orthod 1989; 11:325–331.

98. Vincent SD, Lilly GE. Incidence and characterization of temporomandibular joint sounds in adults. J Am Dent Assoc 1988; 116:203–206.

99. Bay R, Timmis D, Helmy E, Sharawy M. Histopathology of human TMJ disc perforation after anterior repositioning splint therapy (abstract). J Dent Res 1989; 68:1004.

100. Akerman S, Kopp S, Rohlin M. Histological changes in temporomandibular joints from elderly individuals. Acta Odontol Scand 1986; 44:231–239.

101. Baldioceda F, Bibb C, Pullinger A. Morphologic variability in the human TMJ disc and posterior attachment (abstract). J Dent Res 1989; 68:229.

102. Blaustein DI, Scapino RP. Remodeling of the temporomandibular joint disk and posterior attachment in disk displacement specimens in relation to glycosaminoglycan content. Plast Reconstr Surg 1986; 78:756–764.

103. Hall MB, Brown RW, Baughman RA. Histologic appearance of the bilaminar zone in internal derangement of the temporomandibular joint. Oral Surg 1984; 58:375–381.

104. Salo L, Raustia A, Pernu H, Virtanen K. Internal derangement of the temporomandibular joint:A histochemical study. J Oral Maxillofac Surg 1991; 49:171–176.

105. Scapino RP. Histopathology associated with malposition of the human temporomandibular joint disc. Oral Surg 1983; 55:382–397.

106. Solberg WK, Hansson TL, Nordstrom B. The temporomandibular joint in young adults at autopsy: A morphologic classification and evaluation. J Oral Rehabil 1985; 12:303–321.

107. Solberg WK, Bibb C, Nordstrom BB, Hansson TL. Malocclusion associated with temporomandibular joint changes in young adults of autopsy. Am J Orthod 1986; 89:326–330.

108. Kirk WS. Magnetic resonance imaging and tomographic evaluation of occlusal appliance treatment for advanced internal derangement of the temporomandibular joint. J Oral Maxillofac Surg 1991; 49:9–12.

109. Tallents RH, Katzberg RW, Machen DJ, Roberts CA. Use of protrusive splint therapy in anterior disk displacement of the temporomandibular joint: A 1 to 3 year followup. J Prosthet Dent 1990; 63:336–341.

110. Okeson JP. Management of Temporomandibular Disorders and Occlusion, ed 3. St Louis: Mosby Year Book; 1993.

111. Friedman MH, Weisberg J. Temporomandibular Joint Disorders: Diagnosis and Treatment. Chicago: Quintessence; 1985.

112. Gelb H (ed). Clinical Management of Head, Neck and TMJ Pain and Dysfunction, ed 2. Philadelphia: WB Saunders; 1985.

113. Morgan DH, House LR, Hall WP, et al (eds). Diseases of the Temporomandibular Apparatus, ed 2. St Louis: CV Mosby; 1982.

114. Sarnat BG, Laskin DM (eds). The Temporomandibular Joint, ed 4. Springfield, Ill: Charles C Thomas; 1992.

14

Other Musculoskeletal Pains

For purposes of description, pains that emanate from musculoskeletal structures of the mouth and face have been divided into separate groups: periodontal and odontogenous pains (see Chapter 11), pains of muscle origin (see Chapter 12), temporomandibular joint pains (see Chapter 13), and other musculoskeletal pains of the mouth and face. All such musculoskeletal pains display the clinical characteristics of deep somatic pain, of which they constitute a major subdivision. In addition, they display features that identify them as being of musculoskeletal origin: the pain relates reasonably to the demands of biomechanical function, and manual palpation (or functional manipulation) induces a graduated response. The other musculoskeletal pains of the face and mouth include osseous pains, periosteal pains, and soft connective tissue pains (Fig 14-1). Since osseous structures and soft connective tissue are less intimately related to biomechanical function, they are less well-innervated proprioceptively and therefore are less localizable subjectively. Also, pains emanating from such structures are less likely to induce muscle effects.

Osseous Pains

Pains that emanate from the bony structures of the mouth and face exclusive of the periodontal structures and the temporomandibular joints constitute another subdivision of musculoskeletal pain. Pains from this source are predominantly inflammatory as a result of injury, infection, or surgical intervention.

Osseous pain are more constant than myogenous pains and they typically follow an inflammatory time frame. They usually differ from cellulitic pains in that initially pain alone dominates the complaint. Osseous pains also show less evidence of other inflammatory symptoms. Due to the rigid unyielding structure of the tissues involved, inflammatory swelling may not be observed until surrounding structures become involved. During this phase, the pain relates especially to three factors: the susceptibility of inflamed osseous tissue to environmental noxious irritation such as mechanical encroachment, movement of fractured or injured parts, and contact with saliva; the confinement of inflammatory exudate; and the type and virulence of the contaminating organism. The pain level usually drops

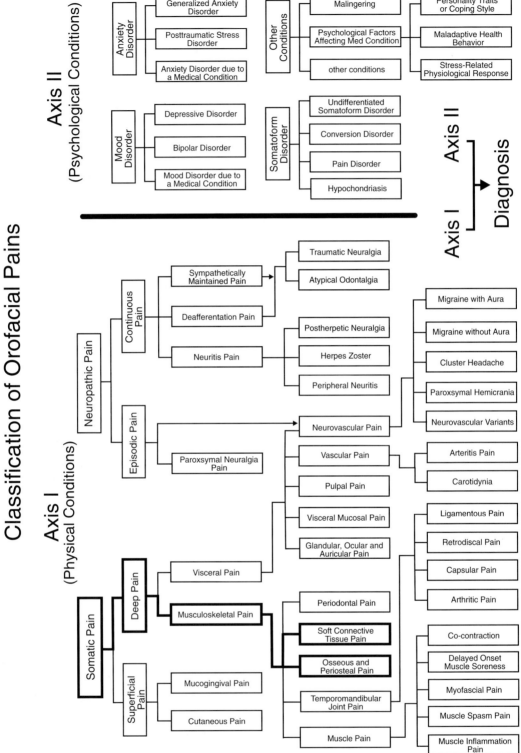

Fig 14-1 Pain classification chart highlighted to show the relationship of osseous, periosteal, and soft connective tissue pains to other orofacial pain disorders.

rapidly as these factors are obtunded by natural resolution or therapy. Final relief of pain follows a protracted inflammatory time frame. There is minimal dysfunction other than that due to the inhibitory influence of pain. Secondary factors, however, such as muscle co-contraction, local muscle soreness, myospasm, or cellulitis may contribute to some dysfunction.

By definition, *osteitis* denotes inflammation of bone involving the haversian spaces, canals, and medullary spaces.[1] Acute septic osteitis is usually designated osteomyelitis. The inflammatory reaction occurs in the soft tissues confined within the rigid osseous compartments, a condition that in some ways simulates pulpal inflammation. Congestion within such rigidly confined areas may cause pain out of proportion to that experienced when such confinement is not present. This may give the pain a throbbing quality. It induces necrosis by pressure against the unyielding walls. Thus, the inflammatory condition spreads through the bone by following paths of least resistance.

When the cortex is penetrated, the inflammatory process is considerably less confined, and the pain intensity decreases. Subperiosteal spreading occurs with surface swelling and pain, which is readily identifiable by manual palpation. Subperiosteal spreading may proceed until a barrier is reached, such as a muscle attachment. At that point it may rupture through and the inflammation may spread to the overlying soft tissues. Confined acute subperiosteal inflammation may be extremely painful due to sensitivity of the periosteum to pain.[2]

When confinement is released by rupture or surgical drainage, the pain intensity drops dramatically, and the throbbing quality disappears. In turn, cellulitic involvement accompanies the osteitis, and further spreading takes place along natural barriers such as the fascial planes. The degree of pain again is determined largely by confinement imposed by the relation of the anatomic features to the quantity of exudate and degree of purulence. Tissues offering little resistance to swelling provide less intense pain, whereas tissues that tightly contain the inflammatory process increase the pain level and incidence of throbbing. Surface rupture and fistulization (or surgical drainage) reduce pain intensity, and the throbbing usually disappears.

It should be evident therefore that the pain behavior is determined by several factors including the type of injury, virulence and behavioral characteristics of the invader, resistance of the host, and anatomic conditions imposed at the site of inflammation. Nonseptic inflammatory conditions are less painful. Chronicity may cause the pain to disappear entirely or to remain as only low-grade tenderness. Accompanying cellulitis, regional lymphadenitis, and systemic symptoms are valuable clues to the progress and resolution of all such inflammatory conditions.

Dry-Socket Pain

A frequent osteitic involvement of the mouth is *acute dental alveolitis* or the so-called *dry-socket* that follows tooth extraction. This condition is the result of inflammation of remnants of the periodontal ligament and cortical bone of the alveolus. Being components of a fibrous joint, these structures are richly innervated with both mechanoreceptors and nociceptors. They therefore have the propensity to initiate reactive muscle effects and considerably more nociceptive response than do other osseous structures. Protective muscle co-contraction as well as secondary central excitatory effects are frequent complications. Referred pain involving many teeth, spots of touchy gingiva or skin, areas of deep palpable tenderness, and secondary masticatory muscle soreness may be displayed. Dry-socket pain may also initiate a myofascial trigger point pain mechanism especially affecting the masseter and temporalis muscles. The referred pain from such trigger points may be felt at or near the site that initiated the mechanism. It therefore may be mistaken for continuing primary pain from the extraction site. Accurate differentiation between primary pain input and its secondary effects is essential for effective management.

Since confinement usually is not present, spreading of infection from the dental alveolus into the deeper osseous tissue is rare. If deep-seated infection or excessive surgical trauma complicates the problem, osteomyelitis may result. As soon as the exposed surface becomes covered with granulation tissue, the pain subsides and healing usually proceeds uneventfully.

Osseous pains of inflammatory origin should be differentiated from other less common pains such as those that stem from cysts and tumors. Radiographic evidence is essential with most osseous lesions.

Periosteal Pains

The periosteum, in contrast to bone, is richly innervated with sensory receptors. It is particularly sensitive to pressure and impact stress. The mechanoreceptors in periosteal tissue supply proprioceptive input for underlying bony structures. Noxious stimulation of the periosteum therefore has a high potential for reactive muscle effects and nociception. The pain that emanates from the periosteum is disproportionately greater than the initiating noxious stimulus.

Inflammatory conditions of the periosteum are common. Periosteitis may occur as a primary osseous condition due to injury or superficial infection. Acute suppurative periosteitis may be painful. Subperiosteal spreading occurs with involvement of the surface cortical layer of bone, which is relatively insensitive to pain.[2] If it penetrates more deeply, osteomyelitis may develop. Periosteitis is frequently encountered in the mouth due to the vulnerability presented by prominent bony contours and exostoses. Edentulous ridges are vulnerable.

Injury or infection that penetrates sufficiently to involve the periosteum and osseous cortex may occur as a result of dental appliances and accidental injuries from such causes as toothbrushing, foods, burns, and objects held in the mouth. The tongue may rub through and expose prominences, especially along the mandibular internal oblique ridge. If the overlying tissues are thin, full-thickness ulceration including the periosteum may occur, with the cortical bone becoming exposed. The pain arises chiefly from the margins of the ulcer. Since there is no confinement, spreading beneath the periosteum and into the cancellous bone is limited, and the condition usually remains localized. Elimination of the cortical bone by back-resorption may be slow and healing delayed.

Periosteitis may arise from contiguous obscure dental sepsis and involve the adjacent bony structure extensively. Such subperiosteal abscess formation may be attended by deeper osteomyelitic and superficial cellulitic development, thus presenting a rather complex clinical problem that generates considerable pain. Muscle attachments that penetrate the periosteum and attach directly to the bone form barriers to subperiosteal spreading. An intimate knowledge of such attachments is extremely valuable to the examiner.[3]

Chronic forms of periosteitis may become troublesome management problems but do not present a diagnostic challenge as far as pain is concerned. Local tenderness evident to manual palpation and other clinical signs usually make the diagnosis simple.

Soft Connective Tissue Pains

Pain that emanates from the soft connective tissue structures of the mouth and face constitutes a major subdivision of musculoskeletal pain. Pains from these structures are predominantly inflammatory and relate to other signs of inflammation by which the source of pain may be identified.

The pain is considerably more constant than muscle pain and it usually follows an inflammatory time frame. When the inflammatory exudate is confined, the pain develops a pulsatile quality and increases in intensity. When evacuated by penetration, rupture, or surgical drainage, pain intensity drops dramatically, and the pulsatile quality disappears. Dysfunction is due chiefly to inflammatory swelling.

By definition, *cellulitis* denotes an acute, diffuse, spreading, edematous, suppurative inflammation of the deep subcutaneous tissues.[2] Most purulent inflammatory conditions involving the deeper soft tissues of the face and mouth are designated as cellulitis.

Specific terms may designate certain types and locations of cellulitic involvement. The intensity of pain depends largely on the acuity, rate of spreading, distension of tissues, and confinement of inflammatory exudate. Manual palpation gives essential information, as do concomitant regional lymphadenitis and systemic effects. Spreading follows the fascial planes.

Acute cellulitis is usually evident from the swelling and pain, and no diagnostic problem occurs as long as the inflammation is located in accessible regions. When this condition involves the sublingual area, its location relative to the mylohyoid muscle largely determines its clinical features and behavior. Supramylohyoid cellulitis lifts the tongue and interferes with speech and swallowing. Inframylohyoid cellulitis causes external swelling in the submental and submandibular areas and may embarrass respiration if it encroaches on the glottis. Palatal cellulitis causes swelling that interferes with speech and swallowing. In the buccal regions it usually causes external swelling of the face that spreads readily to the eyelids. Confinement, spreading, and location of the swelling relate to the anatomic arrangement of facial muscles and to the anchorage of fascial barriers. Cellulitis in the pterygomandibular space causes trismus due to medial pterygoid muscle involvement. Similar inflammation adjacent to the masseter muscle does the same. Cellulitis in the infratemporal fossa area causes characteristic facial swelling above the zygoma and trismus due to temporal muscle involvement.

Subacute and chronic cellulitis is less dramatic and may present diagnostic problems of differentiation from cysts and tumors.[4] The history and clinical course plus manual palpation and surgical aspiration are the usual means of establishing the diagnosis.

Pain of cellulitic origin should be differentiated from muscle pain, vascular pain, and glandular pain. Other conditions that may initiate soft connective tissue pain are cysts and tumors, both benign and malignant.

Differential Diagnosis

The primary deep somatic musculoskeletal pains that emanate from the osseous, periosteal, and soft connective tissue structures of the orofacial area should be distinguished diagnostically from the following conditions:

1. Odontogenous pains
2. Orofacial myalgia and arthralgia
3. Neoplastic and cystic pains
4. Vascular, neurovascular, and other visceral pains
5. Heterotopic referred pains and secondary hyperalgesias due to other deep pain input
6. Heterotopic projected neuropathic pains
7. Somatoform pain disorders
8. Heterotopic pains of central origin

Therapeutic Options

For the management of primary deep somatic musculoskeletal pains that emanate from osseous, periosteal, and soft connective tissue structures, the following therapeutic options are available (see Chapter 9):

1. Analgesics for palliative relief, reduction of functional demands, and counseling
2. Cause-related therapy consisting of the identification and treatment of causative factors and contributing conditions, and general medical and surgical supportive care including antibiotics, anti-inflammatory agents, and deep heat therapy

References

1. Dorland's Illustrated Medical Dictionary, ed 28. Philadelphia: WB Saunders; 1994: 1198.
2. Dorland's Illustrated Medical Dictionary, ed 28. Philadelphia: WB Saunders; 1994: 294.
3. DuBrul EL. Sicher's Oral Anatomy, ed 7. St Louis: CV Mosby; 1980.
4. Kaplan JN, Cummings CW. Pain in the ear, midface, and aerodigestive tract. In Bonica, JJ (ed): The Management of Pain, ed 2. Malvern, Pa: Lea and Febiger; 1990: 769–783.

15 | Visceral Pains

Primary deep somatic pain emanates from either the musculoskeletal structures or the visceral structures of the body. Musculoskeletal pain derives from the structures that give physical form and stability to the body as well as provide for the biomechanical functions that accomplish posture, locomotion, and other useful working movements. Visceral pain derives from components of the supply and maintenance system that subserve the musculoskeletal structures. The visceral system has to do with oxygen supply, nutrition, metabolism, detoxification, and elimination of waste products. It is composed of organs of many different types, glandular structures, and a network of vessels of different kinds to transport substances throughout the body. Whereas sensation emanating from the musculoskeletal structures relates to more or less conscious volitional biomechanical functions, sensation initiated in visceral structures is largely unconscious and serves to facilitate ongoing automatic metabolic functioning of the body. Pain of musculoskeletal origin therefore relates to biomechanical function as a graduated response, while pain of visceral origin commands attention only to warn that all is not well within. The clinical symptoms displayed by the two kinds of deep somatic pain are sufficiently different to make them identifiable. This is of considerable importance diagnostically.

In addition to the clinical characteristics of deep somatic pain, all such visceral pains display features by which they may be recognized: the pains are of threshold type and do not yield graduated responses, and the pains are influenced very little by biomechanical function. Visceral pains are usually not accompanied by distinct evidence of dysfunction other than that induced by the inhibitory influence of pain. Cervero[1] described visceral pain as being accompanied frequently by generalized increased excitability of the central nervous system (CNS) that is expressed as general discomfort, tenderness of the skin, skeletal muscle spasms, and autonomic reflexes. He confirmed that visceral pain was mediated by visceral afferents in sympathetic nerves.

Behavior of Visceral Pains

The mechanism of visceral pain has been described by several authors.[2-6] Ordinarily, sensory information transmitted by afferent neurons of the visceral nervous system remains well below conscious levels. It serves to monitor the involuntary muscle action of vessels, glands, and organs. It reports unusual sensation occurring in the lining membranes of organs and cavities. It helps regulate the automatic functioning of the body by supplying the CNS with a constant inflow of information. When such sensation becomes noxious, pain is felt. Visceral afferent fibers of both the sympathetic and parasympathetic type are known to mediate pain.[5] Visceral pain usually has a distinct stinging or burning quality. It is said that protracted visceral pain[6] tends to provoke vasomotor effects, local edema, and trophic changes.

It appears that conscious visceral sensation is normally of a very low order of intensity, the visceral afferents having high-threshold receptors. However, the presence of inflammation may reduce this threshold considerably so that conscious pain becomes evident with little added provocation. For example, the stomach yields minimal sensation other than when it is very empty or very full. But an inflamed gastric mucosa causes the normal stomach contents to excite painful sensation, usually described as heartburn.

Visceral pain in the maxillofacial region is not rare. Esophagitis and pharyngitis have the dull, diffuse, burning quality of visceral pain. Nasal and ostium maxillare mucosa pain has a similar burning quality. The major salivary glands as well as the numerous glands of the lymphatic system, the skin, and the mucous membranes are other sources of this type of pain.

Some pains arising in the maxillofacial region are mediated by sympathetic afferent fibers that do not enter the CNS via any cranial or cervical nerve sensory root. Rather, these visceral fibers leave the orofacial structures and pass through the cervical sympathetic chain and finally enter the CNS via the sensory roots of the upper thoracic spinal nerves. Head and neck pains mediated by this route cannot be arrested by division of any or all cranial and cervical spinal sensory roots. Such pains are arrested by analgesic blocking of the stellate ganglion through which such afferents pass, even though they undergo no synapse prior to reaching the CNS.[6,7]

Analgesic blocking of the stellate ganglion does not necessarily arrest some of these vascular pains. This strongly suggests that the cranial parasympathetics constitute the mediating pain pathway. No parasympathetic afferent fibers pass through the dorsal root of the trigeminal nerve. Rather, they leave this nerve and enter the CNS via the seventh and ninth cranial nerve dorsal roots. Thus division of the trigeminal sensory root will not arrest pains from the trigeminal area that are mediated by parasympathetic afferent fibers.

Visceral pain input tends to provoke central excitatory effects. Referred pains, secondary hyperalgesias, and localized autonomic effects may accompany visceral pains. Sometimes they dominate the symptom picture and constitute the patient's complaint. The so-called sinus headache typifies this clinical behavior.

For purposes of description, visceral pains have been separated into three groups: pulpal odontogenous pains; vascular pains of the mouth and face; and other visceral pains, including those of mucosal, glandular, ocular, and auricular origin. Pulpal pains have already been reviewed in Chapter 11. Since vascular pains are a common and important type of pain originating from the orofacial structures, an entire chapter will be devoted to them (see Chapter 16). This chapter will review visceral pains that have their origin in mucosal tissues of the pharynx, nose, and paranasal sinuses. This chapter will also review pains from glandular, ocular, and auricular structures (Fig 15-1).

Pains Eminating from Visceral Mucosa

While pain emanating from the oral mucogingival tissues is exteroceptive in character and displays clinical characteristics of the superficial somatic type, pain from other mucosal structures of the face is definitely interoceptive in character and exhibits the clinical characteristics of deep pain of the visceral type. This refers particularly to the mucosal linings of the pharynx, the nasal cavity, and the paranasal sinuses.

Ordinarily, sensory perception of visceral mucosa linings remains below conscious levels. This rule applies especially to the more deeply situated structures. The closer such tissues are located to external environmental sources of stimulation, however, the more responsive they are to all stimuli, and the more conscious such sensation becomes. For example, the nasal mucosa is more sensitive to low-level stimulation than is the pharyngeal mucosa, while that of the esophagus is less reactive. The fine sensibility of nasal mucosa applies also to the ostium maxillare, but the lining membrane of the maxillary sinus remains resistant to all stimuli. The external portion of esophageal mucosa is highly responsive to stimuli of

threshold intensity, but the more deeply situated portion is nearly insensible to all noxious stimuli. There is a transitional zone where the oral mucogingival tissue joins the pharyngeal mucosa and symptoms of both superficial somatic and deep visceral pain categories may be displayed.

An appreciation of the different types and degrees of sensibility of the lining membranes of the oral, nasal, and pharyngeal structures is needed to understand the nociceptive sensations that emanate from these tissues.

The normal inflow of sensation from visceral mucosa serves to regulate automatic functioning. Several reflex mechanisms are recognized: irritation of the nasal mucosa excites the sneeze reflex, the pharyngeal mucosa initiates the swallowing and gag reflexes, upper esophageal mucosa may induce esophageal spasm, and upper tracheal and laryngeal irritation stimulates the cough reflex. When mucosal stimulation becomes noxious, burning pain is felt.[2-5] It is said that continuing visceral pain tends to provoke vasomotor effects, local edema, and trophic changes.[6] The normally high threshold level of sensibility is lowered in the presence of inflammation so that nociceptive impulses may be generated by otherwise nonnociceptive stimuli.

Nociceptive pathways from orofacial mucosal structures likely involve afferent elements of both the somatic and the visceral nervous systems. Somatic afferents are mediated by the fifth, seventh, and ninth cranial nerves. Parasympathetic visceral afferents are mediated by the seventh and ninth cranial nerves only. Sympathetic visceral afferents do not enter the CNS by way of cranial nerves. Instead, they leave the head and travel the cervical sympathetic chain to

Classification of Orofacial Pains

Fig 15-1 Pain classification chart highlighted to show the relationship of visceral mucosal, glandular, ocular, and auricular pains to other orofacial pain disorders.

enter through the upper thoracic spinal nerves. Pain mediated by sympathetic visceral afferents can be arrested by analgesic blocking of the stellate ganglion, through which such pathways pass even though they undergo no synapse prior to reaching the CNS.[7]

Like other forms of deep pain, visceral mucosa pain tends to initiate central sensitization or excitatory effects. Many times, the secondary symptoms predominate while the primary pain input remains silent or goes unnoticed. Some orofacial pain disorders are almost exclusively expressed as secondary central excitatory effects. Caution should be exercised in differentiating such effects from the true source of primary input.

Pharyngeal Mucosa Pain

Inflammatory conditions of the pharyngeal mucosa expressed as a sore throat point out the marked difference between nociceptive conditions involving the oral mucogingival tissues and the visceral mucosa of the pharynx. While the pharyngeal mucosa is quite susceptible, the oral lining membranes are resistant.

Nonspecific Pharyngitis. Ordinary pharyngitis is usually viral in origin and occurs in conjunction with nasal and laryngeal symptoms. Pain on swallowing is characteristic. Central excitatory effects include referred pain, especially with swallowing. The reference zone is usually deep in the ear, and the pain is sensed as sharp and lancinating. Secondary hyperalgesia may be felt as a deep palpable tenderness in the throat, larynx, neck, or face or as superficial touch-

iness of the facial skin or scalp. Secondary autonomic symptoms may include puffy swelling of the eyelids, lacrimation, and nasal secretion. Sneeze and cough reflexes are active. Referred headache is common.

Streptococcal Pharyngitis. Streptococcal pharyngitis is typified by sore throat, fever, acutely inflamed pharyngeal mucosa, and referred pains, including headache. Cervical and submandibular lymphadenitis is present. Laryngitis, coughing, and nasal congestion are not due to streptococcal infection. When present, other etiologic agents coexist. Definitive diagnosis rests on laboratory examination to identify the group A beta-hemolytic organism.

Tonsillitis. Tonsillitis is an acute inflammation of the palatine tonsils that is due usually to viral and/or bacterial infection. Severe pain on swallowing, fever, malaise, headache, and regional lymphadenopathy are common. A differential diagnosis includes diphtheria, Vincent's angina, and infectious mononucleosis, each of which requires laboratory examination for identification.

Diagnostic Considerations. Pharyngeal mucosa pain should be differentiated from Eagle's syndrome, glossopharyngeal neuralgia, geniculate neuralgia, and Ramsay Hunt syndrome. Eagle's syndrome is due to an elongated styloid process or calcification of the stylohyoid ligament. The symptoms are persistent raw throat, ear pain, pain and difficulty with swallowing, and limited jaw movement.[8,9] Glossopharyngeal neuralgia is typical neuropathic pain of the paroxysmal neuralgia type that is triggered by throat movement incidental to swallowing, talking,

Fig 15-2 Points stimulated on turbinates, indicated by large crosses, cause referred pain to be felt in all maxillary teeth as well as in the face. (From Wolff HG. Headache and Other Head Pain, ed 2. New York: Oxford University Press; 1963. Used with permission.)

and chewing food. Geniculate neuralgia is an extremely rare neuropathic pain of the paroxysmal neuralgia type that is felt as sharp lancinating pain within the depths of the ear. It is triggered by touching the external ear canal or by movement of the auricle. Ramsay Hunt syndrome is herpes zoster of the nervus intermedius portion of the seventh cranial nerve. It is felt as ongoing burning pain deep in the ear and is accompanied by herpetic lesions in the external auditory canal and sometimes on the soft palate as well.

Nasal Mucosa Pain

Pain that emanates from the nasal mucosa is typically a dull, burning sensation that exhibits the clinical characteristics of visceral mucosa pain. Pain arising from the external lining of the nasal ala exhibits features of the superficial somatic category. When the deeper nasal mucosa is irritated as a result of viral or bacterial infection or as an expression of allergic rhinitis, typical deep visceral pain along with a variety of central excitatory effects may occur spontaneously or with the normal passage of air through the nose. The primary pain may go unnoticed

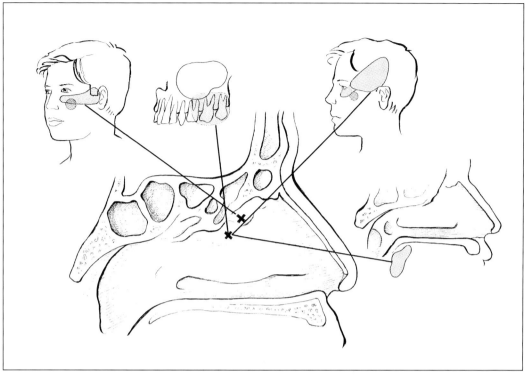

Fig 15-3 Stimulation of the ostium maxillare causes referred pain to be felt in the maxillary molar teeth and in the face. (From Wolff HG. Headache and Other Head Pain, ed 2. New York: Oxford University Press; 1963.)

because of the predominance of secondary effects such as referred pain, secondary hyperalgesia, and autonomic symptoms.

Primary pain in the inferior turbinate area has secondary reference zones that include all the ipsilateral maxillary teeth and areas of the face (Fig 15-2). Pain from the region of the ostium maxillare induces referred pain in the maxillary molar teeth and on the face (Fig 15-3). The referred pain may be sensed as a spontaneous toothache (Case 16). Secondary hyperalgesia may be felt as tender teeth or areas of touchy gingiva. Pain emanating from the nasal mucosa may induce referred pain throughout the entire upper part of the face. It may be sensed as a headache. Secondary hyperalgesia may be felt as areas of deep palpable tenderness in the upper portion of the face or as superficial touchy areas of skin, scalp, or mucogingival tissue.

Central excitatory effects are frequently expressed as autonomic symptoms. This includes puffy swelling of the eyelids and other loose facial tissue, injection of the conjunctiva, lacrimation, nasal secretion, and nasal congestion. When such symptoms occur in conjunction with diffuse maxillary pain, the condition is usually thought to be due to maxillary sinusitis. When compli-

Case 16	Heterotopic pain felt as toothache and referred from an inflamed nasal mucosa (so-called sinus headache)

Chief Complaint

Non-localizable maxillary toothache.

History

A 56-year-old man with mild-to-severe continuous but recurrent episodes of steady dull aching pain diffusely located bilaterally in the upper face and described as maxillary "toothache" that spreads to the zygomatic and orbital areas. The pain is accompanied by sensations of stopped-up ears and nose, swelling of the eyelids, tenderness of the scalp, and discomfort in the masseter and temporal areas with chewing. The episodes are irregular and fairly frequent, lasting from a few hours to 1 or 2 days. The pain is increased with lowering of the head position. He sometimes reports a mandibular toothache also.

The complaint began about 6 to 8 years ago and has been recurrently present ever since in spite of treatment by dentists, oral surgeons, internists, otolaryngologists, orthopedists, and neurosurgeons for dental disease, chronic sinusitis, temporomandibular arthropathy, nasal obstruction, neuralgia, and Meniere's syndrome, all without success. The TM joints have been injected with corticosteroid many times and he has taken nicotinic acid for 6 years. Presently he takes codeine for pain and nicotinic acid 150 mg twice a day.

Examination

Intraoral: Clinically and radiographically negative for cause of pain.

TM Joints: Clinically and radiographically normal.

Muscles: Palpable tenderness in the masseter and temporal muscles bilaterally and discomfort with firm contraction of these muscles but no masticatory dysfunction of any kind.

Cervical: Within normal limits.

Cranial Nerves: Within normal limits.

Diagnostic Tests: Withdrawal of nicotinic acid, 5-day trial of ergotamine tartrate, and 7-day trial of diphenylhydantoin sodium did nothing. Referral to neurologist cleared any neurologic or medical cause. Allergic rhinitis was confirmed by allergist. Topical application of local anesthetic to nasal passages relieved all pain except the muscle tenderness.

Impression

No dental, oral, or masticatory cause for the complaint. It appears that all pains and muscle effects are expressions of central excitation that arise from the nasal mucosa as a result of deep somatic nasal mucosa pain due chiefly to allergic rhinitis.

Diagnosis

So-called "sinus toothache" resulting from expression of allergic rhinitis.

cated by a spontaneous maxillary toothache or tender teeth (see Chapter 11), the condition may cause doctor and patient alike to think that it constitutes a dental problem, a sinus problem, or both. Not finding adequate dental cause, the dentist may refer the patient for ear, nose, and throat evaluation—or vice versa.

When the referred pain is sensed as a headache, the condition is popularly known as sinus headache. This is especially so when allergic rhinitis is the precipitating cause.

Upper Respiratory Infections. Upper respiratory infections frequently involve the nasal and pharyngeal mucosa as well as that of the larynx and upper part of the trachea. The inflammatory reaction is of the serous type that produces serous exudate on the surface. When the nasal mucosa is inflamed, the secondary effects of referred pain, secondary hyperalgesia, or autonomic symptoms may be displayed throughout the maxillary region and upper part of the face. Such symptoms frequently include aching or tender teeth. The differential diagnosis depends on distinguishing between the primary pain and its secondary effects. A topical anesthetic applied to the nasal mucosa will arrest a spontaneous referred toothache but will not arrest stimulus-evoked tenderness of the teeth, which is a heterotopic expression of secondary hyperalgesia. Analgesic blocking of the tooth may reduce but does not arrest the symptoms of secondary hyperalgesia. (Note that if the tooth were the primary source of pain, analgesic blocking would arrest it.)

With such conditions, the question may arise as to whether it represents a complication of maxillary sinusitis. The symptoms as described do not emanate from maxillary sinusitis except insofar as the ostium maxillare, nasal mucosa, or both are involved by direct extension from the antrum. The lining membrane of the maxillary sinus does not initiate appreciable secondary excitatory effects of any kind. Whether the antrum is truly involved in such conditions requires radiography and other specific examining techniques.

Paranasal Sinus Pain

Inflammatory conditions of the maxillary antrum and other paranasal sinuses are generally misunderstood. The syndrome of symptoms usually thought to be clinically indicative of sinusitis are chiefly secondary autonomic and sensory effects induced by primary pain emanating from the nasal mucosa as previously described. Whether such symptoms occur in conjunction with antral disease depends chiefly on patency of the ostium maxillare. Inflammatory exudate that accumulates in the antral cavity remains below the opening of the antrum into the middle meatus of the nose as long as the head is erect. Bending forward, however, permits the fluid to wash over the pain-sensitive tissue around the ostium, thus eliciting pain. If the ostium is open, antral inflammation can spread to the nasal mucosa and thereby initiate the symptoms as described previously. If the ostium is closed by swollen membrane or mucous polyps, the maxillary sinus may remain essentially non-symptomatic. This is because the lining membrane is nearly insensible to pain. This is altered very little even when the sinus is inflamed. Contrary to popular belief, pain is not a highly characteristic symptom of paranasal sinusitis, and chronic sinusitis seldom gives rise to facial pain or a headache.[10] Waltner[11] stated that in his experience no more than 20% of patients treated for sinus disease had any disease of the sinus at all. Chronic obstructive sinusitis exhibits symptoms of fullness or pressure, but not pain or headache, unless the nasal mucosa is conjointly affected.[12]

The question may arise whether the teeth and the maxillary sinus are affected in a common disease process. Sinusitis, of course, can result from dental sepsis just as antral disease can spread to involve teeth. A determination, however, of which is the primary source cannot be made from the clinical symptoms alone. If the cause of the sinusitis is dental, adequate clinical and radiographic evidence of the dental sepsis should be forthcoming. If the teeth are secondarily involved by direct extension of prior antral disease, the dental pain will be sensed initially as periodontal in type, with pulpal pain coming later. This, it should be noted, is the reverse of what takes place in the usual temporal sequence of pain of odontogenic origin.

Neuritic Toothache. Referred spontaneous toothache and secondary hyperalgesia involving the teeth and mouth do not arise as a result of antral inflammation. There is, however, a condition that does cause tooth pain. This is neuritic neuralgia that occurs as a result of inflammation of elements of the superior alveolar plexus by direct extension of antral inflammation. The neuritic symptoms occur in the peripheral distribution of the affected nerve. Thus, any ipsilateral maxillary tooth can be painful. The quality and character of the pain, however, is that of the neuritic type of neuropathic pain (see Chapter 17). It is also accompanied by other sensory symptoms that may go unnoticed. These include hyperesthesia, hypoesthesia, paresthesia, and anesthesia of other maxillary teeth, the adjacent gingiva, or the tissues around the infraorbital foramen. To confirm the diagnosis, clinical or radiographic evidence of preexistent antral disease is needed. Positive confirmation can be obtained by surgical aspiration of the maxillary sinus (see Case 26, page 426).

Glandular Pains

Primary visceral pain that emanates from glandular structures of the mouth and face is not uncommon. A diagnostic problem may occur especially when heterotopic pains, secondary muscle co-contraction, autonomic symptoms, or a combination are displayed. The source of such pain includes the major salivary glands, mucous and sebaceous glands, lacrimal and oil glands, and especially the lymph glands.[13]

Most glandular pain is inflammatory and therefore relates to infection, trauma, or sialolithiasis. Cystic degeneration or tumor formation may be present. Lymphadenitis results primarily from infection. Infectious mononucleosis and neoplasia may be other causes. The major salivary glands are subject to the irritating effects of mineral deposits and retrograde infection through the ducts that communicate with the oral cavity. Distension and compression may accentuate the pain. Salivary gland pain usually increases at mealtime and therefore may be associated with mastication. Submandibular salivary gland pain is frequently accentuated by chewing and swallowing movements. It may be mistaken for masticatory pain (Case 17).

Case 17

Heterotopic pain felt as preauricular pain and referred from an inflamed submandibular gland

Chief Complaint

Left TMJ and facial pain.

History

A 38-year-old man with mild continuous protracted steady dull aching pain located diffusely in the left preauricular and facial area, aggravated by chewing and opening widely but without any accompanying masticatory dysfunction.

The complaint began about a year ago as intermittent pain in the left face. It continued to increase in frequency and severity until about 6 months ago. It was constant but variable. During the last 6 weeks it has become severe enough to seek medical aid. His ENT physician found nothing wrong with the ear and advised a dental examination. His dentist removed the left mandibular third molar, injected the left TM joint with corticosteroid, and then prescribed a narcotic analgesic, all without benefit. He then referred him to another dentist who made a occlusal appliance which seemed to aggravate the complaint. He was then referred for a temporomandibular disorder examination. No medications are presently being taken.

Examination

Intraoral: Although the patient is missing three of the first molar teeth, the remaining teeth are clinically and radiographically negative for cause of pain. No occlusal instabilities are noted. All jaw movements are adequate in amplitude and symmetric. Tongue movements are normal. There is no palpable tenderness except in the left submandibular triangle where an indurated mass is felt and acute pain is elicited on firm palpation. An occlusal radiograph revealed a large irregular calcific mass in the region of the left submandibular salivary gland and this was seen also in the left lateral oblique film of the mandible. This mass was interpreted to represent massive sialolithiasis. Manipulation of the left submandibular gland seemed to increase the left facial and preauricular pain.

TM Joints: Normal structurally and functionally.

Muscles: Negative for pain and dysfunction.

Cervical: Within normal limits.

Cranial Nerves: Within normal limits.

Impression

The patient's masticatory discomfort appears to be a secondary manifestation of primary pain arising from the left submandibular gland presumably from the sialolith radiographically observed. The primary pain apparently is largely inhibited except when stimulated by firm manual palpation. Normal mandibular movements seem sufficient to induce impulses that are felt as referred pain in the left preauricular area and face.

Diagnosis

Masticatory pain referred from primary sources in the submandibular gland.

Because most painful glands are inflammatory, the pain can be localized quite well by manual palpation and by the presence of other signs of inflammation. Secondary central excitatory effects may complicate the symptom picture. Occasionally, heterotopic pains constitute the entire complaint. Careful diagnostic identification of the pain source is important. Lymphadenopathy, especially of the low-grade or chronic type, may be mistaken for a cyst or tumor.

Ocular Pains

Primary pains emanating from the nonmuscular structures of the orbit are mediated by the trigeminal nerve. Ocular muscle pain displays the clinical characteristics of musculoskeletal pain, while pain from the eye proper is chiefly visceral in type. All such pains should be managed by a competent ophthalmologist.

Heterotopic pain felt in the eye is frequently of muscle origin. Eye pain is usually accompanied by a headache. Although retro-orbital pain is sometimes attributed to masticatory causes, it is usually referred from nonmasticatory muscles. The occipital portion of the occipitofrontalis, the splenius cervicis, and the sternocleidomastoid muscles are the chief sources of such pain. It occurs frequently in conjunction with tension headache. Careful diagnostic identification of the pain source is needed to avoid therapeutic errors.

Auricular Pains

Since the ear is innervated by several different cranial and cervical nerves, the symptom earache can be quite misleading. Primary pain emanating from the ear may arise from different causes and be mediated by different nociceptive pathways. All such complaints should be managed by a competent otolaryngologist.

External auditory canal pain is of considerable interest to the dentist. Such pain is usually inflammatory and causes heterotopic symptoms in the face as well as deep in the ear and throat. Since it usually is accentuated by swallowing, it may be mistaken for masticatory pain or glossopharyngeal neuralgia. Otitis externa may be mistaken for temporomandibular joint arthralgia. One difference, however, is that ear pain is accentuated by movement of the auricle.

Since it is common practice to palpate the mandibular condyle through the external auditory canal, consideration should be given to the condition of the ear prior to inserting the finger. It should be inspected visually by using a speculum and direct light if an otoscope is not available.

Earache, like headache and retro-orbital pain, is frequently a heterotopic manifestation of deep somatic pain located elsewhere. Frequent sources of such pain are the deep masseter and the clavicular portion of the sternocleidomastoid muscle (Case 18). Earache may be referred from inflamed dental pulps and from the pharyngeal mucosa. Such ear pain is a dominant symptom of a sore throat. Preauricular pain is frequently referred from the lateral pterygoid muscle.

Ear pain such as that of otitis media has the propensity to induce a variety of central excitatory effects including co-contraction of masticatory muscles, thus often producing a restriction in the range of mandibular movement. In this sense the clinician can easily mistake the condition for a TM disor-

Case 18   Heterotopic pain felt as preauricular pain due to a trigger point affecting the sternocleidomastoid muscle

---

Chief Complaint   Left ear pain.

History   A 46-year-old man with intermittent short periods of mild-to-severe steady dull aching pain diffusely located in the left auricular and preauricular area, lasting a few minutes each time, and vaguely related to head and jaw movements.

The complaint began about 2 years ago following a severe upper respiratory infection and was initially diagnosed as otitis media. The periods of increased discomfort had been such that he sought only medical attention for his "bad ear." Recently, he went to an ENT physician who found the ear to be normal and suggested it to be a "bite problem." His dentist was unable to find any cause, so returned him to the physician who then prescribed therapy for "neuralgia" without benefit. He was then returned to his dentist to "take care of this dental problem" and was promptly referred for a TMD examination. Presently he is taking no medications.

Examination   **Intraoral:** There is no apparent dental or oral cause of pain. The occlusal condition is within normal limits. All mandibular functioning is well within normal limits. No discomfort of any kind is elicited by mandibular movements.

TM Joints: Both joints are clinically and radiographically normal.

Muscles: The masticatory muscles are entirely negative for cause of pain or dysfunction. There is palpable tenderness in the midbody of the left sternocleidomastoid muscle which when squeezed causes acute pain to be felt in the left ear and preauricular area.

Cervical: Bending and rotation of the head seems to increase the pain felt in the ear.

Cranial Nerves: Within normal limits.

Diagnostic Tests: Analgesic blocking of the left sternocleidomastoid muscle trigger point arrested all local tenderness as well as the induced ear and preauricular pain.

Impression   The present pain complaint does not originate from masticatory, dental, or oral cause. It appears to be referred pain arising from stimulation of the painful myofascial trigger point in the left sternocleidomastoid muscle.

Diagnosis   Preauricular nonmasticatory pain referred from myofascial pain originating in the sternocleidomastoid muscle.

---

der. Careful diagnosis as to cause is therefore essential for effective management of the condition. If the ear pain is protracted, the cycling nature of muscle pain may perpetuate the muscle disorder long after the initiating deep pain input has disappeared. Such a complaint now constitutes a true masticatory muscle disorder requiring treatment (see Chapter 12).

Since ear pains and masticatory pains have an intimate interrelationship, it is important that the pain source be accurately identified prior to definitive therapy by either dentist or otolaryngologist.

Differential Diagnosis

Primary deep somatic pains arising from visceral structures of the orofacial area other than blood vessels should be distinguished diagnostically from the following conditions:

1. Odontogenic pains of pulpal origin
2. Vascular and neurovascular pain disorders
3. Eagle's syndrome and carotodynia
4. Primary pains of musculoskeletal, neoplastic, or cystic origin
5. Heterotopic referred pains and secondary hyperalgesias due to other deep pain input
6. Heterotopic projected neuropathic pains
7. Somatoform pain disorders
8. Heterotopic pains of central origin

Therapeutic Options

For the management of primary deep somatic pains that emanate from visceral structures of the orofacial area other than blood vessels, the following therapeutic options are available (see Chapter 9).

1. Analgesics for palliative relief and counseling
2. Medications such as antihistamines, decongestants, antimicrobial agents, vasoconstrictors, and cough suppressants
3. Vaporizers for nasopharyngeal mucosa complaints
4. Referral for specialized medical care of the eye, ear, nose, and throat disorders
5. General supportive medical care

References

1. Cervero F. Visceral pain. Pain 1987 (suppl 4); 31:1.
2. Bonica JJ. The Management of Pain. Malvern, Pa: Lea & Febiger; 1990: 168–169.
3. Procacci P, Zoppi M. Pathophysiology and clinical aspects of visceral and referred pain. In: Bonica J, Lindblom U, Iggo A (eds). Advances in Pain Research and Therapy. New York: Raven Press; 1983: 643–658.
4. Wall PD, Melzack R. Textbook of Pain. New York: Churchill Livingstone; 1984: 309–392.
5. Abram SE. Sympathetic pain. In: Raj PP (ed). Practical Management of Pain. Chicago: Year Book; 1986: 209–214.
6. Gross D. Pain and autonomic nervous system. In Bonica JJ (ed): Advances in Neurology, vol 4. New York: Raven Press; 1974: 93–103.
7. Verrill P. Sympathetic ganglion lesions. In: Wall PD, Melzack R (eds). Textbook of Pain. New York: Churchill Livingstone; 1984: 581–584.
8. Lawrence FR, Cornielson E. Eagle's syndrome. J Oral Maxillofac Surg 1982; 40:307–309.
9. Correll RW, Wescott WB. Eagle's syndrome diagnosed after history of headache, dysphagia, otalgia, and limited neck movement. J Am Dent Assoc 1982; 104:491–492.

10. Mahan PE, Alling CC. Facial Pain, ed 3. Philadelphia: Lea & Febiger; 1991: 311–322.

11. Waltner JG. Otolaryngeal sources of pain. J Am Dent Assoc 1955; 51:417–419.

12. Druce HM, Slavin RG. Sinusitis: Critical need for further study. J Allergy Clin Immunol 1991; 88:675–677.

13. Procacci P, Zoppi M. Pathophysiology and clinical aspects of visceral and referred pain. In Bonica JJ, Lindblom U, Iggo A (eds): Advances in Pain Research and Therapy, vol 5. New York: Raven Press; 1983: 643–658.

16 Vascular and Neurovascular Pains

Primary deep somatic pain of visceral type may arise from the pulps of the teeth (see Chapter 11) or from other visceral structures (mucosa of the pharynx, nose, and paranasal sinuses; from the glandular, ocular or auricular structures; see Chapter 15). Probably one of the most common sources of visceral face pain, however, is vascular pain.

Behavior of Vascular and Neurovascular Pains

Vascular pain can be a very debilitating pain condition for many patients. The distinctive feature of vascular pain is its primary pulsatile or throbbing quality. The pulsations match the heart beat and no doubt stem from the cardiac systoles. The greater the amplitude of vascular dilation, the more pronounced the throbbing quality of the pain. This quality may be very slight at times and may be masked by coexistent muscle pain. The pulsatile feature of a vascular pain syndrome is not constant but is usually present during exacerbations. Between such peaks of discomfort, the pulsations may diminish in intensity or be imperceptible.

The throbbing quality of true vascular pain must be distinguished from other throbbing pains. Inflammatory pains, especially those confined in such a way that the pulsating vessels in the inflamed area cause noxious stimulation, have a throbbing quality. Examples of such inflammatory pains frequently encountered by the dentist are pulpitis, osteitis, periosteitis, and confined cellulitis. Usually differentiation can be made on the basis of other clinical signs of inflammation. Some neoplastic lesions have a pulsatile quality.

For the purpose of discussion in this text, vascular pains will be divided into two categories: those pains that actually have their origin in the vascular tissues (vascular pains) and those vascular pains that were initiated by neurovascular mechanisms (neurovascular pains). This division is made because etiologies, diagnoses, and therapies are different. Since the etiology of neurovascular pains is related to neural mechanisms, these pains is also related to the category of neuropathic pains.

Neurovascular Pains of the Mouth and Face

Probably the most commonly known neurovascular pain in the mouth and face is migraine. Until recently migraine pain had not been well understood. Wolff[1] explored these pains in depth, and his investigations indicated that pain occurred as a result of the dilation of arteries, which distort and noxiously stimulate the sensory receptors and afferent fibers in the vascular and perivascular tissues. When a vasoconstricting medication such as ergotamine tartrate reduced the dilation and amplitude of pulsation of such arteries, the pain decreased. He also demonstrated that pressure on the carotid artery diminished the pain. More recently, however, it has been demonstrated that the pain does not always relate to cerebral blood flow or vessel dilation.[2] With these findings and other research investigations, the profession has had to reevaluate the prevailing thoughts regarding the mechanisms of neurovascular pain. It became clear that the vascular changes that had been observed to be associated with the pain were merely a result of the condition and not the actual cause of the pain. The actual mechanism appears to be more closely related to a neurogenic phenomenon, thus, the term neurovascular pain.

Neurovascular pains are a group of visceral pain disorders that are generally characterized by episodic pains accompanied by neurologic, gastrointestinal, and psychologic changes (Fig 16-1). These pains are commonly unilateral with varying duration and can greatly debilitate the patient. Neurovascular pains can be divided into the following categories: *(1)* migraine, with or without aura, *(2)* cluster headache, *(3)* chronic paroxsymal hemicrania, and *(4)* neurovascular variants. Included in this section will be a fifth category, tension-type headache. Although tension-type headache is not thought to be primarily neurovascular in origin, there is certainly a neurovascular component and it is best discussed in this section.

Migraine (with or without aura)

Clinical Characteristics. Migraine is a severe type of headache that affects approximately 16% of the population. It is more commonly found in women, affecting 25%, while only 8% of men are affected.[3] Of patients with migraine, 15% report having a migraine headache between 8 to 10 days per year, while 9% report having the pain more than 14 days per year. Eighty-five percent of patients report the headache as being severe. The ratio of men:women is about 1:3. It appears that there exists a predisposition to migraine pain making some people more susceptible to this condition.[4] Earlier studies suggest that migraine susceptibility is related to genetic factors. These studies[5-7] report that between 50% and 60% of patients with migraine have parents that also experience migraines. In one study by Dalsgaard-Nielsen,[8] 90% of 100 women with migraine had an immediate family member that also experienced migraine. Although this evidence is strong, some[9] have recently questioned whether this relationship is actually inherited or environmentally influenced.

Migraine most often develops in the first three decades of life. The episodes may occur at any time of the day or night but most frequently on arising in the morning.

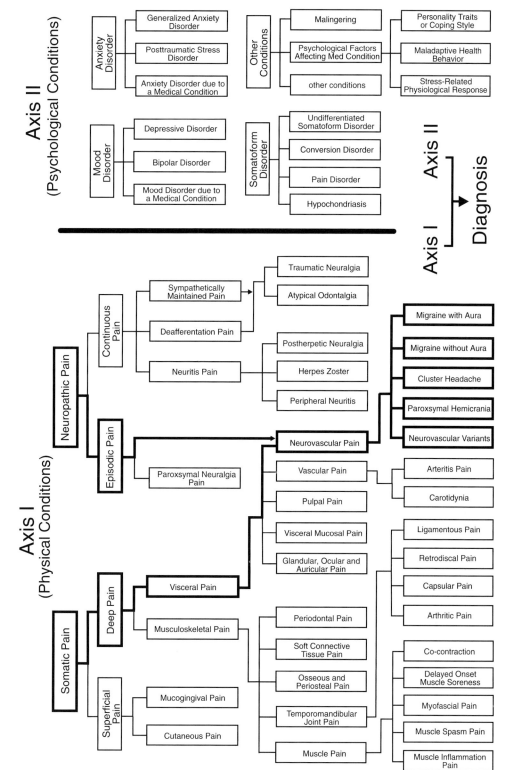

Fig 16-1 Pain classification chart highlighted to show the relationship of neurovascular pains to other orofacial pain disorders.

The pain onset is usually gradual, peaking and then subsiding. The pain episode commonly lasts 4 to 72 hours in adults and 2 to 4 hours in children.[10] The headache is unilateral in 60% of the cases and consistently occurs on the same side of the head in only 20% of the patients.[11] The pain can vary greatly from mild to very intense. When mild, the pain maybe constant and described by the patient as tight or band-like. At this level, the headache takes on the clinical characteristics of a tension-type headache. (Tension-type headache will be discussed later in this section.) When the headache is severe, it assumes a throbbing quality that may move from one part of the head to another and even radiate down to the neck and shoulder. The pain is commonly aggravated by physical activity or simple head movement.[12] Scalp tenderness occurs in two thirds of the patients during or after the headache.

Stages of Migraine. Blau[13] has divided the migraine attack into five phases: the prodrome, the aura, the headache itself, the headache termination, and the postdrome. The *prodrome* is the time that occurs hours or even days before the headache is felt. It can consists of mental, neurologic, and general symptoms that relate to autonomic and constitutional factors. Mental symptoms may include depression, euphoria, irritability, restlessness, mental slowness, hyperactivity, fatigue, and drowsiness. Neurologic symptoms may consist of photophobia, phonophobia, and hyperosmasis. Other general symptoms may include stiff neck, diarrhea, constipation, fluid retention, and food cravings.

The migraine *aura* is a complex of focal neurologic symptoms that immediately precede the headache. The aura usually develops in 5 to 20 minutes and lasts less than 1 hour. The aura is commonly characterized by visual, sensory, or motor phenomena and may even include language and brain stem disturbances. The visual aura is commonly characterized by a zigzag, flashing colored phenomenon that migrates across the visual field. This is known as *teichopsia*. Scotoma usually accompanies these visual disturbances. Sensory symptoms may include paresthesias in the hands, elbows, arms, and neck. These symptoms may migrate to the tongue and lips. Motor effects may present as focal fatigue or difficulty with speech. On occasion, the patient may have difficulty understanding language.

Not all patients who experience migraine headaches report an aura before their pain begins. Migraine therefore can be divided into two types, migraine with aura and migraine without aura. Earlier terminology referred to migraine with aura as *classic migraine* and migraine without aura as *common migraine*. At this time it appears that these two headaches originate by the similar mechanisms and therefore are likely to represent variations of the same condition.

The clinical characteristics of migraine headache pain have been reviewed in an earlier section. The pain is characterized by severe, throbbing, often debilitating pain. The patient will often report photophobia, phonophobia, and osmophobia, and will seek a dark, quiet room.[14] Some patients report lightheadedness and vertigo.[15] Anorexia is common and food cravings may occur. Nausea is typical and vomiting is frequent.[16] Some patients may have nasal stuffiness during the migraine attack followed in some by profuse nasal secretion as the attack terminates.[17]

Once the headache pain has terminated (postdrome), the patient will feel very tired, listless, and washed out. The patient may also be irritable and lack the ability to concentrate. Muscle weakness and aching is common. Anorexia and food cravings can occur.[18]

Pathophysiologic Migraine. Understanding the pathophysiologic features of migraine begins with a reminder that the brain is a visceral organ and, like all visceral organs, has a pain signaling mechanism. Like most other structures of the head, the trigeminal nerve carries nociceptive input from the innervated intracranial structures to the brain stem by way of the trigeminal spinal tract nucleus. This system of neural innervation of the intracranial structures is called the *trigeminovascular system.*

Not all brain structures are innervated with nociceptors. The cortex, for example, appears to be without nociception. All of the supratentorial pain-sensitive structures, such as the meninges and intracranial vessels, are innervated by the trigeminovascular system.[19] Pain sensation from the posterior fossa structures is carried centrally by the vagus nerve, the upper three cervical nerves, and the trigeminal nerve. It becomes obvious that the trigeminal nerve is an extremely important nerve involved in migraine pain.

The trigeminovascular system can be stimulated by both neural (electrical) and chemical activators (neurotransmitters). Once activated, a cascade of events can take place that result in migraine pain. It appears at this time that the mechanism of neurogenic inflammation is a significant contributor to migraine. When stimulated, the C fibers in the trigeminal nerve an-

tidromically release tachykinins, such as substance P and calcitonin gene-related peptide (CGRP) into the dural and meningeal blood vessels. These substances cause the degranulation of mast cells, releasing histamine and causing vasodilatation and plasma extravasation into the tissues. The release of substance P also results in inflammation and swelling of the blood vessel walls. To further compound this condition, serotonin (5-hydroxytrypamine, or 5-HT) is released from the platelets. Although serotonin in the brain stem is generally an inhibitory neurotransmitter, in the peripheral structures it has excitatory effects. The release of serotonin, therefore, seems to play a significant role in this condition.[20-25] This local inflammation and the resultant sensitization of polymodal nociceptors by substance P are thought to cause the pain associated with migraine.[26]

The action of histamine in initiating attacks of neurovascular pain applies only to so-called "migraine patients"; it does not act in this way with healthy subjects.[27] It has also been shown that attacks of migraine without aura display an increase in electromyographic (EMG) activity in pericranial muscles.[28,29] Masticatory muscle pains occur frequently with migraine headaches. They usually do not constitute a clinical complaint, however, because of the limited duration. Most migraine sufferers know that discomfort is a part of the headache problem and give it no thought. Therapeutic mistakes in this regard are usually those of the doctor who mistakenly thinks the headaches are due to a dental or masticatory cause. Moss[30,31] reported that migraine without aura and migraine with aura appear to be dissimilar phenomena etiologically. Migraine without aura is largely muscular pain and responds to muscular relaxation techniques.[32] Clinically there appears to be a relationship between neurovascular headaches and tension-type headaches.[33] It is likely that the underlying systemic factors stem from a common cause. Currently, it is believed that systemic factors, complex as they are, exercise a dominant role in neurovascular pain disorders.

A major advancement in the understanding of migraine has come with studies of the serotonin (5-HT) receptors.[34] It is now known that there are at least five serotonin receptor subtypes: 5-HT$_{1A}$, 5-HT$_{1D}$, 5-HT$_{1C}$, 5-HT$_2$, and 5-HT$_3$. The 5-HT$_{1D}$ receptors are widespread in the human brain. Studies have implicated this receptor in the constriction of cerebral blood vessels and arteriovenous anastomoses.[35] It has also been found that 5-HT$_{1D}$ receptor agonists can block trigeminovascular neurogenic inflammation but will not prevent inflammation caused by systemic substance P.[36] The 5-HT$_{1A}$ receptor has been shown to mediate serotonin-induced contractions of the basilar artery in dogs.[35] Additionally, 5-HT$_{1A}$ receptor agonist inhibits raphe cell firing.[35] The 5-HT$_2$ receptor has been shown to mediate smooth muscle contraction in many vascular beds. Serotonin, probably via 5-HT$_2$ receptors, can stimulate production of prostacyclin and other products of arachidonic acid metabolism in smooth muscle cells. Theoretically, 5-HT2 antagonists are able to inhibit serotonin from inducing an arachidonic acid–derived inflammatory state. It quickly becomes evident that understanding the function of these receptors can open pharmacologic avenues of therapies for the management of migraine pain. This aspect will be discussed further in the section on management.

To assume that only the primary afferents in the trigeminal nerve are involved in migraine pain is quite naive. The autonomic nervous system, as well as several brain stem structures, also affect cranial vessel function and have been implicated in migraine pain. The parasympathetic fibers arise in the superior salivatory nucleus of the brain stem and accompany the facial nerve to traverse the sphenopalatine ganglion and otic ganglion on to the intracranial vessels including the internal carotid artery (Fig 16-2). The parasympathetic fibers are thought to contribute to migraine by the release of substances such as acetylcholine, vasoactive intestinal polypeptide, and peptide histidine isoleucine. Sympathetic fibers ascend from the superior cervical ganglion to form a plexus in the walls of both the internal and external carotid arteries. These sympathetic fibers can contribute to migraine by the release of norepinephrine, neuropeptide Y, and peptide YY.

Located in the wall of the fourth ventricle in the upper pons is the locus ceruleus. This nucleus is made up of cells that contain the highest concentration of noradrenaline in the brain. It receives afferent fibers from the cortex, amygdala, hypothalamus, reticular formation, raphe, vestibular nucleus, and tractus solitarius. All these areas relate to the internal and external sensory stimuli or to the affective state. The locus ceruleus also projects to the thalamus, geniculate nuclei, facial nerve nucleus, and the trigeminal spinal tract nucleus. It has been found in monkeys that stimulation of the locus ceruleus decreases cerebral blood flow and increases vascular permeability.[37] Not only can the locus ceruleus directly affect intracranial vessels but it can cause the release of norepinephrine from the adrenal

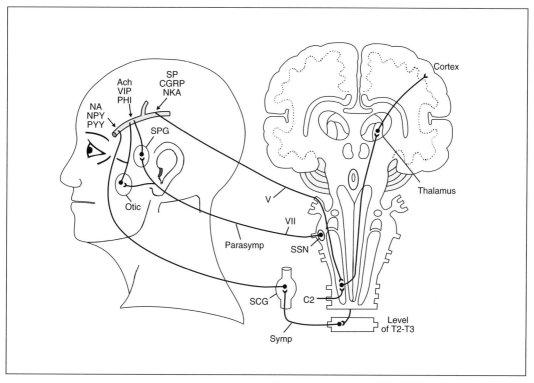

Fig 16-2   The central pain pathways and neurotransmitters with afferent and efferent pathways in the trigeminovascular system. Vascular afferent are carried by the trigeminal nerve *(V)* and descend into the trigeminal spinal tract to synapse with the second-order neuron in the nucleus caudalis. Input from the cervical neurons *(C2)* also synapse in the region and can influence ascending input onto the thalamus. Sympathetic nerve fibers *(Symp)* leave the spinal cord at the level of T2 and T3 to joint the sympathetic cervical chain to ascend to the superior cervical ganglion *(SCG)*. Sympathetic fibers then leave the ganglion to innervate the cranial vessels. The parasympathetic neurons leave the superior salivatory nucleus *(SSN)* and travel by way of the facial nerve *(VII)* to the sphenopalatine ganglion *(SPG)* and the otic ganglion *(Otic)*. From these ganglioa the parasympathetic fibers move on to the cranial vessels. Each type of neuron is responsible for the release of neurotransmitters that can play an active role in neurovascular pain disorders. Abbreviations for these neurotransmitters are: Afferent: Substance P *(SP)*; calcitonin gene–related peptide *(CGRP)*; neurokinin A *(NKA)*. Parasympathetic: acetylcholine *(Ach)*; vasoactive intestinal polypeptide *(VIP)*; peptide histidine isoleucine *(PHI)*. Sympathetic: norepinephrine (noradrenaline, *NA*); neuropeptide Y *(NYP)*; and peptide YY *(PYY)*. (Adapted from Goadsby PJ, Zagami AS, Lambert GA. Headache 1991; 31:365–371.)

gland by its connection with the intermediolateral cell column of the thoracic cord. This norepinephrine along with serotonin releasing factor causes a platelet release reaction. Free serotonin released from the platelets increases the sensitivity of vascular receptors thus augmenting the afferent inflow through the trigeminal nerve, increasing the cascade of events leading to the migraine pain.

Studies that investigate cerebral blood flow during migraine attacks reveal a decrease in flow during certain phases of the attack. Several studies[38,39] have demonstrated that in the early stages of migraine there may be patchy areas of increased cerebral blood flow just prior to a systematic decrease in blood flow. Diminution of the flow starts in the occipital region and extends forward as a spreading oligemia.[38] This wave of oligemia progresses over the cortex at a rate of 2.2 mm/min and stops short of the central and lateral sulci. The spreading oligemia typically begins before the patient notices any local neurologic symptoms, reaching the sensorimotor area only after the appropriate symptoms have started and outlasts these symptoms. Oligemia lasts for several hours and is followed by delayed hyperemia. The headache usually starts while the cerebral blood flow is diminished.

This spreading oligemia seems to follow a pattern that was first described by Laeo in 1944.[40] Laeo observed in animal brains a pattern of activity that slowly progressed as a wave over the cortex, starting in the posterior region and migrating anteriorly at a rate of 3 mm/min. This phenomena was known as the *spreading depression of Laeo* and is likely to be associated with the wave of decreased blood flow just described.

It appears that the focal neurologic symptoms associated with migraine are accompanied by diminished cortical perfusion of the appropriate part of the opposite cerebral hemisphere. On some occasions, a wave of hypoperfusion may advance slowly over the cortex in association with a slow march of visual or other neurologic symptoms. However, this is not always the case. It is not possible to deduce with certainty from current techniques whether constriction of the cortical microcirculation precedes or follows diminution in cortical neuronal activity. Adams et al[41] found that stimulation of the locus ceruleus at frequencies that reduced cerebral blood flow in the cat had no consistent effect on the resting discharge of neurons in the visual cortex, suggesting that an important action of this brain stem area was constriction of the microcirculation. It is clear that cortical blood flow does not always dictate the presence or absence of headache, but dilation of the middle cerebral artery and possibly other intracranial arteries may certainly contribute to the perception of pain.

Summary. Migraine is a neurovascular pain disorder that appears to be related to a trigeminovascular reflex involving both peripheral and central mechanisms. Stimulation of the trigeminovascular reflex by either excessive afferent or central input can create excessive discharge of part of the spinal tract nucleus of the trigeminal nerve and its thalamic connections. This discharge can produce a neurogenic inflammation of the primary afferents that innervate the intracranial vessels resulting in an antidromic release of excitatory neurotransmitters. This begins a cascade of events that produce the migraine pain. Accompanying this trigeminovascular reflex activity is the effect of the locus ceruleus on the cerebral cortex that initiates cortical oligemia and possibly spreading depression. This activity could account for the migrainous aura that often occurs prior to the headache. The end result is a complex interaction between the brain stem, cranial nerves, and the cranial blood vessels, with the afferent impulses from the latter intensifying pain perception through the trigeminovascular system. It is reasonable to assume that patients with unstable trigeminovascular reflexes are more susceptible to migraine disorders.

Precipitating Factors (Triggers). The combination of trigeminal nerve input along with the parasympathetic, sympathetic, and brain function activities makes up what has been suggested to be a trigeminovascular reflex that is responsible for migraine pain.[42] It has been found that a number of different factors can activate this reflex and precipitate a migraine attack. Factors that stimulate the cascade of events leading to migraine are called *triggers*.

Some common triggers are certain food products. Foods that contain nitrites[43] such as hot dogs, monosodium glutamate,[44] red wines,[45] or any type of alcohol[43] may frequently trigger migraine attacks. Sometimes changes in normal sleep patterns can trigger a migraine.[12] These may represent either too little or too much sleep. Work shift changes or even jet lag may be responsible. In other cases, environmental conditions may be triggering factors. Bright or flashing lights, weather changes, pungent odors, or high altitudes may trigger a migraine.[46] Hormonal changes can also trigger migraines. Menstrual migraines attacks are linked to the period of menses in 60% of women and exclusively to this period in 14%.[47] Migraines

may worsen in the first trimester of pregnancy but significantly improve during later pregnancy. This is thought to relate to high levels of estrogen during this time.[7,48] Another common trigger is emotional stress and anxiety. This may be especially true of the poststress letdown period.[17,49,50]

Diagnostic Considerations. According to the International Headache Society's Classification for Headaches[51] (see Table 7-1), migraine headache can be diagnostically divided into migraine without aura and migraine with aura.

Migraine without Aura. Migraine without aura is a recurring headache disorder manifest by attacks that last 4 to 72 hours. Typical characteristics of the headache are unilateral location; pulsating quality; moderate or severe intensity; aggravation by routine physical activity; and association with nausea, photophobia, and phonophobia. The International Headache Society[51] specifically states that the patient must experience at least five attacks of the above described headache to be classified as having migraine without aura.

Migraine with Aura. Migraine with aura is a recurring headache disorder manifest by attacks of neurologic symptoms unequivocally localizable to the cerebral cortex or brain stem, usually gradually developed over 5 to 20 minutes and usually lasting less than 60 minutes. Headache, nausea, and/or photophobia usually follow neurologic aura symptoms directly or after a free interval of less than an hour. The headache usually lasts 4 to 72 hours. The International Headache Society[51] specifically states that the patient must experience at least two attacks of the above described neurologic symptoms plus the headache to be classified as having migraine with aura. On occasion a patient may experience an aura but never develop a headache. These patients are considered in the classification of migrainous aura unaccompanied by headache.[51]

Management. The management of migraine with or without aura can be divided into (1) patient education and trigger avoidance, (2) nonpharmacologic methods, and (3) pharmacologic methods. Pharmacologic methods can be subdivided into those drugs that abort the migraine and those that prevent the migraine.

1. Patient Education and Trigger Avoidance. Patients who experience migraine headaches need to understand basic information regarding their pain condition. They need to know that even though the pain is very severe, it is still benign and not an aggressive tumor such as cancer. (Of course, if other neurologic symptoms are present, additional tests must be performed to rule out any aggressive diseases.) Assuring the patient that the pain is not life threatening often assists them in coping with the pain attacks. Probably the most important aspect of education, however, is in having the patient identify any triggering factors that initiate the migraine attack. Often patients may have no appreciation for triggers. If the patient can identify a trigger, then proper avoidance can be instituted. The best way to identify triggers is to ask the patient to develop a pain diary. The patient should keep a record of any and all headaches along with the circumstances that were present prior to or during the onset. With time the patient is often able to identify factors that

are associated with the headache. Once these factors are identified, an effort should be made to avoid them, to reduce the number of episodes of migraine. Factors that relate to diet can usually be quickly controlled. Sometimes environmental factors such as light, weather changes, and pungent odors may be more difficult to avoid. Other factors such as fatigue, sleep patterns, and stress need to be identified and addressed appropriately. Nothing is more satisfying to the patient than his or her own ability to control the number of migraine attacks. This, of course, can only occur with patient education.

2. Nonpharmacologic Methods. Patients with migraine should be encouraged to maintain a regular schedule of events through their day. Changes in routine should be avoided since they may precipitate attacks.[50] Patients should be encouraged to participate in regular exercise, good health practices, regular mealtimes, and good sleep hygiene. The patient should go to sleep and arise in the morning at the same time each day. This same schedule should be maintained even on the weekends when often the individual can sleep longer. Migraine attacks frequently begin in the last hour of sleep when the regular sleep duration has been lengthened.

Other nonpharmacologic methods of managing migraines are relaxation training,[52,53] biofeedback,[54] hypnosis, cognitive-behavioral therapy,[55] and sometimes even formal psychotherapy. These therapies are oriented toward stress management by decreasing the autonomic nervous system responsiveness.

3. Pharmacologic Methods. Pharmacologic management of migraine with and without aura can be divided into two types: medications that are used to abort a migraine at its start and medications that are used to prevent migraine attacks. The choice of which type of management approach lies in the frequency of the migraines. As a general rule, migraines that occur less than twice a week are managed with abortive medications so that treatment is provided during the onset of the attack. If migraines occur more frequently than twice a week, the patient should be managed with preventive medications.

Abortive Medications. In a small number of patients, analgesic medications such as aspirin, acetaminophen, and nonsteroidal anti-inflammatory drugs (NSAIDs, ie, ibuprofen) can be useful in aborting migraine. When these medications are helpful they should be used because of their low toxicity and side effects. Unfortunately these medications are not commonly effective once a migraine has begun. A standard class of medications that have been used are the ergotamine derivatives. The ergotamines are known vasoconstrictors and have for years been thought to counter the effects of vasodilatation associated with the migraine. Ergotamine can be given in a 2-mg tablet sublingually at the onset of the headache. Preparations of 1-mg ergotamine tartrate and 100-mg caffeine take as an oral tablet can also be helpful. If the patient is nauseated, a rectal suppository of 2-mg ergotamine tartrate and 100-mg caffeine can be used.

In recent years, there have been significant advances in abortive medications. Dihydroergotamine (DHE) and even more recently sumatriptan (Imitrex) have proven to be quite helpful for migraine suffers. DHE can be administered either intravenously,[56] intramuscularly,[57] subcutaneously,[58] or even by an intranasal formulation.[59] Sumatriptan is normally given subcutaneously,[60] but can be given orally[61] or intranasally.[62] It is even packaged so the patient can administer the drug himself or herself so that an office visit is not needed. (The first administration should be in the office so the patient can be observed for any side effects.) Both of these medications work at the 5-HT$_{1D}$ and the 5-HT$_{1A}$ receptor sites to block the trigeminovascular neurogenic inflammation associated with migraine. Generally speaking, medications that act as 5-HT$_{1D}$ and the 5-HT$_{1A}$ agonists decrease neurogenic inflammation and are therefore abortive medications. Medications that have antagonist activity at the 5-HT$_2$ and the 5-HT$_{1C}$ receptor sites provide prophylactic migraine activity.[63]

Preventive Medications. Frequent migraine attacks are best managed with medications that, when taken regularly, decrease the likelihood of the next attack. As just mentioned, these medications seem to provide antagonist activity at the 5-HT$_2$ and the 5-HT$_{1C}$ receptors. One group of such medications is the beta-adrenergic agents (beta blockers). Medications such as propranolol (Inderal), metoprolol (Lopressor), timolol (Blocadren), nadolol (Corgard), and atenolol (Tenormin) reduce the attack frequency in patients with and without aura.[64,65] Along with the beta blocker effect on the 5-HT receptors, they also act centrally to inhibit the central beta receptors and decrease the enhancing adrenergic pathways.

Another group of medications used to prevent migraine attacks are the calcium channel blockers. These medications were originally developed as a cardiovascular agent but were later found to be useful in preventing migraines. Not only do these medications act on the 5-HT receptors but they also inhibit contraction of vascular smooth muscle, inhibit prostaglandin formation and prevent hypoxia of cerebral neurons. The most common calcium channel blockers used in migraine are nifedipine (Procardia), verapmil (Calan, Isoptin), diltiazem (Cardizem), and nimodipine (Nimotop).

Another group of prophylactic migraine medications are the serotonin antagonists. The most commonly used is methysergide (Sansert). Methysergide is a semisynthetic ergot 5-HT$_2$ receptor antagonist that displays affinity for the 5-HT$_1$ receptor. Its chronic administration blocks the development of neurogenic inflammation.[66] Another serotonin antagonist is periactin (Periactin).

Still another group of prophylactic migraine medications are the tricyclic antidepressants. These medications have proven to be most helpful in the management of many chronic pain disorders at dosages that are far below antidepressive levels. The tricyclic antidepressants increase the availability of synaptic serotonin and norepinephrine by inhibiting its reuptake. They also seem to downregulate the 5-HT$_2$ receptors and decrease beta receptor density. Some of the more common tricyclic antidepressants used for prevention of migraine are amitriptyline (Elavil, Endep), nortriptyline (Pamelor), doxepin (Sinequan), desipramine (Norpramin), and protriptyline (Vivactly). Preventive dosages for migraines may be as little as 25 to 50 mg before sleep. It is not thought that this dosage has any antidepressant effects.

Many of the drugs used to manage migraine have significant side effects, especially on the cardiovascular system. Although most are quite safe in a healthy patient, the medically compromised patient may experience significant problems that will need to be properly managed. Before any medication is used, the clinician should be well informed of the patient's medical condition and have a good understanding of the medication that will be used. When any question arises, appropriate medical personnel should be consulted.

Cluster Headache

Clinical Characteristics. Cluster headache is a neurovascular disorder that is far less common than migraine. Cluster headache has also been referred to as migrainous neuralgia, Raeder's syndrome, sphenopalatine neuralgia, ciliary neuralgia, histamine cephalalgia and Sluder's headache. It affects men more than women at a ratio of 6:1. Although most patients begin experiencing headache between the ages of 20 and 50 years (mean, 30 years), the disorder may begin as early as the first decade and as late as the eighth decade. Unlike migraine, there does not appear to be a significant hereditary factor in cluster headache. Kudrow[67] reported that only 18 of 495 patients with cluster headache reported a family history of the disorder. Migraine headache occurred no more frequently among the cluster headache population than among random populations.[68]

The pain of cluster headache commences quickly, without warning, and reaches a crescendo within 2 to 15 minutes. It is often excruciating in intensity and is deep, nonfluctuating, and explosive in quality. Only occasionally is it pulsatile, which is not typical of neurovascular pains. Approximately

10% to 20% of the sufferers will report superimposed paroxysms of stabbing, ice pick–like pains in the periorbital region that last for a few seconds and may occur once or several times in rapid succession. The pain usually begins in, around, or above one eye or the temple. It is always unilateral and generally affects the same side in every episode. Each attack of cluster headache is usually accompanied by ipsilateral lacrimation and nasal drainage, lid drooping, pupillary change, and conjunctival injections. Focal neurologic symptoms as seen in migraine are very uncommon in patients with cluster headache; however, on occasion patients may experience typical photopsia, teichopsia, facial paresthesia, and vertigo at the time of the attack.

The attacks last from 30 minutes to 2 hours in about 75% of the cases. A patient will experience a group or cluster of these headaches as frequently as 6 per day to once a week. These attacks will cycle for 4 to 8 weeks and then 90% of the patients will experience a pain-free period of remission. This pain behavior is how the disorder received it name. Most patients experience one or two bouts of the pain each year but some may be pain-free for years.

Periodicity is a characteristic feature in 85% of the cases, meaning that the pain occurs at the same time of the day. About 75% of the attacks occur between 9 PM and 10 AM.[69] A common time to experience the pain is between 1 and 2 AM[70] with the patient waking up with the paroxysms of pain in 50% of the cases, usually within 2 hours of falling asleep.[71] One to 3 PM seems to be another common time period for the onset of cluster headache.

Pathophysiologic Features. In earlier studies it was suggested that cluster headaches resulted from a dilation of the external carotid artery.[72] Because of the retro-orbital pain, investigators have more recently looked at the possibility of changes in the internal carotid artery. Ekbon and Greitz[73] found a segmental luminal narrowing of the ipsilateral internal carotid artery in the region of the carotid canal as well as a significant dilation of the ipsilateral ophthalmic artery. Along with these changes is an increase in the cerebral blood flow in the central, basal, and parietotemporal regions during the attack.[74] Further investigations have revealed that, as with migraine, these vascular changes may be the result of this pain disorder and not actually the cause. It is now thought that these vascular changes are related to an autonomic nervous system dysfunction.[75,76] This sympathetic activity is responsible for the ipsilateral lacrimation, nasal drainage, lid drooping, pupillary change, and conjunctival injections seen during the attack.

It appears that histamine may play a significant role in pathophysiology of cluster headache. The level of histamine found in the blood is greatly increased during the attack.[77,78] As with migraine, the increased level of histamine is related to mast cell degranulation in the area of the involved vessels. The interesting clockwork periodicity phenomenon of cluster headache may also shed light on its pathophysiology. Cluster headache may be the result of a central nervous system discharge in the region of the hypothalamus containing the posterior cells that regulate autonomic functions and anterior nuclei that serves as the major circadian pacemaker in mammals.[79] The biologic clock is serotonergically modulated and is connected anatomically to the eye.[80] Perhaps cluster headache is the result of an antidromic discharge of the biologic pacemaker.[81]

Precipitating Factors. A common triggering factor in cluster headache is alcohol. This trigger is present in approximately 50% of the patients. Patients who are sensitive to alcohol note that drinking alcohol will trigger an attack in 70% to 80% of the times they are exposed. The attacks are triggered within 5 to 45 minutes after ingesting even a very small amount of alcohol. Other common triggers are emotional stress, relaxation following stressful times, exposure to heat or cold, glare, hay fever attacks, and occasionally the ingestion of specific foods (ie, eggs, dairy products, chocolate).

There is some evidence that head trauma can precipitate the disorder.[82] Among 180 patients studied by Manzoni et al,[70] previous head injury was reported by 41, with loss of consciousness occurring in 20. This is significantly more frequent than observed among patients with other types of headaches. Other studies have not found this relationship.

Certain medications can trigger cluster attacks in susceptible patients. One milligram of nitroglycerin sublingually can initiate an attack.[83] In approximately 70% of patients, an attack can be initiated with subcutaneous histamine.[84]

Diagnostic Considerations. According to the International Headache Society,[51] cluster headache is a headache characterized by attacks of severe strictly unilateral pain orbitally, supraorbitally, and/or temporally, lasting 15 to 180 minutes and occurring from once every other day to eight times a day. The headache is associated with one or more of the following: conjunctival injection, lacrimation, nasal congestion, rhinorrhea, forehead and facial sweating, miosis, ptosis, and eyelid edema. Attacks occur in series lasting for weeks or months separated by remission periods usually lasting months or years. To be classified as cluster headache, there must be at least five attacks with the symptoms.

Most cluster headaches have periods of remission as just described. About 10% of the patients, however, may experience chronic symptoms with no periods of remission. This condition is called *chronic cluster headache.*

Management

1. Patient Education and Trigger Avoidance. As with migraine, patients who experience cluster headaches need to understand basic information regarding their pain condition. They need to know that even though the pain is very severe, it is still benign and not an aggressive disease. Probably one of the most important aspects of education is in having the patient identify any triggering factors that initiate the attacks. Often patients may have no appreciation for triggers. If the patient can identify a trigger, then proper avoidance can be instituted. Since the attack usually occurs shortly after the trigger, it may be easy for the patient to recognize the trigger.

Since cluster headache is related to the "biologic clock," changes in sleep pattern can affect the attacks. The patient should be encouraged to maintain good sleep hygiene and avoid any afternoon naps. Any change in the sleep cycle, such as vacation schedule, work shift changes, studying habits, or jet lag can precipitate an attack. Patients who experience long periods of stress, anger, rage, worry, or frustration often experience an attack after the event has passed. Patients should be aware of these factors and minimize them as much as possible.

2. *Nonpharmacologic Methods.* Ekbom[85] found that compression of the superficial temporal artery provided relief for about 40% of his patients but he also found this worsened the pain in another 40%. Carotid compression reduced the pain half the time, while worsening the pain in 25%. Vigorous physical exertion at the earliest sign of an attack can, in some cases, be remarkably effective in amelioration or even aborting an attack.[86,87] Ice can also be placed over the painful area. Because the attack comes on so quickly, the pain is very severe before any therapy can begin. These therapies are not tremendously effective, but even the smallest pain reduction is appreciated by the patient.

3. *Pharmacologic Methods.* Pharmacologic management of cluster headache can be divided into two types: medications that are used to abort the headache and medications that are used to prevent attacks.

Abortive Medications. Since the headaches come on so fast, it is difficult to get adequate relief from oral medications. Instead inhalants can be used. One of the most effective inhalants is 100% oxygen.[88,89] The patient should breathe pure oxygen via a tight-fitting mask at a flow rate of 8 to 10 L/min for 10 to 15 minutes. This therapy can be 80% effective in those patients that find this approach feasible. Since the attacks can occur frequently during the cluster period, oxygen must be made available to the patient in the home or workplace. Oxygen inhalation is especially helpful in nocturnal attacks.

Other inhalants that can be effective in aborting a cluster headache are ergotamine and lidocaine. Ergotamine aerosol at a dosage of 0.36 to 1.08 mg (one to three inhalations) produces peak plasma levels of ergotamine within 5 minutes[90] and is effective in 80% of the patients.[67,91] Kittrelle et al[92] demonstrated that intranasal administration of 1 mL 4% topical lidocaine was effective in terminating attacks in four of five patients. These patients were instructed to lie supine, with their heads extended backward 45 degrees and rotated 30 to 40 degrees toward the side of the headache. One milliliter of lidocaine was slowly dropped into the nostril ipsilateral to the pain while the patient was maintained in that position for several minutes. These investigators believe that the lidocaine reached the sphenopalatine fossa and anesthetized the sphenopalatine ganglion.

Another abortive medication is dihydroergotamine (DHE). DHE can be given intravenously and usually will abort the headache. The only difficulty with this therapy is that the patient must be in the doctor's office for administration. This limits its use as an abortive medication.

Preventive Medications. The most appropriate management of cluster headache is to prevent the attacks especially during the cluster period. Medication should be provided to the patient during the entire cluster period. Once the cluster period has resolved, the medication can be withdrawn. Therapeutically it may be difficult to know exactly when to begin or stop the medications since the onset is quick and the duration of cluster period may vary greatly. This often becomes a management problem.

Oral administration of 2 mg of ergotamine tartrate 1 to 2 hours before bedtime can be very effective in preventing nocturnal attacks.[93] However, when a patient is experiencing long periods of cluster attacks, the ergotamine can produce rebound attacks. Therefore short time use is advised. Cluster attacks during the day are best prevented by the prophylactic use of agents such as methysergide, verapamil, lithium, DHE, or prednisone. The use of methysergide, verapmil, and DHE have already been reviewed in the section on migraine. Lithium can be used for chronic cluster headache but side effects may limit its use. Prednisone has been shown to be 75% effective for the episodic form of cluster headache.[94] The dosage may vary from 10 to 80 mg daily for 7 days with a tapering off over the next 6 days.[17] The paroxysmal pain should cease within hours of the first dose. If it does not, the prednisone should be discontinued. Prolonged or repeated use of prednisone is not advised due to its general effects on the immune system.

Indomethacin can be a very helpful drug for the prevention of cluster headache. Indomethacin can be given at dosages of 25 to 50 mg three times a day. Stomach irritation is a common side effect that should be monitored. Indomethacin is a very specific drug used in the treatment of paroxysmal hemicrania, a very similar condition to cluster headache that will be discussed in the next section.

Chronic Paroxysmal Hemicrania

Clinical Characteristics. Chronic paroxysmal hemicrania (CPH) has many clinical characteristics that are similar to cluster headache. Both conditions are characterized by episodes of severe unilateral pain that is consistently reported on the same side. Accompanying the headache is ipsilateral nasal stuffiness and rhinorrhea, along with lacrimation and conjunctival injection. Forehead perspiration may also accompany the severe pain. An aura is rarely present with either cluster or chronic paroxysmal hemicrania. Nocturnal attacks are common with both headaches and the mean age of onset is between 30 and 34 years.

Because of these similarities, diagnosis can be confusing. Since treatment for these two headaches is different, one must focus on their differences. There are five differences that help distinguish CPH from cluster headache:

1. While cluster headache is more common in men, CPH is five times more common in women than men.[95] This statistic is not helpful when establishing a diagnosis for one patient, but it may be considered.
2. Chronic paroxysmal hemicrania attacks occur much more frequently than cluster, with a mean number of attacks being 10.8 during a 42-hour period.[96]
3. Attacks of CPH are shorter in duration (mean, 13.3 minutes) than cluster headaches (mean, 49 minutes).[97]
4. Attacks of CPH may be mechanically precipitated, with 10% of the attacks related to flexing or rotating the head.[97] This is not common with cluster headache.
5. Unlike cluster headaches, CPH has a prompt, dramatic, and lasting response to indomethacin. This characteristic is almost pathognomonic of the disorder.

The location of CHP headache is usually described as being in the temple, forehead, eye, or periaural areas and occasionally in the occiput. The pain can be excruciatingly severe, but there is a continuous fluctuation between severe and moderate attacks. In the worst periods, there may be a continuous, sore feeling in the usually painful areas between attacks. The pain usually has a piercing, boring, or claw-like character, but in the initial stages, especially in precipitated attacks, it may be pulsating.

Pathophysiologic Features. The pathophysiologic features of chronic paroxysmal hemicrania are not well understood. It can probably be viewed as a disorder that is closely related to cluster headache, yet some distinct differences exist. During the PHC attack, there is an increase in the intraocular pressure of the eye on the symptomatic side along with an rise in the temperature of the cornea. These findings suggest a marked increase in vasodilatation within the eye.[98,99] Forehead sweating increases on both sides with CPH yet with cluster, sweating is unilateral. This suggests that the pathophysiologic features may be different.[100]

CPH attacks can be abruptly precipitated by applying pressure to certain particularly sensitive points in the neck or by neck flexion. In only a few seconds, tears appear and the intraocular pressure is increased on the symptomatic side. Obstructing the flow in the common or internal carotid artery on the symptomatic side does not initiate an attack, nor does rubbing these arteries. The pathway from the neck to the eye would therefore appear to be neurogenic rather than vascular.[101] Although autonomic symptoms predominate during the attacks, they do not seem to cause the pain.[101] The fact that nocturnal attacks are common also suggests a central mechanism or at least a central influence. Perhaps, as with other neurovascular disorders, there is a peripheral mechanism that is influenced by a central dysregulation. The precise mechanism has eluded researchers.

Precipitating Factors. As previously mentioned, neck movements seem to be a precipitating factor in some patients. At this time, other trigger factors have not been well described. It would not be surprising to learn that common factors that trigger other neurovascular disorders may also trigger chronic paroxysmal hemicrania.

Diagnostic Considerations. According to the International Headache Society[51] chronic paroxsymal hemicrania is a headache characterized by attacks with largely the same characteristics of pain and associated symptoms and signs as cluster headache, but the attacks are shorter in duration, more frequent, occur mostly in women, and there is absolute effectiveness of indomethacin.

Management. As mentioned in the diagnosis section, chronic paroxysmal hemicrania can be eliminated by continuous administration of adequate doses of indomethacin.[96,102,103] The dosage may vary greatly from patient to patient and even from attack to attack in the same individual depending upon severity. Indomethacin is easily titrated and dosage may vary from 25 to 250 mg/day. Indomethacin is tolerated well although it may cause dyspepsia. If dyspepsia occurs, a histamine H_2 receptor blocking agent or indomethacin suppositories can be used.

Neurovascular Variants

Neurovascular variants are pain disorders that have neurovascular origins but their clinical presentations are different than those of migraine, especially in location. Neurovascular variants may be easily mistaken for neuropathic pain disorders. It is important, therefore, that a thorough history and examination be completed so that these conditions can be differentiated from the episodic neuropathic pains, such as paroxsymal neuralgia and the constant neuropathic pains, such as neuritis or deafferentation pain (see Chapter 17).

Clinical Characteristics. The neurovascular pain disorders are of deep somatic origin, not neurogenous. Neurovascular variants differ from those of neural origin in the following ways[20]:

1. Pain is not limited to the peripheral distribution of a nerve but may spread beyond neurologic boundaries following the vascular arborization.
2. Pain is not precisely controlled by division of the sensory root of a single nerve.
3. Pain is steady, diffuse, aching, and usually throbbing, with milder dull, diffuse, nonpulsatile discomfort bridging the more severe exacerbations. It may last for hours, days, or weeks.
4. Summation effects such as triggering from slight stimulation are not observed.
5. The disorder occurs in younger age groups.
6. Attacks of pain are not induced by stimulation of superficial sensory receptors.
7. Vasoconstricting medications usually decrease the intensity of the throbbing component of pain.

Pathophysiologic Features. Little is known regarding the pathophysiologic features of neurovascular variants. As with other neurovascular disorders, there are likely to be both central and peripheral mechanisms that precipitate the attacks. Perhaps continued research investigations will help the profession better understand these disorders and may even lead to new approaches to classification and management. At this time, this category is used for those disorders that have clinical symptoms that more closely resemble neurovascular disorders than any other pain disorders. This is a very naive approach to pain classification but has some use since their response to treatment seems to be similar.

Types of Neurovascular Variants. The location of pain felt with a neurovascular variant varies according to the vascular tissue that is involved. The location of the pain does not affect the quality or characteristics of the pain, but it may greatly influence how the clinician views the condition. If the pain is felt in a tooth, it may become a diagnostic problem for the dentist. When the pain is felt in the sinus area, it now becomes a diagnostic problem for the otolaryngologist. Pain felt in the face or cheek may be called atypical facial pain,[104] which is a catch-all term for facial pain of unknown etiology. It is the clinician's duty to thoroughly assess the condition before any therapy begins. As one can imagine, this condition can be easily mistreated.

Neurovascular (Migrainous) Toothache. When a neurovascular variant is felt primarily in a tooth, it is referred to as a neurovascular toothache or sometimes a migrainous toothache. This type of pain is most commonly felt in the maxillary canine and premolar area (Case 19). The initiating pain is sufficiently similar to true pulpal toothache to convince the patient, and perhaps the dentist as well, that a dental cause is present and dental treatment indicated. Unfortunately such dental treatment may be instituted prior to an accurate diagnosis and followed by still other forms of therapy. For example, such a tooth may be prepared and filled (when minor caries is identified or the tooth has been previously treated) only to be then followed by endodontic treatment and finally extraction. Then treatment may begin on adjacent teeth, and sometimes extensive procedures are attempted. Because of the accompanying nasal symptoms, the patient may be treated for sinusitis, then allergic rhinitis. Finally, the patient may be branded as neurotic. As treatment progresses, so does spreading of the complaint. As rapport between patient and doctor breaks down, the patient may blame the initial or subsequent dental treatment for his or her predicament.

The ability of the dentist to recognize and identify this pain condition is extremely important and only the dentist can do it. Differential diagnostic criteria include the following:

1. The aching tooth is free of reasonable dental cause for the pain.
2. The toothache has a persistent, episodic, recurrent behavior.
3. Analgesic blocking of the tooth proper may stop the pain in some instances and lead the dentist to assume that the source is of dental origin. At other times

its effect is not precise or conclusive and may even aggravate the pain.
4. Definitive therapy such as endodontic treatment or extraction may give temporary, transitory benefit, only to be followed in time by recurrence of the complaint.
5. Frequently, there are accompanying ipsilateral autonomic signs involving the eye and nose.
6. With time, the complaint spreads to involve wider areas of the face and neck, even the shoulder. Frequently, occipital muscle effects are observed, with symptoms suggestive of tension-type headache. Very frequently, chewing pains occur due to secondary hyperalgesia or muscle co-contraction of masticatory muscles. Efforts to manage a masticatory muscle disorder may follow.
7. Early in the disorder, the pain complaint may be favorably influenced by carotid pressure or administration of ergotamine tartrate, which helps identify it as a vascular pain. This effect diminishes as secondary muscle involvement occurs.

Although a neurovascular variant may frequently occur initially as a toothache, it may spread to involve the entire maxilla, side of the face, ear, neck, and shoulder. It is episodic and recurrent. Its throbbing quality and muscular component may simulate both odontogenous and masticatory pains. Its extreme variability and sudden exacerbations give it a neuralgic quality that may be mistaken for trigeminal neuralgia (tic douloureux). The acute pains may occur rather regularly at night. As spreading occurs, the accompanying autonomic effects; ie, edema of the eyelids and face, lacrima-

Case 19	Heterotopic pain felt as a toothache secondary to a neurovascular pain source

Chief Complaint

Maxillary right first premolar toothache.

History

A 46-year-old woman with recurrent episodes of mild-to-severe variable intermittent dull aching throbbing pain diffusely located in the right first premolar tooth, aggravated by tension and fatigue, and accompanied by nasal congestion.

The complaint has been recurrently present for 4 to 5 years, each episode lasting a few weeks, followed by a remission of several months. The present one began about a month ago. There is mild constant aching in the face and some also in the occipital area with severe exacerbations described as throbbing toothache lasting up to an hour occurring once or twice daily, sometimes at night. She has lacrimation and congestion of the nose on the right side that increases when the pain is severe. It was initially treated as sinusitis, then as trigeminal neuralgia, and more recently as allergic rhinitis, all without benefit. Dental treatments have included occlusal adjustments, endodontics, and extraction of the maxillary right second premolar. She has been cleared neurologically. The internist wants the dental problem cleared.

Examination

Intraoral: There is no clinical or radiographic evidence of any dental, oral, or masticatory cause for the complaint. The quality of the previous dental care is excellent. Oral hygiene is good. There is no occlusal instability. Masticatory functioning appears to be normal in all respects.

TM Joints: Both joints are structurally and functionally normal.

Muscles: There is no palpable tenderness of any masticatory muscles and no muscular dysfunction. There is vague occipital discomfort that seems to parallel the dental and facial pain.

Diagnostic Tests: A sublingual trial therapy with ergotamine tartrate gave noticeable relief during a spontaneous exacerbation of tooth pain. The occipital discomfort and constant mild aching sensation in the face were not affected.

Impression

There is no dental, oral, or masticatory cause for the complaint. By history, clinical course, present behavioral characteristics, and trial therapy, the entire pain problem suggests a neurovascular pain disorder. The dental, nasal, and ocular symptoms are very likely secondary central excitatory effects of the deep pain that presumably involves the right maxillary artery. Management should be on a medical level.

Diagnosis

Toothache secondary to a neurovascular pain disorder.

tion, and nasal congestion, may be confused with allergic rhinitis and sinusitis.[105] The component of occipital pain that secondarily refers to the frontal region may induce tension-type headache.

When expressed as a direct central excitatory effect, the muscle symptoms almost invariably occur in the masticatory muscles because these are innervated by the trigeminal nerve that mediates the pain input. Actual masticatory muscle co-contraction causing true masticatory pain and representing a masticatory muscle disorder can therefore be a direct secondary effect of persistent neurovascular pain. When this is true, both the initiating primary neurovascular pain and the secondary masticatory pain should be identified, and therapy for both pain problems is required for adequate management. This immediately becomes a multidisciplinary effort. If only the masticatory component is treated, a prompt relapse occurs when active therapy ceases. If only the neurovascular component is treated, the secondary masticatory muscle component remains as a complaint. Proper management depends on diagnostic identification of the dual phenomena present and simultaneous therapy administered (Cases 20 and 21).

Neurovascular Variants Reported as Atypical Facial Pain. When a neurovascular variant is felt in the face or cheek region it is frequently referred to as atypical facial pain. Atypical facial pain is a general term often used to describe facial pain of unknown origin. Although this term is used to describe many different conditions, it is included in this section since neurovascular variants felt in the face are often misunderstood or misdiagnosed.

Diagnostic Considerations. The clinician needs to be very familiar with the behavior of facial neurovascular pains. Definite similarities exist between neurovascular variants and masticatory muscle pain since both are representative of deep somatic pain. Both conditions are episodic or recurrent, the pains are steady not paroxysmal, the pains have a dull aching quality, the pains are very poorly localized or frankly diffuse, and both conditions readily induce central excitatory effects. The following points should serve as guidelines to help differentiate them:

1. Neurovascular variants usually have a characteristic pulsatile, throbbing quality.

2. Neurovascular variants follow the vascular arborization and therefore violate neuroanatomic boundaries. Frequently the pain is simultaneously felt in the side of the neck, sometimes in the shoulder. Vessel wall edema may occur and is identified as palpable tenderness along the superficial arteries. Occipital muscular discomfort may be present.

3. Neurovascular variants vary in intensity from low to high—low enough almost to go unnoticed followed by a sudden exacerbation of high-intensity pain. This gives it a neuralgic quality, but the pains are not truly paroxysmal, and the intermissions are not completely pain-free. The low-intensity pain is predominantly myalgic and nonpulsatile, whereas the high-intensity exacerbations are usually more characteristically vascular and throbbing. The intense exacerbations may have a temporal regularity unrelated to functioning. These attacks are frequently nocturnal.

Case 20   Cyclic masticatory muscle pain in the masseter secondary to neurovascular pain

Chief Complaint

Left face and ear pain.

History

A 60-year-old man with mild-to-severe continuous protracted steady dull aching pain diffusely located in the left auricular and preauricular area, aggravated by mandibular movement, associated with a continuous but quite variable high- and low-intensity throbbing pain in the left maxillary teeth, face, orbit, and neck. When the pain is intense it is accompanied by tearing, swelling, and redness of the left eye, left nasal congestion, and flushing of the left face.

The complaint began about 2 years ago as a recurrent throbbing pain in the left maxillary teeth, several of which were treated dentally without lasting benefit. He was then unsuccessfully treated for sinusitis and allergic rhinitis. About a year ago, the pain became continuous and soon spread to involve the masticatory system. He has been examined medically, neurologically, and otolaryngologically and the consensus was that he had a temporomandibular disorder. The complaint has remained the same for several months. No medications are presently being taken.

Examination

Intraoral: The teeth and mouth are essentially negative clinically and radiographically. There is pain in the left masseter area with opening beyond 24 mm, with chewing eccentrically, and with clenching the teeth. The mandible deflects to the left after about 24 to 25 mm of opening. The maximum opening is about 30 mm. The occlusal condition appears stable

> **TM Joints:** Both joints are clinically normal except for left side restriction of opening. Radiographically, the left joint is normal structurally and functionally except for evidence of extracapsular restriction of translatory movement with opening.
>
> **Muscles:** There is palpable tenderness in the left masseter muscle.
>
> **Cervical:** Within normal limits.
>
> **Cranial Nerves:** Within normal limits.

Diagnostic Tests: Analgesic blocking of the left masseter muscle arrested the masticatory component of the complaint but did not affect the diffuse throbbing pain. Ergotamine tartrate temporarily reduced the throbbing component when used during a period of high-intensity pain.

Impression

It appears that a neurovascular pain disorder preceded the masticatory complaint and as such represented the primary pain that secondarily induced muscle pain in the left masseter muscle. Cycling has no doubt occurred. The resulting cyclic masticatory muscle pain was induced by nonmasticatory causes.

Diagnosis

Cyclic masticatory muscle pain of the left masseter muscle, secondary to preexistent neurovascular pain.

Case 21 Neurovascular pain disorder mistaken for masticatory pain

Chief Complaint

Left occipital and face pain.

History

A 36-year-old woman with recurrent episodes of continuous mild protracted steady dull aching pain diffusely located in the left occipital and preauricular areas. The pain is aggravated by head movements and hard chewing, punctuated several times daily by spontaneous periods of high-intensity throbbing pain located in the left maxillary teeth and jaw and associated with ipsilateral lacrimation and nasal congestion, sometimes with noticeable nausea. Each episode lasts several weeks separated by irregular intervals of several months.

The complaint began about 2 years ago and was treated as tension-type headache. When the chewing discomfort occurred, the physician thought it was due to a "TM joint syndrome" and promptly referred the patient for dental treatment. This has consisted of refilling several left maxillary teeth and adjustments of the occlusion, all without benefit. At times, the remissions were attributed to medical and/or dental therapy. The present episode has lasted 5 weeks without responding favorably to any treatment. No medications are presently being taken.

Examination

Intraoral: No dental or oral cause for the complaint is found clinically or radiographically. Masticatory function is entirely normal in all respects. No occlusal instability is identified clinically. There is some minor preauricular and temporal discomfort with hard chewing.

TM Joints: Both joints are normal clinically and radiographically.

Muscles: There is a slight palpable tenderness in the left masseter, temporal, occipital, and trapezius muscles but no dysfunction of any kind.

Cervical: Slight restriction to rotational movement with a soft end feel.

Cranial Nerves: Within normal limits.

Diagnostic Tests: Sublingual ergotamine tartrate was administered several times during the severe episodes. Each time it arrested the throbbing maxillary component within 30 minutes but it had no noticeable effect on the preauricular and occipital discomfort. Nighttime use of amitriptyline seem to reduce the episodes and intensity of the pain.

Impression

The history, clinical course, and present behavioral characteristics of the pain complaint are highly suggestive of a neurovascular pain disorder accompanied by muscular, cervical, and occipital pain. The left masticatory muscles have become secondarily involved, probably as a central excitatory effect, causing discomfort with hard chewing but no masticatory dysfunction of any kind.

Diagnosis

Neurovascular pain disorder with a secondary muscle component mistaken for a masticatory muscle pain disorder.

4. Neurovascular variants are prone to occur in episodes lasting several weeks and separated by pain-free remissions of several weeks or months. Sometimes they occur in clusters of short painful episodes followed by long periods of remission. The episodes relate more to emotional stress and fatigue than to functional demands.

5. Neurovascular variants do not cause appreciable dysfunction unless there is a dominant component of secondarily induced muscle co-contraction. Since such effects involve chiefly the masticatory muscles, the symptoms of a masticatory muscle disorder may become evident, and the underlying important neurovascular pain disorder may go unnoticed. The only indication of its presence may be recurring exacerbations of throbbing pain, a phenomenon wholly inconsistent with true masticatory pain.

6. Neurovascular variants frequently present characteristic autonomic effects; ie, nasal congestion, lacrimation, injection of the conjunctiva, edema of the eyelids and face–on the affected side. These central excitatory effects may be confused with allergic rhinitis and sinusitis clinically. However, allergic rhinitis is always bilateral.

7. When a neurovascular variant is suspected, the throbbing component (but not the muscle component) may be reduced by applying pressure to the carotid artery manually or by administration of ergotamine tartrate.

8. Differentiation between neurovascular variants and true masticatory pain is best made by the accumulation of positive evidence of the presence of neurovascular pain on one hand or of masticatory pain on the other.

9. When the two conditions occur simultaneously, therapeutic trials may be required to confirm the diagnosis.

Neurovascular variants may follow facial trauma, including tooth extraction and other minor oral surgery. As such, it may be confused with other posttraumatic pain problems. Because of the extreme versatility of this type of neurovascular pain and its propensity to simulate other facial pain disorders, especially those involving dental practice, errors in diagnosis may be made. The dental examiner should be constantly alert to these possibilities because neurovascular pain is very common.

The examiner should have at his command sufficient understanding to identify pains of this type. He should be especially cautious in advising definitive therapy either of the teeth or the masticatory apparatus until a confirmed diagnosis is established.

Management. Neurovascular variants are managed, in part, according to the clinical characteristics. If the pain is only occasional, abortive medications are used. If the pain is prolonged, preventive medications may be in order. Severe pain is treated more aggressively than mild pain.

When a neurovascular variant has a periodic presentation, ergotamine can be given in a 2-mg tablet sublingually at the onset of the pain. If relief is achieved, it is quite indicative of a neurovascular origin and therefore can assist in diagnosis. Preparations of

1 mg ergotamine tartrate and 100 mg caffeine taken orally can also be helpful. If the patient is nauseated, a rectal suppository of 2 mg ergotamine tartrate and 100 mg caffeine can be used.

For some patients, analgesic medications such as aspirin, acetaminophen, and NSAIDs can be useful in controlling the pain. When these medications are helpful they should be used because of their low toxicity and side effects. Low-dose tricyclic antidepressants, such as amitriptyline (25 to 50 mg) may be helpful in some neurovascular variants. When the pain condition persists, medications used to manage migraine, such as dihydroergotamine and sumatriptan, may be helpful. Medications used for the prevent of migraine may also be tried (see section on migraine management).

Tension-Type Headache

Clinical Characteristics. Tension-type headache is a very common source of head pain. The headache is described as a dull, nonpulsing pain. Often patients will use the terms tightness, pressure, or soreness. Some will describe the feeling of a tight headband compressing their head as if they were wearing a tight cap. Most tension-type headaches are of mild or moderate intensity, rarely becoming debilitating as with migraine. In 90% of the cases the pain is felt bilaterally.[106] The typical location of tension-type headache is in the occipital, parietal, temporal, and frontal regions.[107]

In a cross-sectional population study of 740 adult subjects, 74% had experienced tension-type headache within the previous year, while as many as 31% of the same population had more than 14 days of this type of headache during the previous year.[106] In another study, a 1-year prevalence rate for tension-type headache in men was 63% and in women, 86%.[108] Friedman et al[109] found a positive family history in 40% of the patients with tension-type compared to 70% in the patients with migraine.

Most tension-type headaches are episodic, lasting an average of 12 hours. The duration can vary greatly from 30 minutes to 72 hours.[107] The onset of the headaches is usually between 20 and 40 years of age.[109] If the headaches last more than 15 days a month, the condition is considered to be a chronic tension-type headache. Nausea and vomiting are rare with episodic tension-type headache. However, with chronic tension-type headache, the pain can become moderate to severe and nausea and vomiting have been reported.[107] Phonophobia and photophobia can also be associated with severe chronic tension-type headache but are rare with episodic tension-type headache.[106,107]

Pathophysiologic Features. For many years it was thought that this very common headache was directly related to muscle tension. In fact, for years this headache was referred to as a muscle contraction or muscle tension headache. More recently it has been demonstrated that although some muscle tenderness is commonly present, increased levels of electromyographic activity are not always associated with the condition.[110] Some studies[111,112] do suggest that patients with tension-type headache have increased EMG responses to emotional stressors as compared to those in control subjects. It has been suggested, however, that this increase in EMG activity may not be the cause of the pain but in fact a response to the pain.[113] Although muscle pain does seem to play a part in the etiology of this headache, it certainly does not offer a complete explanation. Central factors are also likely to contribute, especially related to limbic system activities. Emotional stress, anxiety, and depression seem to present causal relationships with tension-type headaches.[114,115] Olesen[33,116] has proposed a model that describes tension-type headaches occurring as a result of an interaction between changes in the descending inhibitory system, which controls nociceptive brain stem neurons and peripheral input coming from myofascial and vascular sources. The input from each of these sources combines to influence the characteristics of the headache. Significant myofascial input may produce the referred tension-type headache[117] described in Chapter 12. Greater input from vascular sources may reflect a headache more similar to migraine. Significant input from the limbic structures (ie, anxiety, depression) may greatly affect descending inhibitory function and produce a more chronic tension-type headache.

Many researchers now believe that migraine and tension-type headache are two different presentations of the same pathophysiologic mechanism. Perhaps migraine represents a pain condition with a significant vascular input while tension-type headache represents a pain condition with more myofascial input. Careful patient interviews will often reveal that many patients experience both of these headaches. Commonly they will report a tension-type headache for several hours or days and then develop a migraine. Once the migraine has resolved, the tension-type headache will linger for a few more hours or days. This pain condition is referred to as a *mixed*

headache. Mixed headaches are common and reflect a unified pain mechanism.

Precipitating Factors. As just mentioned, factors that influence either the limbic, myofascial, or vascular structures can be important in precipitating a tension-type headache. It is for this reason that tension-type headache needs to included in this section as well is in the chapter on muscle pains (see Chapter 12). Obvious precipitating factors are emotional stress, anxiety, depression, and myofascial pain. There are also other factors that influence or cause tension-type headaches. Some of these are daily hassles,[118] unphysiologic working position, muscle strains,[119] sleep deprivation,[120] severe snoring,[121] weather changes,[122,123] and menstruation.[122] Chronic tension-type headache can also be induced by analgesic abuse. Patients who have overused or abused drugs, even over-the-counter analgesics, can have what is called a *rebound headache* when the medication is withdrawn.[124-126] These patients need to be educated to the problem, which may seem foreign at first. Then the medications must be slowly reduced.

There is some evidence that masticatory muscle activity may play a role in some tension-type headaches.[127] Masticatory muscle disorders seem to be related to tension-type headaches in a number of studies.[128-131] Tension-type headaches can sometimes be precipitated by clenching the teeth or introducing a high occlusal contact.[132] Although this relationship is not clear, the dentist needs to be aware of any increased masticatory muscle activity that may be contributing to a tension-type headache. When this is suspected, proper therapy to reduce muscle activity should begin.

Diagnostic Considerations. According to the International Headache Society's Classification,[51] tension-type headache is a recurrent episodic headache lasting minutes to days. The pain is typically pressing/tightening in quality, of mild or moderate intensity, bilateral in location, and does not worsen with routine physical activity. Nausea is absent, but photophobia or phonophobia may be present. A patient who experiences the headache less than 15 days per month is diagnosed as having episodic tension-type headaches. If the patient experiences the headaches more than 15 days per month, for longer than 6 months, the condition is classified chronic tension-type headache.

Management. Like many pain disorders, management of tension-type headache begins with patient education. The patient needs to know those factors that are aggravating the condition as well as those that might be helpful in relieving symptoms. It is often helpful to have the patient maintain a headache diary so that factors that are not always easy to identify might be recognized. The patient should be encouraged to decrease intake of caffeine (coffee, tea, soft drinks) and alcohol, as well as any medications that have been chronically used by the patient for the headache. The patient should be informed that eliminating these substances may at first increase the frequency and intensity of the headaches. After 1 to 2 weeks, the withdrawal effects should subside.

Since emotional stress plays an important role in tension-type headache, the patient should be assessed for any significant stressors. This is of course a difficult task since one's perception and response to stress is very individual. When significant stressors are identified, corrective behaviors or when possible avoidance should be encouraged. Stress management skills can be important therapies with tension-type headache. Relaxation training and biofeedback techniques[133] can also be very helpful. The patient must be willing to take the time to work with these therapies. This will only happen if the clinician educates the patient on their importance and the patient is willing to actively participate in the treatment. Success in managing tension-type headaches often resides in the hands of the patient. If a major depression disorder or anxiety disorder is present, these conditions need to be managed by the proper medical personnel.

Judicious use of mild analgesics may be needed, but the patient should be aware of the potential complications. NSAIDs are often helpful, especially if the patient has not been using them previously. When a previous NSAID has been occasionally used, change to another. Often low dosages of a cyclic antidepressant, such as amitriptyline, can be helpful in managing the headache. When tricyclic antidepressants are used they are best taken before bedtime because of their sedative effects. These effects are often beneficial when a coexistent sleep disorder is present. When a mixed headache is present, anti-migraine medications may be useful, as described in the earlier sections.

When tension-type headache is present in association with a masticatory muscle disorder, the muscle disorder should be managed.[134] Headache on awaking may be related to nocturnal bruxism. In such instances, an occlusal appliance that is directed toward reducing bruxism can be very helpful. This appliance is best worn only at night, when the bruxism occurs. During the day the patient should be taught cognitive awareness so that he or she becomes aware of the bruxing or clenching habit and subsequently learns to stop it. The dentist should be aware that not all morning headaches are caused by bruxism. A good history and dental examination should be completed before an appliance is fabricated.

Often tension-type headache is a heterotopic pain originating in the cervical muscles. When a cervical myofascial pain disorder is present, treatment should be oriented toward resolving this disorder. Physical therapy modalities such as spray and stretch can be helpful. Heat, ultrasound, and deep massage may also be used. On occasion, trigger point injections may be therapeutic. These therapies have been reviewed in Chapter 12.

Vascular Pains of the Mouth and Face

Vascular pains are those pains that originate from the tissues that make up the vessel walls. These pain conditions are far less common than the neurovascular pains discussed in the previous section. Vascular pain originating from inflammation of the vessel wall is referred to as either *arteritis*, in the case of an artery, or *phlebitis*, in the case of a vein. There are many different types of vascular conditions that can produce head and neck pain. Some of these conditions are arterial hypertension, cerebral venous thrombosis, ischemic stroke, vascular malformation, and intracranial hematoma. Most of these conditions do not refer pain to the orofacial structures, and

therefore will not be reviewed in this text. There are two vascular pain conditions, however, that can produce pains in the orofacial regions and therefore will be reviewed (Fig 16-3). These conditions are cranial arteritis and carotidynia.

Cranial Arteritis

Clinical Characteristics. The term cranial arteritis suggests that an artery in the cranial region has become inflamed. The most common artery to be involved is the temporal artery, which is therefore referred to as *temporal arteritis*. Because of its cause, this condition is also sometimes referred to as giant cell arteritis or polymyalgia rheumatica. The incidence of temporal arteritis increases greatly after the age of 50. It is rarely seen before this age. It is nine times as frequent in the ninth decade as the sixth.[135] It appears to be a disease of whites and is rarely seen in Asians and blacks.[136] Temporal arteritis commonly presents as a severe headache in the temporal region. It is usually unilateral, affecting only one artery, but on occasion can present bilaterally. The pain is often throbbing and boring.[137] It may be felt superficially as burning pain with a superimposed lancinating quality. The intensity may range from mild to severe. In half the cases, the pain is constant with the other half intermittent.[138] Palpation of the temporal region will usually reveal a prominent, tortuous, very tender and enlarged temporal artery.[139] Minor jaw movement will not produce pain; however with increased use of the jaw, pain will increase significantly (jaw claudication). Blood studies reveal an elevated erythrocyte sedimentation rate (ESR), often greater than 100 mm/hr.

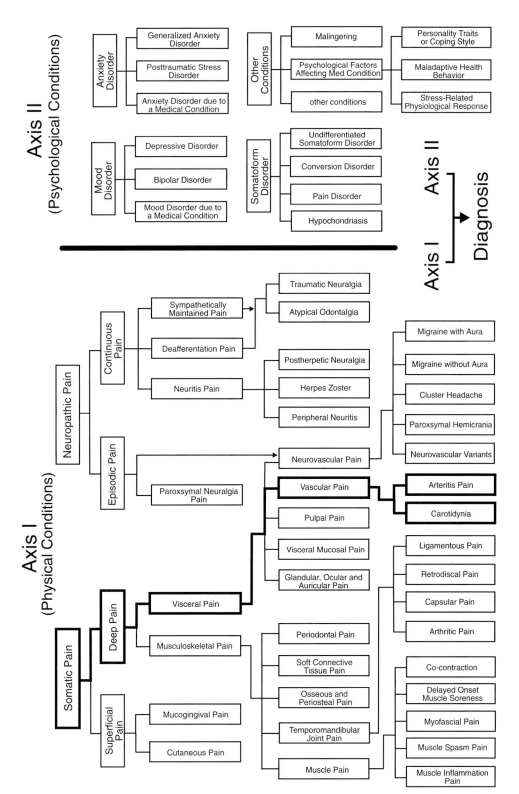

Fig 16-3 Pain classification chart highlighted to show the relationship of vascular pains to other orofacial pain disorders.

The disease is confirmed by results of biopsy of the artery confirming a giant cell arteritis.

Because of the pathophysiologic features of temporal arteritis, other pains may be present such as shoulder or hip pain, diplopia, malaise, weakness, weight loss, anorexia, and fever.[140] Complete or partial loss of vision is the most serious consequence of temporal arteritis. This occurs in at least one-third of all cases.[141,142] Blindness can occur when the temporal arteritis produces a granulomatous inflammation of the posterior ciliary arteries resulting in an anterior ischemic optic neuropathy.[143]

Pathophysiologic Features. The pathophysiologic features of cranial arteritis are unknown. It is very similar in clinical presentation to polymyalgia rheumatica, which also has an unknown etiology. These disorders may in fact be the same disorder presenting in different regions. These disorders seem to present with a common inflammatory process and the clinical picture may reflect certain host responses to an inciting agent. The inflammatory phase often appears to be self-limiting but because of the possibility of blindness and stroke, immediate management is essential.

Precipitating Factors. At this time, there are no known precipitating factors of cranial arteritis. Local provocation of the involved artery will greatly increase the pain but this does not seem to be due to anything more than local stimulation.

Diagnostic Considerations. According to the International Headache Classification[51], cranial arteritis is diagnosed by a swollen and tender scalp artery (usually the superficial temporal artery) with an elevated ESR and confirmed by results of artery biopsy, revealing a giant cell arteritis. The diagnosis is also confirmed by disappearance of the headache within 48 hours after the beginning of steroid treatment.

Management. Since cranial arteritis is considered a semiacute inflammatory disease, it demands rapid treatment. Because temporal arteritis can quickly threaten vision, it can be considered a medical emergency. If symptoms are progressing rapidly, hospitalization may be indicated. The treatment of choice is 40 to 60 mg of prednisone daily.[140] This dosage may be rapidly tapered to a maintenance level, depending on the relief of symptoms and the decline in the ESR toward normal. The duration of treatment is uncertain. It may be necessary to continue corticosteroids for months although eventually it is possible to discontinue treatment in almost all patients.

Carotidynia

Clinical Characteristics. Carotidynia is a pain condition that arises from the cervical carotid artery resulting in unilateral neck pain that frequently radiates to the ipsilateral face and ear and sometimes to the head. Facial pain is a common primary symptom and carotid artery tenderness and overlying soft tissue swelling are the major physical findings. There appear to be two forms of this disorder, an acute form and a chronic form. The acute form seems to be the result of a monophasic illness usually lasting for a week or two and tends not to recur. The chronic form is likely to be a neurovascular variant.[144]

Roseman[145] found that carotidynia seems

to affect both sexes equally while Lovshin[146] found women to be affected more than men at a ratio of 4 to 1. Although this condition can present at any age, middle age seems to be the most common. Palpation of the neck reveals tenderness, swelling, and sometimes conspicuous pulsation of the common carotid artery on the affected side.[147] If the thumbs are placed on the common carotid arteries just below the bifurcation and the structures are pressed back against the transverse cervical processes with a rolling movement, a severe pain is produced. Pain originating from the carotid artery is often referred to the eye, deep in the malar region, and spreading back to the ear. Pressure on a painful carotid artery will often increase this referred pain pattern.

Pathophysiologic Features. Acute carotidynia appears to be associated with an acute inflammatory response in the carotid artery. The cause of this inflammation is unknown but it appears to be self-limiting and usually resolves in 1 to 2 weeks. There is also no evidence that it recurs. The chronic form does recur and can be associated with migraine attacks.

Precipitating Factors. There are no known precipitating factors associated with acute carotidynia. Since chronic carotidynia is associated with a neurovascular mechanism, precipitating factors may be similar to those of migraines.

Diagnostic Considerations. According to the International Headache Classification,[51] carotidynia is diagnosed by either tenderness, swelling, or increased pulsations overlying the carotid artery with no other structural findings to explain the pain. The pain is over the affected side of the neck and may project to the ipsilateral side of the head.

Management. Acute carotidynia is a self-limiting disorder and therefore conservative therapy is all that is indicated. Patient education is helpful especially in explaining the natural course of the disorder. Mild analgesics may be useful in making the patient more comfortable. If the degree of pain warrants more treatment, 30 mg of prednisone given for 2 days and tapered over the next 4 days is usually helpful.[148]

For chronic carotidynia, medications used for migraine are usually the treatment of choice. Since these pains are neurovascular in origin, migraine therapies are the most appropriate method of intervention.

Differential Diagnosis

Primary deep somatic visceral pain expressed as a vascular and neurovascular pain disorders should be distinguished diagnostically from the following conditions:

1. Odontogenous pains
2. Primary musculoskeletal pains, especially myalgia of cervical, occipital, or masticatory origin, and temporomandibular arthralgia
3. Posttraumatic headaches[149]
4. Heterotopic referred pains and secondary hyperalgesias due to other deep somatic pains
5. Heterotopic projected neuropathic pains
6. Heterotopic pains of central origin
7. Psychologic factors in Axis II

References

1. Wolff HG. Headache and Other Head Pain. New York: Oxford University Press; 1947.

2. Olesen J, Tfelt-Hansen P, Henricksen L, Larsen B. The common migraine attack may not be initiated by cerebral ischaemia. Lancet 1981; 2:438-440.

3. Rasmussen BK, Jensen R, Schroll M, Olesen J. Epidemiology of headache in a general population - A prevalence study. J Clin Epidemiol 1991; 44:1147-1157

4. Walters WE, Silberstein SD, Dalessio DJ. Inheritance and Epidemiology of Headache. In Dalessio DJ, Silberstein SD (eds): Wolff's Headache and Other Head Pain, ed 6. New York: Oxford University Press; 1993: 42-58.

5. Selby G, Lance JW. Obsevations on 500 cases of migraine and allied vascular headache. J Neurol Neurosurg Psychiatry 1960; 23:23-32.

6. Ely FA. The migraine-epilepsy syndrome. Arch Neurol Psychiatry 1930; 24:943-949.

7. Lance JW, Anthony M. Some clinical aspects of migraine. A prospective survey of 500 patients. Arch Neurol 1966; 15:356-361.

8. Dalsgaard-Nielsen T. Migraine and heredity. Acta Neurol Scand 1965; 41:287-300.

9. Ziegler DK. Genetics of migraine. In Rose FC (ed): Handbook of Clinical Neurology, vol 48. Amsterdam: Elsevier Science Publishers; 1986: 23-30.

10. Headache Classification Committee of the International Headache Society. Classification and diagnosis criteria for headache disorders, cranial neuralgia, and facial pain. Cephalalgia 1988 8(suppl 7): 1-96.

11. Selby G, Lance JW. Observations on 500 cases of migraine and allied vascular headache. J Neurol Neurosurg Psychiatry 1960; 23:23-32.

12. Silberstein SD, Saper JR. Migraine: Diagnosis and treatment. In Dalessio DJ, Silberstein SD (eds): Wolff's Headache and Other Head Pain ed 6. New York: Oxford University Press; 1993: 96-170.

13. Blau JN. Migraine prodromes separated from the aura: Complete migraine. Br Med J 1980; 281:658-660.

14. Drummond PD. A quantitative assessment of photophobia in migraine and tension headache. Headache 1986; 26:465-469.

15. Kuritzky A, Ziegler KE, Hassanein R. Vertigo, motion sickness and migraine. Headache 1981; 21:227-231.

16. Olesen JA. Some clinical features of the acute migraine attack. An analysis of 750 patients. Headache 1978;18:268-271.

17. Raskin NH. Headache, ed 2. New York: Churchill Livingstone; 1988.

18. Blau JN. Resolution of migraine attacks: Sleep and the recovery phase. J Neurosurg Psychiatry 1982; 47:223-226.

19. Coffey RJ, Rhoton AL. Pain-sensitive cranial structures. In Dalessio DJ, Silberstein SD (eds): Wolff's Headache and Other Head Pain ed 6. New York: Oxford University Press; 1993: 19-41.

20. Ferrari MD. Systemic biochemistry. In: Olesen J, Tfelt-Hansen P, Welch KM (eds). The Headaches. New York: Raven Press; 1993: 179-183.

21. Dvilansky A, Rishpon S, Nathan I, et al. Release of platelet 5-hydroxytryptamine by plasma taken from patients during and between migraine attacks. Pain 1976; 2:315-318.

22. Anthony M, Hinterberger H, Lance JW. Plasma serotonin in migraine and stress. Arch Neurol 1967; 16:544-552.

23. Anthony M, Hinterberger H, Lance JW. Plasma serotonin in migraine and stress. Arch Neurol 1967; 16:544-552.

24. Moss RA, Lombardo TW, Cooley JE, et al. Effects of sleep duration on classic migraine and depression headache pain: Case reports. J Craniomand Pract 1987; 5:88-94.

25. Govitrapong P, Limthavon C, Srikiatkhachorn A. 5-HT$_2$ serotonin receptor on blood platelet of migraine patients. Headache 1992; 32:480-484.

26. Moskowitz MA. Brain mechanisms in vascular headache. Neurol Clin 1990; 8:801-815.

27. Krabbe AA, Olesen J. Headache provocation by continuous intravenous infusion of histamine: Clinical results and receptor mechanisms. Pain 1980; 8:253-259.

28. Clifford T, Lauritzen M, Bakke M, et al. Electromyography of pericranial muscles during treatment of spontaneous common migraine attacks. Pain 1982; 14:137-147.

29. Bakke M, Tfelt-Hansen P, Olesen J, et al. Action of some pericranial muscles during provoked attacks of common migraine. Pain 1982; 14:121-135.

30. Moss RA. Oral behavioral patterns in common migraine. J Craniomand Pract 1987; 5:197-202.

31. Moss RA. A structural imbalance/muscular hyperactivity interactional theory of common migraine pain. J Craniomand Pract 1988; 6:87-89.

32. Lapeer GL. Reduction of the painful sequelae of migraine headache by use of occlusal diagnostic splint: An hypothesis. J Craniomand Pract 1988; 6:83–86.

33. Olesen J. Clinical and pathophysiological observations in migraine and tension-type headache explained by integration of vascular, supraspinal and myofascial inputs. Pain 1991; 46:125–132.

34. Solomon GD. Therapeutic Advances in Migraine. J Clin Pharmacol 1993; 33:200–209.

35. Peroutka S. Developments in 5-hydroxytryptamine receptor pharmacology in migraine. Neurol Clin 1990; 8:829–839.

36. Buzzi MG, Moskowitz, MA. The antimigraine drug, sumitriptan specifically blocks neurogenic plasma extravasation from blood vessels in dura mater. Br J Pharmacol 1990; 99:202–206.

37. Hartman BK, Swanson ME, Raichle et al. Central adrenergic regulation of cerebral microvascular permeability and blood flow, anatomic and physiologic evidence. Adv Exp Med Biol 1980; 131:113–126.

38. Olesen J, Larsen B, Lauritzen M. Focal hyperemia followed by spreading oligemia and impaired activation of rCBF in classical migraine. Ann Neurol 1981; 9:344–352.

39. Friberg L, Olsen TS, Roland PE, Lassen NA. Focal ischaemia caused by instability of cerebrovascular tone during attacks of hemiplegic migraine. A regional cerebral blood flow study. Brain 1987; 110:917–934.

40. Laeo AAP. Spreading depression of activity in the cerebral cortex. J Neurophysiol 1944; 7:359–390.

41. Adams RW, Lambert GA, Lance JW. Stimulation of brain stem nuclei in the cat: Effect on neuronal activity in the primary visual cortex of relevance to cerebral blood flow and migraine. Cephalalgia 1989; 9:107–118.

42. Lance JW. The pathophysiology of migraine. In Dalessio DJ, Silberstein SD (eds): Wolff's Headache and Other Head Pain, ed 6. New York: Oxford University Press; 1993: 59–95.

43. Raskin NH. Chemical headaches. Annu Rev Med 1981; 32:63–71.

44. Schaumberg HH, Buckley CE, Gerstl R, Mashman JH. Monosoduim L-glutamate: Its pharmacology and role in the Chinese restaurant syndrome. Science 1969; 163:826–828.

45. Littlewood JT, Glover V, Davies PTG, et al. Red wine as a cause of migraine. Lancet 1988; 1:558–559.

46. Van den Bergh V, Amery WK, Waelkens J. Trigger factors in migraine: A study conducted by the Belgian migraine society. Headache 1987; 27:191–196.

47. Epstein MT, Hockaday JM, Hockaday TDR. Migraine and reproductive hormones throughout the menstrual cycle. Lancet 1975; 1:543–548.

48. Ratinahirana H, Darbois Y, Bousser MG. Migraine and pregnancy: A prospective study in 703 women after delivery. Neurology 1990; 40:437.

49. Lance JW. Mechanisms and Management of Headache, ed 4. Boston: Butterworth; 1982: 16–21.

50. Saber JR. Headache Disorder: Current Concepts in Treatment Strategies. Litteton, Mass: Wright-PSG; 1983.

51. Olesen J. Classification and Diagnosis Criteria for Headache Disorders, Cranial Neuralgias and Facial Pain. Cephalalgia 1988 (suppl 7);8:81–96.

52. Larsson B, Melin L. Follow-up on behavioral treatment of recurrent headache in adolescents. Headache 1989; 29:249–253.

53. Blanchard EB, Appelbaum KA, Radnitz CL, et al. A placebo-controlled evaluation of abbreviated progressive muscle relaxation and relaxation combined with cognitive therapy in the treatment of tension headache. J Consult Clin Psychol 1990; 58:210–215.

54. Richter IL, McGrath PJ, Humphreys PJ, et al. Cognitive and relaxation treatment of paediatric migraine. Pain 1986; 25:195–203.

55. Andrasik F. Psychological and behavioral aspects of chronic headache. Neurol Clin 1990; 8:961–976.

56. Saddah H. Abortive headache therapy in the office with intravenous dihydroergotamine plus prochlorperazine. Headache 1992; 23: 143–146.

57. Mondell B, Giuliano R. A prospective evaluation of intramuscular dihydroergotamine for the control of acute migraine in the office setting: Preliminary findings. Headache 1992; 32:251–252.

58. Freitag F, Diamond M, Urban G, Diamond S. Subcutaneous dihydroergotamine in the acute treatment of menstrual migraine. Headache 1992; 32:252–253.

59. Mondell B, DiSerio F, Friedman A. Dihydroergotamine nasal spray in the acute treatment of migraine headache. Clin Pharm Ther 1989; 45:161.

60. Cady R, Wendt J, Lirchner J, Sargent J, Rothrock J, Skaggs H. Treatment of acute migraine with subcutanous sumatriptan. JAMA 1991; 265:2831–2835.

61. Goadsby P, Zagami A, Donnan G, et al. Oral sumatriptan in acute migraine. Lancet 1991; 338:782–783.

62. Finnish Sumatriptan Group. A placebo-controlled study of intranasal sumatriptan for the acute treatment of migraine. Eur Neurol 1991; 31:332–338.

63. Peroutka S. 5-Hydroxytryptamine receptor subtypes. Ann Rev Neurosci 1988; 11:45–60.

64. Andersson K, Vinge E. Beta-adrenoceptor blockers and calcium antagonists in the prophylaxis and treatment of migraine. Drugs 1990; 39:355–373.

65. Diamond S, Medina JL. Double blind study of propranolol for migraine prophylaxis. Headache 1976; 16:24–27.

66. Moskowitz MA. Basic mechanisms in vascular headache. Neurol Clin 1990; 8:801–815.

67. Kudrow L. Cluster Headache: Mechanisms and Management. New York: Oxford University Press; 1980: 53–70.

68. Andersson PG. Migraine in patients with cluster headache. Cephalalgia 1985; 5:11–16.

69. Russell D. Cluster headache: severity and temporal profile of attacks and patient activity prior to and during attacks. Cephalalgia 1981; 1:209–219.

70. Manzoni GC, Terzano MG, Bono G, et al. Cluster headache - Clinical findings in 180 patients. Cephalalgia 1983; 3:21–30.

71. Lance JW, Anthony M. Migrainous neuralgia or cluster headache? J Neurol Sci 1971; 13: 401–414.

72. Horton BT, MacLean AR, Craig WM. A new syndrome of vascular headache: Results of treatment with histamine: Preliminary report. Mayo Clin Proc 1939; 14:257–260.

73. Ekbom K, Greitz T. Carotid angiography in cluster headache. Acta Radiol (Stockh) 1970; 10:177–186.

74. Aebelholt-Krabbe A, Henriksen L, Olesen J. Tomographic determination of cerebral blood flow during attacks of cluster headache. Cephalalgia 1984; 4:17–23.

75. Salvesen R, Bogucki A, Wysocka-Bakaowska MM, et al. Cluster headache, pathogenesis: A pupillometric study. Cephalalgia 1987; 7:273–284.

76. Boccuni M, Morace G, Pietrini U, et al. Coexistence of pupillary and heart sympathergic asymmetries in cluster headache. Cephalalgia 1984; 4:9–15.

77. Anthony M, Lance JW. Histaminic and serotonin in cluster headache. Arch Neurol 1971; 25:225–231.

78. Dimitriadou V, Henry P, Brocher B, et al. Cluster headache: Ultrastructural evidence for mast cell degranulation and interaction with nerve fibers in the human temporal artery. Cephalalgia 1990; 10:221–228.

79. Moore-Ede MC, Czeisler CA, Richardson GS. Circadian timekeeping in health and disease. N Engl J Med 1983; 309:469–479.

80. Sadun AA, Schaechter JD, Smith LEH. A retinohypothalamic pathway in man: Light mediation of circadian rhythms. Brain Res 1984; 302:371–377.

81. Raskin NH. Headache, ed 2. New York: Churchhill Livingstone; 1988: 236–240.

82. Turkewitz LJ, Wirth O, Dawson GA, Casaly JS. Cluster headache following head injury: A case report and review of the literature. Headache 1992; 32:504–506.

83. Ekbom K. Nitroglycerine as a provocative agent in cluster headache. Arch Neurol 1968; 19:487–493.

84. Horton BT. Histamine cephalgia. Md State Med J 1961; 10:92–98.

85. Ekbom K. Some observations on pain in cluster headache. Headache 1975; 14:219–225.

86. Atkinson R. Physical fitness and headache. Headache 1977; 17:189–195.

87. Ekbom K, Lindahl J. Effect of induced rise in blood pressure on pain in cluster headache. Acta Neurol Scand 1970; 46:585–600.

88. Kudrow L. Response of cluster headache attacks to oxygen inhalation. Headache 1981; 21:1–4.

89. Fogan L. Treatment of cluster headache. A double-blind comparison of oxygen vs air inhalation. Arch Neurol 1985; 42:362–363.

90. Ekbom K, Krabbe AA, Paalzow G, et al. Optimal routes of administration of ergotamine tartrate in cluster headache patients. A pharmacokinetic study. Cephalalgia 1983; 3:15–20.

91. Speed WG. Ergotamine tartrate inhalation: A new approach to the management of recurrent vascular headaches. Am J Med Sci 1960; 240:327–331.

92. Kittrelle JP, Grouse DS, Seybold ME. Cluster headache: Local anesthetic abortive agents. Arch Neurol 1985; 42:496–498.

93. Kudrow L, McGinty DJ, Phillips ER, Stevenson M. Sleep apnea in cluster headache. Proceedings of the 12th Scandinavian Migraine Society Meeting, Helsinki, June 17-18, 1984.

94. Kudrow L. Comparative results of prednisone, methysergide, and lithium therapy in cluster headache. In Greene R (ed): Current Concepts in Migraine Research. New York: Raven Press; 1978: 159–163.

95. Raskin NH. Headache, ed 2. New York: Churchill Livingstone; 1988: 255–268.

96. Sjaastad O, Dale I. Evidence for a new (?) clinical headache entity "chronic paroxysmal hemicrania." Acta Neurol Scand 1976; 54:140–149.

97. Russel D. Chronic paroxysmal hemicrania: Severity, duration and time of occurrence of attacks. Cephalalgia 1984; 4:53–56.

98. Horven I, Sjaastad O. Cluster headache syndrome and migraine, Ophthalmological support for a two-entity theory. Acta Ophthalmol 1977; 55:35–50.

99. Horven I, Russel D, Sjaastad O. Ocular blood flow changes in cluster headache and chronic paroxysmal hemicrania. Headache 1989; 29:373–376.

100. Sjaastad O. Chronic paroxysmal hemicrania. In Vinken PJ, Bruyn GW, Klawans HI (eds): Handbook of Clinical Neurology. Netherlands: Elsevier; 1986: 257–266.

101. Sjaastad O. Chronic paroxsymal hemicrania and similar headaches. In Dalessio DJ, Silberstein SD (eds): Wolff's Headache and Other Head Pain, ed 6. New York: Oxford University Press; 1993: 198–202.

102. Sjaastad O, Dale I. Evidence for a new (?) clinical headache entitiy chronic paroxysmal hemicrania. Headache 1974; 14:105–108.

103. Delcanho RE, Graff-Radford SB. Chronic paroxysmal hemicrania presenting as toothache. J Orofacial Pain 1993; 7:300–306.

104. McArdle MJ. Atypical facial neuralgia. In Hassler R, Walker AE (eds): Trigeminal Neuralgia. Stuttgart: Georg Thieme Verlag; 1970: 35–42.

105. Campbell JK. Cluster headache. J Craniomandib Disord Facial Oral Pain 1987; 1:27–33.

106. Rasmussen BK, Jensen R, Olesen J. A population-based analysis of the criteria of the International Headache Society. Cephalalgia 1991; 11:129–134.

107. Iversen HK, Langemark M, Andersson PG, Hansen PE, Olesen J. Clinical characteristics of migraine and tension-type headache in relation to new and old diagnostic criteria. Headache 1990; 30:514–519.

108. Rassmussen BK, Jensen R, Schroll M, Olesen J. Epidemiology of headache in a general population–a prevalence study. J Clin Epidemiol 1991; 44:1147–1157.

109. Friedman AP, Von Storch TJC, Merritt HH. Migraine and tension headaches, A Clinical study: 2000 cases. Neurology 1954; 4:773–788.

110. Pikoff H. Is the muscular model of headache viable? A review of conflicting data. Headache 1984; 24:186–198.

111. Feuerstien M, Bush C, Corpisiero P. Stress and chronic headache: A psychophysiological analysis of mechanisms. J Psychosom Res 1982; 26:176–182.

112. Schoenen J, Gerard P, De Pasqua V, Juprelle M. EMG activity in pericranial muscles during postural variation and mental activity in healthy volunteers and patients with chronic tension-type headaches. Headache 1991; 31:321–324.

113. Schoenen J. Neurophysiology: Tension-type headache, cluster headache and miscellaneous headaches. In Olesen J, Tfelt-Hansen P, Welch KMA (eds): The Headache. New York: Raven Press; 1993: 463–470.

114. Blanchard EB, Kirsch CA, Appelbaum KA, Jaccard J. The role of psychopathology in chronic headache: Cause and effect. Headache 1989; 29:295–301.

115. Schulman B. Psychiatric management of the headache patient. In Diamond S, Dalessio DJ (eds): The Practicing Physician's Approach to Headache, ed 5. Baltimore: Williams & Wilkins; 1992: 217–223.

116. Olesen J, Schoenen J. Synthesis, tension-type headache, cluster headache and miscellaneous headaches. In Olesen J, Tfelt-Hansen P, Welch KMA (eds): The Headache. New York: Raven Press; 1993: 493–496.

117. Bovim G. Cervicogenic headache, migraine, and tension-type headache. Pressure-pain threshold measurements. Pain 1992; 51:169–173.

118. Andrasik F, Passchier J. Psychological aspects, tension type-headache, cluster headache and miscellaneous headaches. In Olesen J, Tfelt-Hansen P, Welch KMA (eds): The Headache. New York: Raven Press; 1993: 489–492.

119. Jensen R, Paiva T. Episodic tension-type headache. In Olesen J, Tfelt-Hansen P, Welch KMA (eds). The Headache. New York: Raven Press; 1993: 497–502.

120. Blau JN. Sleep deprivation headache. Cephalalgia 1990; 10:157–160.

121. Sahots PK, Dexter JD: Sleep and the headache syndromes: A clinical review. Headache 1990; 30:80–84.

122. Rasmussen BK. Migraine and tension-type headache in a general population: Precipitating factors, female hormones, sleep pattern and relation of lifestyle. Pain 1993; 53:65–72.

123. Solomon S, Lipton RB, Newman LC. Clinical features of chronic daily headache. Headache 1992; 23:325–329.

124. Baumgartner CP, Wessely P, Bingol C, Maly J, Holzner F. Long term prognosis of analgesic withdrawal in patients with drug induced headaches. Headache 1989; 29:510–514.

125. Mathew NT, Reuveni U, Perez F. Transformed or evolutive migraine. Headache 1987; 27: 102–106.

126. Diener HC, Tfelt-Hansen P. Headache associated with chronic use of substances. In Olesen J, Tfelt-Hansen P, Welch KMA (eds). The Headache. New York: Raven Press; 1993: 721–727.

127. Jensen R, Olesen J. Oromandibular dysfunction, tension type-headache, cluster headache and miscellaneous headaches. In Olesen J, Tfelt-Hansen P, Welch KMA (eds): The Headache. New York: Raven Press; 1993: 479–482.

128. Forssell H, Kangasniemi P. Mandibular dysfunction in patients with muscle contraction headache. Proc Finnish Dent Soc 1984; 80: 211–216.

129. Gelb H, Tarte J. A two year clinical dental evaluation of 200 cases of chronic headache: The craniocervical-mandibular syndrome. J Am Dent Assoc 1975; 91:1230–1236.

130. Heloe B, Heloe LA, Heiberg A. Relationship between sociomedical factors and TMJ symptoms in Norwegians with myofascial pain-dysfunction syndrome. Commun Dent Oral Epidemiol 1977; 5:207–212.

131. Jensen R, Rasmussen BK, Pedersen B, Olsen J. Muscle tenderness and pressure pain thresholds in headache. A population study. Pain 1993; 52:193–199.

132. Magnusson T, Enbom L. Signs and symptoms of mandibular dysfunction after introduction of experimental balancing side interferences. Acta Odontol Scand 1984; 42:129–135.

133. Andrasik F, Gerber WD. Relation, biofeedbak and stress-coping therapies. In Olesen J, Tfelt-Hansen P, Welch KMA (eds): The Headache. New York: Raven Press; 1993: 833–842.

134. Okeson JP. Management of Temporomandibular Disorders and Occlusion, ed 3. St Louis: Mosby Year Book; 1993: 381–400.

135. Bengtsson BA, Malmvall BE. Gaint cell arteritis. Acta Medica Scand 1982; 658:1–102.

136. Liang GC, Simlin PA, Hunder CC, et al. Familiar aggregation of polymyalgia rheumatica and giant cell arteritis. Arthritis Rheum 1974; 17:19–24.

137. Scheitler LE, Balciunas BA. Carotidynia. J Oral Maxillofac Surg 1982; 40:121–122.

138. Solomon S, Cappa KG. The headache of temporal arteritis. J Am Geriatr Soc 1987; 35:163–165.

139. Dalessio D. Evaluation of the patient with chronic facial pain. Am Fam Physician 1977; 16;84–92.

140. Dalessio DJ, Williams GW. Giant cell arteritis and polymyalgia. In Dalessio DJ, Silberstein SD (eds): Wolff's Headache and Other Head Pain, ed 6. New York: Oxford University Press; 1993: 262–275.

141. Powers W, Britton BH. Nonotogenic otalgia: Diagnosis and treatment. Am J Otol 1980; 2:97–104.

142. Acetta D, Kelly J, Tubbs R. An elderly black woman with a painful swollen face. Ann Allergy 1985; 55:819–823.

143. Wall M, Corbett JJ. Arteritis. In Olesen J, Tfelt-Hansen P, Welch KMA (eds): The Headache. New York: Raven Press; 1993: 653–662.

144. Murray TJ. Carotidynia: A cause of neck and face pain. Can Med Assoc J 1979; 120:441–443.

145. Roseman DM. Carotidynia. A distinct syndrome. Arch Otolaryngol 1967; 85:81–84.

146. Lovshin L. Carotidynia. Headache 1977; 17: 192–195.

147. Troiano MF, Gaston GW. Carotid system arteritis: An overlooked and misdiagnosed syndrome. J Am Dent Assoc 1975; 91:589.

148. Bank H. Idiopathic carotiditis. Lancet 1978; 1:726.

149. Campbell JK. Posttraumatic headaches. J Craniomandib Disord Facial Oral Pain 1987; 1:75–77.

17 Neuropathic Pains

Neuropathic pain is due to an abnormality in components of the nervous system itself rather than to noxious stimulation of otherwise normal neural structures as with superficial and deep somatic pain disorders. The cause of neuropathic pain lies within the nerves, and its clinical significance relates to such abnormality. Whereas somatic pains are predominantly a warning system that noxious stimulation is present, neuropathic pain is symptomatic of a structural abnormality in the peripheral or central nervous system.

Behavior of Neuropathic Pains

Neuropathic pains can be divided into two broad categories according to their clinical characteristics: those that are episodic and those that are continuous. These categories are diagnostically helpful and will therefore be used in this text. *Episodic neuropathic pains* are pains of neurogenous source that have periods of complete remission between the episodes. The episodes may be frequent or separated by long periods. Episodic neuropathic pains are normally triggered by some event or stimulus. There are two categories of episodic neuropathic pains: neurovascular pains and neuralgic pains. Neurovascular pains have been discussed in the previous chapter. They are considered in this chapter because their etiology is tied to a neurovascular mechanism that triggers the cascade of events already presented in Chapter 16. They will not be discussed further in this chapter.

The second type of episodic neuropathic pain is that associated with a neuralgia. *Neuralgic pain* is characterized by sudden volleys of electrical-like pain. This paroxsymal pain is quite characteristic of the neuralgias, assisting greatly in diagnosis.

Continuous neuropathic pains present with periods of high and low intensity but no periods of total remission. They may be felt as dull aching or sharp and burning. They are often provocated or aggravated by relatively normal sensory stimuli. These clinical characteristics make it difficult to differentiate them from other pain conditions. The key identifying factor is the lack of any somatic source for the pain. Continuous neuropathic pains are divided into three categories: neuritis pains, deafferentation pains, and sympathetically maintained pains. Each type of neuropathic pain will now be discussed.

Episodic Neuropathic Pains

Paroxsymal Neuralgia

Clinical Characteristics. Paroxysmal neuralgia (Fig 17-1) is characterized by sudden bursts of electric-like pain that projects heterotopically along the course of a nerve. The pains are bright and stimulating. They are usually described as burning, hot, or shocking and can be accurately located by the patient. There is typically a peripheral site on the face that when lightly touched, triggers the paroxsymal pain. The relationship between the initiating stimulus or trigger and location of the pain is anatomically accurate. The relationship between the initiating stimulus and intensity of the pain, however, is inaccurate in that the pains are extremely intense compared with the degree of stimulation. In fact, the pains occur spontaneously from the normal stimulation induced by ordinary functioning, and frequently the patient will refrain from actions that excite the pains. Such activities as eating, talking, washing the face, and shaving may become too painful to bear. The impulses from surface stimulation or movement received by the sensory receptors of the nerve are painless until they summate to the threshold level, then they burst through as excruciating pain. There may be delays of up to half a minute between stimulation and pain response. Frequently after a period of severe pain, there may be an interval during which pain cannot be induced, a so-called refractory period.

There are no central excitatory effects, no referred pains or secondary hyperalgesias, no autonomic effects, and no secondary muscle effects. There are usually no sensory changes or muscle effects other than the hard contractions induced by the paroxysms of pain and some residual muscular soreness incidental to such contractions. Both the pain and the triggering are promptly arrested by analgesic blocking of the sensory pathways that conduct impulses from the peripheral receptors of the affected nerve. If such impulses arise in the oral mucosa, application of a topical anesthetic at that site likewise may arrest the pain and triggering.[1]

Most neuralgias occur after the age of 50. The typical pains last only seconds, but on occasion they may last up to 20 or 30 seconds. The pains are unilateral and felt in the precise distribution of the involved nerve. They present as rapidly repeated volleys or jabs separated by pain-free intermissions. This feature is characteristic; however, not all neuralgias present with a completely pain-free intermittent behavior. In addition to the paroxysms, some patients with true neuralgia may have a mild, steady, background aching sensation that usually is bearable.[2]

In summary, paroxysmal neuralgias are characterized by the following features[3]: severe paroxysmal pain; unilateral location; and initiation of the pain by minor superficial stimulation in the peripheral distribution of sensory fibers of the same nerve that is affected.

Types of Cranial Neuralgias. Although the clinical characteristics of most cranial neuralgias are similar, the location is dependent on the nerve that is affected. This section will review the unique features and locations of the following cranial neuraglias: trigeminal neuralgia, glossopharyngeal neuralgia, geniculate neuralgia, superior laryngeal neuralgia, and occipital neuralgia.

Trigeminal neuralgia,[4-9] sometimes called

Fig 17-1 Pain classification chart highlighted to show the relationship of paroxysmal neuralgia pains to other orofacial pain disorders.

tic douloureux, has been known for centuries and is one of the most painful afflictions of humanity. Only recently has it been identified as a true neuropathy. It occurs predominantly during middle and old age, the incidence increasing with age. It occurs more frequently in women. A single nerve branch may be affected without involving other branches, the entire division, or other divisions of the nerve. The pains and triggering occur in the receptor area of the affected nerve so precisely that analgesic blocking to interrupt the passage of impulses from the superficial peripheral receptors accurately arrests both pain and triggering. This effect is diagnostic. Yet the peripheral receptors are not hyperalgesic. The stimulus for pain is the normal sensation induced by surface stimulation due to such factors as movement, contact, and thermal change, which gives the paroxysms a spontaneous character. Triggering may occur from a light touch or movement of the same receptor areas.

The pain usually is unilateral and remains in the anatomic distribution of the affected nerve regardless of intermissions or remissions. Sometimes it may slowly spread to involve more extensive portions of the nerve, even sometimes affecting all divisions of the nerve simultaneously. There have been reports of pain occurring bilaterally but not at the same time. Rapid-spreading, bilateral involvement or simultaneous involvement with other nerve trunks should suggest a systemic involvement such as multiple sclerosis or expanding cranial tumor (to be discussed under pathophysiologic features). Examples of simultaneous involvement with other major nerve trunks are *tic convulsif,*[9] which afflicts both the fifth and seventh cranial nerves, and occurrence of symptoms in

both the trigeminal and glossopharyngeal areas, a condition that is not rare (to be discussed).

Usually, the longer the condition lasts, the more typical it becomes. Sometimes incipient trigeminal neuralgia has rather atypical features and is difficult to diagnose accurately. Occasionally only the auriculotemporal branch may be involved. The pains and triggering are located in the auricle as well as in the temple region. This entity may be confused with geniculate and glossopharyngeal neuralgias (to be discussed). Analgesic blocking clearly differentiates them (Case 22).

Since triggering may relate to facial and tongue movements incidental to chewing and swallowing, trigeminal neuralgia must be differentiated from masticatory pain that has the clinical characteristics of deep somatic rather than neuropathic pain. Masticatory pain is induced by jaw movements, and it may be intense, but true triggering by a light superficial touch and slight movement does not occur. Masticatory pain is not arrested by a conventional mandibular local anesthetic block because the nerves mediating the pain from the joint or the masticatory muscles are not anesthetized (Case 23).

Neuropathies such as trigeminal neuralgia can cause tooth pains of nondental origin that at times may be difficult to identify properly. In the past it has not been unusual to examine a patient with obvious trigeminal neuralgia who had lost some or all the teeth to the midline on the side of pain. Such cases bear witness that true neuralgia of the maxillary or mandibular divisions of the trigeminal nerve causes pain that may be felt as a toothache of sufficient intensity to induce the patient to demand removal of

Case 22   Paroxysmal neuralgia of the auriculotemporal nerve

Chief Complaint

Sharp burning pain in the left temple.

History

A 75-year-old woman with recurrent episodes of mild to severe continuous protracted steady bright burning pain localized in the left auricular, periauricular,
and temporal areas, aggravated by jaw movements as well as by superficial
touch and movement of the painful structures. Exacerbations are nearly paroxysmal.

The complaint has been recurrent for several years in irregular episodes of several weeks or months separated by pain-free remissions of several months' duration. The discomfort is of low intensity except when stimulated by opening, chewing, or touching the left ear, periauricular structures, and temple. Such stimulation
causes a sudden volley of paroxysmal pain. She has been treated with vitamins,
B-12, iron, and liver extract. She has been cleared medically for sinusitis, allergies, nutritional deficiency, anemia, and diabetes. Her complaint was presumed
to be of masticatory origin. Her dentist has adjusted the occlusion, altered her
partial dentures, and extracted several teeth without benefit. He referred the patient for a TMD examination. The present episode began 6 months ago.

Examination

Intraoral: There is no dental or oral cause for the complaint. The masticatory
system functions normally and no pain results from any mandibular movement except when the speed and amplitude causes movement of the temporal and auricular structures.

TM Joints: Both joints are structurally and functionally normal.

Muscles: There is no palpable tenderness in any masticatory muscle and no
muscular dysfunction of any kind.

Cervical: Within normal limits.

Cranial Nerves: Present of mild hyperesthesia, especially following an
episode of pain. All other functions are normal.

Diagnostic Tests: Intraoral analgesic blocking of the left inferior alveolar nerve
did not affect the pain. Blocking of the left auriculotemporal nerve where it
crosses the zygomatic arch anterior to the tragus promptly and completely arrested all pain and triggering for the duration of anesthesia.

Impression

There is no dental, oral, or masticatory cause for the pain complaint. The history,
clinical course, behavioral characteristics, and effect of analgesic blocking are indicative of neural pain involving the auriculotemporal branches of the left trigeminal nerve. The complaint probably should be classified clinically as an atypical
trigeminal neuralgia.

Diagnosis

Auriculotemporal paroxsymal neuralgia mistaken for masticatory pain.

Case 23	Paroxysmal neuralgia of the maxillary branch of the trigeminal nerve

Chief Complaint

Severe left face pain.

History

A 63-year-old woman with recurrent episodes of frequent intermittent short paroxysms of severe bright burning pain located in the left face, upper lip, nose, and lower eyelid, occurring both spontaneously and triggered by light touch to the upper lip and nose and by movement of the face and jaw, especially opening widely, chewing food, and touching the palate with the tongue.

The complaint began about 2 years ago. It was diagnosed as a left TM joint pain and treated by injections with corticosteroids. During the pain-free remissions, it was thought that the injections had been beneficial. The present episode began about 2 months ago and has continued despite joint therapy. Another dentist has given her muscle relaxants without benefit. Her physician thought the complaint consisted largely of "nerves" and prescribed phenothiazine therapy. Since the complaint has persisted, she was referred for a TMD examination.

Examination

Intraoral: The mouth is completely edentulous and patient is wearing artificial dentures that appear to be satisfactory. There is no hyperemia or palpable tenderness. Masticatory function is entirely normal in all respects. The severe face pain is triggered by light touch, face and lip movement, and extended mandibular movements. Episodes are accompanied by contraction of the facial muscles The pain continues even though the mandible is stabilized by biting against a bite block.

TM Joints: Both joints are structurally and functionally normal.

Muscles: There is no palpable tenderness in any masticatory muscle and no muscular dysfunction.

Cervical: Within normal limits.

Cranial Nerves: Within normal limits.

Diagnostic Tests: Analgesic blocking of the left infraorbital and anterior palatine nerves promptly and completely arrested both the pain and the triggering for the duration of anesthesia.

Impression

By the history, clinical course, behavioral characteristics, and effect of analgesic blocking, it is concluded that no masticatory pain is present. Rather, the complaint is that of neuropathic origin, likely trigeminal neuralgia of the maxillary division of the left trigeminal nerve.

Diagnosis

Trigeminal neuralgia (tic douloureux) mistaken for masticatory pain.

the painful tooth (Case 24). Unfortunately, the following characteristics of true neuralgia contribute to this situation:

1. Stimulation of a tooth by percussion or other means may trigger the neuralgia paroxysm, or a spontaneous paroxysm may be felt in the tooth. This is because the teeth are part of the sensory receptor system of the affected nerve trunk.
2. The pain is immediately and completely arrested by analgesic blocking of the tooth that hurts, which leads the dentist and patient to believe that the proper offending tooth has been identified.
3. Extraction of the tooth, or for that matter any surgery or even the analgesic block itself, may interrupt the neuralgic paroxysms for days or weeks, thereby convincing both patient and dentist that the offending cause has been found and removed.

These characteristics of the usual behavior of neuralgia should be well known to the dentist so that he or she may guard against being deceived by them and be able to convince the patient that such dental treatment is unnecessary and futile.

Glossopharyngeal neuralgia or ninth cranial nerve neuralgia[1,3,6,10–12] is characterized by severe pain in the region of the tonsil and ear. It has similar clinical features as those of trigeminal neuralgia but the pain is initiated by yawning and swallowing or contact of food with the tonsillar region. Since the pain relates to jaw use, it may easily be confused with pain emanating from the temporomandibular joint or masticatory muscles (Case 25). Patients suffering with glossopharyngeal neuralgia will often refrain from any food or drink, which compromises their health quickly. The pain of glossopharyngeal neuralgia can be provoked by touching the lateral aspect of the throat. A second episode cannot be immediately provoked because of the refractory period associated with paroxysmal neuralgias.

Glossopharyngeal neuralgia can occur in conjunction with trigeminal neuralgia. Unless they are separate entities, a neurologic search should be made to determine whether a common lesion is responsible.

Sometimes the pain is felt deeply in the ear only, and when this occurs, it is usually designated as *tympanic plexus neuralgia.* The ear pain may be excruciating. Such neuralgia may be indistinguishable from geniculate neuralgia when that disorder occurs only in the ear. Precise differentiation may at times require surgical exposure of these nerves under local anesthesia and direct stimulation to determine which nerve is involved.[3,12]

Glossopharyngeal neuralgia may be accompanied by vagal symptoms, and the examiner should be watchful for such signs. Syncope, arrhythmia, and even cardiac arrest may accompany the paroxysms of glossopharyngeal neuralgia.[12]

Clinical differentiation of glossopharyngeal neuralgia from masticatory pain may be made by the following criteria:

1. Masticatory pain has the clinical features of deep somatic pain, whereas the neuralgia is neuropathic.
2. Masticatory pain is arrested or decreased by immobilization of the mandible with a bite block. This does not prevent triggering of neuralgia by tongue movement and swallowing.
3. Masticatory pain is not arrested by application of a topical anesthetic to the pharyngeal mucosa.

| Case 24 | Paroxysmal neuralgia of the mandibular branch of the trigeminal nerve |

Chief Complaint

Severe left mandibular toothache.

History

A 65-year-old woman with severe intermittent momentary paroxysms of bright burning pain localized to the left mandibular teeth, jaw, tongue, and lower lip. The paroxysms sometimes occur so frequently as to cause nearly continuous pain for up to 5 minutes. It is spontaneous and triggered by light touch and movement of the lower lip, sometimes also the tongue. The pains are accompanied by muscular contractions of the face that leave minor discomfort between attacks. Otherwise, the intermissions are entirely pain-free.

The pains began about 3 weeks ago and have increased slightly in frequency and severity. She has on the average about five severe paroxysms daily, none at night. She promptly went to her dentist because of the dental pain but when he was not been able to decide which tooth was responsible for the pain he referred her for a more complete diagnostic evaluation. No medications are presently in use since analgesics seem to do no good.

Examination

Intraoral: There is no clinical or radiographic evidence that the pain originates from the teeth or mouth. All the teeth are asymptomatic and there is no evidence of any occlusal problems. The pain may sometimes be triggered by very light touch or minor movement of the lower lip. Manual palpation, pressure, and gross movement do nothing.

TM Joints: Both joints are clinically within normal limits.

Muscles: There is no palpable tenderness in any masticatory muscle and no discernible muscular dysfunction.

Cervical: Within normal limits.

Cranial Nerves: Although light touch seems to initiate the pain, there is no hyperesthesia, hyperalgesia, or paresthesia.

Diagnostic Tests: Analgesic blocking of the left mandibular nerve promptly and completely arrested all pain and triggering for the duration of anesthesia. Trial therapy with diphenylhydantoin sodium, 110 mg, three times a day, reduced the pain to limits readily controllable with simple analgesics in about 3 days.

Impression

No dental, oral, or masticatory cause is present for the pain complaint. The behavioral characteristics and results of trial therapy are indicative of typical paroxysmal neuralgia of the mandibular division of the left trigeminal nerve.

Diagnosis

Trigeminal neuralgia with referring pain to the teeth and other orofacial structures.

Paroxysmal neuralgia of the glossopharyngeal nerve

Chief Complaint

Severe throat, ear, and tongue pain.

History

A 61-year-old woman with recurrent episodes of mild to severe intermittent short paroxysms of bright burning pain located in the right ear, postmandibular area, throat, and tongue, occurring both spontaneously and triggered by jaw movements, talking, and swallowing.

The complaint began 5 years ago as sharp pains in the right ear, throat, and tongue induced by jaw use. Her ENT physician found no aural cause and thought it was neuralgia. Her neurologist thought the pain was TMJ arthralgia. So her dentist remade her dentures to "correct the bite." Soon a pain-free remission occurred and lasted 3 years with only minor breakthrough. Two years ago, it recurred as before. The neurologist treated with B-12, nicotinamide, alcohol injection of the right mandibular nerve, corticosteroids, and various injections. An oral surgeon was than consulted. He did several TM joint injections, used ethyl chloride spray, physical therapy, and finally did a right condylectomy. After 3 months another remission of 7 months occurred after which the present episode began. Another oral surgeon again blocked the right mandibular nerve with alcohol, then referred her for TMD exam.

Examination

Intraoral: The mouth has been edentulous for 8 years with satisfactory dentures. There is no oral cause for the pain. She has right TMJ hypomobility and localized tenderness due presumably to the surgery. This is not her chief complaint. There is mandibular anesthesia from the alcohol blocks. All other functions are normal.

TM Joints: Radiographically, a surgical defect in the right condyle is seen and there is condylar fixation due presumably to cicatrization. Left is normal. There is palpable tenderness over the right condyle.

Muscles: There is palpable tenderness over the masseter muscle presumably secondary to the arthralgia.

Diagnostic Test: Neurologic consultation was requested to differentiate between very likely paroxsmal neuralgia and TM arthralgia which was presumed to reflect only the surgical interference, numerous injections, and cicatrization. His diagnosis based chiefly on cocainization of the throat was glossopharyngeal neuralgia. Complete relief followed 9th nerve rhizotomy.

Impression

No doubt the recurrent glossopharyngeal neuralgia was the chief complaint during the five years. Unfortunately, triggering from jaw movements misled all concerned and was diagnosed repeatedly as masticatory pain. Only the failure of TM therapy was neuropathic pain considered. Then it was diagnosed as trigeminal instead of glossopharyngeal.

Diagnosis

Glossopharyngeal neuralgia mistaken for masticatory pain.

Glossopharyngeal neuralgia has pain characteristics similar to those of trigeminal neuralgia, but the location of the initiating stimulus for both spontaneous and triggered pain is different. This distinction can be made by immobilizing the mandible and face by having the patient bite on a bite block, which minimizes stimulation of the trigeminal structures, and by noting whether pain still occurs from tongue movement and swallowing. A more positive means of distinguishing between the two neuralgias is by application of a topical anesthetic to the pharyngeal mucosa. This arrests glossopharyngeal neuralgia triggering but does not affect that of trigeminal neuralgia.

Nervus Intermedius Neuralgia. The sensory component of the facial nerve that innervates the external auditory meatus, parts of the pinna of the ear, and a small zone of skin beneath and behind the lobe of the ear is called the nerve intermedius. When a paroxysmal neuralgia affects this nerve it is called nervus intermedius neuralgia.[1,3,6,7,12] This condition is also referred to a *geniculate or VII nerve neuralgia.* The pain is felt in the tympanic membrane, walls of the auditory canal, the external auditory meatus, and the external structures of the ear. On occasions the pain may be felt in the palate, tongue, and even deep in the facial musculature. When the triggering is caused by touching the ear, topical anesthesia of the external auditory canal may arrest it.

In the neuralgic process, one part of the afferent distribution may be involved without implication of the whole nerve, and the site of pain varies accordingly. Since fibers of the facial nerve innervate the anterior two-thirds of the tongue and part of the soft palate, the actual propensity for numerous sites of pain and triggering is great indeed.

The pains, although typically those of neuralgia, are not especially dramatic, and the diagnosis may not be evident. Neurosurgical exposure of the cerebellopontine angle under local anesthesia allows the accurate identification of the affected nerve prior to sectioning. The nervus intermedius can be isolated so that no facial paralysis results from rhizotomy to control nervus intermedius neuralgia.

Nervus intermedius neuralgia may sometimes be clinically confused with a migraine variant. The following conditions may be helpful in differentiate these conditions:

1. Neurovascular pain has deep somatic-category characteristics, usually with a component of throbbing. The pain distribution often follows the vascular arborization. Neuralgia is neuropathic and has a precise though widespread distribution that makes anatomic sense to a knowledgeable examiner.
2. Neurovascular pain is often accompanied by central excitatory effects not evident with neuralgia.
3. If a surgical approach is contemplated and positive identification of the affected nerve is required, this can be done by a neurosurgical suboccipital exposure under local anesthesia for direct stimulation of the nervus intermedius.[3,12]

This condition may be associated with a herpes zoster infection of the geniculate ganglion, which will be reviewed under the category of neuritis.

Superior Laryngeal Neuralgia. The superior laryngeal nerve is a branch of the vagus and innervates the cricothyroid muscle of the larynx, which stretches, tenses, and adducts the vocal cord. Paralysis of this nerve causes hoarseness and fatigued voice, with altered pitch. The clinical characteristics of superior laryngeal neuralgia are periodic, unilateral submandibular pain radiating through the ear, eye, or shoulder. It is sometimes difficult to differentiate this condition from glossopharyngeal neuralgia. The pain is paroxsymal, lasting momentarily, and may be provoked by swallowing, straining the voice, turning the head, coughing, sneezing, yawing, or blowing the nose. The patient may report an irresistible urge to swallow. A trigger is frequently present just superior and lateral to the thyroid cartilage.[13]

Occipital Neuralgia. The greater occipital nerve is a continuation of the dorsal ramus of the second cervical nerve. It moves superiorly between the sternocleidomastoid and trapezius muscles to innervate the posterior scalp. Compression of this nerve induces paresthesiae or dysesthesiae in the back of the head. True occipital neuralgia is rare but, when it is present, the paroxsymal pains are felt in the posterior occipital region radiating up the back of the head. The pain may also be felt in the cervical region.

Most pain and tenderness felt in the posterior occipital region is not neuralgic pain but instead musculoskeletal. Many of these conditions are secondary to trauma such as a cervical strain. When evaluating the cervical region, the clinician needs to be constantly aware of the difference in clinical characteristics of neuropathic pains and musculoskeletal pains.

Pathophysiologic Features of Neuralgic Pain

Until recently, the mechanism of neuralgic pain was not known. Kerr and Miller[14,15] have shown that significant pathologic change occurs in the myelin sheath of fibers in the ganglion, dorsal root, or both. This change, recognizable by both light and electron microscopy, consists of disintegration of the myelin sheath-demyelination. There is some evidence that demyelination results from a progressive degenerative process.[4] Demyelination affects the fibers in such a way as to permit ephaptic exchange of neural signals at the site of neuropathy.

There are likely to be several reasons for demyelination of the nerve fiber. One reason seems to be associated with a structural abnormality whereby an adjacent structure applies constant force to the nerve root. In the case of trigeminal neuralgia, the nerve root can be affected in the posterior fossa as it exits the pons before reaching the gasserian ganglion. One source of such compression is an aberrant loop of the superior cerebellar artery that lie on the nerve root and produces a significant microvascular compression.[10,16,17] This compression is thought to cause the demyelination of the nerve.

Other sources of compression that need to be considered are space occupying lesions in this region of the brain, the most frequent of which is a cerebellopontine angle tumor.[18] Posterior fossa tumors or basilar artery aneurysms are also possible sources as well as a meningioma of Meckel's cavity or an epidermoid cyst. It is established that malignant tumors that initiate pain are extramedullary.[3,9] Destructive lesions of the nerve located within the brain tissue from the entrance of the trigeminal nerve into the pons throughout the numerous sensory circuits to the cortex do not cause neuralgia.[19]

Nerve fiber demyelination of the trigeminal nerve may result from a systemic condition such as multiple sclerosis.[3,5,6,9,20] Approximately 1 of every 100 patients with multiple sclerosis suffers from trigeminal neuralgia. Multiple sclerosis may present with pain as the initial symptom that, once established, may continue throughout the course of the disease. Occasionally the pain may be paroxysmal trigeminal pain associated with trigeminal neuralgia. At autopsy, sclerotic plaques have been found at the root entrance zone of the trigeminal nerve when trigeminal neuralgia had been present. Such plaques in the descending root and sensory nucleus have been observed without associated paroxysmal pains.

When trigeminal neuralgia occurs in a patient with known multiple sclerosis, several features can help determine the etiology. If it is the initiating symptom, the patient's age may be important since multiple sclerosis is most likely to develop between the ages of 20 and 40. Neuralgia from this cause may be bilateral, which is rare with other causes of trigeminal neuralgia.

In a recent paper, Rappaport and Devor[21] proposed a hypothesis for the mechanism of trigeminal neuralgia, and for that matter any neuralgia. They suggested that the compression and demyelination of the nerve root causes ectopic firing of a focal group of trigeminal ganglion neurons. This causes this same cluster of neurons to become hyperexcitable. When this activity is supplemented by activity evoked from a peripheral trigger, especially light touch, the aggregate focus activity produces a chain reaction spread of activity to passive neighboring cells in the ganglion. After a brief period of autonomous firing, activity is quenched and a refractory period is initiated by an intrinsic suppressive (hyperpolarizing) process engaged as a result of the rapid firing. Since

the primary abnormality resides in the trigeminal ganglion and nerve root, normal sensation is present in the periphery between periods of ectopic paroxysmal discharges.

The International Headache Society[22] has classified neuralgias into two categories according to etiology. Neuralgias associated with compression of the nerve root or systemic cause, such as multiple scerlosis, are considered *symptomatic neuralgias*. Neuralgias of unknown cause are called *idiopathic neuralgias*.

Precipitating Factors. As discussed, precipitating factors of neuralgic pains are often a relatively innocuous peripheral stimulation. A light touch to the face or facial movement associated with smiling or swallowing may be enough to evoke the pain. The location of the trigger shows no evidence of tissue abnormality, which is diagnostic of the disorder. The patient will go to great effort not to stimulate the trigger area. Local and sometimes topical anesthetic in the location of the trigger area will temporarily stop the pain episodes.

Diagnostic Considerations

Considerations for Symptomatic Neuralgias. About 2% of the paroxysmal neuralgias of the orofacial region result from pathologic lesions. Although such symptomatic neuralgias are only rarely encountered, they must be considered in the diagnosis of neuropathic pains around the face and mouth. Symptomatic neuralgias usually present certain clinical features that indicate the presence of some pathologic lesion. When one or more of the following features are observed by the clinician, referral for a neurologic consultation is indicated:

1. Atypical manifestations such as prolonged or nearly continuous paroxysms of pain.
2. Definite bridging of paroxysms with a more continuous aching or burning pain
3. Bilateral neuralgic pains
4. Neuralgic involvement of two or more cranial nerves simultaneously
5. Neuralgia accompanied by other sensory manifestations such as hypoesthesia, paresthesia, dysesthesia, or anesthesia
6. Neuralgia accompanied by muscular weakness or paralysis or by unusual autonomic signs
7. Rapid or significant change in behavior of the symptom complex
8. Failure of the complaint to respond to reasonable therapy
9. Typical paroxysmal neuralgia in young people

Neuralgia vs Masticatory Pain. Neuropathic pains in the orofacial region that are influenced by jaw movement may be mistaken for masticatory pain. It is necessary that they be clearly differentiated. The examiner can distinguish between paroxysmal neuralgic pains of all types and true masticatory pain by remembering that neuralgia is a precisely localized, bright, stimulating, burning pain occurring in spontaneous or triggered paroxysms induced by normal functioning, light touch, superficial stimulation, or movement, the pain being wholly disproportionate to the stimulus and exhibiting characteristics of temporal and spatial summation. Masticatory pain, in contrast, is a poorly localized, dull, depressing, aching pain, sometimes punctuated by sharper lancinating pain or having a minor burning component. It is more consistently related to functional demands and is not so clearly intermittent or triggered by insignificant stimulation. The pain is more proportional to the stimulus and does not exhibit characteristics of summation. Neuralgia is not accompanied by dysfunction other than muscular contractions with severe paroxysms or the inhibitory influence of fear of the pain. Masticatory pain is usually related to symptoms of masticatory dysfunction and commonly induces secondary referred pains and cyclic muscle pain.

Neuralgia is promptly and completely arrested by interrupting the input from the sensory receptors of the affected nerve. This can be done by analgesic blocking. Mucosal triggering can be arrested by application of a topical anesthetic. Masticatory pain is arrested by analgesic blocking of the source only, which is either the temporomandibular joint or the masticatory muscles. In differentiating glossopharyngeal neuralgia from masticatory pain, both of which are stimulated by mastication, it is well to insert a small bite block between the teeth to restrain movements of the masticatory muscles and joints. With the mandible thus stabilized, if throat stimulation and tongue movements continue to trigger the pain, it is probably of glossopharyngeal origin. Analgesic blocking of the joint, masticatory muscles, or both does not arrest glossopharyngeal pain. Topical anesthesia of the throat does.

The best differentiation between masticatory pain and the paroxysmal neuralgias is by identification of positive evidence of masticatory pain by completing an adequate examination and applying trial palliative therapy to arrive at a confirmed working diagnosis. The International Headache Society has published criteria[22] and a classification number for each neuralgia mentioned in this section. To assist in diagnosis and for consistency between health professions, the classification is listed in Table 17-1.

Management of Paroxsymal Neuralgias. There are several approaches to the management of paroxsymal neuralgias. Since trigeminal neuralgia is the most common neuralgia, it will be highlighted in this section. Similar approaches are indicated for the other neuralgias.

Treatment considerations should begin with knowledge of the etiology. When a systemic condition such as multiple sclerosis is responsible, treatment is directed toward the disease itself. Likewise, if a space-occupying lesion is found in the posterior fossa, it needs to be appropriately managed. The remaining treatments can be divided into two categories: pharmacologic and neurosurgical.

Pharmacologic Management of Paroxsymal Neuralgias. The most effective drug used to treat trigeminal neuralgia is carbamazepine (Tegretol). In fact this drug is so effective that when it is tried and effectively eliminates the symptoms, it confirms the diagnosis of trigeminal neuralgia. Carbamazepine is an anticonvulsant medication that is thought to inhibit or reduce synaptic transmission. It has been shown to depress the post-tetanic potentiation at the spinal cord level in animals and significantly inhibit polysynaptic reflex activity in the spinal cord.[23] Unfortunately this medication does not address the etiology of the neuralgia and therefore may need to be taken long-term. Although it is very effective, long-term use is not without medical complications.

Table 17-1 The International Headache Society's Classfication of Headaches (Category for Neuropathic Pains)

12. Cranial Neuralgias, Nerve Trunk Pain, and Deafferentation Pain
   12.1 Persistent (in contrast to tic-like) pain of cranial nerve origin
      12.1.1 Compression or distortion of cranial nerves
      12.1.2 Demyelination of cranial nerves
      12.1.3 Infarction of cranial nerves
      12.1.4 Inflammation of cranial nerves
      12.1.5 Tools-Hunt syndrome
      12.1.6 Neck-tongue syndrome
      12.1.7 Other causes of persistent pain of cranial nerve origin
   12.2 Trigeminal neuralgia
      12.2.1 Idiopathic trigeminal neuralgia
      12.2.2 Symptomatic trigeminal neuralgia
   12.3 Glossopharyngeal neuralgia
      12.3.1 Idiopathic glossopharyngeal neuralgia
      12.3.2 Symptomatic glossopharyngeal neuralgia
   12.4 Nervus intermedius neuralgia
   12.5 Superior laryngeal neuralgia
   12.6 Occipital neuralgia
   12.7 Central causes of head and facial pain other than tic douloureux
      12.7.1 Anesthesia dolorosa
      12.7.2 Thalamic pain
   12.8 Facial pain not fulfilling criteria in groups 11 or 12

From Olesen J. Classification and diagnostic criteria for headache disorders, cranial neuralgias and facial pain. Cephalalgia 1988;8:7–97. Used with permission.

Initial side effects may include ataxia, drowsiness, and fatigue. Idiosyncratic side effects include leukopenia, agranulocytosis, and aplastic anemia. It is therefore advisable to obtain pretreatment baseline values of blood and platelets, and to repeat these tests at regular intervals (eg, monthly) during treatment. The medication should be begun slowly and titrated to the minimal dosage that is needed to eliminate the paroxysms.

Another drug that can be helpful is baclofen (Lioresal). Baclofen depresses excitatory synaptic transmission in the spinal trigeminal nucleus. It has been shown to increase the latency of response and decrease the number of spikes in trigeminal nucleus neurons elicited by maxillary nerve stimulation.[24] Although baclofen is not as effective as carbamazepine, it is associated with fewer side effects especially associated with blood disorders. Patients may, however, report significant drowsiness, weakness, nausea, and vomiting.

Other medications used to treat trigeminal neuralgia are phenytoin (Dilantin), chlorphenesin, and even in mild, early cases, a tricylic antidepressant such as amitriptyline (Elavil). Since the medications used to treat paroxsymal neuralgias may have significant medical side effects, the clinician needs to be well versed in managing these complications. Appropriate plans for the long-term treatment of the patient need to be considered.

Neurosurgical Management. Since trigeminal neuralgia is such a painful and debilitating condition, patients have been willing to submit to a variety of surgical procedures in hopes of eliminating their pain. Unfortunately between 25% and 50% of the patients treated pharmacologically report unsatisfactory results.[6] Before a neurosurgical procedure is attempted, the patient must be completely and clearly informed of the nature of the operation, the procedures to be

undertaken, possible side effects, costs, morbidity, and mortality.

In early years, aggressive ablative procedures were attempted. Peripheral neurosurgical procedures such as peripheral neurectomy and neurolytic block are now less enthusiastically undertaken because of better understanding of the problems that attend deafferentation of peripheral nerves. The benefit of such procedures must be weighed against the possibility of dysesthesia and anesthesia dolorosa (to be discussed). Although such procedures do provide long-term relief from pain, the benefit is not lasting.

Another temporary alternative to invasive neurosurgery for trigeminal neuralgia is radiofrequency thermolysis of the peripheral nerve. Although pain threshold and tolerance are significantly raised, it is said that the sensory threshold to tactile-discriminative stimuli is not permanently altered. This suggests that the method is somewhat selective for small myelinated and unmyelinated fibers.[25] These procedures may be useful instead of a more definitive neurosurgical approach to the problem, particularly in medically compromised patients.

Today there are two types of neurosurgical procedures that are commonly used for trigeminal neuralgia: rhizotomy and microvascular decompression. *Rhizotomy* is a neurosurgical procedure by which selected nerve fibers near or within the gasserian ganglion are either traumatized or destroyed. This is accomplished by placing a needle guided by radiographic fluoroscopy into the foramen ovale of the sedated patient. After careful manipulation and feedback from the patient, the selected nerve fibers involved in the pain condition are located. At that time the selected nerve fibers are destroyed by either radiofrequency thermocoagulation (called radiofrequency rhizotomy[20]) or by depositing a toxic substance such as glycerol (called glycerol rhizotomy[26]). A third type of rhizotomy can be used which merely traumatizes the nerve fibers by inflating a tiny balloon in the area of the involved nerves fibers (called percutaneous microcompression[27]). This procedure appears to be effective without risking neural destruction.

Rhizotomy procedures can generally be accomplished on an outpatient basis and therefore do not incur major hospital expenses. Although the effectiveness of the procedure is good, there may be a return of symptoms in 1 to 2 years. Complications of these procedures are loss of facial sensation and occasionally masseter muscle weakness. The most significant complication is corneal anesthesia that may eventually lead to blindness.

An alternative to rhizotomy is the *decompression* of the trigeminal ganglion and dorsal root. This was first described in 1952 by Taarnhoj[28] in Denmark and by Love[29] in the United States. More recently Janetta[30] refined and popularized this operation. This procedure involves a craniotomy in which the posterior fossa is opened and explored. The cortex is carefully lifted, exposing the root entry zone of the trigeminal nerve. The offending vessel or lesion is located that is producing the compression on the nerve root. The superior cerebellar artery is the most common offending vessel. When this is the case, the vessel is carefully dissected from the trigeminal nerve and a sponge is placed between the structures. Remarkable success immediately follows this procedure.[31]

Although this neurosurgical procedure appears to have great long-term success, a major surgical procedure is required. Patient selection is therefore extremely important. Relatively young, healthy patients are obviously the best candidates. The neurosurgeon must select the appropriate patients for this procedure.

Continuous Neuropathic Pains

Continuous neuropathic pains are pain disorders that have their origin in neurostructures and are expressed as constant, ongoing, unremitting pain. They will often have high and low intensity but no periods of total remission. The category of continuous neuropathic pain is used in this text to merely assist the clinician in the diagnosis of the pain condition.

Mechanisms of Continuous Neuropathic Pains

Recent investigations have lead to a new understanding of continuous neuropathic pain. Animal studies[32,33] have demonstrated that a barrage of deep pain nociceptive input can alter the excitability of the second-order neuron. Prolonged deep pain input seems to enhance the release of excitatory amino acids into the synapse between the primary and secondary neuron. Some of the specific neurotransmitters are aspartate and glutamate.[34,35] These neurotransmitters in turn bind to the N-methyl D-aspartate (NMDA) receptor sites on the second-order neuron (ie, wide dynamic range), producing an increase in the sensitization of this neuron. As this neuron becomes more sensitized, additional primary afferent input is enhanced or misinterpreted

(Figs 17-2a, 17-2b). Once the central neuron becomes sensitized, little and often innocuous stimulation from the primary neuron can result in the initiation of nociceptive input, which is transferred to the higher centers. This condition is called *neuroplasticity* and has been discussed in Chapter 4. Once a second-order neuron has become sensitized, even normally nonnoxious A-beta input, such as light touch, can be perceived as painful. This condition is called *allodynia* (Fig 17-2d).

Another feature of central sensitization involves the other afferent neurons that converge on the sensitized secondary neuron. This condition is characterized by spreading or a widening of the receptive field. Clinically this presents as a neuropathic condition that is far greater in area than the original location.

Once neuroplasticity has occurred, the original source of pain can resolve, leaving a neuropathic pain disorder that seems to have no apparent clinical source (Fig 17-2c). This can be extremely frustrating to the clinician who does not appreciate this condition. All of the pain disorders reviewed in this section produce continuous pain and therefore may be the results of neuroplastic-

ity. This central sensitization only complicates the condition and explains why local treatment often fails to relieve the pain.

Preventing Central Sensitization. Understanding this mechanism of neuropathic pain introduces some very interesting clinical implications. If a constant barrage of nociceptive input carried by the C-fiber can sensitize the second-order neuron then it would make clinical sense that if known tissue damage were planned, blocking nociceptive input to the second-order neuron would lessen the likelihood of central sensitization. An example of known trauma is surgery. With most dental procedures, local anesthesia is performed before tissue damage is begun. In this instance the C-fibers are blocked before there is any chance of nociception reaching the second-order neuron. When this is done, the chances of any central sensitization are minimal. If, on the other hand, a patient receives a surgical procedure under general anesthesia, a different condition exists. General anesthesia blocks neural impulses from reaching the cortex at the level of the brain stem or higher. Surgery under general anesthesia would allow nociceptive input to reach the

Fig 17-2 *(See following page)* Continuous neuropathic pain may develop with a sensory barrage of afferent input in the central nervous system. *(a)* Trauma to an orofacial structure produces a barrage of nociceptive input carried by the primary afferent neuron (C fiber) to the second-order neuron (wide dynamic range neuron, WDR). The WDR neuron then carries the input to the thalamus, which sends it to the cortex for interpretation (pain). *(b)* If the sensory input is great or persistent, the second-order neuron may become sensitized, lowering its action potential threshold. This is known as neuroplasticity. *(c)* If the WDR neuron remains sensitized, the original nociceptive input may stop; however, pain may still be perceived by the cortex as a result of the altered plasticity of the WDR. *(d)* Even light touch, which only activates the normally nonnociceptive A-beta afferent fibers, can elicit a pain response (known as allodynia).

17-2a

17-2b

17-2c

17-2d

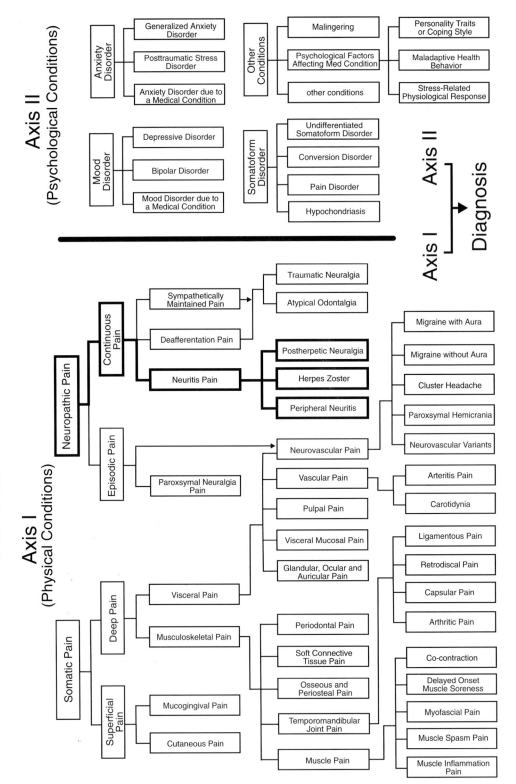

Fig 17-3 Pain classification chart highlighted to show the relationship of neuritic pains to other orofacial pain disorders.

dorsal horn and therefore, sensitization could still occur. This is likely demonstrated by studies that report patients who received local anesthesia prior to surgery have less postoperative pain than those who receive general anesthesia and no local tissue blockade.[36-39] Preemptive analgesia may be an important consideration in the prevention of some neuropathic pains. These same management considerations may be equally important in managing any acute musculoskeletal pain disorder.[40]

Continuous neuropathic pains can be classified into one of three categories: neuritis, deafferentation, or sympathetically maintained (Fig 17-3).

Neuritis

Neuritic pain[6,41,42] sometimes referred to as neuritic neuralgia, occurs as the result of alteration of the afferent fibers in a nerve trunk. It is felt as projected heterotopic pain in the peripheral distribution of the affected nerve. Presumed to be inflammatory due to traumatic, bacterial, viral, or toxic causes, the process alters the fibers that mediate pricking and burning pain and elevates the threshold for pricking pain but lowers it for burning pain.[6] This gives the pain a characteristic burning quality along with the other characteristics of neuropathic pain, such as a bright, stimulating, precisely localizable pain that is accurately related in location to the site of inflammation as far as the anatomic distribution of those fibers is concerned. It is inaccurately related, however, to the intensity of the stimulus. In fact, the pain persists regardless of added stimulation, only increasing when stimulated. No secondary excitatory effects are seen.

Although variable in degree, neuritic pain has a strange constancy that relates to the incidence and resolution of the inflammatory process. Its temporal behavior is less dramatic than that of other neuropathic pains.

The clinical symptoms of neuritis relate to which fibers are affected and to what degree. This gives neuritis important identifying characteristics. Neuritis may also present with other sensory effects such as hyperesthesia, hypoesthesia, paresthesia, dysesthesia, and anesthesia. If motor efferent fibers are present in the nerve trunk and are also affected, then muscular signs become evident such as muscular tic, weakness, or paralysis. If autonomic fibers are present, various autonomic effects become clinically evident. The symptom complex therefore depends on the types of fibers affected, the degree of change, the peripheral distribution of the affected fibers, and the state of the inflammatory process. A knowledgeable examiner can utilize these clinical symptoms to locate the site of inflammation. When the inflammatory process occurs within a bony canal, compression effects from the inflammatory exudate may occur. The relationship between the clinical symptoms and inflammatory process is strictly anatomic. The effects are directly the result of peripheral fiber involvement and do not represent central excitatory phenomena.

Neuritic pains of the mouth and face may be classified as follows: peripheral neuritis, herpes zoster, and postherpatic neuralgia.

Peripheral neuritis

Clinical Characteristics. Peripheral neuritis is a pain condition that relates to the entire peripheral nerve trunk, not just nerve endings and terminal branches. Sensory, motor, and autonomic symptoms may be present, depending on the fiber content of the affected nerve. Neuritic pain has a persistent, unremitting, burning quality that is fairly characteristic.

Trigeminal neuritis most frequently involves branches of alveolar nerves. More centrally located inflammatory lesions may induce pain that is more widely located peripherally. With the mandibular division, it may be accompanied by weakness or paralysis of masticatory muscles. Some salivary gland and taste effects may occur, depending on the location of the inflammation. Auriculotemporal neuritis deserves special attention since it can be mistaken for masticatory pain.

Toothache and other pains felt in and around the teeth, periodontal structures, and oral mucogingival tissues may be due to neuritis. The pain is a direct neurologic manifestation of a nerve trunk, and the symptoms relate to the types of nerve fibers thus inflamed and to the precise anatomic distribution of those fibers. Referred pains and other central excitatory effects do not occur. Therefore a direct organic relationship exists between the toothache and its neuritic cause, and the symptoms presented identify this relationship. For example, if dental pain is the only symptom, the location of the neuritis should be sought in the terminal dental branches of the maxillary or mandibular nerves (ie, the superior alveolar plexus above and the inferior alveolar nerve below). If the neuritis is more centrally located, sensory symptoms in other areas would be expected along with muscular and autonomic signs when such fibers are present in the nerve trunk at the site of inflammation.

A toothache from neuritic cause would be expressed as discomfort that differs considerably from a typical odontogenous toothache. Perhaps more important is that neuritis almost invariably causes sensory symptoms other than hyperalgesia, especially paresthesia or anesthesia. Such symptoms occur in the peripheral distribution of the affected nerve so that other teeth may feel strange or dead and may thus respond to electric pulp testing. Either pain, dysesthesia, paresthesia, or anesthesia may occur in the superficial soft tissues supplied by the affected nerve. This would include not only the cutaneous distribution of the infraorbital and mental nerves above and below, respectively, but also the areas of mucogingiva supplied by the affected nerves. A good understanding of the local neuroanatomy therefore is essential in the diagnosis of neuritic symptoms.

Pathophysiologic Features. The assumed cause of peripheral neuritis is an inflammatory processes along the course of a nerve trunk secondary to traumatic, bacterial, viral, or toxic causes. The inflammation process alters the fibers that mediate pricking and burning pain and elevates the threshold for pricking pain but lowers it for burning pain.[6] The cause of a neuritic toothache arising from the dental branches of the maxillary and mandibular nerves should be well understood. Neuritis of the superior dental plexus occurs most frequently as a result of contiguous inflammation in the maxillary sinus. The dental nerves frequently lie just below the lining mucosa or are separated by very thin osseous structure. They are vulnerable to involvement by direct extension. This is not a tooth-root relationship but a neural relationship. When antral disease causes inflammation of the dental nerve plexus, a neuritic toothache may occur in any maxillary tooth on that side. The symptoms may be pain, hypoesthesia, paresthesia, and/or anesthesia of a tooth, several teeth, mucogingiva, or the cutaneous area supplied by the infraorbital nerve. When anterior teeth are thus affected, and they frequently are, especially when the antral symptoms are silent due to the relative insensibility of the antral mucosa, a very real diagnostic problem confronts the dentist. Many teeth so affected have been treated endodontally and even extracted, only for the pain to continue. For example, such a tooth endodontally treated may not only continue to ache, the pain may actually be excited by electric stimulation—a condition anatomically impossible from pulpal sources. Therefore, a diffuse maxillary toothache occurring as a direct result of maxillary sinusitis may be neuritic if its behavior follows the rules that apply to neuritis. This should be well understood by all dentists and otolaryngologists (Case 26).

A neuritic toothache arising from inflammation of the inferior dental nerve occurs most frequently from contiguous inflammation in the mandibular canal, usually from trauma or infection. The most common source is surgery involving deeply embedded mandibular third molars. However, spreading of dental sepsis to the mandibular canal is also a cause of this condition (Fig 17-4). Sometimes such neuritic pain involves all mandibular teeth to the midline. Frequently, paresthesia or anesthesia of the lower lip is encountered. Paresthesia sensed as tightness of dental contacts and various dead feelings may be described. Mucogingival pain and sensations of swelling in the peripheral distribution of the inferior

Fig 17-4 Radiograph of a mandibular third molar showing extensive radiolucency indicative of an interradicular abscess that communicated with the mandibular canal. The patient's clinical symptoms were those of localized periodontal odontogenous pain in the third molar region accompanied by neuritic pain in other mandibular teeth, with paresthesia and hypoesthesia of the structures supplied by the mental nerve.

alveolar nerve are common. All such mandibular toothache complaints due to inferior alveolar neuritis follow the rules that apply to neuritis (Case 27).

Facial Nerve Neuritis (Bell's Palsy) results from inflammation of the facial nerve. The location is usually but not necessarily within the facial canal. Although some deeply situated neuritic pain along with a persistent burning pain of the auricular area is noticeable, the predominant effects are weakness or paralysis of facial muscles because efferent fibers to the muscles of facial expression are numerically greater. Other sensory effects, autonomic effects, and taste aberrations also may be recognized.

Compression effects due to angioneurotic edema within the facial canal can also cause facial paralysis that may be indistinguishable from true facial neuritis. Clinically it may be assumed that sudden painless and

425

Case 26 Peripheral neuritis secondary to a maxillary sinusitis that is expressed as toothache

Chief Complaint

Right maxillary toothache.

History

A 65-year-old woman with mild to severe variable but protracted continuous steady bright burning pain located in the right maxillary teeth and gingiva, accompanied by some sensations of hyperesthesia, and paresthesia. The pain is located in the right maxillary canine and incisor region where the teeth have recently been extracted.

The complaint began 3 months ago as intermittent burning pain in the maxillary anterior teeth which were treated endodontically without benefit. After about 30 days, she had some burning pain and sensations of swelling of the right labial and buccal maxillary mucogingival tissues. This has persisted as a variable tingling and numb sensation. About 6 weeks ago, the dental pain became severe and more constant. A few days ago the right maxillary canine and lateral incisor were extracted in a futile attempt to control the patient's pain.

Examination

Intraoral: The right maxillary canine area shows evidence of recent operation for removal of the canine and incisor teeth. No surgical complications are evident. The remaining right maxillary teeth appear to be normal clinically and radiographically except for decreased response to pulp testing of the right maxillary first and second premolars.

TM Joints: Entirely negative.

Muscles: Entirely negative.

Cervical: Within normal limits.

Cranial Nerves: Sensory alterations in the region of the extraction sites, especially to light touch. The presence of hyperesthesia, and paresthesia in this region.

Diagnostic Tests: Local anesthetic infiltration of the extraction region failed to arrest the pain. Right second division analgesic block nearly completely arrested the pain for the duration of anesthesia.

Impression

The persistent bright burning pain accompanied by other definite sensations, especially in the absence of central excitatory effects such as referred pain and secondary muscle symptoms, is highly suggestive of neuropathic pain rather than true odontalgia. A presumptive diagnosis, therefore, is superior alveolar neuritis probably secondary to antral. Subsequent consultation with an otolaryngologist confirmed the diagnosis.

Diagnosis

Superior alveolar neuritis due to maxillary sinusitis, felt as neuritic toothache.

Case 27	Neuritis of the inferior alveolar nerve that is expressed as a mandibular toothache

Chief Complaint

Burning pain in the left mandibular teeth.

History

A 45-year-old woman with mild continuous but variable protracted steady bright burning pain located in the left mandibular teeth, accompanied by some paresthesia described as a tingling sensation. The discomfort increases with firm biting pressure on the teeth and when she is tired and nervous.

The complaint began about 4 months ago following the extraction of the mandibular left third molar tooth about 2 months before. The immediate postoperative pain was intense for several days. This was followed by a period of numbness that lasted several weeks and then subsided. As the numbness decreased, the present mild burning pain was felt in several left mandibular teeth, especially the second molar. The "toothache" has been more annoying than actually painful. It worries her and makes her nervous. The last few weeks the complaint seems to be decreasing gradually. Medically negative for cause. No medications presently being taken.

Examination

Intraoral: The left mandibular teeth are clinically and radiographically free of obvious cause for the complaint. The left mandibular alveolus appears to be healing satisfactorily. The root ends appear to have been in close proximity to the mandibular canal. There is no palpable tenderness. All the teeth respond within normal limits to pulp testing.

TM Joints: Within normal limits.

Muscles: Within normal limits.

Cervical: Within normal limits.

Cranial Nerves: Sensory alterations in the region of the extraction sites, especially to light touch. The presence of hyperesthesia, and paresthesia in this region.

Impression

The descriptive behavior of the complaint from its inception is highly suggestive of neuropathic pain of neuritic type rather than any form of true odontogenous pain. It appears that the inflammatory process incidental to the surgery and the healing process enveloped the mandibular neurovascular bundle causing first severe pain, then anesthesia, and subsequently neuritis. The dental pain and tingling sensation seem to be subsiding as the inflammatory process resolves naturally.

Diagnosis

Neuritic toothache due to postoperative neuritis of the left inferior alveolar nerve.

otherwise nonsymptomatic facial paralysis of a transitory type that accompanies other allergic manifestations results from angioneurotic edema rather than facial neuritis.

Glossopharyngeal neuritis is characterized by neuritic pain in the throat and postmandibular and auricular areas. The pain may be aggravated by throat and mandibular movement and therefore may be mistaken for masticatory pain. Traumatic involvement of a prominent styloid process may cause glossopharyngeal neuritis that may be confused with masticatory pain because of its relationship with mandibular functioning (Case 28). Styloid process pain usually can be identified by manual palpation through the tonsillar fossa, pressure being directed laterally toward the styloid process. Elongation of the styloid process and/or calcification of the stylohyoid ligament is commonly known as Eagle's syndrome.[43] The symptoms are those of glossopharyngeal neuritis and sometimes of carotidynia.

Tools-Hunt syndrome is a rare and relatively poorly understood disorder that is thought to arise from inflammation of the third, fourth, or sixth cranial nerves. It can originally present as intermittent pain in the region of the orbit but when progressive leads to constant pain. It often leads to paralysis of the one or more of the third, fourth, or sixth cranial nerves, leading to the inability to move the eye.

Precipitating Factors. Often neuritis begins associated with local trauma or inflammation. Once present the pain is constant, burning, and is located in the distribution of the involved nerve. Since the pain is constant, there are no precipitating factors. The pain, however, is usually accentuated by local stimulation of the involved area.

Diagnostic Considerations. Analgesic blocking peripheral to the site of neuropathy may reduce discomfort by shutting off the input of noxious impulses received by the sensory receptors, but it does not arrest the ongoing burning pain that characterizes neuritis. Analgesic blocking central to the site of neuropathy arrests the neuritic pain.

Since peripheral neuritis can present as toothache, the clinician needs to be aware of the proper differential diagnosis. The following characteristics are associated with neuritic toothache and therefore can be helpful in differentiating it from odontalgic toothache:

1. The pain is less variable, is more persistent, has more of a burning quality, and is less likely to be accompanied by central excitatory effects than is true odontogenous pain.
2. The pain is likely to be accompanied by other sensory effects such as hypoesthesia, dysesthesia, paresthesia, or anesthesia in other teeth or in the superficial mucogingival and cutaneous tissues innervated by fibers of the affected nerve.
3. More centrally located inflammation involving a nerve trunk may cause motor or autonomic symptoms if efferent somatic and visceral fibers are present in the nerve trunk at the site of inflammation.
4. Electric pulp testing may give results indicative of the varied sensory responses characteristic of neuritis.
5. Neuritis of the superior dental plexus may be confirmed by evidence of antral disease. In the absence of clinical or ra-

Case 28	Neuritis of the glossopharyngeal nerve due to a fractured styloid process mistaken for masticatory pain

---

Chief Complaint Left ear and throat pain.

History History A 44-year-old woman with mild continuous variable protracted steady bright aching, stinging and burning pain located in the left ear and throat, aggravated by chewing, talking and swallowing, and accompanied by rawness of the throat and a sensation of "wetness" in the left ear.

The complaint began about 30 days ago following a severe blow to the left face. That evening she had pain in the left ear and postmandibular area that increased with opening the mouth. Her ENT physician found no aural cause for the complaint and advised a corticosteroid injection of the left TM joint. This was vetoed by her internist pending a dental examination. Her dentist found no dental or oral cause for the pain. Open and closed TM joint radiographic visualization of the left styloid process shows a long process with an overriding fracture in its midbody.

Examination ***Intraoral:*** No dental or oral source of pain.

TM Joints: Both joints are structurally and functionally normal.

Muscles: There is no palpable tenderness in any masticatory muscle and no muscular dysfunction of any kind.

Cervical: Cervical muscle palpation is negative but palpation of the sternocleidomastoid muscle increases the pain. Swallowing also increases the pain.

Cranial Nerves: Within normal limits.

Diagnostic Tests: Topical anesthetic applied to the throat did not arrest the pain. Analgesic blocking of the left mandibular nerve intraorally and of the left TM joint proper extraorally did not arrest the pain.

Impression The only masticatory relationship is extensive mandibular movement that stretches the stylomandibular ligament. The behavioral characteristics are highly suggestive of neuropathic pain involving the left glossopharyngeal nerve. Radiographic evidence of fracture of the left styloid process should confirm a diagnosis of glossopharyngeal neuritis induced by trauma. Eagle syndrome is ruled out due to the constancy of the pain and neuropathic quality of the pain.

Diagnosis Glossopharyngeal neuritis mistaken for masticatory pain.

---

diographic evidence of maxillary sinusitis, direct surgical aspiration of the antrum may be done. This is a simple intraoral procedure accomplished by infiltrating a small amount of local anesthetic in the canine fossa area superior to the premolar teeth and drilling a small hole through the facial wall of the antrum superior to the premolar root ends (as guided by the dental radiograph). A No. 1 round bur may be used. An aspiration needle is then inserted into the cavity of the antrum and its contents aspirated. A normal antrum contains only air. Fluid aspirated is positive evidence of antral disease, and the patient should be transferred to the care of an otolaryngologist. Such a test is harmless if properly done. The information obtained more than justifies its use when the cause of a maxillary neuritic toothache is in doubt.

Management. The management of peripheral neuritis begins with understanding the etiology of the inflammation. When a bacterial source is suspected, antibiotics are indicated. Other treatments needed to eliminate the infection should be undertaken. When a viral infection is suspected, antiviral medications such as acyclovir can be helpful.

When no obvious infection exists, administration of steroids should be considered. Steroids can reduce swelling of the nerve tissue which may be extremely important when neuritis effects a nerve that exits a cranial foramen. It is thought that this swelling is responsible for the paralysis seen in Bell's palsy and Tools-Hunt syndrome. Early treatment with steroids in these conditions may spare the patient permanent paralysis.

Herpes Zoster

Clinical Characteristics. Herpes zoster is an acute neuritis of viral source that presents with severe pain in the exact distribution of the involved nerve. The viral infection often causes production of tiny vesicles in the peripheral distribution of the nerve. These vesicles usually present 4 to 5 days after the onset of the pain and typically burst open to produce surface lesions. The most typical areas of involvement in the head and neck are in the distribution of the ophthalmic division of the trigeminal nerve and the occipitocervical junction. Most attacks are unilateral.

Pathophysiologic Features. Acute herpes zoster[3,4,6] is a self-limiting viral infection of the ganglion, sensory root, or medullary tract of a nerve. The cause of the infection is the varicella-zoster virus of chickenpox. It is unlike the virus of herpes simplex. The heterotopic neuritic pain and herpetic eruptions are located superficially in the exact anatomic peripheral distribution of the affected nerve. Strong evidence supports the hypothesis that herpes zoster occurs as the result of reactivation of the virus after having remained inactive and latent since the initial varicella infection.[44] Ordinarily, one attack renders the subject immune. Sometimes, however, recurrences do occur. It may persist in chronic form as postherpetic neuralgia, especially in the elderly. Although most patients recover within 6 weeks, immunocompromised patients may develop serious infections that can become life-threatening.[45]

Trigeminal herpes zoster may involve any of the nerve divisions but most frequently the ophthalmic. The maxillary and mandib-

a

b

Fig 17-5 *(a)* Herpes zoster involving all divisions of the right trigeminal nerve. Note that cutaneous herpetic lesions are confined to the peripheral distribution of the nerve on the right side of her face. *(b)* Herpes zoster involving only the ophthalmic division of the right trigeminal nerve. (*b* is courtesy of Dr Donald E. Falace, Lexington.)

ular divisions may be affected individually, in conjunction with each other, or with the ophthalmic. The cutaneous and mucosal eruptions are located in the superficial peripheral sensory distribution of the particular nerve affected, and the pain is felt in exactly the same area (Fig 17-5). Intraoral lesions may be the only eruptions and are therefore confused with aphthous stomatitis or herpes simplex. The diagnostic clue that the condition is herpes zoster is the anatomic location of the lesions, which is identical to that of the peripheral superficial distribution of the sensory nerve mediating the pain. Herpes zoster pain is not arrested by the application of a topical anesthetic or by regional block anesthesia. Sometimes it may occur before or after the appearance of the mucosal or cutaneous lesions and occasionally without superficial lesions (Case 29).

Ramsay Hunt syndrome is herpes zoster of the nervus intermedius, the sensory component of the facial nerve. This rare syndrome causes neuritic pain and superficial herpetic lesions in the external ear, auditory canal, and mastoid area and even on the tympanic membrane. Intraorally, the heterotopic pain and herpetic lesions affect the fauces, soft palate, and anterior part of the tongue.[3] Herpes zoster does not display muscle symptoms.

Geniculate herpes involves the viral infection of the facial nerve and geniculate ganglion. The pain is often felt deep in the ear and is referred to the retro-orbital, posterior nasal, malar, and palatal regions of the face. There may also be a loss of taste. Vesicles may appear on the face and also in the external auditory canal.

Precipitating Factors. There are no other precipitating factors other than the viral infection itself. Once the pain is present, any sensory stimulation such as light touch exacerbates the pain. Even clothing that touches the involved area is not tolerated.

Case 29	Herpes zoster involving the mandibular nerve and expressed intraorally

Chief Complaint

Left lower jaw pain.

History

A 66-year-old woman with moderately severe steady bright burning pain located in the left lower jaw from the mental foramen to the ear and in the lower lip and labial gingiva from the mental foramen to the mandibular symphysis.

The pain began without apparent cause about 4 to 5 days ago and has continued as a protracted complaint ever since. She had a similar but milder attack about 10 months ago. It lasted 5 to 6 weeks and finally disappeared without therapy. Her dentist has checked her dentures and prescribed a muscle relaxant without benefit. There appears to be no history of prior illness, infection, trauma, or allergy. Simple analgesics only are presently being used but they are not very helpful.

Examination

Intraoral: The mouth is edentulous and the dentures appear to be satisfactory. There is no hyperemia or ulceration seen. The tissues around the mental foramen and the entire lower lip are hyperalgesic.

TM Joints: Negative.

Muscles: Negative.

Cervical: Within normal limits.

Cranial Nerves: Tissues innervated by the mandibular branch of the left trigeminal nerve were very hyperalgesic and hyperesthetic. All other sensory and motor functions were within normal limits.

Diagnostic Tests: Local anesthetic mandibular block caused a mild burning sensation in the left lower lip prior to anesthesia. A few hours later, patient noticed some superficial swelling of the lower lip. This was followed by some vesiculation of the inner mucosa of the lip. About two days later, herpetic type ulceration became evident located precisely in the peripheral distribution of the left mental nerve.

Impression

This complaint presents the features of neuritic pain of herpetic origin. Probably recurrent.

Diagnosis

Herpes zoster involving the mandibular division of the left trigeminal nerve.

Diagnostic Considerations. Herpes zoster may be difficult to diagnose in the very early stage when pain is the only symptom. Once the vesicles appear, the diagnosis becomes more obvious. Laboratory examination of spinal fluid shows elevated protein levels and pleiocytosis.

Management. Since herpes zoster is usually a self-limiting disease, treatment is normally directed toward making the patient comfortable during the painful stage. Unfortunately this is not always easy with neuritic pain. Education and reassurance are important. Mild analgesics may be useful while topical anesthetics do not usually provide much help.

Postherpetic Neuralgia

Clinical Characteristics. Some cases of acute herpes zoster persist as postherpetic neuralgia. This rarely occurs prior to 40 years of age. The incidence of postherpetic neuralgia is about 10% at the age of 40 and increases dramatically with older people, reaching an incidence of about 75% at the age of 90.[46] Postherpetic neuralgia occurs as an intractable, chronic, burning pain. The heterotopic pain of postherpetic neuralgia is felt superficially in the area affected by the acute attack. If it lasts as long as a year, it is likely to persist indefinitely, and to resist all therapy. The pain is usually accompanied by other sensory symptoms such as dysesthesia, hypoesthesia, and hyperesthesia in the cutaneous distribution of the affected nerve. The syndrome may display episodes of exacerbated symptoms. Occasionally, spontaneous pain reduction occurs. Usually the pain remains moderate in intensity, but the constancy and intractability may render it intolerable.

Pathophysiologic Features. Like herpes zoster, postherpetic neuralgia is caused by the varicella zoster virus. It occurs in patients who have been exposed to herpes zoster and the virus lies dormant in the nerve ganglion cell bodies. In approximately 10% of the infected patients, the virus will become active and produce the postherpetic neuralgia.[47] Sixty percent of those affected are over the age of 45 years.

It is thought that one reason for the extreme difficulty in managing this syndrome, even by trigeminal deinnervation, is that the virus involves central pathways in the brain stem and cerebral hemispheres.[48] It is thought that the virus destroys the large inhibitory fibers, opening the spinal gate, allowing smaller fibers to predominate the input.[49] This would increase the C-fiber nociceptive input.

Precipitating Factors. Postherpetic neuralgia is caused by the reactivation of the herpes virus that is dormant in the nerve ganglion. The precipitating factors that may reactivate the virus are not completely known. Some possible factors are re-exposure to the virus, stress and fatigue, immunosuppression, and Hodgkin's disease.

Diagnostic Considerations. A prior infection of the varicella zoster virus is required but this may not always be a significant finding in the history. If the patient had experienced an episode of herpes zoster, the history will likely reveal this finding. However, even a childhood infection of chickenpox can leave the dormant virus.

Management. The management of postherpetic neuralgia is very difficult. Analgesics can be given but they provide little relief.

Classification of Orofacial Pains

Fig 17-6 Pain classification chart highlighted to show the relationship of deafferentation and sympathetically maintained pains to other orofacial pain disorders.

Amitriptyline[50] can be helpful in enhancing the descending inhibitory system so that central pain modulation can be most effective. The topical application of capsaicin cream (0.025% or 0.075%) can also be helpful in reducing the pain.[47] Sometimes antineuralgic agents and even repeated intravenous infusions of procaine or lidocaine may be helpful.[50] Suzuki et al[51] reported the use of cryocautery of sensitized skin areas in refractory postherpetic neuralgia. Their success rate was reported to be good. Spinal trigeminal nucleotomy has been used to control the pain of postherpetic neuralgia, painful dysesthesia, and some deafferentation disorders with variable levels of success.[52-54]

Deafferentation Pains

Deafferentation means that there is a loss of normal afferent input to the central nervous system. Earlier it was thought that if a painful condition could not be managed, simply cutting the nerve was a logical treatment. Although this assumption seemed logical at first, we have now learned that deafferentation can itself produce pain. Of the neuropathic pains that afflict the mouth and face, the deafferentation pain disorders (Fig 17-6) are likely to be the most important to the practicing dentist, not only because they are numerous but also because they are very difficult to manage. They constitute a serious medicolegal problem because they can occur as a result of otherwise innocent and wholly innocuous dental treatment.

Deafferentation symptoms in the orofacial region are common. Only a few such conditions, however, elicit pain. The most frequent complaint is anesthesia and paresthesia following injury of the mandibular nerve that is incidental to the removal of teeth. Despite considerable regeneration, some sensory abnormality may persist. Being nonpainful, such conditions are beyond the scope of this text. The painful deafferentation disorders of the mouth and face may be classified as either traumatic neuralgia or atypical odontalgia.

Traumatic Neuralgia

Clinical Characteristics. Crushing and lacerating injuries of the mouth and face as well as surgery and deinnervation procedures interrupt the flow of normal afferent impulses in sensory neurons. Damage to peripheral nerves causes reactions not only in the central terminals but also in other peripheral and central cells that are functionally related. Such deafferentation therefore may initiate a variety of symptoms including pain. Such pains arise within the nervous system itself and are not significantly influenced by the subject's activities nor effectively controlled by measures that reduce peripheral nociceptive stimulation. Some deafferentation symptoms may remain even when considerable regeneration takes place. Thus, sensory symptoms including anesthesia, hypoesthesia, paresthesia, dysesthesia, hyperesthesia, hyperalgesia, and spontaneous pain may be felt in the region innervated by an injured nerve. These strange sensations may be felt in an area larger than that subserved by the injured nerve because deafferentation causes an enlargement of the receptive field. Such symptoms may persist indefinitely. Deafferentation symptoms may follow such simple surgical procedures as tooth extraction and pulp extirpation[55] (Case 30).

Persistent conditions around the mouth and face that follow as complications of trauma or surgery are usually divided into hyperalgesia, in which dysesthesia and pain predominate, and anesthesia dolorosa, in which a deinnervated area continues to hurt even though it is anesthetic.

It has been demonstrated that deeply located, permanent, degenerative change may take place in the afferent neurons following peripheral nerve trauma.[56] It is now recognized that varying degrees of anesthesia, paresthesia, dysesthesia, and hyperalgesia characterize such deafferentation, and it is only when regeneration is sufficient and orderly that the return of normal sensibility effectively masks otherwise abnormal sensations. A relative deficiency in the regeneration mechanism leaves a residual of altered sensations that may range from numbness to severe pain.

Perhaps the most frequent of such disorders is the familiar paresthesia that may follow the surgical removal of impacted mandibular third molars. Either the inferior alveolar or the lingual nerve may be involved. But posttraumatic hyperalgesia may develop and persist following the extraction of teeth and other minor surgical procedures including gingivectomy and endodontic therapy. Major surgical intervention and maxillofacial trauma present more serious hazards.

Posttraumatic trigeminal neuralgia presents features that identify it as neuropathic. It combines the characteristics of both painful neuritis and paroxysmal neuralgia so that the examiner may be unable to clearly call it one or the other. The disorder has the persistent, unremitting, although variable, bright, burning pain that suggests painful neuritis, and it may be accompanied by other sensory, motor, and/or autonomic effects that characterize a neuritic manifestation. These effects are anatomically direct and do not behave as central excitatory effects. This basic background neuritic pain may be interrupted by paroxysms of neuralgic pain. The term atypical trigeminal neuralgia has been used to designate this syndrome.

Deafferentation may induce anesthesia of the area innervated by the severed or damaged nerve. This may be accompanied by paresthesia. If the abnormal sensation becomes unpleasant, dysesthesia complicates the symptom picture. Hyperesthesia also may occur, or hyperalgesia and spontaneous pain. When pain occurs in an anesthetic area, the condition is termed *anesthesia dolorosa*. Such pain may follow trauma or surgery involving facial structures. It is also one of the hazards of rhizotomy for the control of facial pain. Anesthesia dolorosa is a chronic intractable pain syndrome that may persist indefinitely. It is a hazard of peripheral neurectomy and neurolytic alcohol or glycerol blocks for the control of trigeminal neuralgia. Sometimes the deafferentation syndrome plagues the patient more than the condition for which treatment was instituted.

Pathophysiologic Features. Traumatic neuralgia is the result of an injury to a nerve that causes either partial or complete differentiation. If the injury is minor, the nerve tissue may gradually repair, resulting in a return of normal neural function. When injury is significant, total repair may not be possible. Injuries that result in significant crushing of the nerve or complete severing and nerve displacement are especially difficult to heal. A cut nerve will sprout a new nerve

Case 30 — Deafferentation pain expressed as toothache

Chief Complaint

Left mandibular toothache.

History

A 42-year-old woman with mild continuous protracted steady bright burning pain located in the left mandibular teeth and accompanied by paresthesia described as a sensation of "high teeth" and recently as "gingival swelling."

The complaint began 5 years ago following the surgical removal of an impacted mandibular left wisdom tooth. After a few months, dental pain began in the left mandibular first molar which was extracted and replaced with a fixed bridge that felt "too high" in spite of repeated occlusal adjustment and finally remaking. A year later, the left mandibular second molar was treated endodontically because of pain and later the left mandibular first and second premolars as well. The fixed partial denture was replaced after the second premolar and first molar were extracted with a removable partial denture that could not be tolerated because of pain. Then some diffuse temporal discomfort began which lead to muscle therapy by first a periodontist and then an oral surgeon unsuccessfully. Presently she has an excellent prosthesis but she cannot wear it because of pain and a sensation of gingival swelling. It feels no better when she leaves it out.

Examination

Intraoral: The missing left mandibular teeth were replaced with an excellent removable partial denture which she does not wear. No dental cause is evident either clinically or radiographically. There is an acutely tender spot to finger pressure located in the mucosal scar residual to the surgery for removal of the left mandibular third molar.

TM Joints: The joints were clinically and radiographically normal.

Muscles: There was minor tenderness in the left temporal muscle area which was interpreted to be a secondary response to the chronic pain condition. Analgesic blocking of that muscle arrested the muscle pain only.

Cervical: Within normal limits.

Cranial Nerves: Hyperalgesia, paresthesia, and dysesthesia noted at the gingival tissue over the former extraction sites.

Diagnostic Tests: Injection of a local anesthetic into the mucosal scar immediately gave considerable relief of pain and, therefore, it was presumed to represent a painful neuroma. Excision, however, gave only transitory relief and after a few weeks all pain was as before.

Impression

The behavioral characteristics of this pain problem suggest a posttraumatic peripheral neuritis based on degenerative neural changes located centrally in either the somatic or visceral pain conduction system. There is no evidence that the pain originates from dental, oral, or masticatory causes.

Diagnosis

Deafferentation toothache caused by a previous nerve injury.

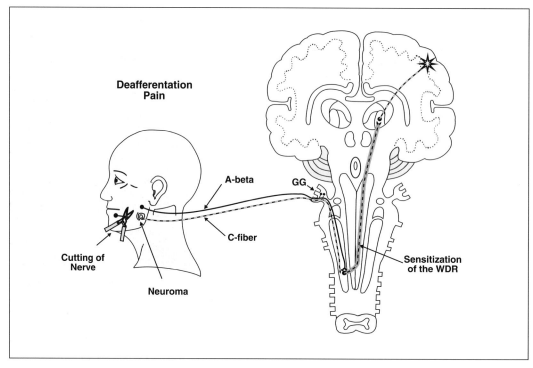

Fig 17-7 *Deafferentation Pain:* When a peripheral nerve is damaged or cut, there is a loss of afferent input to the CNS. The cut neuron sprouts in an attempt to reinnervate the area. If the neurolemma sheath is damaged or displaced, a neuroma may form. The newly developed neural tissue is sensitized to norepinephrine resulting in spontaneous ectopic nociceptive impulses. The cell bodies of the deafferent neurons in the gasserian ganglion *(GG)* can also produce ectopic nociceptive impulses. These impulses excite the second-order neuron (drawn here as the *WDR* neuron), which carries the impulse on to the higher centers for interpretation, often felt as pain. As this afferent barrage continues, the WDR neuron can become sensitized (neuroplasticity) producing a continuous neuropathic pain felt in an anesthetic tissue area.

ending. If the neurolemma sheath is present, the nerve sprout is directed by the sheath to the peripheral distribution of the nerve and reinnervation can occur with time. If the nerve sheath has been damaged or displaced, the sprouting neurons will likely growth haphazardly into a small growth called a *neuroma*. Traumatic neuromas are not true neoplasms. Rather, they consist of a random overgrowth of inter-

twined extraneural and intraneural tissues and Schwann's cells that develops as part of the regeneration process after a nerve is cut. This disorganized mass of young nerve sprouts are extremely sensitive to norepinephrine, which is released by the sympathetic fibers in the area. The result is an ectopic firing of the neurons that make up the neuroma, creating a source of nociceptive input carried centrally to the second-order neuron. This condition seems to be further aggravated by ectopic impulses that seem to be generated by the cell bodies of these injured neurons found in the dorsal (gasserian) ganglion[57] (Fig 17-7). Traumatic neuromas can therefore produce spontaneous pain. Other factors that can aggravate or extenuate the pain are pressure, impingement, or stretching.

Large traumatic neuromas are not reported in the oral structures, presumably due to the size of the nerve trunks that may be sectioned. Many sensory nerves are situated within bony canals where they are protected from injury, and if sectioning should occur and a neuroma develop, it is unlikely that pain would occur due to the protection of overlying osseous tissue. Following fracture of facial bones and deep lacerations, one should be alert to the inherent possibility of neuroma formation as a cause of posttraumatic pain. The oral surgeon especially should know the characteristic features of this source of neuropathic pain.

Of considerable importance is the formation of minute neuromas in scar tissue because these may be a cause of painful scars.[7] Microscopic examination of painful scar tissue excised from the mouth is not remarkable, and the pathologist should not expect to find typical end-bulb neuromas. Usually, considerable fibrous tissue is seen with small nerve fibers that appear thicker than normal and nodular and terminate in little whorls. The time between wound healing and the development of a painful scar varies considerably. Once a painful neuroma becomes clinically evident, the complaint will continue until the mass is surgically excised.

Precipitating Factors. The most important precipitating factor associated with trau-

Fig 17-8 A panoramic radiograph of a gunshot injury to the right angle of the mandible. One month following this injury the patient began complaining of constant burning pain in the region of the injury. Mechanical allodynia is present even though the patient reports the area as numb. This condition reflects a deafferentation pain disorder secondary to a traumatic neuroma.

matic neuralgia is a significant history of trauma (Fig 17-8). Most patients have no difficulty relating the onset of their pain disorder with a traumatic event. Other precipitating factors may be locally associated with provocation of the injured tissue or neuroma by touch, pressure, or any form of local irritation.

Diagnostic Considerations. Traumatic neuralgias are characterized by continuous neuropathic pain associated with prior trauma. Mucogingival scars following minor oral surgical procedures such as extraction of teeth and alveoloplasty can elicit typical neuropathic pain. This type of mucogingival scar reveals increased pain when the finger

439

pressure is applied over the area or when compressed by a denture base. Such minute painful spots can easily be overlooked by the examiner (Case 31).

The following features of mucogingival scars with neuroma formation are diagnostic: history of surgery or lacerating injury at the site of pain; usually no visible or palpable mass; no complaint of pain except when the site is aggravated by pressure or stretching; and decisive arrestment of pain for the duration of anesthesia by injection of a drop of anesthetic at the pain site.

Traumatic neuromas may form in temporomandibular joint adhesions and contractures that result from an operation or lacerating trauma (Case 32). Pain from this source must be differentiated from arthralgia due to inflammatory conditions of the joint. Such pains also may be confused with neuralgic pains of the trigeminal and glossopharyngeal nerves. True paroxysms of the spontaneous type do not occur, and triggering from slight stimulation of the peripheral sensory receptors does not take place.

The following features that differentiate the pain of traumatic neuromas in TM joint adhesions from inflammatory arthralgia: ·

1. History of surgery or lacerating trauma
2. Clinical characteristics of neuropathic rather than deep somatic pain
3. Evidence that adhesions restrain joint movements
4. No complaint of pain except at the moment that such adhesion is stretched

Management. In cases of traumatic injury, microsurgical repair of injured peripheral sensory nerves of the face has been accomplished successfully. Trauma-induced paresthesia and lacerated nerves offer opportuni-

ties for oral surgery of this type. Regeneration of afferent fibers may be sufficient to restore useful sensation.[58] Surgical decompression and other microneurosurgical techniques may be helpful in the treatment of mandibular nerve paresthesia and neuritis due to surgical trauma to the inferior alveolar nerve or to accidental involvement of the nerve canal during endodontic procedures.[59-66]

A relatively conservative approach to treating traumatic neuralgia is the application of topical medications to the painful area. In some instances topical application of local anesthetic can assist in reducing the ongoing nociceptive input and improve the condition. Any decrease in nociceptive input lessens the barrage of afferent input that may be responsible for the neuroplasticity. Capsaicin (Zostrix) can also be used to desensitize the primary afferent neurons. Capsaicin is the active ingredient in hot chilli peppers and has been shown to stimulate the primary afferent neuron to release substance P into the synapse at the second-order neuron.[67] At first, application of capsaicin causes an increase in pain. It has been found, however, that repeated applications of capsaicin can deplete the primary afferent neurons of substance P, decreasing their influence on the second-order neuron. It is thought that this shut down of the primary afferents may provide an opportunity for the desensitization of the second-order neuron. The capsaicin should be applied five times a day to the affected area for the first week and three times a day for the next 3 weeks. If this treatment is too painful for the patient, the cream can be mixed with 5% lidocaine ointment.

In some instances, a low dosage of tricyclic antidepressant (amitriptyline, 25 to 50 mg daily) may help reduce the pain ex-

Chief Complaint   Constant denture ridge pain.

History   A 65-year-old woman with mild-to-severe bright steady burning pain induced momentarily by denture or finger pressure at a point in the maxillary right edentulous ridge area about halfway between the crest of the ridge and the mucobuccal
fold. The pain is proportionate to the pressure. There is no spontaneous or triggered pain. Location is precise and the pain predictable.

Complaint began about 30 years ago following the extraction of the anterior
maxillary teeth and has remained the same ever since. Many doctors have been
consulted and therapy of different types unsuccessfully tried, including all types of
topical applications, systemic medications, denture adjustments, and surgically
smoothing the underlying alveolar bone. No medications are presently being
taken.

Examination   **Intraoral:** The mouth is edentulous with no evidence of hyperemia, ulceration,
or palpable tenderness other than precisely at the "spot" in question. That site appears normal radiographically and there is no abnormal prominence of the bone
beneath. Pain is readily elicited when this site is pressed with the finger.

TM Joints: Within normal limits.

Muscles: Within normal limits.

Cervical: Within normal limits.

Cranial Nerves: Extreme hyperalgesia and hyperesthesia in the central area
of pain. All other sensory and motor functions are normal.

Diagnostic Tests: Application of a topical anesthetic to the painful site did not
prevent pain when pressed. Injection of a drop of local anesthetic directly into
the painful site immediately arrested all pain from pressure for the duration of
anesthesia.

Impression   The complaint is typical of that elicited by pressing upon a painful neuroma located in the mucoperiosteum. Full-thickness excision of the painful site was done
and the pathologic diagnosis obtained by biopsy of the excised tissue was:
"Neuromatous formation, benign, involving skeletal muscle tissue." The pain did
not return following excision.

Diagnosis   Painful neuroma (traumatic neuralgia) located in the mucoperiosteum of edentulous right maxillary alveolar ridge.

| Case 32 | Traumatic neuroma pain located in the temporomandibular joint as a result of trauma |

Chief Complaint

Sharp momentary left TMJ pain.

History

A 27-year-old man with mild-to-severe momentary intermittent steady bright burning pain located in the left temporomandibular joint area, induced by mandibular movements, and accompanied by some restriction of jaw movements.

The complaint began about 6 months ago and has remained much the same ever since. Some 12 months prior, the patient sustained bilateral mandibular condylar fractures in an automobile accident. Reduction was closed via intermaxillary fixation for 6 weeks. When fixation was released, his opening was said to have been about 15 mm. This increased to about 32 mm during the ensuing year with little or no change since. Although he has some restriction of mandibular movements and definite malocclusion, his chief complaint during the last 6 months has been the acute burning pain that occurs almost every time he tries to open the mouth to chew. Presently, he is wearing an occlusal applicance that seems to have improved his occlusion but it has not altered the sharp pains.

Examination

Intraoral: There is malocclusion which seems to have been very well corrected with an occlusal appliance. All mandibular movements are restricted, with lateral and protrusive movements less than 2 mm. He has some mild dull constant discomfort in the left masseter and joint area but this does not seem to constitute his chief complaint. There is sharp burning pain when he opens 32 mm and with extended protrusive and lateral excursions. This pain does not occur in the occlusal position, with eccentric biting, or with actual chewing.

TM Joints: Both joints show evidence of malposition presumed to be due to the trauma and cicatrization. The condyles are radiographically normal in appearance.

Muscles: There is palpable tenderness in the left masseter muscle.

Cervical: Within normal limits.

Cranial Nerves: Within normal limits.

Diagnostic Tests: Analgesic blocking of the left masseter muscle reduced the discomfort only partially. Trial therapy consisting of one corticosteroid injection into the left TMJ did nothing to reduce the pain complaint.

Impression

Since the sharp burning pain does not originate from the muscles or inflamed adhesions and since the behavioral characteristics are those of neuropathic pain, it is presumed that the pain arises from a painful neuroma formation associated with the cicatrization sequential to trauma. Surgical management is suggested.

Diagnosis

Painful neuroma formation in scar tissue of the left TM joint secondary to trauma.

perienced with traumatic neuralgia but this rarely totally controls the condition. New medications are being developed at this time to block the NMDA receptor, which it is hoped will help manage this and other neuropathic pain conditions.

Atypical Odontalgia. Probably one of the most frustrating conditions that plagues the dental practitioner is atypical odontalgia. By definition atypical odontalgia means tooth-ache of unknown cause.[68] This condition has also been referred to as phantom tooth pain.[69,70] Most patients who suffer with atypical odontalgia will have had multiple dental procedures completed before the diagnosis is established. The reason for these unnecessary procedures is that the patient is often totally convinced that the pain is coming from a tooth. When the treatment fails, the patient will often encourage or sometimes even demand that the dentist continue with additional therapy. The dentist will often closely evaluate the last treatment and critically look for reasons to explain the failure. For example, if the last treatment was an endodontic procedure, the dentist may closely evaluate the radiograph and often find that the filling was not perfect. Another root canal will be tried or perhaps even an apicoectomy. When this treatment fails, the frustration increases for both the patient and the clinician. Acknowledging the existence of this condition is the first step in diagnosis.

Clinical Characteristics. Atypical odontalgia is felt as a toothache and often with no other symptom. The patient can usually locate the exact tooth that is responsible or at least thought to be responsible for the pain. The pain is felt as dull, aching, and persistent. Often the toothache has been present for months or even years with no significant change in clinical characteristics. It may increase and decrease in intensity but rarely resolves. The most common area affected is the maxillary premolar or molar regions. It appears to occur more frequently in women in their fourth or fifth decade of life. There is no explanation for this prevalence. Although the pain is felt in the tooth or alveolar process, there is no local pathosis present to explain the pain. Local provocation of the tooth or surrounding tissues does not alter the pain.

Pathophysiologic Features. In past years, there has been some controversy regarding the etiology of atypical odontalgia. Earlier this condition was thought to be associated with a vascular pain condition.[71,72] Later a neurovascular etiology was suggested.[73] The clinical characteristics of the condition do not meet the criteria for either vascular or neurovascular origin. For example, the pain is continuous, which is unlike vascular and or neurovascular pain. Also, the pain does not respond to vascular or neurovascular therapies.

Another theory suggested was that atypical odontalgia has a psychogenic etiology.[71,74,75] This theory was proposed when it was observed that many patients with atypical odontalgia also had common psychopathologic disorders. For example, in one study[76] depression was found to be present in 42% of the patients with atypical odontalgia. In this study, however, it was pointed out that this percentage was very similar to the percentage of patients found with depression in any medical population seeking treatment for pain conditions.[77] The question must then be asked is whether the depression had caused the pain condition or the pain condition caused the depression. The general opinion at this time is that more evidence exists to suggest that the presence of chronic pain is likely to be associated with the development of depression.[78] This relationship, however, is not a simple one. There is little doubt in my mind that psychologic factors do contribute to the pain of atypical odontalgia. As previously discussed, all pain is influenced by Axis II factors. Since atypical odontalgia is a chronic pain condition, Axis II factors can become a significant portion of the condition. On the other hand, little evidence exists to support the concept that this condition is caused by psychologic factors.

The clinical characteristics of this pain disorder more closely place it in the category of deafferentation pain. As with other deafferentation pains, the pain is constant, sometimes even described as burning or pressure. It does not present with periods of remission. Often a history of trauma or deafferentation is present. The clinician should remember that removal of pulpal tissue or extraction of teeth represent deafferentation procedures.

Precipitating Factors. Some patients with atypical odontalgia will report in the history that the onset was associated with prolonged pain felt in the region of the pain; eg, an endodontic procedure with persistent pain. Perhaps this pain experience, in combination with the deafferentation associated with pulp removal, resulted in the condition. There are, however, many patients who report no past or present trauma associated with the onset of the pain. At this time there is no explanation for this condition.

Diagnostic Considerations. It is extremely important to differentiate atypical odontalgia from toothache of pulpal source. The following characteristics are common to atypical odontalgia and not pulpal toothache:

1. There is constant pain in the tooth with no obvious source of local pathosis.
2. Local provocation of the tooth does not relate consistently to the pain. Hot, cold, or loading stimulation does not reliably affect the pain.
3. The toothache is unchanging over weeks or months. Pulpal pain tends to worsen or improve with time.
4. Repeated dental therapies fail to resolve the pain.
5. Response to local anesthesia is equivocal.

A condition that may lead to diagnostic confusion is that atypical odontalgia may be associated with neurogenic inflammation leading to secondary hyperalgesia. Since the pain is felt in the tooth, the neurogenic inflammation may present as secondary hyperalgesia in the periodontal ligament. The clinical presentation is an increased response to local provocation of the tooth. This can often lead the clinician to assume that the etiology is pulpal. The clinician always needs to be suspicious of atypical odontalgia, especially when local cause is not obvious.

Management. Like other deafferentation pains, management of atypical odontalgia can be difficult. There is some evidence that tricyclic antidepressants may be of some benefit.[71,72,75,76] It is likely that this effect is not related to the management of depression but instead to the analgesic effects of relatively low doses of the tricyclic antidepressants. These medications inhibit the reuptake of serotonin and norepinephrine, thus increasing the effectiveness of the descending inhibitory system. Doses ranging from 25 to 75 mg seem to be adequate for pain relief; however, total pain elimination is rare.

There may also be some use for the topical application of capsaicin to the site of the painful tooth.[79] As previously discussed, capsaicin applied to the painful tissue appears to deplete the C-fiber of substance P, thus reducing its ability to further stimulate the second-order neuron.[80,81] Capsaicin ointment should be applied to the area 4 times a day for 4 weeks.[79] If this treatment is too painful, the capsaicin ointment can be mixed with a topical anesthetic.

At this time, there is no suitable medication that reliably reduces the pain of atypical odontalgia. The future holds promise that new medications will better address this pain condition.

Sympathetically Maintained Pains

Clinical Characteristics. In recent years, it has been recognized that the continuous neuropathic pain disorders (ie, deafferentation) can be maintained by activity of the sympathetic nervous system. These pain conditions are therefore referred to as sympathetically maintained pains. These pains are often characterized by constant burning sensations that are frequently associated with a history of tissue damage. There are several different terms that have been used to describe pain conditions that involve the sympathetic nervous system. One of the original terms is causalgia. Causalgia was

first reported in 1872 by Mitchell[82,83] as a condition associated with nerve damage to limbs of injured soldiers during the Civil War. Causalgia was described as a painful burning condition usually felt in a limb that had received the trauma. The pain may appear immediately or be delayed for weeks or months. More recently, causalgia has been defined as burning pain, allodynia, and hyperpathia, usually in the hand or foot after partial injury of a nerve or one of its major branches.[84]

Another term used to describe a pain condition associated with the sympathetic nervous system is reflex sympathetic dystrophy.[85,86] Reflex sympathetic dystrophy (RSD) is described as continuous pain in a portion of an extremity after trauma that does not involve a major nerve and is associated with sympathetic hyperactivity.[59] Other terms that have been used are minor causalgia, posttraumatic pain syndrome, posttraumatic spreading neuralgia, and chronic traumatic edema. RSD usually involves the distal extremities adjacent to the traumatized area. The main clinical features are pain described as burning, continuous, exacerbated by movement, cutaneous stimulation, or stress, with onset usually weeks after injury. There are certain physical signs that are seen in association with RSD. These signs include initial vasodilatation with an increase in temperature, hyperhidrosis, and edema. Atrophy of skin appendages, cool, red clammy skin are variably present, disuse atrophy of deep structures may be progressive. The pain is aggravated by movement and relieved by immobilization. Later vasospastic symptoms become prominent with persistent coldness of the affected extremity, pallor, cyanosis, Raynaud's phenomenon, atrophy of the skin and nails, loss of hair, atrophy of soft tissue, and stiffness of joints.[84]

In 1986, Roberts[87] proposed a hypothesis that attempted to explain the mechanism behind these pain conditions. He coined the term *sympathetically maintained pain* to include this group of pain disorders that seem to be influenced by activity of the sympathetic nervous system. According to Roberts, sympathetically maintained pain (SMP) is characterized by past physical trauma in the painful area, continuous burning pain, mechanical hyperalgesia, and allodynia. Also included in his description was the relief of pain following a sympathetic blockade. If a patient has all of the symptoms but did not respond to a sympathetic block, the pain is called *sympathetically independent pain* (SIP).

Sympathetically maintained pains are characterized by pain in an area that is associated with prior trauma. The pain may not begin immediately following the trauma but in fact present several weeks or months later. SMP is typically a constant, diffuse, intense, burning sensation, not necessarily confined to the sensory distribution of the injured nerve. The skin is usually sensitive and excruciatingly painful even to innocuous stimulation such as touch, air drafts, thermal changes, vibration, noise, or emotional stress. Autonomic symptoms are often seen as changes in cutaneous temperature, color, texture, and perspiration. Trophic changes in the skin, muscles, and bones also followed with time. When significant cutaneous changes are noted, the term RSD is often used.

Cutaneous tissue changes are not often observed in the head and face region and therefore one might question the term RSD for the face region. SMP, however, may occur with some frequency in the face. SMP may follow nerve injury incidental to trauma, surgery, or infection. Since this condition may follow minor oral surgery or postsurgical infection, the history of a dental relationship may be misunderstood by patient and dentist alike.

Pathophysiologic Features. Sympathetically maintained pain seems to begin with trauma to peripheral tissues and/or peripheral nerves. The primary afferent neuron carries the nociceptive input into the dorsal horn and synapses with the second-order neuron (Fig 17-9a). With time this input can centrally sensitize the second-order neuron (ie, wide dynamic range neuron) as discussed in an earlier section. As the wide dynamic range neuron becomes sensitized, even normal mechanical input from the A-beta fibers can produce a nociceptive response (alloydynia)[88] (Fig 17-9b). It appears that changes may occur at the original site of tissue damage that maintains activity of the primary afferents to continue the sensitization of the second-order neuron.[89] It is thought that following the trauma, alpha-1 adrenoreceptors are expressed on the primary afferent nociceptors and that these receptors are activated by norepinephrine released by the sympathetic efferents in the area[90,91] (Fig 17-9c). It also appears that even normal activity of the postganglionic sympathetic neurons is adequate to fire these altered primary afferents. Since normal activity of the sympathetics can activate the primary afferents, nociceptive input becomes constant, which further enhances the central sensitization of the second-order neuron. A self-maintaining loop is established, which is known as SMP.

Further contributing to this pain condition is evidence that sympathetic activity may directly affect the second-order neuron in the dorsal horn and nucleus caudalis, contributing to the neuroplasticity and sensitization.[92] The findings that sympathetic activity can influence painful conditions both centrally and peripherally add to the understanding of many painful conditions and will hopefully lead to more effective therapies.

Precipitating Factors. As already stated, trauma to peripheral tissues seems to be a precipitating factor to SMP. Fortunately not all trauma results in this pain condition. At this time we do not know what unique characteristics are present to initiate this condition. In some instances the trauma may be minor and not even associated with the condition. This is further complicated by the fact that SMP may not present immediately.

Since this condition is maintained and enhanced by sympathetic activity, it is not surprising to find that any condition that increases the sympathetic system will likely increase the pain experience. Increased levels of emotional stress and even visual or auditory stimuli can markedly increase the pain intensity.

Diagnostic Considerations. Sympathetically maintained pains are best diagnosed by the pain characteristics and clinical presentation. Confirmation of SMP is achieved by regional blockade of the sympathetic nerve input to the painful region. In the case of the orofacial structures, this is accomplished with a stellate ganglion block. Anesthetic blocking of the stellate ganglion should immediately reduce or eliminate the pain condition.

Although rare, SMP may cause a toothache of nondental origin. Toothache from this cause has descriptive characteristics that differ from those of true pulpal pain. The pain is described as a persistent, unremitting, only slightly variable, burning sensation in and around the tooth. It is characterized by a neuritic quality and not characteristic of an odontogenous toothache (Case 33).

Sympathetically maintained pains may be confused with masticatory pain (Case 34). They may be differentiated from masticatory pain by the following criteria:

1. The underlying ongoing, persistent, constant, diffusely located, burning sensation should never suggest masticatory pain, which is characterized by variability linked to functional demands and by an aching quality that can be clinically identified as to source by manual palpation and analgesic blocking.
2. SMP can be differentially diagnosed by a stellate ganglion block.
3. True masticatory pain should be identified by positive evidence, as obtained by a satisfactory and exacting examination by the examiner.

Management. Managing sympathetically maintained pain is no easy task. Much confusion still exists regarding cause and pathophysiologic factors and without this knowledge, treatment is quite lacking. It is believed that the earlier the condition is treated, the better the results. This likely involves the reduced sensitization or neuroplasticity of the central neurons. Medications such as clonidine have been suggested[91,93] as a topical agent that may reduce the sympathetic activity in the region

447

Fig 17-9 *Sympathetically Maintained Pain: (a)* Trauma to facial tissues excites the C fibers that carry nociceptive impulses to the second-order neuron (WDR), which then relays the impulse to the higher centers resulting in pain. Note that the sympathetic fibers *(Symp)* have been included in this diagram. The sympathetic fibers descend from the hypothalamus to the dorsal horn in the region of T2 and T3 where they exit the spinal column to enter the sympathetic chain. From there they ascend to the superior cervical ganglion *(SG)* and exit to innervate the facial tissues. *(b)* The afferent sensory input can lead to a sensitization of the WDR neuron (neuroplasticity) thus resulting in light touch (A-beta fiber stimulation) producing pain (allodynia). *(c)* Norepinephrine released by the sympathetic fibers in the area of the peripheral injury can excite the A-beta fibers resulting in continued input to the sensitized second-order neuron. This establishes a self maintaining loop known as sympathetically maintained pain.

17-9a

17-9b

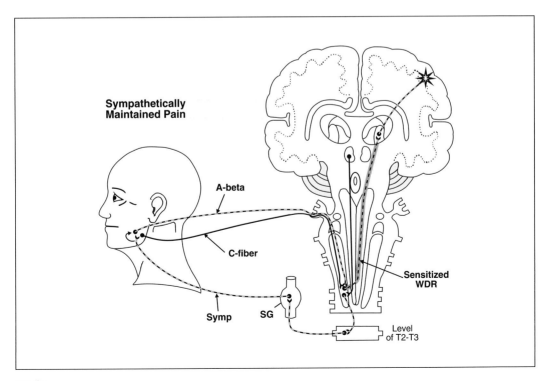

17-9c

Sympathetically maintained pain felt in a tooth

Right mandibular toothache.

History

A 45-year-old woman with mild-to-severe variable but continuous steady dull burning pain diffusely located in the right mandibular teeth and edentulous area described as persistent toothache in the remaining teeth as well as phantom toothache in the right mandibular teeth and edentuous area.

The complaint began following an automobile accident in which the patient sustained injuries to the back and head. A neurologic examination at the time indicated a cerebral concussion and fracture of T-11, plus complaints including transient leg numbness, headaches, facial paresthesias, and visual disturbance even though there were no abnormal sensory or motor nerve findings. All the cranial nerves were said to be intact.

After the accident, the patient felt toothache in the right mandibular first and second molars which after 2 weeks were extracted without benefit. Two months later, the right mandibular second premolar was also extracted, but the complaint contunued as before. Percodan is used to control the pain.

Examination

Intraoral: Recent extraction of the mandibular teeth is evident. Healing appears to be normal. Remaining teeth and mouth are clinically and radiographically negatve for cause of the pain.

TM Joints: Clinically normal.

Muscles: No tenderness or dysfunction noted.

Cervical: Marked pain to palpation of cervical muscles and right trapezius. Restriction to head rotation and bending.

Cranial Nerves: Marked dysesthesia, hyperalgesia and allodynia noted directly over the edentulous area. All other sensory and motor functions within normal limits.

Diagnostic Tests: Analgesic blocking of the right mandibular and maxillary teeth did not arrest the pain even though satisfactory anesthesia was promptly obtained. The patient was referred for a neurologic consultation and diagnostic analgesic blocking of the right stellate ganlion. This block arrested the mandibular pains.

Impression

There does not appear to be any dental, oral, or masticatory cause for the complaint. The toothache and other pains appear to be mediated by afferent sympathetic fibers from the head. The stimulus appears to arise central to the level of intraoral analgesic blocking of the mandibular nerve. The neuritic-like pain appears to be part of a posttraumatic condition.

Diagnosis

Sympathetically maintained pain referred as a toothache.

Case 34   Deafferentation pain being maintained by sympathetic activity

Chief Complaint

Left face and jaw pain.

History

A 41-year-old woman with mild continuous protracted steady dull burning pain diffusely located in the left jaw and face and aggravated by peripheral stimulation of the entire painful area as well as by masticatory movements.

The complaint began about 6 months ago as pain following the extraction of several left mandibular posterior teeth. Initially, it was treated as an acute alveolitis but the pain persisted after healing occurred. Soon it was felt as earache. Her ENT physician found the ear to be normal and advised that the dentist "raise her bite." Her dentist repaced the missing teeth without benefit. As the pain spread to the masseter, temporal, and orbital areas, the dentist adjusted the occlusion several times, prescribed ibuprofen and muscle relaxants, remade the partial denture, tried an anterior repositioning, appliance and injected corticosteroid into the left joint. When the complaint presisted, she was referred for a TM disorders evaluation. Presently, the patient is only taking the ibuprofen.

Examination

Intraoral: The teeth and mouth are clinically and radiographically negative for cause of pain. The left mandibular edentulous area is hypersensitive to touch. There is subjective increase in discomfort with all mandibular movements but there is no identifiable masticatory dysfunction of any kind. The auricular, masseter, temporal, and orbital areas all seem to be hyperalgesic to touch.

TM Joints: Both joints are clinically and radiographically normal.

Muscles: There is vague subjective discomfort in the masseter and temporal muscles with manual palpation but no muscular dysfunction of any kind.

Cervical: Within normal limits.

Cranial Nerves: Marked dysesthesia, hyperalgesia, and allodynia noted directly over the edentulous area. All other sensory and motor functions within normal limits.

Diagnostic Tests: Analesic blocking of the left masseter and temporal muscles, followed by blocking of the left TM joint proper, did not arrest the complaint. Consultation with an anesthesiologist was requested for the purpose of making an analgesic block of the left stellate ganglion. This block arrested all left orofacial pain and subsequently two more similar blocks eliminated the complaint without relapse.

Impression

The history, clinical course, and present behavioral characteristics suggested an autonomic involvement. This presumptive diagnosis was confirmed by analgesic blocking of the stellate ganglion.

Diagnosis

Deafferentation pain felt in the teeth and being maintained by sympathetic activity.

of the peripheral generator. Clonidine is an alpha-2 agonist, which suppresses norepinephrine release. Clonidine has also been used orally. Although it does provide some reduction in sympathetic activity as demonstrated by decreased vasoconstrictor ice response, the reduction of pain may not be much better than that with a placebo.[94]

Alpha-1 and alpha-2 agonists, such as phentolamine, have also been suggested to decrease the sympathetic activity and reduce the pain.[95] These medications are infused intravenously and therefore must be administered under proper supervision. Sometimes repeated infusions may gradually reduce the pain condition and therefore become of therapeutic benefit. For those patients who experienced a significant reduction of pain during a diagnostic stellate ganglion block, repeated blocks may also result in gradual pain reduction. These blocks can be repeated weekly until the pain is eliminated or until no more reduction is achieved.

Since sympathetically maintained pains are very difficult to manage, they are often best treated by a trained chronic pain specialist such as an appropriately trained anesthesiologist. It is most important for the clinician to recognize this type of pain condition so that inappropriate treatments are avoided and the patient can be quickly treated by trained personnel. Remember, the sooner appropriate therapy is introduced, the more successful the results.

Summary

At this time the management of neuropathic pains is both an exciting and frustrating area of study. The excitement stems from the recent significant research investigations into this most complex type of pain. Each day new research provides a clearer understanding of the mechanisms responsible for this source of chronic suffering. The frustration felt by the clinician, however, stems from the present inability to effectively manage the neuropathic pain. Each day new mechanisms, neurotransmitters, and receptor sites are being uncovered. It takes additional research, however, to discover a safe and effective manner to interrupt these pain processes. The development of effective treatment follows the understanding of etiology. The delay, however, is very frustrating to the suffering patient and the concerned clinician. Presently researchers are working on both peripheral and central methods of interrupting this type of pain. I believe the profession is on the verge of making major impact on this most common source of chronic pain and suffering.

References

1. Walker AE. The differential diagnosis of trigeminal neuralgia. In Hassler R, Walker AE (eds): Trigeminal Neuralgia. Stuttgart: Georg Thieme Verlag; 1970: 30–34.

2. McArdle MJ. Atypical facial neuralgia. In Hassler R, Walker AE (eds): Trigeminal Neuralgia. Stuttgart: Georg Thieme Verlag; 1970: 35–42.

3. Stookey B, Ransohoff J. Trigeminal Neuralgia. Springfield, Ill: Charles C Thomas; 1959: 85–111.

4. Kerr FWL. Evidence for a peripheral etiology of trigeminal neuralgia. J Neurosurg 1967 (suppl 126):168–174.

5. Jensen TS, Rasmussen P, Reske-Nielsen E. Association of trigeminal neuralgia with multiple sclerosis: Clinical and pathological features. Acta Neurol Scand 1982; 65:182–189.

6. Dalessio DJ, Silberstein SD. Wolff's Headache and Other Head Pain, ed 6. New York: Oxford University Press; 1993: 345–364.

7. Rovit RL, Murali R, Jannetta PJ. Trigeminal Neuralgia. Baltimore: Williams & Wilkins; 1990: 1–77.

8. Earl C. Disorders of cranial nerves V, VII, IX, X, XI, XII. In Asbury AK, McKhann GM, McDonald WI (eds). Diseases of the Nervous System: Clinical and Neural Biology, vol 1. Philadelphia: Saunders; 1986: 577–579.

9. Gardner WJ. Trigeminal neuralgia. In Hassler R, Walker AE (eds): Trigeminal Neuralgia. Stuttgart: Georg Thieme Verlag; 1970: 162–165.

10. Stevens JC. Cranial neuralgias. J Craniomandib Disord Facial Oral Pain 1987; 1:51–53.

11. Gorlin RJ, Pindborg JJ. Syndromes of the Head and Neck (ed 2). New York: McGraw-Hill; 1976: 201–203.

12. Walker AE. Neuralgia of the glossopharyngeal, vagus, and intermedius nerves. In Knighton RS, Dumke PR (eds): Pain. Boston: Little, Brown; 1966: 421–429.

13. Saper JR, Silberstein S, Gordon CD, Hamel RL. Handbook of Headache Management. Baltimore: Williams & Wilkins; 1993: 128–129.

14. Kerr FWL, Miller RH. The pathology of trigeminal neuralgia: Electron microscopic studies. Arch Neurol 1966; 15:308–319.

15. Kerr FWL. Fine structure and functional characteristics of the primary trigeminal neuron. In Hassler R, Walker AE (eds): Trigeminal Neuralgia. Stuttgart: Georg Thieme Verlag; 1970: 11–21.

16. Dandy WE. Concerning the cause of trigeminal neuralgia. Am J Surg 1934; 24:447–455.

17. Jannetta PJ. Neurocompression in cranial nerve and systemic disease. Ann Surg 1980; 192:518–525.

18. Youmans JR. Neurological Surgery, vol 5. Philadelphia: WB Saunders; 1973: 2959–3003.

19. Kaemmerer EF. A review of the etiologic factors in trigeminal neuralgia. In Hassler R, Walker AE (eds): Trigeminal Neuralgia. Stuttgart: Georg Thieme Verlag; 1970: 175–179.

20. Sweet WH, Wepsic JG. Controlled thermocoagulation of trigeminal ganglion and rootlets for differential destruction of pain fibers: I. Trigeminal neuralgia. J Neurosurg 1974; 39:143–156.

21. Rappaport ZH, Devor M. Trigeminal neuralgia: the role of self-sustaining discharge in the trigeminal ganglion. Pain 1994; 56:127–138.

22. Olesen J. Headache Classification Committee of the International Headache Society: Classification and diagnosis criteria for headache disorders, cranial neuralgia, and facial pain. Cephalalgia 1988 (suppl 7); 8:1–96.

23. Fromm GH. Pharmacological consideration of anticonvulsants. Headache 1969; 9:35–41.

24. Fromm GH, Terrence CF, Maroon JC. Trigeminal neuralgia. Current concepts regarding etiology and pathogenesis. Arch Neurol 1984; 41:1204–1207.

25. Gregg JM, Banerjoe T, Ghia JN, et al. Radiofrequency thermoneurolysis of peripheral nerves for control of trigeminal neuralgia. Pain 1978; 5:231–243.

26. Young RF. Glycerol rhizolysis for treatment of trigeminal neuralgia. J Neurosurg 1988, 69:39–45.

27. Meglio M, Cioni B. Percutaneous procedures for trigeminal neuralgia: Microcompression versus radiofrequency thermocoagulation. Pain 1989; 38:9–16.

28. Taarnhoj P. Decompression of the trigeminal root as treatment in trigeminal neuralgia: Preliminary communication. J Neurosurg 1952; 9:288–298.

29. Love JG. Decompression of the gasserian ganglion and posterior root. A new treatment for trigeminal neuralgia: Preliminary report. Proceeding of a Staff Meeting of the Mayo Clinic; July 2, 1952; p 27.

30. Jannetta PJ. Treatment of trigeminal neuralgia by suboccipital and transtentorial cranial operations. Clin Neurosurg 1977; 24:538–549.

31. Bederson JB, Wilson CB. Evaluation of microvascular decompression and partial sensory rhizotomy in 252 cases of trigeminal neuralgia. J Neurosurg 1989; 71:359–367.

32. Dubner R, Hylden JLK, Nahin RL, Traub RJ. Neuronal plasticity in the superficial dorsal horn following peripheral tissue inflammation and nerve injury. In Cervero F, Bennett GJ, Headley PM (eds): Processing of Sensory Information in the Superficial Dorsal Horn of the Spinal Cord. New York: Plenum; 1989: 429–442.

33. Torebjork HE, Lundeberg L, LaMotte RH. Central changes in processing of mechanoreceptive input in capsaicin-induced secondary hyperalgesia in humans. J Physiol 1992; 448: 765–780.

34. Coderre TJ, Katx J, Vaccarino AL, Melzack R. Contribution of central neuroplasticity to pathological pain: Review of clinical and experimental evidence. Pain 1993; 52:259–285.

35. Woolf CJ, Thompson WN. The induction and maintenance of central sensitization is dependent on N-methyl-D-aspartic acid receptor activation: Implications for the treatment of postinjury pain hypersensitivity states. Pain 1991; 44:293–300.

36. Ejlersen E, Anderson HB, Eliasen K, et al. A comparison between preincisional and postincisional lidocaine infiltration and postoperative pain. Anesth Analg 1992; 74:495–498.

37. Jebeles JA, Reilly JS, Gutierrez JF, et al. The effect of pre-incisional infiltration of tonsils with bupivacaine on the pain following tonsillectomy under general anesthesia. Pain 1991; 47:305–308.

38. McQuay HJ, Carroll D, Moore RA. Postoperative orthopedic pain: the effects of opiate premedication and local anesthetic blocks. Pain 1988; 33:291–295.

39. Ringrose NH, Cross MJ. Femoral nerve block in knee joint surgery. Am J Sports Med 1984; 12:398–402.

40. Linton SJ, Hellsing AL, Andersson D. A controlled study of the effects of an early intervention on acute musculoskeletal pain problems. Pain 1993; 54:353–359.

41. Agnew DC. Painful neurological disorders. In: Aronoff GM (ed). Evaluation and Treatment of Chronic Pain. Baltimore: Urban & Schwarzenberg; 1985: 65–67.

42. LaBanc JP, Epker BN. Serious inferior alveolar nerve dysesthesia after endodontic procedure: Report of three cases. J Am Dent Assoc 1984; 108:605–607.

43. Eagle WW. Elongated styloid process: Further observations and a new syndrome. Arch Otolaryngol 1948; 47:630–640.

44. Straus SE, Reinhold W, Smith HA, et al. Endonuclease analysis of viral DNA from varicella and subsequent zoster infections in the same patient. N Engl J Med 1984; 311:1362–1364.

45. Shepp DH, Dandliker PS, Meyers JD. Treatment of varicella-zoster virus infection in severely immunocompromised patients. N Engl J Med 1986; 314:208–212.

46. De Marages JH, Rierlord BP. The outcome of patients with herpes zoster. Arch Dermatol 1957; 75:193–196.

47. Peters C, Watson N, Evans R, et al. Post-herpetic neuralgia and topical capsaicin. Pain 1988; 3:333–340.

48. Sweet WH. Trigeminal neuralgia. In Alling CC, Mahan PE (eds): Facial Pain, ed 2. Philadelphia: Lea & Febiger; 1977:71–93.

49. Watson C, Morshead C, Van der Kooy D, et al. Post-herpetic neuralgia: Post-mortem analysis of a care. Pain 1988; 34:129–138.

50. Watson CPN, Evans RJ. Post-herpetic neuralgia: A review. Arch Neurol 1986; 43:836–840.

51. Suzuki H, Ogawa S, Nakagawa H, et al. Cryocautery of sensitized skin areas for the relief of pain due to postherpetic neuralgia. Pain 1980; 9:355–362.

52. Kunc Z. Vertical trigeminal partial nucleotomy. In Bonica JJ, Liebeskind JC, Albe-Fessard DG (eds): Advances in Pain Research and Therapy, vol 3. New York: Raven Press; 1979: 325–330.

53. Schvarez JR. Stereotactic spinal trigeminal nucleotomy for dysesthetic facial pain. In Bonica JJ, Liebeskind JC, Albe-Fessard DG (eds): Advances in Pain Research and Therapy, vol 3. New York: Raven Press; 1979: 331–336.

54. Tasker RR. Surgical approaches to the primary afferent and the spinal cord. In Fields HL, Dubner R, Cervero F (eds): Advances in Pain Research and Therapy, vol 9. New York: Raven Press; 1985: 799–824.

55. Gobel S, Binck JM. Degenerative changes in primary trigeminal axons and in neurons in nucleus caudalis following tooth pulp extirpation in the cat. Brain Res 1977; 132:347–354.

56. Gregg JM. Posttraumatic pain: Experimental trigeminal neuropathy. J Oral Surg 1971; 29:260–267.

57. Wall PD, Devor M. Sensory afferent impulses originate from dorsal root ganglia as well as from the periphery in normal and nerve injured rats. Pain 1983; 17:321–339.

58. Mozsary PG, Middleton RA. Microsurgical reconstruction of the infraorbital nerves. J Oral Maxillofac Surg 1983; 41:697–700.

59. Merrill RG. Oral neurosurgical procedures for nerve injuries. In Walker RV (ed): Oral Surgery. London: Livingstone; 1970: 131–140.

60. LaBanc JP, Epker BN. Serious inferior alveolar dysesthesia after endodontic procedure: Report of three cases. J Am Dent Assoc 1984; 108: 605–607.

61. Wessberg GA, Wolford LM, Epker BN. Experiences with microsurgical reconstruction of the inferior alveolar nerve. J Oral Maxillofac Surg 1982; 40:651–655.

62. Mozsary PG, Syers CS. Microsurgical correction of the injured inferior alveolar nerve. J Oral Maxillofac Surg 1985; 43:353–358.

63. Noma H, Kakizawa T, Yamane G, et al. Repair of the mandibular nerve by autogenous grafting after partial resection of the mandible. J Oral Maxillofac Surg 1986; 44:31–36.

64. Kaban LB, Upton J. Cross mental nerve graft for restoration of lip sensation after inferior alveolar nerve damage: Report of case. J Oral Maxillofac Surg 1986; 44:649–651.

65. LaBanc JP, Epker BN, Jones DL, et al. Nerve sharing by an interpositional sural nerve graft between the great auricular and inferior alveolar nerve to restore lower lip sensation. J Oral Maxillofac Surg 1987; 45:621–627.

66. Mozsary PG, Middleton RA. Microsurgical reconstruction of the lingual nerve. J Oral Maxillofac Surg 1984; 42:415–420.

67. Epstein JB, Marcoe JH. Topical application of capsaicin for treatment of oral neuropathic pain and trigeminal neuralgia. Oral Surg 1994; 77:135–140.

68. Rees RT, Harris M. Atypical odontalgia: Differential diagnosis and treatment. Br J Oral Surg 1978; 16:212–218.

69. Marbach J, Hulbrock J, Hohnn C, Segal AG. Incidence of phantom tooth pain: An atypical facial neuralgia. Oral Surg 1982; 53:190–193.

70. Marbach JJ. Phantom tooth pain. J Endod 1978; 4:362–371.

71. Rees RT, Harris M. Atypical odontalgia. Br J Oral Surg 1979; 16:212–218.

72. Brooke RI. Atypical odontalgia. J Oral Surg 1980; 49:196–199.

73. Moskowitz MA. The neurobiology of vascular head pain. Ann Neurol 1984; 16:157–168.

74. Lascelles RG. Atypical facial pain and depression. Br J Psychiatry 1966; 112:651–659.

75. Kreisberg MK. Atypical odontalgia: Differential diagnosis and treatment. J Am Dent Assoc 1982; 104:852–854.

76. Graff-Radford SB, Solberg WK. Atypical odontalgia. J Craniomandib Disord Facial Oral Pain 1992; 6:260–266.

77. Smith DP, Pilling LF, Pearson JS, Rushton JG, Goldstein NP, Gibilisco JA. A psychiatric study of atypical facial pain. Can Med Assoc J 1969; 11:286–291.

78. Magni G, Moreschi C, Rigatti-Luchini S, Merskey H. Prospective study on the relationship between depressive symptoms and chronic musculoskeletal pain. Pain 1994; 56:289–297.

79. Epstein JB, Marcoe JH. Topical application of capsaicin for treatment of oral neuropathic pain and trigeminal neuralgia. Oral Surg 1994; 77:135–140.

80. Rumsfield JA, West DP. Topical capsaicin in dermatologic and peripheral pain disorders. Ann Pharmacother 1991; 25:381–387.

81. Bernstein JE, Bickers DR, Dahl MV, Roshal JY. Treatment of chronic postherpetic neuralgia with topical capsaicin. J Am Acad Dermatol 1987; 17:93–96.

82. Mitchell SW. Injuries of Nerves and Their Consequences. Philadelphia: JP Lippincott; 1872.

83. Livingston WK. Silas Weir Mitchell and his work on causalgia. In Knighton RS, Dumke PR (eds): Pain. Boston: Little, Brown; 1966: 561–572.

84. International Association for the Study of Pain (IASP). Classification of chronic pain. Descriptions of chronic pain syndromes and definitions of pain terms, ed 2. Prepared by the Subcommittee on Taxonomy. Pain 1986; (suppl 3).

85. Bonica JJ. The Management of Pain, ed 2. Philadelphia: Lea & Febiger;1990: 230–243.

86. Bonica JJ. Management of intractable pain. In Way EL (ed): New Concepts in Pain. Philadelphia: FA Davis; 1967: 155–167.

87. Roberts WJ. A hypothesis on the physiological basis for causalgia and related pains. Pain 1986; 24:297–311.

88. Campbell JN, Raja SN, Meyer RA, et al. Myelinated afferents signal the hyperalgesia associated with nerve injury. Pain 1988; 32:89–94.

89. Gracely RH, Lynch SA, Bennett GJ. Painful neuropathy: Altered central processing maintained dynamically by peripheral input. Pain 1992; 51:175–194.

90. Campbell JN, Meyer RA, Raja SN. Is nociceptor activation by alpha-1 adrenoreceptors the culprit in sympathetically maintained pain? Am Pain Soc J 1992; 1:3–11.

91. Raja SN, Davis KD, Cambell JN. The adrenergic pharmacology of sympathetically maintained pain. J Reconst Microsurg 1992; 8:63–69.

92. Gillette RG, Kramis RC, Roberts WJ. Sympathetic activation of cat spinal neurons responsive to noxious stimulation of deep tissues in the low back. Pain 1994; 56:31–42.

93. Davis KD, Cambell JN, Raja SN, Treede RD, Lin C, Meyer RA. Topical application of an alpha-2 adrenergic agonist relieves hyperalgesia in sympthetically maintained pain. Pain 1990; (suppl 5):S421.

94. Glynn C, Jones P. An investigation of the role of clonidine in the treatment of reflex sympathetic dystrophy. In Stanton-Hicks M, et al. (eds): Reflex Sympathetic Dystrophy. Boston: Kluwer; 1990:187–196.

95. Raja SN, Treede RD, Davis K, Cambell JN. Systemic alpha-adrenergic blockade with phentolamine: A diagnostic test for sympthetically maintained pain. Anesthesiology 1991; 74:691–698.

18 | Psychologic Factors and Orofacial Pain: Axis II

In recent years, the advancement of medical science has been phenomenal. We know more today about disease processes than ever before. As we study a disease and begin to understand the mechanisms responsible for its development, we learn ways of interrupting its progression, thereby terminating the disease. This new knowledge has certainly improved the health and well-being of the human race. This processing of information, however, can pose some interesting conflicts in the understanding and management of pain.

Most of the medical community acquire a belief that every disease has a physical condition associated with it. Once the physical condition that is responsible for the disease is found, it can be corrected and the disease is terminated. This mechanistic model of disease makes complete sense for some diseases, such as pulpitis. When a carious lesion nears the dental pulp, the pulpal tissues become inflamed and painful symptoms begin. If the carious lesion is removed, and the pulpal tissues recover, the symptoms resolve. The successful management of this type of pulpal disease occurs everyday in the practice of dentistry. If removal of the carious lesion does not resolve the pain

symptoms, it is assumed that the pulpal tissues are necrotic and a new therapy (endodontics) is performed. When this disease process is present, the removal of the pulp eliminates the painful symptoms. These clinical findings reinforce the physical cause and effect (mechanistic) approach to treating pulpal pain. Since pulpal pain fits this model so well, it perfectly supports the mechanistic approach to disease.

Taking this example one step further, however, helps demonstrate the limitations of the mechanistic model of disease. Assume that after the endodontic procedure was completed, the pain continued. The mechanistic approach would suggest that the endodontic therapy has failed, even though no clinical evidence of failure exists, and the tooth would logically be extracted. Unfortunately it is found that after extraction of the tooth, the pain continues. Since there is no longer evidence of disease, the mechanistic approach to the disease fails to explain the pain. It is at this time the clinician will often blame the pain on some psychologic factor. Since the condition is now psychologic, the clinician who is not trained in managing psychologic issues will likely feel inadequate and not have any treatment strategies. A common occurrence at this time is for the clinician to brand the patient as neurotic. This type of thinking greatly limits the clinician's ability to manage pain.

Every clinician who manages pain needs to appreciate that no pain is without some influence of psychologic factors. As nociception enters the brain stem, it ascends to the higher centers for interpretation and evaluation. As it reaches the thalamus, the nociceptive input is influenced by neural interaction between the limbic structures, the cortex, and the hypothalamus. It is at this level that the nociceptive input is given meaning. The limbic structures add instincts, drives, and emotions to the input. The cortex adds the influence of experiences and present environment conditions to the input. The hypothalamus prepares the body to react to the input through responses of the autonomic nervous system (blood pressure, heart rate, vigilance, etc). It is this unique response at the thalamic level that makes the experience of pain so individual and personal. It is at this level that one can begin to understand why the experience of pain is dependent on the attention drawn to the injury and the consequence of the injury (see Chapter 1).

As discussed in the first chapter, nociception is merely the mechanism by which noxious information is carried into the central nervous system. Pain is an unpleasant sensation perceived in the cortex usually as a result of incoming nociceptive input. The presence or absence of nociceptive input, however, does not always relate closely to pain. The term suffering refers to even another phenomenon. Suffering refers to how the human reacts to the perception of pain. It is at this level that the complex interaction of the cortex, thalamus, hypothalamus,

and limbic structures become evident. Suffering, therefore, may not be proportionally related to nociception or pain. Patients experiencing little pain may suffer greatly while others with significant pain may suffer less. Pain behavior is still something different. Pain behavior refers to the individual's audible and visible actions that communicates his suffering to others. Pain behavior is the only communication the clinician receives regarding the pain experience. This behavior is as individual as people themselves.

When one appreciates the complexity of the pain experience, it becomes evident that the mechanistic model of disease is inadequate in the management of pain conditions. A more suitable model is the biopsychosocial model of disease (Fig 18-1). The "bio" represents the nociceptive input arising from the somatic tissues and the "psychosocial" component represents the influence of the interaction between the thalamus, cortex, and limbic structures. The neurotransmission of impulses between all these higher centers is responsible for what we call the psychologic aspects of pain. In fact, like all neural functions, psychologic factors and moods are based on neurotransmitter activity. Although some clinicians cling to the notion that psychologic activity somehow operates independently of somatic structures, there is a preponderance of evidence that points to an organic neural basis for all such activity. Receptors, neurons, synapses, electric charges, and neurochemicals are the structural elements that underlie all functional activities, psychologic as well as physiologic. Neurochemistry seems to be the key to such mechanisms. As mentioned in Chapter 5, psychology could be construed as really neurology that is not

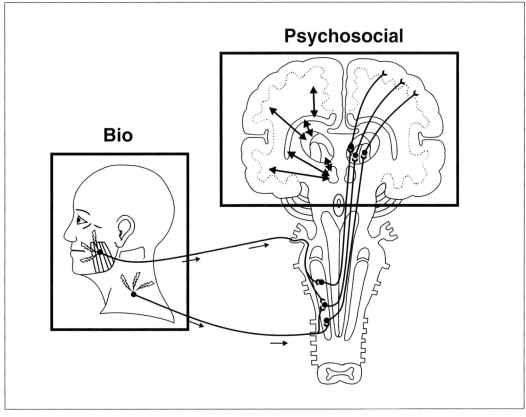

Fig 18-1 A graphic depiction of the biopsychosocial model of disease. Nociceptive input is arising from the masseter and the trapezius muscles. This input represents the *Bio* portion of model. Once the nociceptive input enters the CNS and ascends to the higher centers the interaction of the thalamus, limbic structures, hypothalamus, and cortex interpret the input and label it as painful or not. This higher center interaction represents the *Psychosocial* portion of the model. Both areas are equally important in the pain experience.

yet fully understood. No doubt, as these mechanisms are better understood, we shall know a great deal more about suffering and pain behavior.

It is with this appreciation of pain that a dual Axis classification of orofacial pain has been developed for this text. Axis I represents those conditions that have a physical basis. A detailed review of these conditions has been presented in Chapters 9 through 17. The clinician must appreciate that each Axis I diagnosis is likely to be influenced by the presence of an Axis II diagnosis. For complete patient treatment, the presence and influence of each Axis must be assessed for proper diagnosis. In some pain conditions, treating only Axis I factors will fail to treat the patient's complaints. Unfortunately, this concept is foreign to many health professionals.

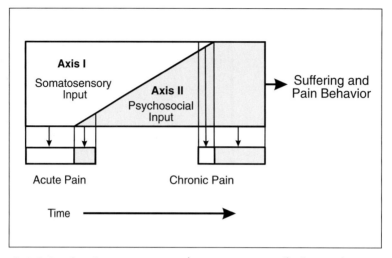

Fig 18-2 Axis I input represents the somatosensory (bio) input that contributes to the patient's pain and suffering. Axis II represents the psychosocial input that contributes to pain and suffering. Both Axis I and Axis II factors must be considered when evaluating the patient's pain and suffering. Early in the pain experience, Axis I input often dominates the degree of pain and suffering. As the condition becomes chronic, Axis II factors often become the dominant input. Understanding this relationship is important in therapy.

Acute Pain vs Chronic Pain and the Biopsychosocial Model

As discussed in Chapter 5, acute pains are of short duration and are often closely related with somatic tissue changes such as those produced by trauma or disease. Chronic pain refers to pains of long duration and these pains take on a different therapeutic meaning. Most clinicians use the term chronic pain to describe any pain that has lasted longer than 6 months regardless of its origin. Although this is the classic definition, perhaps a better concept of chronic pain would be pains that last longer than normal healing time. It is expected that tissue damage will produce nociception and pain but when healing is complete, pain should subside. If pain continues after normal healing time, the origin of the pain is in doubt. One reason for continued pain is the influence of the Axis II psychologic factors. As pain becomes protracted, a shift in the origin of the pain can be expected from primary somatosensory input to the affective, cognitive, and behavioral inputs of pain. As the duration of pain input continues, the level of suffering increases even when the intensity of somatosensory input remains the same (Fig 18-2). In fact, chronic pain can be sustained at a high level of discomfort even though the intensity of the somatosensory input may decrease or disappear altogether. As pain becomes chronic, management options shift from local to systemic modalities. Pain that could initially be managed on a purely Axis I level may require extensive and coordinated interdisciplinary therapy to be effective.

When considering the effects of acute and chronic pains on the biopsychosocial model one realizes that early in the pain experience the somatosensory input (bio) often has the greatest influence on the pain experience. As pain becomes protracted, the influence from the higher centers (psychosocial) will likely become predominant. As already stated, this has therapeutic significance.

Psychologic intensification of pain is a normal modulating effect peculiar to humans and has to do with their evaluation of the consequences attending the experience. All pains are subject to some degree of intensification. It is only when psychogenic factors (Axis II) dominate the complaint that it becomes a significant therapeutic consideration. Since duration increases pain intensification, a component of Axis II factors become an ingredient in the development of chronicity.

Another element that appears to be important in the development of chronic pain is the continuity of nociceptive input. Intermittency lessens the likelihood of the development of pain chronicity as is seen in such conditions as trigeminal neuralgia and migraine. Even though persisting and recurring indefinitely, such disorders usually do not change appreciably in their response to therapy and therefore are not likely maintained by Axis II factors. Pain disorders that have a constant input, even though of variable high and low intensity, are more likely to develop symptoms of chronicity. A combination of duration and continuity of nociceptive input predisposes to pain chronicity.

In the past, the term *atypical facial pain* was used to categorize a group of patients who had chronic facial pain of unknown cause. In a study of 34 cases of chronic atypical facial pain, Mock et al[1] reported that all of the patients displayed nonanatomic distribution with no identifiable organic or physiologic cause and complained of symptoms that were not compatible with any known neurologic syndrome. Of the 34 patients, 76.5% were women. More than 50% had had some dental treatment for the pain that made it worse rather than better. Some 38% reported a sensory complaint such as anesthesia, paresthesia, or hyperesthesia; 55% had headaches; and 73% had associated depression, anxiety, or a highly stressed state. Of course these findings would be expected by definition in a population of patients classified as having atypical facial pain. It would appear that this general classification should diminish as the profession becomes more knowledgeable of orofacial pain mechanisms. For this reason, the term atypical facial pain will not be used in this text.

Pain experienced in the orofacial structures may be significantly related to Axis II factors. In a review[2] of 430 patients with psychogenic regional pain, the head and heart regions were the most frequent sites of pain. In a study of 40,000 patients with orofacial pain,[3] 2% to 5% had no organic disease or had exaggerated responses to minimal pathologic conditions. It was noted that depressive illness occurred especially with glossodynia, glossopyrosis, recalcitrant masticatory pain, and atypical facial pain. In one clinic that treated patients with chronic pain of all types,[4] 40% complained of chronic craniofacial and neck pains. In these patients, there was little or no signs of Axis I pathosis, or it was not consistent with the degree of discomfort. The characteristics that these patients displayed included the following:

1. A high level of stress expressed as anxiety and depression
2. A marked tendency toward tolerance, dependence, and addiction, not only to medications but also to surgery and treatments of all kinds
3. A marked dependency on family, friends, and doctors
4. Evidence of loss of self-esteem, impotence, apathy, regressive attitude, and withdrawal behavior
5. Hostility

Moulton[5] identified two types of patients with chronic pain: people who were overtly dependent on someone who was either inadequate, overdominant, or unapproachable and thus became angry and hostile; and unusually competent people who were obsessive and domineering and therefore became hostile secretly. She warned that local treatment in patients with chronic pain may serve to focus their attention on the area treated, with the result that they would continue to seek relief on a purely peripheral level thereafter.

Beck et al[6] associated depression with glossodynia, myofascial pain, and atypical face pains. They listed the symptoms of mild depression as disappointment, lack of self-confidence, and feelings of inadequacy; a desire to be alone and inactive; undue concern for physical appearance; decreased mental and physical alertness; and loss of weight and disturbed sleep. They listed the symptoms of severe and potentially suicidal depression as apathy, self-hate, despondency, immobility, poor posture, decreased muscle tone, insomnia, and fatigue.

Fordyce[7] pointed out that pain behavior, which consists of audible and visible communications that imply suffering, is subject to the influence of conditioning or learning. Examples of such conditioning are the effect of imitating the behavior of others who suffer (social modeling), the reinforcement of the "reality" of pain by medications prescribed to be used as needed as well as by the attention received from others because of suffering, and the indirect reinforcement of pain by avoidance of obligations, commitments, or duties to escape or minimize pain. Pain behavior that is contingent on expectancy or secondary gain may be reinforced by cues in the environment that suffering may be imminent when actually no noxious stimulation is ever sensed. It may be necessary only to anticipate that pain may occur for overt pain behavior to be displayed.

Sternbach[8] observed that subjective improvement in a patient's pain condition follows behavioral improvement. This suggests that pain responses change if the state of mind changes. Thus, if the pain behavior of patients with chronic pain is acquired or learned, it may be unlearned by proper techniques. Chronic pain is modifiable through coping strategies.

Roberts[9] attempted to control chronic pain by focusing on the patient's behavior and not on the source of nociception nor on an attempt to change an alleged emotional state. His objective was to rehabilitate the patient rather than to alleviate the pain. He believed that it is better to teach the patient to live a normal life even though pain may still be present. In chronic pain disorders, treatment measures that are aimed only to alleviate pain tend to reinforce the pain concept that the patient holds.

In patients with chronic pain, the endorphin system does not offer protection of any importance.[10] Perhaps the experience of chronic pain depletes the central nervous system of these pain modulators. Although the action of tricyclic antidepressants in healthy subjects has no greater effect on the pain threshold than placebo,[11] in depressed individuals the analgesic effect parallels the antidepressant action.[12]

Symptoms of Chronicity

It is important that chronicity be identified as early as possible. Even though pains that are truly intermittent are often of greater intensity, they are less prone to be associated with the symptoms of chronicity such as depressive illness. The relief between attacks seems to prevent physical and emotional deterioration. Thus, with paroxsymal neuralgia and neurovascular pain disorders, chronicity seldom becomes a problem. However, the persistence of continuous neuropathic pains such as deafferentation pain or neuritis, or continuous masticatory pains should lead the examiner to identify evidence of chronicity as early as possible. Guidelines based on units of time are not dependable because chronicity is extremely variable. Rather, identification of chronicity depends on such factors as the following:

1. Constancy and continuity of peripheral input
2. Evidence of increased suffering despite of otherwise effective peripheral therapeutic efforts
3. Persistence or prompt relapse of symptoms in spite of different methods of therapy used by different clinicians
4. Increasing anxiety on the patient's part

5. Patient's obsessive concern with his suffering expressed by relief-seeking efforts of all types
6. Progressive depression and withdrawal behavior
7. Physical and emotional deterioration

The Psychologic Significance of Orofacial Pains

All pains carry with them certain importance and meaning. As already mentioned, the attention drawn to the injury and the consequence of the injury directly determine the degree of suffering experienced by the patient. This concept is extremely important when addressing face pain. The clinician should never forget the significant psychologic meaning of pain in this portion of the body. The face and mouth are the primary structures needed for survival. Without these, the individual will not be able to take in food. These structures are basic to life itself. Damage or significant loss of function is a significant threat to the individual.

The orofacial structures are also basic to communication. In our social environment, where communication is so vital, dysfunction of these structures threatens meaningful existence. These structures provide the means by which we relate to others our feelings, goals, opinions, and aspirations. They are a source of gratification and satisfaction both physically, emotionally, spiritually, and sexually. When these structures are threatened by pain or dysfunction, the quality of life can greatly diminish.

Not only do the mouth and face have unusual emotional significance for the individual, but they also relate to concepts of body image in that the individual interprets a damaged face as a damaged self. Distortion of body image results in anxiety that is frequently expressed as pain.[13] This is likely to have an important bearing on the severity and duration of chronic posttraumatic pain syndromes of the maxillofacial region. This trauma may be not only that of actual tissue damage to the face, but also that of emotional trauma such as that associated with physical or sexual abuse.[14–16]

It is wise for the clinician to always be mindful of the unique emotional significance of the orofacial structures. The clinician should always approach the patient with care and respect, never too quickly or abruptly. The successful clinician learns the appropriate examination and management style that gains the confidence of the patient.

Axis II: Classification of Mental Disorders

Understanding the complex neurofunction between the thalamus, cortex, hypothalamus, and limbic structures is indeed a difficult task. Dysfunction of this neural interaction results in what are referred to as *mental disorders*. The study of mental disorders encompasses an enormous body of information. The main purpose of this text is to provide information to the clinician regarding orofacial pain disorders. Although the Axis II conditions described as mental disorders are enormously important, they cannot be completely reviewed in this text. This discussion is limited to a few of the more important mental disorders that may involve orofacial pain conditions. For a thorough discussion of mental disorders, a review of the DSM-IV published by the

American Psychiatric Association[17] is recommended.

There are four general categories of mental disorders that will be reviewed in this chapter. The description of each disorder will be in accord with the DSM-IV[17] publication. The categories that will be discussed are mood disorders, anxiety disorders, somatoform disorders, and a broad category that includes other conditions that may be a focus of clinical attention. Each of these categories will be divided into important subcategories for the purpose of identification. These categories will be discussed strictly for the purpose of identification and not treatment. It is important for the dentist and physician to recognize these conditions so that optimum therapy is provided by appropriate health care personnel.

Mood Disorders

Mood disorders are mental disorders that are characterized by disturbances in the patient's mood. Mood disorders are divided into three categories: depressive disorders, bipolar disorders, and mood disorders due to a medical condition (Fig 18-3).

Depressive Disorders. A depressed mood is characterized by markedly diminished interest or pleasure in all, or almost all, activities most of the day, nearly every day. The depressed mood is described subjectively by the patient as an overwhelming feeling of sadness or emptiness. There is often uncontrolled crying and a common complaint of fatigue or loss of energy nearly every day. Depressive disorders often result in either an increase or decrease in appetite leading to a change of more than 5% of body weight

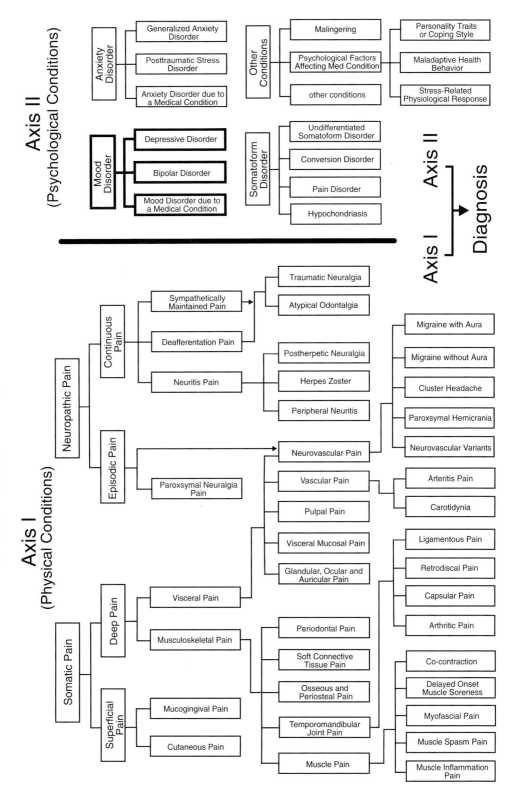

Fig 18-3 Pain classification chart highlighted to show the relationship of mood disorders to the other Axis I and Axis II conditions.

in a month. There is usually a diminished ability to think or concentrate, with much indecisiveness. Insomnia or hypersomnia usually accompanies depressive disorders. Depressive disorders may range in severity from minor to major. In major depressive disorders, recurrent thoughts of death or considerations of suicide are common. When severe depression is suspected, it is important for the clinician to question the patient regarding his or her thoughts regarding suicide. If considerable risk is present, the patient should not be released without proper evaluation.

Bipolar Disorders. Bipolar disorders are characterized by depressive periods followed or preceded by an opposite mood swing called a manic episode. A common term for this disorder is *manic depressive illness*. The manic episode is characterized a distinct period of an abnormally and persistently elevated, expansive, or irritable mood. The mood often includes an inflated self-esteem or grandiosity, decreased need for sleep, pressure of speech, flight of ideas, distractibility, and an increased involvement in goal-directed activities. The expansive quality of the mood is characterized by unceasing and indiscriminate enthusiasm for interpersonal, sexual, or occupational interactions. For example, the person may spontaneously start extensive conversations with strangers in public places. Although the mood may initially have an infectious quality for the uninvolved observer, it is recognized as excessive by those who know the person well. Sometimes the mood becomes irritable rather than elevated or expanded.

A bipolar disorder is characterized by alternating manic and depressive periods. Specific subdivisions are identified accord-

ing to the frequency and severity of the mood changes.[17]

Mood Disorders Due to a Medical Condition. This category of mood disorders is extremely important when considering orofacial pain disorders. Many studies have investigated the common occurrence of depression and chronic pain disorders.[18-21] Although some have concluded that depression can lead to chronic pain, the more convincing evidence suggests that chronic pain can lead to depression.[22] This category of mood disorders is reserved for those patients who experience a prominent and persistent disturbance in mood that is a direct physiologic consequence of a general medical condition. The mood may be depressive or bipolar or any other mood disorder. The physical condition may be a chronic pain disorder or any other medical condition. For example, the condition may be listed as a "depressive disorder due to chronic osteoarthritis of the temporomandibular joint." The common occurrence of both Axis I and Axis II conditions challenges the clinician to astutely evaluate each patient to maximize therapeutic results.

Anxiety Disorders

Anxiety disorders are characterized by an unusual increase in anxiety and worry that lasts longer than a normal or appropriate time. There are three categories of anxiety disorders that will be discussed in this text: generalized anxiety disorders, posttraumatic stress disorders, and anxiety disorder due to a medical condition (Fig 18-4).

Classification of Orofacial Pains

Axis II (Psychological Conditions)

Anxiety Disorder
- Generalized Anxiety Disorder
- Posttraumatic Stress Disorder
- Anxiety Disorder due to a Medical Condition

Other Conditions
- Malingering
- Psychological Factors Affecting Med Condition
- other conditions

- Personality Traits or Coping Style
- Maladaptive Health Behavior
- Stress-Related Physiological Response

Mood Disorder
- Depressive Disorder
- Bipolar Disorder
- Mood Disorder due to a Medical Condition

Somatoform Disorder
- Undifferentiated Somatoform Disorder
- Conversion Disorder
- Pain Disorder
- Hypochondriasis

Axis II / Axis I → Diagnosis

Axis I (Physical Conditions)

Neuropathic Pain

Continuous Pain
- Sympathetically Maintained Pain
  - Traumatic Neuralgia
  - Atypical Odontalgia
- Deafferentation Pain
- Neuritis Pain
  - Postherpetic Neuralgia
  - Herpes Zoster
  - Peripheral Neuritis

Episodic Pain
- Paroxysmal Neuralgia Pain
- Neurovascular Pain
  - Migraine with Aura
  - Migraine without Aura
  - Cluster Headache
  - Paroxysmal Hemicrania
  - Neurovascular Variants
- Vascular Pain
  - Arteritis Pain
  - Carotidynia

Somatic Pain

Deep Pain
- Visceral Pain
  - Pulpal Pain
  - Visceral Mucosal Pain
  - Glandular, Ocular and Auricular Pain
- Musculoskeletal Pain
  - Periodontal Pain
  - Soft Connective Tissue Pain
  - Osseous and Periosteal Pain
  - Temporomandibular Joint Pain
    - Ligamentous Pain
    - Retrodiscal Pain
    - Capsular Pain
    - Arthritic Pain
  - Muscle Pain
    - Co-contraction
    - Delayed Onset Muscle Soreness
    - Myofascial Pain
    - Muscle Spasm Pain
    - Muscle Inflammation Pain

Superficial Pain
- Mucogingival Pain
- Cutaneous Pain

Fig 18-4 Pain classification chart highlighted to show the relationship of anxiety disorders to the other Axis I and Axis II conditions.

Generalized Anxiety Disorders. Generalized anxiety disorders are characterized by excessive anxiety and worry that occurs for more days than not for at least 6 months. The person reveals an intensity, duration, and frequency of the anxiety and worry that is far out of proportion to the actual likelihood or impact of the feared event. The increase in apprehensive and expectation is associated with certain events or activities. These events may be related to work, school, or home functions. The person will often find it difficult to control the worry and be restless or keyed up. The person will often have difficulty concentrating and the mind may suddenly go blank. Generalized anxiety disorders create irritability, muscle tension, and poor quality of sleep. The sleep disturbance is often characterized by either difficulty falling asleep or staying asleep. The anxiety, worry, or physical symptoms will cause clinically significant distress or impairment in social, occupational, or other important areas of functioning.

Posttraumatic Stress Disorders. A posttraumatic stress disorder is a type of anxiety disorder that can develop following an individual's exposure to an extremely traumatic stressor. The stressor may be associated with a direct personal experience that threatened death or serious injury, or threatened one's physical integrity. It may result from witnessing an event that involves death, injury, or threat to the physical integrity of another person. It may even result from learning about an unexpected or violent death, serious harm, or threat of death or injury experienced by a family member or other close associate. The person's response to the event involves intense fear, helplessness, or horror. The person ex-

periencing a posttraumatic stress disorder will often report persistent reexperience of the traumatic event and avoid any stimuli associated with the trauma. The person will reveal a numbing of general responsiveness, yet also show persistent symptoms of increased arousal.

The traumatic event may be reexperienced in various ways. Commonly the person has recurrent and intrusive recollections of the event or recurrent distressing dreams during which the event is replayed. In rare instances, the person may experience dissociative states that last from a few seconds to several hours, even days. During this time, the components of the event are relived and the person may behave as though experiencing the event at that moment. Often intense psychologic distress or physiologic reactivity occurs when the person is exposed to triggering events that resemble or symbolize an aspect of the traumatic event. A well-known example is the combat veteran who overresponds to a loud sound, such as the backfiring of an automobile. Another example is the woman who had been previously assaulted reliving the same fear when approaching her car in a dark parking lot.

It should always be remembered that the traumatic event does not have to appear traumatic to the clinician to be significant. It must only be traumatic to the patient. This is an important concept to remember when obtaining a history from the patient. The clinician should not place his or her own values on the patient.

Posttraumatic stress disorders are likely to represent an generalized upregulation of the autonomic nervous system. As discussed in earlier chapters, stressful events are countered by the fight/flight response. This response is controlled by the autonomic nervous system. In the presence of a sudden environmental challenge, the sympathetic nervous system increases heart rate, blood pressure, and breathing rate while pooling blood to vital organs. This is a normal response to the challenge. When the challenge is eliminated or resolves, the system should return to normal levels of function. In posttraumatic stress disorders, the events are so traumatically imprinted in the person's mind that the autonomic nervous system remains upregulated as if necessary to counter an ongoing challenge. This state of hypervigilance can be seen as irritability, difficulty falling asleep or staying asleep, difficulty concentrating, or an exaggerated startle response.

Often this autonomic upregulation or hypervigilance can lead to subtle changes in peripheral functions. For some patients these persistent changes may present as pain in structures that are free of obvious pathosis. Physical or sexual abuse, especially involving the face, may be common sources of unexplained chronic orofacial pain.[14-16] Patients with histories of physical or sexual abuse often experience posttraumatic stress disorders related to these prior traumatic events. This concept of sympathetic upregulation is important and will be discussed further in the section on therapy.

Anxiety Disorders Due to a Medical Condition. Anyone with a significant medical condition will likely experience some degree of apprehension or anxiety. This is certainly a normal finding. Some patients, however, may reveal that the anxiety produced by the presence of the physical condition is far greater than normal, and in fact may actually impair social, occupational, or other important areas of functioning. When this occurs it represents an anxiety disorder that is due to a general medical condition. Symptoms may include prominent generalized anxiety symptoms, panic attacks, or obsessions or compulsions.

There must be evidence from the history, physical examination, or laboratory findings that the disturbance is the direct physiologic consequence of a general medical condition. The anxiety disorder should not be better explained by some other mental disorder but in fact be related to the physical condition. The relationship between the physical condition and the anxiety disorder may be supported by a temporal association. In other words, there should be an association between the onset, exacerbation, and remission of the general medical condition and the anxiety symptoms.

Somatoform Disorders

Somatoform disorders represent a group of mental disorders in which there is the presence of physical symptoms that suggest a general medical condition and yet there are insufficient positive physical signs to support the diagnosis of a physical condition. Hence the term somatoform. The term *somatization disorder* refers very specifically to a person who is older than 30 years, has had symptoms extending for years and complains of a combination of pain, and gastrointestinal, sexual, and pseudoneurologic symptoms.[17] Since the inclusionary criteria for this category are large, it is not commonly seen in patients with chronic orofacial pain and therefore will not be elaborated in this section. Instead four more common categories seen in patients with

Classification of Orofacial Pains

Axis II (Psychological Conditions)

Anxiety Disorder
- Generalized Anxiety Disorder
- Posttraumatic Stress Disorder
- Anxiety Disorder due to a Medical Condition

Other Conditions
- Malingering
- Psychological Factors Affecting Med Condition
- other conditions

- Personality Traits or Coping Style
- Maladaptive Health Behavior
- Stress-Related Physiological Response

Mood Disorder
- Depressive Disorder
- Bipolar Disorder
- Mood Disorder due to a Medical Condition

Somatoform Disorder
- Undifferentiated Somatoform Disorder
- Conversion Disorder
- Pain Disorder
- Hypochondriasis

Axis II → Diagnosis

Axis I

Axis I (Physical Conditions)

Neuropathic Pain

Continuous Pain
- Sympathetically Maintained Pain
  - Traumatic Neuralgia
  - Atypical Odontalgia
- Deafferentation Pain
- Neuritis Pain
  - Postherpetic Neuralgia
  - Herpes Zoster
  - Peripheral Neuritis

Episodic Pain
- Paroxsymal Neuralgia Pain
  - Neurovascular Pain
    - Migraine with Aura
    - Migraine without Aura
    - Cluster Headache
    - Paroxsymal Hemicrania
    - Neurovascular Variants
  - Vascular Pain
    - Arteritis Pain
    - Carotidynia
  - Pulpal Pain

Somatic Pain

Deep Pain
- Visceral Pain
  - Visceral Mucosal Pain
  - Glandular, Ocular and Auricular Pain
- Musculoskeletal Pain
  - Periodontal Pain
  - Soft Connective Tissue Pain
  - Osseous and Periosteal Pain
  - Temporomandibular Joint Pain
    - Ligamentous Pain
    - Retrodiscal Pain
    - Capsular Pain
    - Arthritic Pain
  - Muscle Pain
    - Co-contraction
    - Delayed Onset Muscle Soreness
    - Myofascial Pain
    - Muscle Spasm Pain
    - Muscle Inflammation Pain

Superficial Pain
- Mucogingival Pain
- Cutaneous Pain

Fig 18-5 Pain classification chart highlighted to show the relationship of somatoform disorders to the other Axis I and Axis II conditions.

orofacial pain will be discussed. They are: undifferentiated somatoform disorders, conversion disorders, pain disorders, and hypochondriasis (Fig 18-5).

Undifferentiated Somatoform Disorders. The clinical features of an undifferentiated somatoform disorder is one or more physical complaints that persist for 6 months or longer. The most frequent complaints are chronic fatigue, loss of appetite, and gastrointestinal or genitourinary symptoms. Of course, pain can also be present but it is not the major complaint in this category. The symptoms cannot be fully explained by any known general medical condition or the direct effects of a substance. The physical complaints or resultant impairment are grossly in excess of what would be expected from the history, physical examination, or laboratory findings. This category is used when the symptoms do not fully meet with all the criteria used for somatization disorders.

Conversion Disorders. Conversion disorders are those mental disorders that are characterized by the presence of symptoms or deficits affecting voluntary motor or sensory function that suggest a neurologic or other general medical condition. Psychologic factors are judged to be associated with the symptom or deficit, a judgment based on the observation that the initiation or exacerbation of the symptom or deficit is preceded by conflicts or other stressors.

Conversion disorders are related to voluntary motor or sensory functioning and are thus referred to as pseudoneurologic. Motor symptoms or deficits include impaired coordination or balance, paralysis or localized weakness, aphonia, difficulty swallowing or a sensation of a lump in the throat, and urinary retention. Sensory symptoms or deficits include loss of touch or pain sensation, double vision, blindness, deafness, and hallucinations.

The diagnosis of conversion disorder can only be made after careful examination has ruled out a neurologic or general medical etiology. Due to the physical symptoms, this may be a very difficult task, taking considerable time. Conversion symptoms are often inconsistent and the astute clinician may be able to diagnose the condition by careful observation. For example, when paralysis is the symptom, small movements of the involved limb may be noticed when dressing or during other activities.

Conversion disorders may also be related to secondary gains, and when so, the clinician needs to be aware. If a conversion disorder results in a paralyzed leg, work becomes impossible. The condition may in fact become the escape from work and the conditions or stressor that are actually responsible for the disorder. The condition, therefore, becomes the treatment that eliminates the etiology. Although this may sound very logical, the clinician should not assume that the patient is actually thinking in this manner on a conscious level. In fact, most conversion disorders are not intentionally produced and therefore the patient is as baffled as the doctor.

Somatoform Pain Disorders. The essential feature of a somatoform pain disorder is pain. Therefore, this disorder is an important condition to recognize in the patient with orofacial pain. In a somatoform pain disorder, pain is the predominant focus of the clinical presentation and is of sufficient severity to warrant clinical attention. The

471

pain is in one or more anatomic sites and causes the person significant distress or impairment in social, occupational, or other important areas of functioning. There is no obvious pathosis present to explain the pain; however, the patient is not intentionally producing the pain (as with a factitious disorder or malingering). Psychologic factors are judged to have an important role in the onset, severity, exacerbation, or maintenance of the pain.

Somatoform pain disorders can certainly pose a significant diagnostic problem for the clinician evaluating orofacial pain complaints. One might be suspicious of this condition if the pain is not associated with any local somatic tissue changes. This statement, however, is very naive when one thinks of the numerous pain disorders that have been described in this text that are not associated with any obvious source of pathosis. For example, most neuropathic pains have no local tissue changes that explain their presence. The clinician must therefore always be mindful of somatoform pain disorders so that an improper diagnosis does not lead to mistreatment. When a patient complains of orofacial pain, always consider all possibilities (Case 35).

Hypochondriasis. Hypochondriasis is a somatoform disorder in which the person is preoccupied with the fears of having, or the idea that one has, a serious disease based on a misinterpretation of one or more bodily signs or symptoms. A thorough medical evaluation does not identify a general medical condition that fully accounts for the person's concerns about disease or for the physical signs or symptoms. The fear or idea of having a disease persists despite medical reassurance that nothing is present. The preoccupation in hypochondriasis may be with bodily functions, with minor physical abnormalities, or with vague and ambiguous physical sensations. The concern may involve several body systems, at different times or simultaneously. Repeated physical examinations, diagnostic tests, and reassurance from the physician do little to allay the concern about bodily disease or affliction. An individual with hypochondriasis may become alarmed by reading or hearing about disease; knowing someone who becomes sick; or from observations, sensations, or occurrences within their own body. The concern about the feared illness often becomes a central feature of the individual's self-image, a topic of social discourse, and a response to life stresses.

Other Conditions that May Be a Focus of Clinical Attention

When developing the Diagnostic and Statistical Manual of Mental Disorders (DSM-IV),[17] the Association thought it was important to include a category recognizing the presence of conditions that do not fully meet the specific criteria for a given disorder but in fact may be a contributing influence on the patient's symptoms. This category is described as "Other conditions that may be a focus of clinical attention." There are numerous possibilities in this category but this text will only review a few. Figure 18-6 reveals a category of other conditions to acknowledge all the other possibilities. There are two categories that should be mentioned in this section: malingering and psychologic factors affecting a medical condition.

Case 35	Clinical presentation of a somatoform pain disorder with some possibility of a posttraumatic stress disorder

Chief Complaint

Bilateral TMJ and tooth pain.

History

A 28-year-old female with protracted continuous mild steady dull aching pain diffusely located in and around the temporomandibular joints and teeth bilaterally. It is described as an itchy uncomfortable sensation punctuated occasionally by lancinating pains through the face. These pains do not seem to relate to masticatory function. Discomfort is worse in early mornings and is accompanied by a "bad taste" in the mouth.

It began some 9 to 10 months ago following her third marriage and at first seemed to involve only the teeth. She wanted them removed but her dentist found no valid reason. Then it spread to involve the entire masticatory system including the teeth, joints, muscles, lips, tongue, and floor of mouth bilaterally. She has been diagnosed by her regular dentist as having a masticatory muscle pain disorder and has been referred for confirmation and therapy.

Due to the vagueness of the complaint, a psychologic survey was done, revealing an emotional overlay that needed further exploration.

Examination

Intraoral: Negative for any cause of the pain.

TM Joints: Clinical and radiographically normal.

Muscles: Some muscle tenderness but not increased with any jaw use.

Cervical: Within normal limits; however, the patient reports pain originating from her neck. No evidence of any pain source.

Cranial Nerves: Within normal limits.

Diagnostic Tests: Further psychologic investigation revealed a traumatic childhood and a sexually traumatic first marriage which ended in divorce. A second marriage was short lived. She then isolated herself from male companions for some time. A third marriage, 11 months ago, seems to have reactivated her old feelings due to what she describes as a very aggressive husband. She seeks ways to avoid sexual relations with him.

Impression

The face pain problem may be related to either a somatoform pain disorder or a posttraumatic stress disorder.

Diagnosis

An Axis II mental disorder clinical manifesting as a masticatory muscle pain disorder.

Classification of Orofacial Pains

Axis II
(Psychological Conditions)

Anxiety Disorder
- Generalized Anxiety Disorder
- Posttraumatic Stress Disorder
- Anxiety Disorder due to a Medical Condition

Other Conditions
- Malingering
- Psychological Factors Affecting Med Condition
- other conditions

- Personality Traits or Coping Style
- Maladaptive Health Behavior
- Stress-Related Physiological Response

Mood Disorder
- Depressive Disorder
- Bipolar Disorder
- Mood Disorder due to a Medical Condition

Somatoform Disorder
- Undifferentiated Somatoform Disorder
- Conversion Disorder
- Pain Disorder
- Hypochondriasis

Axis II

Diagnosis

Axis I

Axis I
(Physical Conditions)

Neuropathic Pain

Continuous Pain
- Sympathetically Maintained Pain →
  - Traumatic Neuralgia
  - Atypical Odontalgia
- Deafferentation Pain
- Neuritis Pain
  - Postherpetic Neuralgia
  - Herpes Zoster
  - Peripheral Neuritis

Episodic Pain
- Paroxysmal Neuralgia Pain →
  - Neurovascular Pain
    - Migraine with Aura
    - Migraine without Aura
    - Cluster Headache
    - Paroxsymal Hemicrania
    - Neurovascular Variants
  - Vascular Pain
    - Arteritis Pain
    - Carotidynia
  - Pulpal Pain

Somatic Pain

Deep Pain

Visceral Pain
- Visceral Mucosal Pain
- Glandular, Ocular and Auricular Pain

Musculoskeletal Pain
- Periodontal Pain
- Soft Connective Tissue Pain
- Osseous and Periosteal Pain
- Temporomandibular Joint Pain
  - Ligamentous Pain
  - Retrodiscal Pain
  - Capsular Pain
  - Arthritic Pain
- Muscle Pain
  - Co-contraction
  - Delayed Onset Muscle Soreness
  - Myofascial Pain
  - Muscle Spasm Pain
  - Muscle Inflammation Pain

Superficial Pain
- Mucogingival Pain
- Cutaneous Pain

Fig 18-6 Pain classification chart highlighted to show the relationship of all the other mental conditions to the other Axis I and Axis II conditions.

Malingering. Malingering is a mental disorder that is characterized by an individual's intentional production of false or grossly exaggerated physical or psychologic symptoms, motivated by external incentives such as avoiding work, military duty, or social encounters. The malingering patient may use the symptoms to obtain drugs or financial compensation such as in a medicolegal issue.

Malingering should be suspected when there is a marked discrepancy between the person's claimed stress or disability and the objective clinical findings or if the person is not cooperative during the diagnostic evaluation. Persons who do not comply with suggested therapies should also be suspected of malingering especially if no logical explanation is given. Of course, ongoing medicolegal issues may also raise suspicion.

Psychologic Factors Affecting a Medical Condition. This category of mental disorders is characterized by the presence of one or more specific psychologic or behavioral factors that adversely affect a general medical condition. These factors may affect the medical condition either by affecting its course, by interfering with the treatment or by constituting an additional health risk for the individual. There are several psychologic factors that may affect a medical condition but only three will be reviewed in this text. They are personality traits or coping style, maladaptive health behavior, and stress-related physiologic responses.

Personality Traits or Coping Style. An individual's personality traits or a maladaptive coping style can sometimes affect the course of treatment of a general medical condition. Some of these traits may actually contribute to the medical condition, such as a type A personality that reveals hostile behavior and continuous pressures affecting coronary artery disease. In some instances, problematic personality traits can interfere with the working relationship of the health care providers, resulting in adverse consequences in treatment.

Maladaptive Health Behavior. Maladaptive health behaviors can greatly affect the outcome of a general medical condition. For example, a sedentary lifestyle, overeating, excessive alcohol and drug abuse can greatly affect the medical condition. Behaviors, such as unsafe sexual practices, also influence medical conditions. These maladaptive health behaviors need to be evaluated and appropriately addressed when treating the general medical condition.

Stress-Related Physiologic Response. Sometimes stress-related physiologic responses can affect the outcome of a general medical condition. This may be seen in an individual who when emotionally stressed, experiences chest pains. As previously discussed, an upregulation of the autonomic nervous system may be responsible, in part, for maintaining some chronic pain conditions. For these patients, treatment to decrease the responsiveness of the autonomic nervous system is in order.

Other Conditions. This category of mental disorders is listed in the flow sheet merely to remind the reader that the mental disorders that have been reviewed in this text are only a few of the many mental disorders that may be present in the patient with orofacial pain. The clinician should be mindful of the possible presence of other disorders such as attention disorders, cognitive disorders, substance-related disorders, psychotic disorders, factitous disorders, eating disorders, sleep disorders, adjustment disorders, and personality disorders. These disorders are best diagnosed and managed by appropriately trained health professionals.

General Therapeutic Considerations

The treatment of chronic orofacial pain is no easy task. Not only is the clinician required to have a sound understanding of the pathophysiology of the somatic and neurogenous structures but also must demonstrate a significant understanding of the Axis II conditions. Most clinical training programs orient their teachings to one or the other but not both. Only recently have programs been developed that emphasize the significance and interaction of both Axis I and Axis II factors. Since it is difficult to master all aspects of pain, a multidisciplinary approach works best in most settings. In a temporomandibular disorders management setting, the minimum support needed is a dentist, a clinical psychologist, and a physical therapist. As the practice expands to include all orofacial pain, the practice should expand to include the appropriate medical personnel to manage the pain conditions. These personnel may include an internist, neurologist, otolaryngologist, rheumatologist, physiatrist, psychiatrist, and a pain management specialist. On occasion, the group may need the expertise of a radiologist, neurosurgeon, or even a pediatrician. This type of interaction may be necessary to manage complex pain conditions.

Although it is difficult for one clinician to manage all pain conditions, each clinician should be aware of certain basic principles in pain management. These principles are based on the understanding of the pain mechanisms that have been presented in this text. Remember, pain is the result of modulated nociception on its way to the cortex. If this modulation can be favorably influenced, the pain experience can be lessened. As mentioned in Chapter 1, the amount of suffering that an individual experiences is not dependent on tissue damage but instead on the amount of attention drawn to the injury and the consequence of the injury. The clinician should always be mindful of the factors that tend to increase the pain experience. Examples of such factors are attention, expectancy, anxiety, fear, and anger. Factors that tend to lessen the pain experience are confidence, self-efficacy, assurance, distraction, relaxation, and positive emotion. The caring therapist will recognize these influencing factors and encourage the patient's behavior to shift away from the exciting factors to more of the inhibitory factors. In many instances, this becomes more of the art of pain management than the science.

All pain management should begin with educating the patient to his or her pain condition. The following suggestions will emphasize the inhibitory pain modulating factors.

Provide a Definitive Diagnosis

Whenever possible, the patient should be given a definitive diagnosis of the pain condition. There is nothing more unsettling to the patient than fear of the unknown. Patients who are not given a diagnosis will often think that their condition is unknown, and unique only to them. Some patients may think that their problem is so unique that no one has ever even seen it before. These feelings will promote fear and anxiety which in turn will likely increase the pain experience.

Provide Assurance

Most pain conditions are not the result of a life-threatening disease. When the condition is not life threatening, the patient should be assured of his or her safety. Certainly the fear of losing one's life increases anxiety, attention, and perhaps even produces anger. When explaining the significance of the disease, care should be taken not to downplay the significance of the pain. The clinician should carefully report that the condition is not life-threatening but, at the same time, show concern for the manner by which the pain is influencing the quality of the patient's life. This reassurance is the foundation of a positive doctor/patient relationship that may greatly influence the success of future treatment.

Explain the Condition in Appropriate Terms

Each patient should be adequately informed regarding the etiology and treatment indicated for his or her pain condition. Often this information provides the patient with an understanding that not only decreases the excitatory pain influencing factors but may also help him or her manage the condition. The clinician should present information regarding the pain condition in a manner that can be understood by the patient.

The patient should be given time to ask the clinician questions to assure maximum understanding. Once the diagnosis is established, too often the clinician will want to move directly into therapy and overlook this important communication. Patient education is extremely important for maximum therapeutic success.

Do Not Deny the Patient's Pain

Too often in the past when the clinician could not find somatic evidence to explain the pain, the patient was thought to have a psychologic problem. Since the clinician assumed the problem was only in the mind, the pain was not real but instead merely fabricated. One of the purposes of this text is to emphasize that all pains are not somatic and therefore the origin may not be obvious on examination. Only in very rare instances is pain fabricated. The clinician should always assume the patient's pain complaints are real and respect his or her report. Absolutely no benefit can be achieved by initially denying the patient's pain or by claiming that it cannot exist. These claims will only create a poor doctor/patient relationship, lessening the likelihood of treatment success.

Provide Realistic Expectations

Unfortunately not all pain conditions can be completely resolved. Pain that has origin in diseased structures that cannot be healed will likely continue, even in the presence of the best medical therapy. There are certain neuropathic pain conditions that are also resistant to therapy. It is important that patients be informed of the likely outcome of their disorder. Many disorders have a natural course that represents a specific time frame with increase of pain and then resolution. When these conditions exist, the patient should be informed of the normal time required for healing and likely outcome. The patient's treatment expectations should be realistic to minimize disappointment. Many patients believe the clinician has all the treatments needed to resolve the pain. When this is not true, the patient needs to appreciate this fact earlier in therapy.

The management of a pain disorder should always begin with conservative therapy. Aggressive treatments should generally be reserved for later considerations. Appropriate pain medications should be used for the condition being treated. With our new understanding of central sensitization, acute pains should be adequately controlled to minimize the afferent barrage to the second-order neuron. This should be accomplished by proper pre-emptive analgesia with local anesthesia as well as oral medications.[23]

An important part of pain management is providing therapies in which the patient can actively participate. A condition that enhances the pain experience is the feeling of helplessness. When a patient can actively participate in his or her treatment, a feeling of control becomes present. This control helps downregulate the pain experience.

One area that can significantly influence many pain conditions is controlling autonomic nervous system activity. As mentioned in many sections of this text, the autonomic nervous system often plays an important role in pain. This is especially true in certain musculoskeletal disorders and in the sympathetically maintained pain conditions. Increased levels of external challenges or emotional stress increase sympathetic nervous system activity. Although this increased activity is certainly appropriate for acute stressors, maintaining this upregulation is not appropriate on a chronic bases. Many patients with chronic pain, however, do just that. These patients are found to maintain a rather rapid rate of breathing from the chest instead of from the diaphragm. Their hand and feet temperatures are colder than normal and their heart rates will increase more rapidly in the presence of stressors.[24] This represents a state of hypervigilance, which increases the pain experience. This is precisely what appears to be present in many posttraumatic stress disorders.

Patients with upregulated sympathetic activity can be trained to manage these activities by using relatively simple techniques. Training the patient to decrease breathing rates and shifting breathing patterns from chest muscles to the diaphragm can be most helpful in beginning to manage the autonomic effects on pain. Training the patient to increase hand temperature or general muscle relaxation techniques can also assist in decreasing autonomic nervous system activity. Many patients who learn these techniques can significantly reduce pain levels at will. When a patient can accomplish this, he or she gains some control of the pain, which ultimately decreases the pain experience.

Perhaps the most important concept for the clinician to remember when managing pain is to: *listen carefully, consider all possibilities, cure if you can, manage if you cannot, but always console.*

References

1. Mock D, Frydman W, Gorden AS. Atypical facial pain: A retrospective study. Oral Surg 1985; 59:472–474.

2. Walters A. The psychogenic regional pain syndrome and its diagnosis: In Knighton RS, Dumke PR (eds): Pain. Boston: Little, Brown; 1966: 439–456.

3. Gerschman J, Burrows G, Reade P. Chronic orofacial pain. In Bonica JJ, Liebeskind JC, Albe-Fessard DG (eds): Advances in Pain Research and Therapy, vol 3. New York: Raven Press; 1979: 317–323.

4. Donaldson D, Kroening R. Recognition and treatment of patients with chronic orofacial pain. J Am Dent Assoc 1979; 99:961–966.

5. Moulton RE. Psychiatric considerations in maxillofacial pain. J Am Dent Assoc 1955; 51:408.

6. Beck FM, Kaul TJ, Weaver JM. Recognition and management of the depressed dental patient. J Am Dent Assoc 1979; 99:967–971.

7. Fordyce WE. Behavior conditioning concepts in chronic pain. In Bonica JJ, Lindblom U, Iggo A (eds): Advances in Pain Research and Therapy, vol 5. New York: Raven Press; 1983: 781–788.

8. Sternbach RA. Fundamentals of psychological methods in chronic pain. In Bonica JJ, Lindblom U, Iggo A (eds): Advances in Pain Research and Therapy, vol 5. New York: Raven Press; 1983: 777–780.

9. Roberts AH. Contingency management methods in the treatment of chronic pain. In Bonica JJ, Lindblom U, Iggo A (eds): Advances in Pain Research and Therapy, vol 5. New York: Raven Press; 1983: 789–794.

10. Lindblom U, Tegner R. Are the endorphins active in chronic pain states? Narcotic antagonism in chronic pain patients. Pain 1979; 7:65–68.

11. Chapman CR, Butler SH. Effects of doxepin on perception of laboratory induced pain in man. Pain 1978; 5:253–262.

12. Ward NG, Bloom VL, Frieder RO. The effectiveness of tricyclic antidepressants in the treatment of coexisting pain and depression. Pain 1979; 7:331–341.

13. Pilling LF. Psychosomatic aspects of facial pain. In Alling CC, Mahan PE (eds): Facial Pain, ed 2. Philadelphia: Lea & Febiger; 1977: 213–226.

14. Wurtele SK, Kaplan GM, Kealrnes M.. Childhood sexual abuse among chronic pain patients. Clin J Pain 1990; 6:110.–113

15. Haber JD, Roos C. Effects of spouse abuse and/or sexual abuse in the development and maintenance of chronic pain in women. In: Fields HL, Dubner R, Cervero F (eds). Advances in Pain Research and Therapy, vol 9. New York: Raven Press; 1985: 889–895.

16. Domino JV, Haber JD: Prior physical and sexual abuse in women with chronic headaches: Clinical correlates. Headache 1988; 27:310–314.

17. Diagnostic and Statistical Manual of Mental Disorders (DSM-IV), ed 4. Washington, DC: The American Psychiatric Association; 1994.

18. Leino P, Magni G. Depressive and distress symptoms as predictors of low back pain, shoulder pain, and other musculoskeletal morbidity. Pain 1993; 53:89–94.

19. Magni G. On the relatiionship between chronic pain and depression when there is no organic lesion. Pain 1987; 31:1–21.

20. Magni G, Caldieron C, Rigatti-Luchini S, Merskey H. Chronic musculoskeletal pain and depressive symptoms in the general population. An analysis of the 1st National Health and Nutrition Examination Survey data. Pain 1990; 43:299–307.

21. Magni G, Marchetti M, Moreschi C, Merskey H, Luchini SR. Chronic musculoskeletal pain and depressive symptoms in the National Health and Nutrition Examination I. Epidemiologic follow-up study. Pain 1993; 53:163–168.

22. Magni G, Moreschi C, Rigatti-Luchini S, Merskey H. Prospective study on the relationship between depressive symptons and chronic musculoskeletal pain. Pain 1994; 54:289–297.

23. Yaksh TL, Abram SE. Preemptive analgesia: A popular misnomer, but a clinically relevant truth? Am Pain Soc J 1993; 2:116–121.

24. Carlson CR, Okeson JP, Falace DA, Nitz AJ. Curran SL, Anderson DT. A comparison of psychological and physiological functioning between patients with masticatory muscle pain and controls. J Orofacial Pain 1993; 7:15–22.

Index